AI for Geriatric Care in an Aging Society:

Ethical, Clinical, and Policy Challenges

Konstantinos Stolakis
https://orcid.org/0000-0002-5497-4172
Geriatric University Clinic of Siena, Greece

Iris Efthymiou
https://orcid.org/0000-0001-9656-8378
University of Greenwich UK

IGI Global
Scientific Publishing
Publishing Tomorrow's Research Today

Vice President of Editorial	Melissa Wagner
Director of Acquisitions	Mikaela Felty
Director of Book Development	Jocelynn Hessler
Production Manager	Mike Brehm
Cover Design	Jose Rosado

Published in the United States of America by
IGI Global Scientific Publishing
701 East Chocolate Avenue
Hershey, PA, 17033, USA
Tel: 717-533-8845 | Fax: 717-533-7115
Website: https://www.igi-global.com E-mail: cust@igi-global.com

Library of Congress Cataloging-in-Publication Data

LCCN: 2025944991 (CIP Data Pending)
ISBN13: 9798337354620
Isbn13Softcover: 9798337354637
EISBN13: 9798337354644

British Cataloguing in Publication Data
A Cataloguing in Publication record for this book is available from the British Library.

Table of Contents

Detailed Table of Contents

predominantly on younger or non-representative data, raising concerns about diagnostic bias, false positives, and underdiagnosis in older adults. The chapter also explores the ethical, practical, and regulatory challenges of implementing AI in clinical environments where human judgment, patient history, and social context remain critical. By focusing on transparency, data quality, and inclusive model design, it argues for a cautious but deliberate rethinking of how AI can serve, not replace, clinical expertise in geriatric care.

This chapter examines the role of Artificial Intelligence (AI) in modern healthcare, focusing on its applications for aging populations and geriatric care. It analyzes how AI enhances diagnostic accuracy, clinical decision-making, and healthcare efficiency while addressing increasing demands due to workforce shortages and demographic changes. The chapter highlights AI's ability to process large and complex datasets from electronic health records, genetic profiles, and wearable devices, as demonstrated in case studies such as Google's Med-PaLM 2 and AI-enabled digital hospitals. Ethical considerations, including data privacy, algorithmic bias, equitable access, and human oversight, are discussed, emphasizing the importance of responsible innovation and representative datasets. The chapter concludes that AI offers transformative potential for improving patient outcomes in older adults and the broader population, but its benefits depend on careful integration with ethical governance and patient-centered practices.

The aging population throws formidable challenges before on-time, effective, and tailored care. Human-AI interaction in aged care environments offers a new solution through intelligent monitoring and preceptive functions as augmenting caregivers' cognition. This paper discusses the deployment of AI-based systems, i.e., Bi-Stacked Artificial Neural Networks (Bi-Stacked ANN), for facilitating monitoring of older adults' physiological, cognitive, and behavioral health parameters. Data were gathered from geriatricians and stakeholders to determine the most prevalent disease conditions in the population, monitoring practices of important signs, and care demands. Ant Colony Optimization (ACO) was implemented in preprocessing and feature selection to provide high-quality and informative input to the model.

This chapter examines how artificial intelligence (AI) is reshaping social dynamics in the context of care for older adults. It focuses on the interplay between technological intervention and human relationships, highlighting both the potential benefits and limitations of AI-driven care. Key issues include autonomy, trust, and the shifting roles of caregivers and recipients. The chapter draws on interdisciplinary evidence to assess how AI systems influence emotional support, decision-making, and social inclusion for ageing populations. It also considers how social representations shape the way individuals and communities perceive and engage with AI in care contexts. It argues that while AI can enhance efficiency and accessibility, it also raises ethical concerns about empathy, responsibility, and the erosion of human contact in care settings.

This chapter attempts to identify the reasons responsible for the present condition of elderly people in India, to empirically investigate with data, about the various challenges faced by them ranging from Emotional, Psychological, Economic, Social and Medical, to investigate various government schemes initiated for their welfare and how much the beneficiaries are actually availing that benefit from different agencies. The findings state that the majority of elders want to be self-employed in order to become self-dependent so that they do not have to depend financially on their next generations. This work would also prove beneficial to the Government, Civil Society, NGOs and the academic world by way of developing their understanding about the needs and wants of these living Gods i.e., Elders. This comprehensive work will help policy builders to frame practical and helpful policies by way of forecasting the status of elders in the coming decade.This comprehensive work will help policy builders to assess and frame practical and helpful policies.

This chapter explores culturally relevant AI strategies for geriatric care in low-resource settings. It focuses on how AI tools can be adapted to local health practices, social norms, and infrastructure limitations. The analysis includes case studies from underserved regions, highlighting the role of AI in extending primary care, supporting informal caregivers, and improving access to diagnostics and monitoring. It discusses the importance of inclusive data, local language processing, and trust-building through community-based models. The chapter also addresses the risks of digital colonialism, poor interoperability, and ethical concerns tied to algorithmic design in non-Western contexts. It concludes with policy recommendations for equitable AI deployment tailored to ageing populations in low-income and rural environments.

The present study provides a comprehensive systematic review of the various studies related to prevalence, risk factors and catastrophic health expenditure associated with non-communicable diseases among older population. This study can help to consolidate and synthesize the multitude of studies which have been done in this field into one cohesive paper. This helps in understanding the current status as well as identifying places for improvement in this purposed field of study. The findings have revealed that the most prevalent NCDs found among older people are cardiovascular diseases such as hypertension, stroke and heart diseases, Type 1 and Type 2 diabetes, cancer, chronic respiratory diseases, neurological and musculoskeletal diseases and mental health issues.The multimorbidity of NCDs was found to be the most significant factor that pushes many households below the poverty line. It was observed that hospitalization due to chronic diseases among elderly was a major factor in for increase in out-of-pocket expenditure leading to catastrophic health expenditure.

This chapter explores the ethical, legal and social issues of the use of artificial intelligence (AI) in geriatrics. With the increasing number of geriatrics in the world, the application of AI, in the form of assistive robotics, predictive health solutions, and digital companions, is growing to assist older adults medically, socially, and emotionally. Although such technologies have potential benefits to increase the efficiency of healthcare, individualize it, and assist caregivers, they give rise to important ethical concerns concerning issues of privacy, autonomy, fairness, and dignity of a human person. This chapter inserts these problems into conventional codes of medical ethics, but at the same time it directs these problems to the risks that are unique to the elderly populations. Specific adversity posed by AI, such as data protection, algorithmic bias, dependency, and accountability, in the course of making crucial decisions using AI, are addressed in detail.

This chapter critically interrogates the integration of AI in geriatric care through the lens of education, positioning learning ecosystems as the foundational infrastructure for ethical, inclusive, and context-sensitive AI deployment. Drawing on global policy frameworks, cross-sectoral case studies, and pedagogical theory, it constructs a multi-tiered roadmap encompassing awareness, skill-building, and professionalisation across stakeholders. The chapter challenges technological determinism by reframing AI not as a neutral tool but as a socially contingent artefact shaped by educational design, equity concerns, and moral responsibility. Case studies from Japan, Finland, India, and South Korea demonstrate that successful AI implementation hinges less on technical sophistication than on educational imagination. It concludes by proposing lifelong, interdisciplinary, and justice-oriented learning strategies as prerequisites for meaningful AI adoption in ageing societies, asserting that without robust education, even the most advanced AI cannot ensure dignified and humane eldercare.

This chapter examines how artificial intelligence (AI) is reshaping ageing healthcare by supporting clinical decision-making and improving outcomes for older adults. It addresses the application of AI in diagnostics, risk stratification, personalised care planning, and resource allocation across geriatric services. The chapter analyses key benefits such as early detection of cognitive decline, fall prediction, medication optimisation, and remote patient monitoring. It also considers ethical and operational challenges, including data bias, patient consent, and the risk of over-reliance on automated systems. Through clinical case examples and policy analysis, the chapter outlines how AI can support ageing populations without replacing the human judgment essential to compassionate geriatric care.

AI-driven food distribution reshapes geriatric care by aligning supply chains, nutrition science, and clinical monitoring to the needs of aging populations.This chapter examines how predictive analytics and personalization engines identify and prevent malnutrition, how intelligent logistics optimize last-mile delivery and reduce waste, and how integration with clinical workflows creates feedback loops for adaptive meal provisioning. It lays out ethical risks—bias, data privacy, consent, and access gaps—and the policy and governance structures needed to mitigate them.The discussion includes operational models from food banks and community services, highlighting scalable AI applications that balance efficiency with impact. The chapter also addresses system resilience: using AI to anticipate demand shocks, ensure continuity in crises, and embed environmental sustainability in food sourcing and distribution, it proposes a framework for aligning clinical standards, data governance, and public policy to support fair, transparent, and accountable AI-enabled food systems for older adults.

Preface

As editors, we are pleased to present *AI for Geriatric Care in an Aging Society: Ethical, Clinical, and Policy Challenges*, a comprehensive exploration of how artificial intelligence (AI) is reshaping the landscape of aging and eldercare. As populations around the world grow older, healthcare systems, economies, and social structures face mounting pressures to provide effective, sustainable, and compassionate care. AI, with its capacity to process complex data, predict health risks, and personalize interventions, offers promising solutions. Yet, its integration into geriatric care raises profound ethical, clinical, and policy questions that must be carefully navigated.

This volume brings together interdisciplinary voices—researchers, clinicians, ethicists, educators, and policymakers—to examine how AI can support healthy, dignified aging. It explores the convergence of technology and humanity, emphasizing that while AI can enhance safety, independence, and clinical precision, it must never come at the expense of empathy, fairness, or social inclusion. Each chapter contributes a unique perspective on the role of AI in supporting older adults, weaving together innovation with ethical reflection and practical insight.

CHAPTER OVERVIEW

Chapter 1: Empowering Elderly Care through Artificial Intelligence

This chapter explores the transformative role of artificial intelligence (AI) in revolutionizing elderly care systems. It illustrates how AI technologies enhance healthcare delivery through remote monitoring, predictive analytics, and emotional support tools such as virtual assistants and socially interactive robots. The authors emphasize both the opportunities and ethical dilemmas that emerge when technology intervenes in deeply human caregiving contexts, particularly the psychological and societal effects of increased automation in elder support.

Chapter 2: Artificial Intelligence in Geriatric Diagnostics

Chapter 2 delves into the application of AI in diagnosing age-related conditions like dementia and frailty. It critically evaluates the limitations of current diagnostic models that rely on data from younger or non-representative populations, raising essential concerns about bias and diagnostic accuracy. The chapter calls for transparent, inclusive, and ethically grounded AI systems that complement, rather than replace, clinical expertise in geriatric healthcare.

Chapter 3: AI in Healthcare: Technological and Ethical Dimensions for Aging Populations

This chapter presents a comprehensive overview of how AI reshapes modern healthcare infrastructures, focusing on its implications for aging societies. Through case studies and real-world examples, it demonstrates the potential of AI to improve diagnostic precision and clinical efficiency. Yet, it cautions against ethical risks related to privacy, equity, and algorithmic bias, underscoring the need for responsible governance and patient-centered design.

Chapter 4: Smart Elderly Care with Integrated Human-AI Decision Support

This chapter investigates intelligent decision-support systems powered by AI, particularly Bi-Stacked Artificial Neural Networks (ANNs) and optimization algorithms. It highlights how such models enable comprehensive monitoring of physiological and behavioral health parameters among older adults. By merging computational intelligence with caregiver expertise, the study demonstrates how data-driven tools can enhance responsiveness and precision in aged care management.

Chapter 5: Social Dynamics and AI-Driven Care for Older Adults

This chapter offers a sociological perspective on AI's influence in geriatric care. It explores how trust, autonomy, and emotional connection are renegotiated as intelligent systems assume greater caregiving roles. Through an interdisciplinary lens, it assesses both empowerment and alienation effects, calling for a careful balance between technological efficiency and the preservation of human relationships in care contexts.

Chapter 6: Scenario of Eldercare in Indian Families: Present Challenges and the Path Ahead

Addressing the sociocultural landscape of eldercare in India, this chapter analyzes the emotional, financial, and medical challenges faced by aging populations. It evaluates the effectiveness of government initiatives and reveals the growing desire among elders for self-reliance. The findings offer vital insights for policymakers and social organizations, advocating for inclusive programs that respect the aspirations and dignity of older adults.

Chapter 7: Culturally Relevant AI Strategies for Geriatric Care in Low-Resource Settings

Chapter 10 explores how AI can be localized and adapted for geriatric care in low-resource regions. Drawing on international case studies, it emphasizes the need for cultural sensitivity, linguistic inclusivity, and ethical AI deployment that aligns with community norms. The authors warn against digital colonialism and propose equitable, context-aware models that empower caregivers and extend healthcare accessibility in underserved areas.

Chapter 8: Ageing Well or Ailing Wallets? Chronic Illness, Risk Factors, and Catastrophic Health Spending among the Elderly

Chapter 12 offers a systematic synthesis of studies on chronic illness and financial vulnerability among older adults. It exposes how multimorbidity and hospitalization costs drive many households into poverty, despite healthcare advancements. The chapter calls for urgent policy reform and preventive health strategies to reduce catastrophic expenditures and protect aging populations from economic distress.

Chapter 9: Navigating Ethical Frontiers in AI-Driven Geriatric Care

Exploring the moral landscape of AI in eldercare, this chapter interrogates issues of privacy, fairness, autonomy, and human dignity. It situates these concerns within established medical ethics frameworks, emphasizing the unique vulnerabilities of elderly populations. The authors propose safeguards to mitigate algorithmic bias, ensure accountability, and preserve trust in AI-mediated healthcare environments.

Chapter 10: Educational, Technological, Epistemic, and Pedagogical Architectures for an Ageing World

This chapter reframes AI integration in geriatric care through an educational lens, arguing that ethical and effective implementation depends on lifelong learning and interdisciplinary collaboration. It critiques technological determinism and presents case studies from multiple countries to demonstrate that equitable AI adoption requires informed, socially conscious education systems. The chapter proposes a global roadmap for human-AI synergy grounded in justice and inclusivity.

Chapter 11: AI in Ageing Healthcare: Improving Decision-Making and Outcomes for Older Adults

Chapter 15 highlights the transformative role of AI in clinical decision-making and personalized care for older adults. It showcases applications in diagnostics, risk assessment, and remote monitoring, while also addressing ethical challenges such as data bias and consent. Through policy insights and case examples, it reinforces the need for AI systems that support rather than supplant human expertise in geriatric medicine.

Chapter 12: Feeding the Future: AI-Driven Food Distribution for Aging Populations

This chapter examines how AI optimizes food distribution networks to meet the nutritional needs of aging populations. It explores predictive analytics for malnutrition prevention, smart logistics for sustainable delivery, and AI-integrated clinical feedback loops. The discussion balances innovation with caution, addressing ethical risks and proposing governance models that ensure fairness, resilience, and environmental sustainability in AI-enabled food systems.

Chapter 13: Devotional Singing and Neurocognitive Resilience: A Non-Pharmacological Approach

Concluding the volume, this chapter introduces a unique, culturally grounded approach to cognitive health through devotional singing. Integrating neuroscientific and psychological perspectives, it reveals how music engages memory, emotion, and reward pathways to foster neuroplasticity and resilience. The authors present devotional singing as a universal, non-pharmacological practice that supports mental well-being and enriches the aging experience across diverse cultures.

This edited volume unites scholars, clinicians, ethicists, and policymakers to explore these intersecting dimensions. It seeks to define the landscape of AI applications in geriatric care, examine the ethical foundations that safeguard older adults' rights, analyze clinical outcomes of AI deployment, and evaluate policy models that promote fairness and sustainability. The book's chapters collectively offer a comprehensive, multidisciplinary view of how AI can serve, not supplant, human-centered geriatric care.

Our aim is not merely to highlight the technological possibilities but to articulate a responsible path forward. Each contribution maps the current state of research, identifies challenges in implementation, and proposes actionable solutions grounded in ethical reflection and clinical pragmatism. Together, these perspectives form a unified framework for understanding AI's role in supporting healthy aging, from bedside care to national health policy.

We envision this book as a resource for geriatricians, healthcare professionals, ethicists, AI developers, and policymakers who seek to integrate innovation with compassion. Clinicians will find guidance on safely incorporating AI into patient care without losing the human connection. Ethicists will gain insight into frameworks for balancing autonomy and protection. Policymakers will find evidence to inform regulation and equitable distribution. AI researchers will be inspired to develop tools that are transparent, explainable, and genuinely responsive to older adults' needs.

Ultimately, this book is a call for collaboration across disciplines. The future of geriatric care depends not only on how advanced our technologies become but also on how thoughtfully we apply them. By aligning ethical principles, clinical practice, and policy foresight, we can ensure that AI serves as an enabler of dignity, independence, and well-being for aging populations worldwide.

Konstantinos Stolakis
Geriatric University Clinic of Siena, Greece

Iris Efthymiou
University of Greenwich, UK

Chapter 1
Empowering Elderly Care Through Artificial Intelligence

Nikhil Kumar Goyal
https://orcid.org/0009-0007-4532-8033
Poornima University, Jaipur, India

Navin Kumar Goyal
https://orcid.org/0009-0006-0901-294X
Poornima Institute of Engineering and Technology, Jaipur, India

Suneel Kumar
https://orcid.org/0009-0005-3063-6813
HyperNex Technologies LLC, Sheridan, USA

Ritam Dutta
https://orcid.org/0000-0003-3089-778X
Poornima Institute of Engineering and Technology, Jaipur, India

Vishal Kothari
https://orcid.org/0009-0002-1568-3847
Poornima Institute of Engineering and Technology, Jaipur, India

Sanjay Kumar Sinha
https://orcid.org/0000-0003-0351-2549
Poornima Institute of Engineering and Technology, Jaipur, India

ABSTRACT

This section discusses how artificial intelligence (AI) can transform the elderly care sector and positively impact how aging populations live. As the world is becoming an aging society increased pressure to ensure patients receive personalised, effective and sustainable healthcare is being placed on traditional healthcare systems. These technologies (AI technologies) are finding innovative solutions to needs in remote health monitoring and wellness, disease prediction, companionship, and rehabilitation, as well as, fall detection. Other ways that AI helps in emotional well-being are besides clinical support by eliminating the feeling of social isolation with the help of virtual assistants and socially interactive robots. The chapter presents a

DOI: 10.4018/979-8-3373-5462-0.ch001

technological overview of AI in elderly care application and indicates its potential advantages, but critically analyzes its ethical consequences, as well as psychological and societal effects.

1. INTRODUCTION

1.1 Needs of the Elderly in Modern Society

The demographic situation in the world is currently undergoing a radical change due to the fact that the life expectancy is growing longer and the number of births is decreasing, which results in an increasingly aging population. The World Health Organization states that the population of people aged 60 and above will be more than doubled in number to nearly 2.1 billion by 2050. Such population change encompasses peculiarities associated with healthcare systems, caregivers and societies in general. Seniors are usually faced with persistent conditions like cardiovascular diseases, diabetes, and dementia among other conditions as well as mobility and sensory loss. The rising prevalence of those conditions makes it obvious that there should be sustainable solutions to caring that suit the demands of the aging population (Ali & Li, 2019).

Figure 1. Need For The Elderly Care

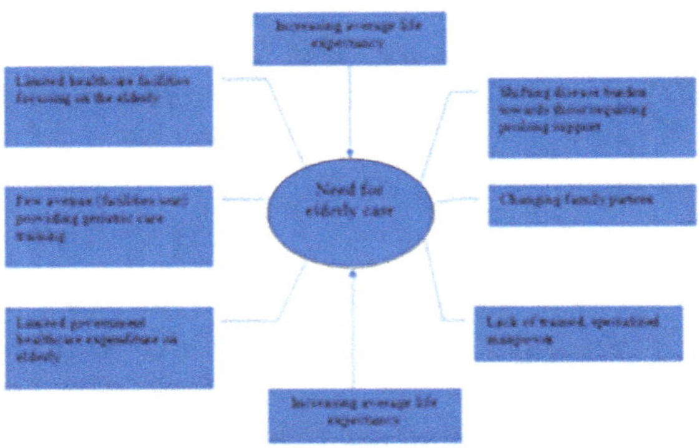

In addition to physical health, aged people also struggle with emotional and mental issues such as loneliness, depression and social isolation. Traditional family-based caregiving is in decline in most societies because of the factors of urbanisation, shift in family model, and migration. This means that older individuals are not so frequently supplied with the much needed social and emotional support, which is the most important to their well-being. The conventional healthcare models do not fit well to address these complex needs; they focus more on giving episodic treatment than continuous monitoring (Efthymiou I., 2026). This discrepancy in between the demand and the capacity of the healthcare systems emphasizes the significance of using technological advances like artificial intelligence.

AI provides an opportunity to fill the existing gaps in dealing with elderly patients by offering them round-the-clock health monitoring, individualized treatment, and interactive companionship. Unlike traditional healthcare services time-limited, place-bound, and human resource-restricted, AI-based tools can be real-time and scalable anytime anywhere and adjustable to the situation. These breakthroughs do not only help medical practitioners in diagnosing and treatment, but enable older adults to take charge of themselves and practice dignity. Therefore, the consideration of the needs of the elderly offers the basis on which AI-powered caring systems are efficiently created and put to play (Amin et al., 2016).

1.2 Role of Technology in Healthcare Transformation

Technology has always served as a revolutionizing factor in the healthcare industry and medical equipment with the introduction of medical imaging devices to electronic health records. Nevertheless, the process of AI integration is a game changer and not an improvement in some way. Adaptability AI technologies like machine learning, natural language processing, and robotics can learn with data and evolve to better fit changing environments and make personalized suggestions (Diareme, K. et al., 2022). The capabilities are especially influential in the context of elderly care because they concern not only medical but also non-medical conditions of aging.

Figure 2. Benefits of Digital Transformation in Healthcare

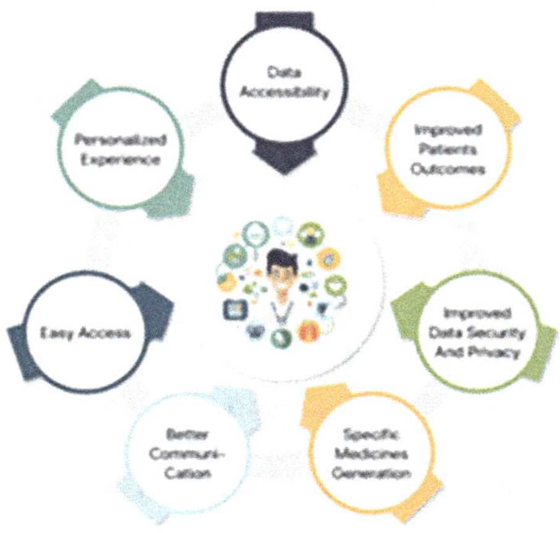
Data Accessibility
Improved Patients Outcomes
Improved Data Security And Privacy
Specific Medicines Generation
Better Communi-Cation
Easy Access
Personalized Experience

The remote health monitoring and predictive analytics is one of the most important contributions of AI. Smart AI-based wearables monitor the body effectively, identifying the early symptoms of health depreciation in order to intervene in time. As an example, it can be said that AI-based tools may be used to track a heart rate variability, identify abnormal walking patterns, or analyze sleep-activity cycles to forecast possible health risks. These preventive insights kill two fowls with one stone as they can reduce hospital admissions, save on healthcare expenses, and enhance the lifestyle. Preventive abilities such as these are essential in dealing with chronic diseases that must be taken care of on an ongoing basis.

Acting beyond health monitoring, AI gives elderly care new social support and companionship technologies. Natural language processing in virtual assistants or companion robots allows having meaningful speech interactions and reminding elderly people to take medications, as well as identifying even the symptoms of depression through speech or behavior patterns. Such tools will hit the psychological aspect of aging by minimizing feelings of loneliness and creating a sense of belonging. People identify that technology can change the very perception of elderly care by making it holistic and personalized through the provision of medical and social care together (Ashfaq et al., 2020).

1.3 Defining the Purpose and Scope

This chapter aims to give a detailed account of how artificial intelligence is reshaping care of the elderly, including both technological developments and their social implications. Although there is a growing body of literature addressing the role played by AI in relation to healthcare, little attention has been paid to the field of elderly care in general, including medical, psychological, ethical and social aspects of which AI is a part of. It does not merely concentrate on describing the existing innovations but gives the critical evaluation of their possible advantages and disadvantages.

The section will present four main areas. First, it highlights underpinnings of AI in healthcare, providing the reader with an insight into the technological basics, including machine learning, natural language processing, and robotics. Second, it will examine practical uses of AI when taking care of the elderly, including health monitoring at a distance and cognitive stimulation. Third, it deals with the ethical, psychological, and social implications of applying the AI systems among the vulnerable population so that the technological solutions are not in opposition to human values. The chapter concludes by examining what may be coming next in the trends and future of AI in shaping the realm of elderly care into the decades ahead.

Notably, the sphere of the discussion is not limited to strictly technical issues. The elderly care includes human aspect, cultural expectations and policy framework which should not be left behind to facilitate effective AI solutions. To this end, although AI-powered robots can technically give someone companionship, their adoption can only be determined by cultural and psychological acceptable availability of the same on the elderly individuals. Likewise, deploying AI in healthcare space needs powerful data governance mechanisms that would ensure the safety of privacy, and trustworthiness. This chapter will capture these wider variables in bringing out a balanced picture of AI in elderly care.

2. FOUNDATIONS OF ARTIFICIAL INTELLIGENCE IN HEALTHCARE

2.1 Overview of Artificial Intelligence Technologies

Artificial Intelligence (AI) is not the technology; it is a toolbox which includes various computational systems copied on the human nature. In healthcare, AI is the ability to analyze information, identify patterns, and make predictions or decisions with little human input. AI systems can improve with additional data unlike more traditional software that follows the predetermined rules, which makes them especially relevant to meet the needs of such a dynamic environment like elderly care (Banner & Olney, 2009).

Figure 3. AI: An Overview

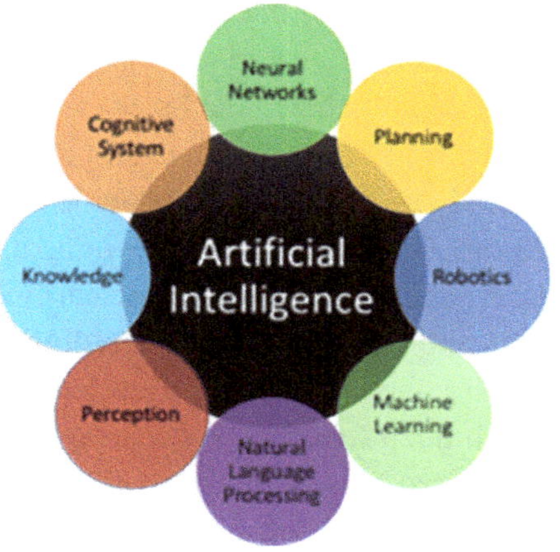

The basic components of AI are algorithms, training data and the computers themselves. Algorithms are the mathematical directions in which data is processed and datasets are the examples of the real-world which permit the algorithms to learn. New breakthroughs in cloud computing and high-performance processors have increased the speed of how quickly AI models can be trained and deployed by several times. It is an indispensable property of the healthcare systems, which operate with huge amounts of data, both medical images and electronic health records, requiring analysis in real time.

At elderly care, the AI technologies have been used in various forms. To illustrate, computer vision can give fall detection systems the ability to keep track of the motions by using cameras or sensors, whereas natural language processing can make useful conversational agents to remind them of the daily reminders, and even provide emotional support. The predictive modeling can determine the possibility of readmission in hospitals using historical data about a patient, and this can prompt the doctor to take corrective measures early. The flexibility of AI is presented in these applications because it is adapted to both non-clinical and clinical aspects of aging (Berridge et al., 2018).

2.2 Machine Learning and Deep Learning in Medical Applications

The central element in contemporary AI is so-called machine learning (ML). The term can be described as the capacity of systems to advance their performance on a task by means of learning (through data) rather than completely by means of programming. L can be partitioned into a number of paradigms: supervised learning, unsupervised learning and reinforcement learning. All these have particular application in healthcare and the care of the elderly (Betriana et al., 2022).

Medical diagnostics is of great interest in supervised learning. The process involves algorithm training using the labeled data sets in which the expected output of an algorithm and the input are known. As an example, an algorithm that would have access to thousands of X-ray pictures with provided names of the conditions (e.g. pneumonia or osteoporosis) might learn to recognize such diseases on new, unexposed X-ray images. In aged care, supervised learning is popularly used in diagnosing chronic diseases and other outcomes including the propensity to fall.

Unsupervised learning In contrast, unsupervised learning concerns unlabeled data and can be used to find hidden structure. As an example, clustering algorithms can be used to classify elderly patients by consulting their similarities in lifestyles, medical history, or gene predispositions and thereby provide personalized healthcare provisions. This is especially useful in treating multi-factorial, complex diseases such as dementia, since different patients can respond to treatments in different ways (Goyal et al., 2025a).

Deep learning Deep learning A which is a subfield of machine learning relies on using artificial neural networks based on the structure of the brain. These networks prove very effective when processing high-dimensional and complex data like medical volumes, audio files or text. In geriatrics, deep learning has been used e.g. to analyze MRI scans to detect early Alzheimer disease or to process speech as an indicator of cognitive impairment. Deep learning also underpins fall-detection systems where video is analyzed in real time to determine whether the person is walking normally or has fallen down.

2.3 Natural Language Processing and Conversational Agents

Another core principle behind AI that can be used greatly in the medical field is Natural Language Processing (NLP). NLP is the concept of computers that know how to process language as human beings do, and interpret as well as produce it. In case of elderly care, NLP is very effective in overcoming communication gaps between old-age people with technology, especially the ones who find it difficult to communicate with complex digital interfaces.

NLP-based use of conversational agents, also known as chatbots, is actively being used to assist elderly people in their everyday routine. These agents have the capability of reminding patients to take their drugs, booking medical appointment or offer companionship through informal typical conversation. State-of-the-art NLP systems are able to infer emotional content in language, like stress or sadness, and provide an emotional response that is supportive, in addition to being more useful than telephonic communication. In the case of socially isolated elderly people, they offer a connection that can increase the emotional condition of people quite substantially (Chen et al., 2020).

NLP is also changing the interaction of patient records with the healthcare provider. The voice recognition systems allow physicians to record their notes that are automatically drafted and organized into electronic health records. In the case of elderly care, this cuts the administration work load on care givers and they are free to give more of their time to the patient. In the same way, unstructured medical information can also be studied using language models trained with AI to find possible health risks that would otherwise not be detected (Conger & Kanungo, 1988).

2.4 AI-Driven Data Analytics for Healthcare Insights

Healthcare produces tremendous amounts of data on a daily basis, including hospital records and laboratory data, as well as data provided by wearable devices and home sensors. The role of data analytics powered by Artificial Intelligence is to help this raw data translate into useful pieces of information that can be acted upon. In elderly care, potential value of such analytics is associated with the fact that it will provide personalized, proactive and predictive interventions.

Predictive analytics can be exceptionally useful in forecasting before health risks get out of hand. To give an example, a heart rate, blood pressure, and activity level of an elderly patient can be put through algorithms and used to predict the probability of occurrence of the events. Equally, AI models are able to predict the evolution of the disease like Parkinson or Alzheimer and enable caregivers to prepare and adjust treatment methods. Such predictive capabilities allow transforming healthcare, which is based on a reactive model in which issues are managed after they have already transpired, into a preventive occupation that focuses on early interventions (de Kervenoael et al., 2020).

Population-level healthcare management is improved with IA-driven analytics as well. By pooling data of thousands of patients at old age, health systems are able to notice some trends, and allocate resources more efficiently. As an example, data analytics could demonstrate that a specific community experiences injuries more often related to mobility, and more specific interventions could be implemented, including fall-prevention programs. AI, in this sense, can help not only individual patients but also help make an informed decision and resource allocation.

Personalization is the other major application of data analytics. Elderly patients posess a variety of health requirements which are not resolvable by a universal approach. By studying trends in diet, medication effects, lifestyle habits, AI-enabled care plans to become individualized and, therefore, more effective. This personalization increases treatment results, patient satisfaction, and aging with dignity and independence (Dilsizian & Siegel, 2014).

3. AI APPLICATIONS IN ELDERLY CARE

3.1 Remote Health Monitoring and Wearable Devices

Remote health monitoring is one of the more important uses of AI in geriatric care and is enabled in large part by wearing sensors and smart devices. The geriatric population may need constant medical monitoring as a result of the fragility of age-related conditions, such as long-term diseases, such as diabetes, high blood pressure and cardiovascular disease. Wearables include smartwatches, fitness trackers, or AI-enabled biosensors, which have converted the way these conditions can be tracked offering real-time data on vital signs (heart rate, oxygen saturation levels, glucose levels, or sleep patterns) (Goyal, 2025a).

The role of AI in such systems is to be the layer of intelligence, that examines data streams and spots departures and anomalies to the norms. To give just one example, when the heart rate of an elderly person changes its regularity, the AI system will be able to issue an urgent notification to caregivers or medical professionals. Early detection can be especially important when it comes to such conditions as atrial fibrillation that are often deprived of attention before the onset of serious complications. In addition, with the help of AI-based predictive models, future risks like a fall or a stroke may be forecasted and preventative measures undertaken prior to the condition escalating (Dill et al., 2014).

In addition to monitoring physiology, wearables are also able to monitor behavioral and mobility characteristics. As an illustration, the gait analysis driven by AI can detect the slight alterations in stride velocity or balance, which could be the symptoms of the development of neurodegenerative diseases like Parkinson. Equally, AI could analyze adherence to the medication schedule by tracking movement patterns relating to the use of a pillbox and make sure that elderly patients do not neglect to take some essential dose.

3.2 AI-Based Diagnostics and Predictive Healthcare

Diagnostics has always been an essential part of healthcare, and AI is introducing a new level to this sector by expediting diagnostic procedures as well as making them more accurate and less invasive. In the elderly care setting, symptoms of conditions tend to be significant late in the process because many of the conditions affect elderly people in silence. Complex data-sets, such as medical imaging or genetic data can be interrogated using AI in order to diagnose diseases earlier than under traditional methods (Fossen & Sorgner, 2022).

So, to continue this example, the scans of the brains suffering Alzheimer disease can be examined by AI-powered imaging tools to identify early stages of the disease because the human eye cannot see the patterns, which the brains exhibit. In the same line, AI can be utilized to detect conditions such as diabetic retinopathy that is predominant amongst diabetes-afflicted elderly individuals long before the condition is obvious. These initial diagnostic strengths promote the effectiveness of treatments as they intervene at earlier stages when the diseases are easier to deal with (Frank et al., 2021).

Another technology that has good prospects of use and considerable success in AI is predictive healthcare. A combination of electronic health records, lifestyle, and wearable data, gives AI systems the ability to create risk scores of a particular condition, such as strokes, heart attacks, or falls. These forecasts enable caregivers to put in place preventive measures including medication adjustment or change of daily activities thus minimizing the chances of hospitalization.

3.3 Virtual Assistants and Companionship Robots

One of the most pertinent problems of the older population across the world is loneliness and social isolation. AI can present new solutions to the problem in terms of virtual assistants and companionship robots as two different forms of helping people by offering functional and emotional assistance. Such technologies are based on using natural language processing, machine learning, and robotics that provide interaction mimicking, help in day-to-day tasks, and companionship.

VR assisted by AI systems like smart speakers or systems would be able to guide adults to take care of their affairs by setting reminders about taking medication, arranging a visit, or asking a question any time. Unlike other digital applications, these helpers are voice-activated, meaning that they are easier to use than smartphones and computers to people who have a hard time using computers. The current hands-free interactions are of great benefit to elderly persons who have visual or motor impairments because they can improve overall autonomy and independence (Gill et al., 2013).

Companionship robots are a further part of the AI-based support. A robotic seal (PARO) has been demonstrated to decrease stress and increase emotional well-being among the elderly, especially among those with dementia patients. Social robots that have the AI incorporated can even hold conversations, identify emotions and react accordingly. These robots also respond to the problem of loneliness in that they, in addition to providing emotional support, provoke intellectual activity and thus slow the development of Alzheimer's and other diseases.

3.4 AI-Powered Rehabilitation and Cognitive Training

To care for the elderly means to rehabilitate them, especially after stroke, surgery or injuries. Cognitive training also plays a significant role in the prevention of decline in memory and reasoning of the age-related reasoning. AI is a major player in both spheres, as it allows the implementation of individual, individually changing, and data-driven interventions.

Physical rehabilitation Physical rehabilitation Rehabilitation for physical problems Rehabilitation Rehabilitation involves the use of AI systems with sensors and computer vision to monitor patients during exercises. These systems are able to give real-time feedback with regard to posture, the accuracy of movement and progress and these systems wether in real life or virtual reality settings fulfill the role of a physical therapist. Take, e.g., the use of AI-powered exoskeletons to help elderly patients reclaim their mobility or robotic rehabilitation devices, which can guide limb motions in the most precise manner and speed up recovery. These technologies not only lead to better rehabilitation results but also they can be used to bring therapy to the home, which means that there would be no need to visit the hospital on a regular basis (Goyal et al., 2025b).

AI-powered cognitive training programs are created to develop cognitive stimulation and delay cognitive deterioration. These are the programs that operate on gamified systems wherein elderly people are provided a challenge with memory, attention and problem solving requirements. AI also adjusts the level of difficulty according to the performance of the user and provides them with a personalized level of challenge that does not exhaust the patients as well. In the case of dementia patients, these adaptive training have been found to help maintain the brainpower longer in comparison to the static programs (Gorla et al., 2010).

4. ENHANCING QUALITY OF LIFE THROUGH AI

The living standard of the aged persons does not confine to the health aspect. It consists of autonomy, security, and psychological well-being, mobility, and social interaction. Artificial intelligence can be used to transform these aspects by integrating intelligence into the daily environment of life, providing individual care, and closing social and emotional gaps. In this section, four major issues in which AI technologies positively affect the lives of the elderly are discussed personal care adaptations, mobility, smart living conditions, and social isolation.

4.1 Personalized Care and Adaptive Interventions

One of the most impressive changes to elderly living with the help of AI is personalized care. Care has traditionally been standardized, and treatment plans and systems of support tend to be accorded to a statistical average rather than by individual needs. AI provides the possibility of paradigm shift as it ensures customising care according to the peculiarities of health conditions of every aged individual, their lifestyle preferences, and psychological condition.

Personalization using AI originates with the massive and varied input of information, such as medical history, real-time health data in wearable devices, and lifestyle factors like food, physical activity and sleep. Care plans that are specific to the individual can then be suggested, with suggestions of dietary changes, physical exercise regimes and prophylactic measures all being suggested by algorithms. To offer one example, an individual with the early stages of arthritis could get AI-created exercise regimens that help them stay mobile without putting the joints through too much stress and a diabetic patient would get some personalized diet suggestions that maintain diet and glucose levels (Hsieh et al., 2018).

Adaptive interventions mark a new development in this area. Unlike predetermined care plans, AI systems continuously assess health related and behavior data and make changes as the situation changes. In an elderly individual whose activity reduces because of tiredness, AI can adjust the exercise plans to inhibit possible injuries, yet promote exercise. This form of care that is responsive, dynamic and effective means that the interventions are always effective and relevant.

4.2 AI for Mobility Support and Fall Detection

Mobility is one of the most common challenges and conditions that afflict the elderly, who face loss of autonomy, hospitalization and long-term disability. The issue of aging and mobility has been becoming increasingly addressed through predictive mobility and fall detection systems in the form of I technologies.

One of the most important applications is the Fall detection. Wearables, cameras and floor sensors reliant on AI are able to see abnormal movement patterns in real-time and make a difference between harmless behaviors and hazardous falls. Whenever a fall is detected, it is able to notify caregivers, family members, or emergency services within seconds, significantly decreasing the time in responding and increasing chances of survival. Next-generation AI systems can make predictions, alerting to a shift in gait or posture that puts patients at a higher risk of falling and sounding an intervention (Junglas & Harris, 2013).

Mobility support is not restricted to detection systems Exoskeletons and walking robots driven by AI would help older people walk safely, regain mobility previously lost and prevent accidents. These devices take computer vision and machine learning and calibrate to help the individual with an optimal degree of assistance. An example is that robotic walking aids have the ability to automatically alter speed and they offer stability in order to negotiate uneven surfaces, and furthermore they have the ability to stop when an obstacle is sensed.

Besides, AI-based navigation systems, incorporated into the smart home or community facilities help aged persons navigate their surroundings with ease. Individuals with eyesight have some kind of aids that can make use of artificial intelligence to create an audible or what we know as a haptic feedback to avoid any kind of an obstacle. Such developments not only make a person safe, but also makes him or her blessed with trust in motion and as a result elderly people get to perform their daily routine without the worry of injuries (Khan et al., 2019).

4.3 Smart Homes and Ambient Assisted Living Systems

The ideology of living at home, instead of being institutionalised in homes, even as elderly people advance in age has caught international speed with what is known as the concept of aging in the place. AI has a central part in enabling such a vision and hence the need to discuss the role of the smart homes and ambient assisted living (AAL) systems. These spaces combine AI with the Internet of Things (IoT), establishing a smart set of environments that focuses on monitoring, modifying and reacting to the demands of older residents.

The AI enabled smart houses are homes with interconnected devices like motion sensors, smart thermostats, voice controlled assistants, and AI-powered appliances. Such systems may automate common activities, like turning the lights on and off with motion, controlling room temperature to stay comfortable, and locking and unlocking doors, relieving elderly people of some of the cognitive and physical strain of their lives. Individuals with movement distortions can have voice-activated programs that enable them to control every capability at home without involving their hands (Laschinger, 2012).

Ambient assisted living systems are an expansion of this functionality where more emphasis is on safety and health. As an example, AI may study the everyday schedule of the person in terms of meals, sleeping, and using the bathroom and establish abnormalities that could indicate health issues. Drastic decline in the activity in the kitchen can be an indication of appetite loss or illness and would trigger interventions on time. In a similar manner, the AI is able to analyze the pills or regimes adherence through the monitoring of the pill dispensers or by noticing that the prescriptions are undertaken.

4.4 Social Inclusion and Reducing Loneliness with AI

Social isolation in ageing populations is an epidemic in silence and its impacts are far reaching with severity in both physical as well as mental health. Long lasting social isolation is attributed to sometimes more depression, cognitive impairment, heart-related illness, and even early death. The AI technologies can provide an innovative means of addressing these risks by means of encouraging social inclusion and offering the possibility to engage in meaningful activity.

One of the most apparent tools here is the use of AI-driven conversational agent. UninsertLike standard virtual assistants, which follow primarily command-based interactions, advanced AI companions also use natural, emotionally receptive dialogue. The systems have the capability of providing communication every day, monitoring emotional well-being, and companionship. In persons with low social interaction, such interactions are comforting and give them a feeling of belongingness (Goyal et al., 2025c).

Social robots built to resemble human or animal behaviors, take it a step further to provide physical presence, as well as emotional attachments. PARO or Pepper has been introduced in facilities caring of the elderly to encourage social interactions, relax the older adults, and exercise the mind. Such robots are able to conduct group activities, games, and promote social engagement and prevent a cycle of isolation, which can be associated with older age.

5. ETHICAL, PSYCHOLOGICAL, AND SOCIAL DIMENSIONS

The involvement of artificial intelligence in taking care of older adults brings about a lot of considerations that extend beyond technological efficiency. Although AI systems are expected to be safer, more personalized, and more companionship, they closely interweave with such delicate aspects as ethics, privacy, dignity, psychological acceptance, and social roles. This section digs deeper into the ethical concerns related to AI-driven elderly care, analyzes the relevance of data confidentiality and security, the psychological attitude of the elderly regarding the AI systems, and the way in which caregivers can play a new role in the human-AI collaboration model in the future (Vousinas, G. et al., 2022).

5.1 Ethical Considerations in AI-Driven Elderly Care

The use of AI in elderly care needs a thorough ethical examination and consideration because the decisions reached by the application have direct impacts on the lives of the sick and frail people. One of the main ethical concerns is the one of autonomy and consent (Efthymiou, I. P. 2024). Aged people tend to lose their agency in healthcare processes through poor mental conditions, or loss of independence, or inefficient structures. Recommendation/making I systems should not rob the elderly the right of making their own decisions but remain active participants in it and not subjects of technological adventures.

The other ethical issue is fairness and equity. The information used by AI systems is data driven, so it can be biased and may underrepresent some age groups, genders, ethnicities, or cultural backgrounds. It can result in inappropriate treatment, miss-diagnosis or even leave certain communities out of the advantages of AI-driven care because of biased algorithms. This necessitates the fairness in AI systems having stringent auditing procedures, clear work processes, and data upon which such systems are based need to be varied and representative (Laschinger et al., 2001).

The ethics of beneficence, that is, acting out what is best in the view of the patient, must also be used to develop AI. Although AI can help enhance medical care and stimulate social interaction, it should never be seen as a way of optimizing processes, to the detriment of human dignity. An example is a robotic caregiver that has the program to lower the costs only, failing to treat the elderly as people and thus disregarding their emotional needs. Ethical AI in old age should promote efficiency within the parameters of treating a person humanely, considering that technology should not be used to dehumanize people.

5.2 Data Privacy and Security Challenges

One of the requirements of elder care systems utilizing AI is the constant gathering of data. Wearable technology, smart homes, conversational agents, and the monitoring of medical conditions are all producing a continuous flow of sensitive personal information, including but not limited to health conditions, daily commitments, and moods. Although these data are vital in bringing the much-needed personalized care, they present tremendous privacy and security risks.

The unauthorized use of medical information can result in identity identity theft, financial exploitation or targeted schemes. Even the health records or daily routines of elderly people can be jeopardized by cybercriminals, which would pose them even greater risks than the aspect of being vulnerable to the cyber community. In addition, the fact that such data is stored in centralized databases makes them pleasant targets to cybercriminals. Just a single breach could jeopardize the privacy of thousands of the elderly persons, which may break trust in AI systems (Leal-Junior et al., 2019).

Beside external dangers, there are some privacy and eavesdropping concerns. The I systems that are integrated into smart homes tend to work twenty-four seven, gathering information about each and every movement, discussion or behavior pattern. On the one hand, it allows creating proactive healthcare interventions; on the other hand, it erodes the distinction between care and surveillance, which can raise concerns related to the concepts of dignity and independence. Aged people will also feel intruded even though they agreed previously and therefore refuse to use such devices.

5.3 Psychological Acceptance of AI among the Elderly

In order to prove their profitability in elderly care, AI technologies will have to become psychologically acceptable as well as to perform well technically. The experience with technology, cultural inclinations and emotional desires influence the perceptions that the elderly people hold about AI. Whereas some accept AI systems as empowering systems that restore independence, others believe them to be fearful, foreign or even dangerous.

One of the major psychological obstacles is that of being replaced. Older people can be afraid that AI, like robot caregivers and virtual assistants, will replace the social relationship with humans and older individuals will be left socially isolated or in need of care. This fear is more dominant in cultures that adhere to intra generational care giving and family orientated support mechanisms. To avoid this, AI has to be positioned not as an alternative but as an accent to human care by turning it into a mechanism that supports against rather than substitutes caregivers (Li et al., 2012).

5.4 Role of Caregivers and Human-AI Collaboration

The uprise of AI in the field of elderly care would not reduce the value of human caregivers; instead, the value would be transferred into an industry partnership where technology is a valued addition. The role of caregivers (both family and professional healthcare personnel) will continue to be invaluable with regard to empathy, cultural considerations, and decision-making which may be too complex to be supported by AI. Nonetheless, AI systems can make their job more fulfilling by decreasing their routine workload, increasing their efficiency, and providing high-quality care.

To cite an example, AI could automate monotonous tasks like monitoring prescriptions, making appointments, and health records so that caregivers could focus on emotional support and making high-level decisions. Predictive analytics has the capability of notifying caregivers of the risks that might come before it is too late so that necessary measures can be taken. Robots may be able to help decrease workload on humans through lifting or mobility support and consequently lower the burden of care on the caregivers and minimize the number of injuries.

Human-AI collaboration can also solve organizational issues of the elderly care sector including the problem of insufficient caregivers. As populations of elderly persons increase everywhere, they sometimes outnumber the number of professionals to provide care to them. The use of AI technologies would allow closing this gap by performing mundane and monitoring and support tasks that do not require advanced human ingenuity as caregivers take care of more complicated or interpersonal requirements (Goyal et al., 2025d).

6. CHALLENGES AND LIMITATIONS OF AI IN ELDERLY CARE

Although the use of artificial intelligence has provided powerful opportunities in old age care, it has been affected by very strong weaknesses and drawbacks. These challenges include technical, economical, cultural and regulatory. As a means to achieve the potential of AI in elderly care, it is necessary to analyze these obstacles with a critical eye and the possibility of mitigating those obstacles. The major constraints, which are discussed in this section, are technical reliability, accessibility and affordability, cultural resistance, and regulatory gaps as key factors that limit the adoption curve of AI to elderly care.

6.1 Technical Barriers and Reliability Concerns

It is imperative that the technologies used to enable AI are reliable and robust in order to be successful in elderly care. The AI systems however are not impeccable and they are affected by a number of technical problems which make them less effective.

The accuracy of AI predictions is one huge problem. Health-monitoring wearable devices, smart gadgets, and diagnostic algorithms use sensor readings and trained algorithms, which are not always capable of representing the complexity of an individual health condition. To give an example, false positive cases can be seen with the fall detection systems once an elderly person sits down too abruptly, and false negative cases also occur when certain slight balance losses are not necessarily detected. Both cases decrease usability and trustworthiness because the old users will be frustrated or unsafe when using such systems (Li et al., 2021).

Another technical obstacle exists in the area of interoperability. Different vendors or device manufacturers deploy devices and platforms that use AI with little standardization. This has made it hard to unify the data collected by various sources by caregivers and healthcare providers. An example in this case is that a wearable heart-rate monitor may not be able to easily spend information with a smart home fall detection system/electronic health record platform, resulting in an inefficient and disjointed care process.

Also, AI systems need extensive amounts of high quality data to train on. The field of elderly care poses some particularities in this respect since health-related data acquired on older populations are mediated by inconsistencies, abnormalities, or unpredictability of health statuses and life approaches. The limited or biased datasets can cause the ineffective models that cannot be generalized in other populations.

6.2 Accessibility and Affordability Issues

Though AI might make care of elderly more efficient, its accessibility is a significant restraint, especially in poorer nations and low-income families. Sophisticated AI systems requiring--such as smart home systems, robotic nurses, or complex diagnostics systems--can have steep upfront purchase prices, continued maintenance, and technical service needs.

To a large number of elderly people especially on fixed pensions, the expenses incurred in purchasing and maintaining AI devices is too high. Even in the more developed countries, AI assisted elderly care solutions may not be covered entirely by insurance and health system, further widening the access gap. This economic obstacle threatens to worsen any social disparities with only those with the greatest wealth enjoying the benefits of the application of AI in elderly care (Moore et al., 2013).

Readability or ease of use is also accessibility. Most AI requires a starting point of digital literacy, like mobile app management, configuration, or alerts. EpixyAi, people who are old and have not been exposed to much technology or quickly destabilizing cognitive abilities may not be able to deal with AI systems well. In underdeveloped regions, or rural areas, the ability to access is also limited by the lack of reliable internet connection since cloud-based AI systems rely on the ability to communicate constantly online (Naim & Lenka, 2018).

6.3 Cultural and Societal Barriers to Adoption

Along with technical and economical elements, cultural and societal predispositions considerably influence the embracement of AI in the care of the elderly. In several societies, the roles of the elderly care are governed by the society and have strong emotional and moral undertone towards intergenerational caregiving. The need to adopt the AI systems in these settings may be seen as a form of ignoring family responsibilities or as abandonment (Petrakaki et al., 2018).

Considering, for example, the collectivism societies in which family values are the top priority, employing robotic caregivers can be seen as a loss of cultural beliefs, which would result in elderly individuals and their family members rebelling against the measure. On the other hand, in relatively more individualistic societies, where being autonomous is highly prized, replacing reliance upon family/external care may be only one of the reasons why AI systems are adopted.

There exist also a generational divide in the way technologies are regarded. A large number of older citizens were socialized when few people had access to digital technologies and may find the process of modernization to the introduction of AI systems unfamiliar. It builds a psychological block, as elder users do not feel empowered by AI, but rather feel intimidated or told they do not need it (Goyal, 2025b).

There is also the stigma that is thus applied on the aged people by using AI in seeking aid, thus lowering the adoption. Others may be afraid of being considered dependent or incapable of handling or operating things on their own, and others may resist the use of technology since they do not wish to be perceived to be vulnerable. Such cultural and societal stumbling block underscores the need to develop AI systems that are culturally-friendly and capitalize on community-based care in elderly people (Rahman et al., 2017).

6.4 Gaps in Policy, Standards, and Regulations

In elderly care, the legal and regulatory environment regarding AI is only in its nascent phase, which presents certain major drawbacks in its use. AI systems usually work in ways that are complicated and adaptive in a way that normal medical device regulations find it difficult to apply. This is unclear to the developers, healthcare providers, and older users hence bringing about uncertainty.

One of the gaps in regulations is an accountability gap. When something (an incorrect diagnosis, failure to detect a fall, violation of privacy) is done by an AI system, there may be no clear understanding of which party is responsible. Lack of liability frameworks may cause older people not to trust AI-driven care and their families (Risling et al., 2017).

There are also underdeveloped standards of safety, interoperability, and quality assurance. As countries start drawing out guidelines on AI in healthcare, there are global differences and thus unequal expectations of AI adoptions. A piece of equipment cleared in one country can easily take longer to roll out in others due to the regulatory differences.

There is even more complication with data protection laws. EU laws like the General Data Protection Regulation (GDPR) place high restrictions on data collection and utilization of personal health data. Though such legislations can protect privacy, they can restrict the flexibility with which AI developers may train and deploy systems, where we want almost constant monitoring in cases of elderly care.

7. FUTURE PROSPECTS AND INNOVATIONS

Artificial intelligence (AI) technology has yet to be fully incorporated into the field of elderly care, but its future looks to be awe-inspiring, with potentially life-altering advances on the horizon that will transform how aging populations live, receive care, and interact with the world around them. Technological changes are accelerating globally in AI, robotics and connected systems, which will play a critical role towards the increasing need in healthcare and elder support as demographic change occur. The section examines the future of AI in elderly care, including integration with the emerging technology, custom medicine in elderly care, case studies around the globe, and the roadmap that research and implementation might require in the global scenario of elderly care through AI applications and developments (Saadatzi et al., 2020).

7.1 Integration of AI with IoT, Robotics, and 5G

The next era of elderly care refers to the introduction and integration of these trending technologies into elderly care, including the Internet of Things (IoT), robotics and high-speed networks like 5G. Such synergy will allow the real-time, and context-sensitive provision of seamless support systems, which is oriented towards the needs of elderly individuals.

With the use of IoT-enabled devices, including smart sensors installed in the homes, the data about the health condition of an elderly person, their mobility, and the conditions around them will be collected continuously. In association with AI, this data can help give predictive warnings of an emergency such as falls, abnormal heart rhythms or unhealthy living conditions. Future AI-IoT environments will provide a more complete picture of real-time information because they will combine the information presented by several separate systems, such as smart watches to smart thermostats and air quality sensors.

Robotics also is going to make a difference as well. Care robots can be robotic assistants that provide mobility support, and socially interactive robots that provide companionship all of which are becoming more adaptive and or human-like over time due to advances in deep learning and AI in natural language processing and emotional intelligence. Obviously, these robots would be physical assistants and emotional support workers as well and decrease the levels of loneliness, assisting with routine tasks like cooking, cleaning, and reminding on medications (Santos et al., 2021).

5G networks deployment will further fuel the rate of innovation. Having 5G with low latency and fast-speed connectivity will enable AI systems to perform calculations in real-time even when they are taking place in the cloud. This is important particularly in old age care as seconds may be the determining factor in the event of emergency detection and response. AI, IoT, robotics, and 5G show promise in providing personalised and real-time care to the worldwide elderly population on a global scale.

7.2 Personalized Medicine and AI in Preventive Care

Probably one of the most attractive opportunities of AI in elderly care is that it allows personalised and preventive medicine. With varied health issues in aged people - be it chronic diseases or even decline in cognitive abilities, AI systems can offer a specific intervention depending on the health history and other factors like DNA, and lifestyle.

Predictive analytics may be used in the future to aid in detection of the early warning symptoms of a condition like dementia, heart disease or diabetes well before it becomes evident. The ability of AI to perform constant analysis of physiological data may push elderly care beyond its treatment model and into prevention, perhaps recommending action in the form of lifestyle changes, adjusting medications, or a routine check-up.

In addition, genomics, and AI-based bioinformatics will make medical interventions more accurate. Elderly patients might get tailor made treatments in relation to genetic predisposition and this will lessen side effects and increase the treatment potency. When it comes to polypharmacy, which is quite prevalent among older people, AI can be used to optimize prescriptions based on the interactional properties and propose safer medication combination.

The preventive care will also be addressed towards mental and emotional health. Brain-stimulating games and cognitive training programs based on AI can assist in the postponement of the onset of cognitive impairment and the enhancement of memory. Emotional wellbeing as well will be enhanced by AI systems that learn to read mood changes and offer the corresponding support in a manner of virtual counseling, companionship robots, or links to human caregivers. In subsequent years, the right and preventative AI systems might add up to elderly people going longer, healthier, and more independently with their lives.

7.3 Global Case Studies and Pilot Projects in Elderly Care

Some of the forms of application of AI in elderly care that characterized the past can be considered as some of the clues that show the future of elderly care and AI.

In Japan that has one of the oldest populations in the world, there is a wide usage of robotic carecler, like Paro, a therapeutic robot seal, and Pepper, a humanoid robot, in the nursing homes to offer companionship and aid. These initial applications can show how social interactive AI can help eliminate the effects of loneliness among the elderly and how it can promote psychological well-being.

In Europe, the smart homes, with the use of AI-controlled sensors and monitoring systems, are being piloted so that they assist independent living. These houses are able to sense abnormal activity patterns - like an elderly person failing to get out of bed within regular time - and automatically send a notice to caretakers. The European Union has sponsored various research projects within the Horizon programs, focusing on hybridization of ambient assisted living (AAL) with AI.

In the United States, care providers are testing AI-driven predictive analytic tools to minimize readmission of elderly patients. These systems analyze medical records, wearable data, life-style behaviors in order to determine which patients are at risk and step in early to prevent the problem. Most concisely, AI-driven chatbots and voice assistants are being created to medically advise and remind the elderly 24/7, making healthcare facilities being more accessible to them.

These case studies not only illuminate the possibility of AI, but also its variability in the elderly care across cultural and economic backgrounds. Large scale projects of this nature are a good way to learn about usability, ethics and shaping the merge between traditional healthcare systems and these projects.

CONCLUSION

One of the most promising ways of addressing the major challenges created by the emerging aging population globally is the infiltration of artificial intelligence into the management of the elderly. As has been described in this chapter, AI projects are not just instrumental in enhancing healthcare results and outcomes but are acting as potential game-changers in the way geriatric people live, communicate with each other, and involve themselves with healthcare services. Whether in the realm of remote monitoring and predictive care, socially interactive robots, and ambient assisted living, technological innovations enabled by AI are promising to meet the demands of medical safety in a broader scope of well-being, including independence, mobility, and social connection.

Simultaneously, the psychological and emotional nature of aging should always be kept at the forefront of these technologies deployment. The older generation is not meant to receive attention but act as a functional part of the process whose cultural beliefs, autonomy, and respect must be given considerations. The future applications of AI are such that a combination of personalization and empathy can lead to a more human-centric approach to the care of elderly people with technology becoming more of an aid to such relationships, instead of functioning as a substitute to personal connection.

Bringing this vision to fruition is, nonetheless, an uphill battle. Ethical concerns like data privacy, transparency of algorithms, risk of over dependence on automation has to be worked upon to enhance trust of not only senior users but also to caregivers. Technical constraints as limits related to interoperability, reliability and affordability are also providing inhibitors to mass adoption. Furthermore, differences in society and culture play a role in the adoption of AI and thus the criticality of designing context-sensitive solutions with the elderly communities and not simply to them.

In perspective, the role of AI in elderly care will rely on inter-stakeholder collaboration. The governments, healthcare institutions, technology companies, and researchers should collaborate with one another by developing standards, regulations, and best practices and maintaining a balance between innovation and accountability. The applicability of AI-enables solutions is empirically proven in most pilot projects and other real-world implementations across the world, however, scale and sustained and inclusive growth is a major challenge that needs to be addressed.

To sum up, AI has potential not only in clinical but also in overall quality of life changes in elderly people. When AI is created with responsibility and inclusivity, it has the potential to enable older people to live longer and healthier lives and to prolong old age with better quality, alleviating the pressure on care givers and healthcare systems. The issue facing researchers, practitioners and policymakers will no longer be whether AI can bring sweeping change in caring for the elderly, but whether this change is ethical, equitable or at all focused on the well-being of humans.

REFERENCES

Ali, H., & Li, H. (2019). Evaluating a smartwatch notification system in a simulated nursing home. *International Journal of Older People Nursing*, *14*(3), e12241. DOI: 10.1111/opn.12241 PMID: 31099184

Amin, M. G., Zhang, Y. D., Ahmad, F., & Ho, K. C. D. (2016). Radar signal processing for elderly fall detection: The future for in-home monitoring. *IEEE Signal Processing Magazine*, *33*(2), 71–80. DOI: 10.1109/MSP.2015.2502784

Ashfaq, M., Yun, J., Yu, S., & Loureiro, S. M. C. (2020). I, chatbot: Modeling the determinants of users' satisfaction and continuance intention of AI-powered service agents. *Telematics and Informatics*, *54*, 101473. DOI: 10.1016/j.tele.2020.101473

Banner, L., & Olney, C. M. (2009). Automated clinical documentation: Does it allow nurses more time for patient care? CIN: Computers, Informatics. *Nursing*, *27*(2), 75–81. DOI: 10.1097/NCN.0b013e3181979e57 PMID: 21685832

Berridge, C., Tyler, D. A., & Miller, S. C. (2018). Staff empowerment practices and CNA retention: Findings from a nationally representative nursing home culture change survey. *Journal of Applied Gerontology*, *37*(4), 419–434. DOI: 10.1177/0733464816653478 PMID: 27566304

Betriana, F., Tanioka, R., Gunawan, J., & Locsin, R. C. (2022). Healthcare robots and human generations: Consequences for nursing and healthcare. *Collegian (Royal College of Nursing, Australia)*, *29*, 767–773. DOI: 10.1016/j.colegn.2022.01.008

Chen, K., Lou, V. W.-Q., Tan, K. C.-K., Wai, M.-Y., & Chan, L.-L. (2020). Effects of a humanoid companion robot on dementia symptoms and caregiver distress for residents in long-term care. *Journal of the American Medical Directors Association*, *21*(11), 1724–1728. DOI: 10.1016/j.jamda.2020.05.036 PMID: 32713772

Conger, J. A., & Kanungo, R. N. (1988). The empowerment process: Integrating theory and practice. *Academy of Management Review*, *13*(3), 471–482. DOI: 10.5465/amr.1988.4306983

de Kervenoael, R., Hasan, R., Schwob, A., & Goh, E. (2020). Leveraging human-robot interaction in hospitality services: Incorporating the role of perceived value, empathy, and information sharing into visitors' intentions to use social robots. *Tourism Management*, *78*, 104042. DOI: 10.1016/j.tourman.2019.104042

Diareme, K. C., Liapakis, A., & Efthymiou, I. P. (2022). Data, sentiment analysis, and examples during the COVID-19 pandemic. *Hellenic Archives of Psychiatry and Clinical Psychology in Behavioral Sciences, 33779*. Advance online publication. DOI: 10.12681/hapscpbs.33779

Dill, J. S., Morgan, J. C., & Weiner, B. (2014). Frontline health care workers and perceived career mobility. *Health Care Management Review, 39*(4), 318–328. DOI: 10.1097/HMR.0000000000000028 PMID: 23989644

Dilsizian, S. E., & Siegel, E. L. (2014). Artificial intelligence in medicine and cardiac imaging: Harnessing big data and advanced computing to provide personalized medical diagnosis and treatment. *Current Cardiology Reports, 16*(1), 441. DOI: 10.1007/s11886-013-0441-8 PMID: 24338557

Efthymiou, I. P. (2024). *Human wellbeing in the age of artificial intelligence*. IGI Global Scientific Publishing.

Efthymiou, I. P. (2026). AI in epidemiology: Predicting the unpredictable leveraging AI to detect outbreaks and predict disease. In *Innovation and transformation of public health* (pp. 281–308). IGI Global Scientific Publishing., DOI: 10.4018/979-8-3693-0000-0.ch012

Fossen, F. M., & Sorgner, A. (2022). New digital technologies and heterogeneous wage and employment dynamics in the United States: Evidence from individual-level data. *Technological Forecasting and Social Change, 175*, 121381. DOI: 10.1016/j.techfore.2021.121381

Frank, B., Herbas-Torrico, B., & Schvaneveldt, S. J. (2021). The AI-extended consumer: Technology, consumer, country differences in the formation of demand for AI-empowered consumer products. *Technological Forecasting and Social Change, 172*, 121018. DOI: 10.1016/j.techfore.2021.121018

Gill, T. M., Murphy, T. E., Gahbauer, E. A., & Allore, H. G. (2013). The course of disability before and after a serious fall injury. *JAMA Internal Medicine, 173*(19), 1780–1786. DOI: 10.1001/jamainternmed.2013.9063 PMID: 23958741

Gorla, N., Somers, T. M., & Wong, B. (2010). Organizational impact of system quality, information quality, and service quality. *The Journal of Strategic Information Systems, 19*(3), 207–228. DOI: 10.1016/j.jsis.2010.05.001

Goyal, N. K. (2025). Security and privacy in IoT, fog, and blockchain networks. In Sathio, A., Rind, M., Awan, S., & Junejo, A. (Eds.), *Energy-efficient deep learning approaches in IoT, fog, and green blockchain revolution* (pp. 371–398). IGI Global Scientific Publishing., DOI: 10.4018/979-8-3373-0300-0.ch015

Goyal, N. K. (2025). Weaponizing misinformation and cyberattacks on supply chains. In Bukhari, S., & Zafar, I. (Eds.), *Mass media and impact of fake news on supply chains* (pp. 177–210). IGI Global Scientific Publishing., DOI: 10.4018/979-8-3373-2175-2.ch007

Goyal, N. K., Dandotiya, M., Kumari, M., Kaloria, S., & Anushya, A. (2025). AI-powered haptic devices for patient rehabilitation. In Mamodiya, U., Kalam, A., Bossoufi, B., Awad, M., & Somwanshi, D. (Eds.), *Integrating AI with haptic systems for smarter healthcare solutions* (pp. 143–170). IGI Global Scientific Publishing., DOI: 10.4018/979-8-3373-2307-7.ch007

Goyal, N. K., Dandotiya, M., Kumari, M., Sheikh, M. F., & Sharma, S. (2025). Emerging job roles in the tourism sector leveraging artificial intelligence. In Silic, M., Luthia, M., Ahmad, F., & Chakraborty, P. (Eds.), *Empowering sustainable performance and competitive advantage in tourism* (pp. 89–126). IGI Global Scientific Publishing., DOI: 10.4018/979-8-3373-4546-8.ch004

Goyal, N. K., Dandotiya, M., Qurashi, J. A., Kumari, M., & Sharma, S. (2025). AI-driven predictive analytics for disease management. In Ouaissa, M., Ouaissa, M., Imad, M., Qurashi, J., & Farooq, M. (Eds.), *Utilizing AI of medical things for healthcare security and sustainability* (pp. 231–276). IGI Global Scientific Publishing., DOI: 10.4018/979-8-3373-0690-2.ch008

Goyal, N. K., Kumari, M., Kushwah, V., Dandotiya, M., & Vijay, A. (2025). Evaluating blockchain security: Trade-offs in consensus mechanisms. *IET Conference Proceedings*, 2024(38), 80–88. https://doi.org/DOI: 10.1049/icp.2025.0775

Hsieh, S. H., Tseng, T. H., & Lee, C. T. (2018). Drivers of online brand community value creation: The role of psychological empowerment. In *Proceedings of the 51st Hawaii International Conference on System Sciences* (pp. 2220–2229). https://doi.org/DOI: 10.24251/HICSS.2018.280

Junglas, I., & Harris, J. (2013). The promise of consumer technologies in emerging markets. *Communications of the ACM*, *56*(5), 84–90. DOI: 10.1145/2447976.2447996

Khan, N., Jackson, D., Stayt, L., & Walthall, H. (2019). Factors influencing nurses' intentions to leave adult critical care settings. *Nursing in Critical Care*, *24*(1), 24–32. DOI: 10.1111/nicc.12348 PMID: 29635820

Laschinger, H. K. S. (2012). Job and career satisfaction and turnover intentions of newly graduated nurses. *Journal of Nursing Management*, *20*(4), 472–484. DOI: 10.1111/j.1365-2834.2011.01293.x PMID: 22591149

Laschinger, H. K. S., Finegan, J., Shamian, J., & Wilk, P. (2001). Impact of structural and psychological empowerment on job strain in nursing work settings: Expanding Kanter's model. *The Journal of Nursing Administration*, *31*(5), 260–272. DOI: 10.1097/00005110-200105000-00006 PMID: 11388162

Leal-Junior, A. G., Díaz, C. R., Leitão, C., Pontes, M. J., Marques, C., & Frizera, A. (2019). Polymer optical fiber-based sensor for simultaneous measurement of breath and heart rate under dynamic movements. *Optics & Laser Technology*, *109*, 429–436. DOI: 10.1016/j.optlastec.2018.08.048

Li, Y., Ho, K., & Popescu, M. (2012). A microphone array system for automatic fall detection. *IEEE Transactions on Biomedical Engineering*, *59*(5), 1291–1301. DOI: 10.1109/TBME.2012.2186446 PMID: 22532430

Li, Y., Zheng, T., Wang, M., Dong, L., Wang, P., & Qin, X. (2021). A coloring and timing brain-computer interface for the nursing bed robot. *Computers & Electrical Engineering*, *95*, 107415. DOI: 10.1016/j.compeleceng.2021.107415

Moore, L. W., Leahy, C., Sublett, C., & Lanig, H. (2013). Understanding nurse-to-nurse relationships and their impact on work environments. *Medsurg Nursing*, *22*(3), 172–179. PMID: 23865278

Naim, M. F., & Lenka, U. (2018). Development and retention of Generation Y employees: A conceptual framework. *Employee Relations*, *40*(2), 433–455. DOI: 10.1108/ER-09-2016-0172

Petrakaki, D., Hilberg, E., & Waring, J. (2018). Between empowerment and self-discipline: Governing patients' conduct through technological self-care. *Social Science & Medicine*, *213*, 146–153. DOI: 10.1016/j.socscimed.2018.07.043 PMID: 30081356

Rahman, S. A., Taghizadeh, S. K., Ramayah, T., & Alam, M. M. D. (2017). Technology acceptance among micro-entrepreneurs in marginalized social strata: The case of social innovation in Bangladesh. *Technological Forecasting and Social Change*, *118*, 236–245. DOI: 10.1016/j.techfore.2017.02.017

Risling, T., Martinez, J., Young, J., & Thorp-Froslie, N. (2017). Evaluating patient empowerment in association with eHealth technology: Scoping review. *Journal of Medical Internet Research*, *19*(9), e329. DOI: 10.2196/jmir.7809 PMID: 28963090

Saadatzi, M. N., Logsdon, M. C., Abubakar, S., Das, S., Jankoski, P., Mitchell, H., Chlebowy, D., & Popa, D. O. (2020). Acceptability of using a robotic nursing assistant in health care environments: Experimental pilot study. *Journal of Medical Internet Research*, *22*(11), e17509. DOI: 10.2196/17509 PMID: 33180024

Santos, N. B., Bavaresco, R. S., Tavares, J. E., Ramos, G., & Barbosa, J. L. (2021). A systematic mapping study of robotics in human care. *Robotics and Autonomous Systems, 144*, 103833. DOI: 10.1016/j.robot.2021.103833

Vousinas, G. L., Simitsi, I., Livieri, G., Gkouva, G. C., & Efthymiou, I. P. (2022). Mapping the road of the ethical dilemmas behind artificial intelligence. *Journal of Politics and Ethics in New Technologies and AI, 1*(1), e31238. DOI: 10.12681/jpentai.31238

Chapter 2
Artificial Intelligence (AI) in Geriatric Diagnostics

Iris-Panagiota Efthymiou
https://orcid.org/0000-0001-9656-8378
Regent College, London, UK

Konstantinos Stolakis
https://orcid.org/0000-0002-5497-4172
University of Patra, Greece

ABSTRACT

The use of Artificial Intelligence (AI) in geriatric diagnostics is expanding rapidly, yet its integration remains uneven and often poorly adapted to the complexities of ageing populations. This chapter examines how AI systems are currently applied in diagnosing age-related conditions such as dementia, frailty, and multi-morbidity. It assesses the strengths and limitations of machine learning models trained predominantly on younger or non-representative data, raising concerns about diagnostic bias, false positives, and underdiagnosis in older adults. The chapter also explores the ethical, practical, and regulatory challenges of implementing AI in clinical environments where human judgment, patient history, and social context remain critical. By focusing on transparency, data quality, and inclusive model design, it argues for a cautious but deliberate rethinking of how AI can serve, not replace, clinical expertise in geriatric care.

1. INTRODUCTION

Geriatric clinical care is a multidisciplinary assessment designed to evaluate older patients' functional ability, physical health, and cognitive well-being. Since elderly

DOI: 10.4018/979-8-3373-5462-0.ch002

patients often present chronic and coexisting conditions that require complex treatments, they frequently suffer from medication- or disease-related problems. Different combinations of diseases frequently result in heterogenous presentations and clinical similarities, requiring special attention to manage and treat these patients. With the increase of public interest in geriatric care, hospitals began utilizing various artificial intelligence (AI) systems to improve clinical care for elderly patients. Research was systematically reviewed on the use of machine learning (ML) in geriatric care to discover ongoing efforts, notable findings, and possible future applications.

Engaging with feedback has significantly stimulated my desire to explore innovative methodologies, particularly the integration of active learning strategies within my sessions, customized to address the diverse requirements of learners. This experience has strengthened my dedication to fostering a collaborative and supportive workplace atmosphere.

Eligibility was assessed based on a published search strategy, resulting in 35 eligible studies classified in three groups: psychological disorder, eye diseases, and others. A majority of research are studies in psychology dealing with screening tools for dementia and other geriatric psychological disorders. These screening tools for dementia are designed to detect early onset mild cognitive impairments, and thus geriatric health problems. One salient finding in this research group is the institutional constraint of fragile population screening tools for dementia that have prompted the emergence of innovative psychological screening instruments. One systematic review of automatic depression identification using photos produced promising results. The study suggested that further provision of a curated dataset improve model performance and generalizability. Eye disease studies deal with image-based classification of age-related macular degeneration, diabetic retinopathy, etc. One notable finding is a new recommended patient-eye image and species-wide model that optimizes prediction accuracy based on multiple parameters. Recently, with the gradual growth of AI applications in the health care industry, it is reasonable to assume a positive impact of AI on geriatric patients. Automated tools may be developed and utilized for offering better prevention, diagnosis, and treatment concerning patients' mental health, physical limitations, and chronic diseases (Kumar, Y., et al., 2022).

2. OVERVIEW OF ARTIFICIAL INTELLIGENCE

Artificial Intelligence (AI) denotes systems that can execute tasks that typically require human intelligence. The core characteristic of AI systems is their capacity to learn from data or improve their performance without being programmed. Geriatric care is a unique area in healthcare, with elderly patients differing from younger patients in their clinical profiles, comorbidities, and social and mental health problems.

Older patients often suffer from chronic diseases requiring additional efforts, such as care management plans, follow-ups, and referrals to specialists (Hansen A. R., et al., 2022; Mbata A., et al., 2024). In response, many hospitals have begun using AI in clinical care. "AI applications" refer to systems that use AI technologies like machine learning, natural language processing, deep learning, computer vision, and automatic speech recognition to perform tasks (Chinnaiyan et al., 2025). Examples include chatbots assisting patients in claiming medical services, machine learning calculating the likelihood of disease progression, or a clinical decision support system providing treatment options. The research questions focus on the applications of AI programs in clinical geriatric care. Key themes are: purposes of AI systems, health conditions for AI screening systems, AI-based decision-support systems, and user involvement. Preliminary information gives a general idea of the importance of the topic and the approach for this research. AI clinical programs are recently adopted as change management actions in hospitals. In some papers, the term Geriatrics encompasses health-related services requiring evaluation and oversight by medical doctors for older patients. AI clinical applications concentrate on two general types of systems: stand-alone screening systems and decision-support systems. An overview and in-depth analysis of AI systems used in clinical geriatric care are provided. Similarities, differences, and future steps with a perspective of humanities in medicine, such as AI ethics, AI behaviours, transparency, and user acceptance issues of AI-based systems are discussed.

3. THE ROLE OF AI IN HEALTHCARE

The advent of artificial intelligence (AI) in healthcare is considerable and presents vast opportunities. AI is often considered a more general category or umbrella term that covers a variety of tools, and in this text 'AI' primarily refers to applications that use machine learning (ML) with neural networks (Goel et al., 2023). The ability of AI algorithms to recognize complex patterns based on training data presents a new set of problems and opportunities across many fields, and perhaps no field is more impacted than healthcare.

Diagnosis is one of the most important and challenging tasks in healthcare. A robust system of diagnostics is needed to screen older people at risk and to enable the identification of conditions earlier in their development. This would allow for routine testing and interactive clinical care, with ongoing improvements from natural language processing (NLP) (Thakur G. K., et al.2024). Accessing routine screening could also support the development of basic social, psychological and physical health fitness outside of interactions with the healthcare system.

Detection of certain conditions is at its most effective when they are still in their earlier phases; thus, other theories of cognitive impairment, such as the social model or the life-course model, are relevant to the fitting of characteristics like health watches to models of the care system. At the same time, there is much greater difficulty in accuracy when trying to interpret single screening stems like the Mini-Mental State Examination (MMSE) (Stefanidis K. B., et al., 2025). There are different stages to cognitive impairment, each with increasing difficulty of prediction. A great burden is placed upon retrospectively trained models trying to detect something not present in the vast majority of the training data, leading to great variability on individual cases.

Long term conditions (LTCs) and multimorbidity are the most common types of health condition in older people. Nearly 7 in 10 people aged over 65 are estimated to live with multiple LTCs, according to the National Institutes of Health (NIH) and the National Council on Aging (NCOA), which can interact in complicated and detrimental ways and contribute to the development of frailty and associated syndromes. New demands facing healthcare systems and the development of preventative strategies and evidence based interventions for the management of LTCs is required.

Numerous healthcare systems in the UK and US are piloting initiatives to introduce self management and decision support to older people. Improved monitoring of LTCs and earlier diagnoses of LTCs and movement disorders, allowing for timely interventions to take place is actively being researched in older populations. Wearable technology including watch or smartphone platforms are now an established prong of health promotion. The potential for near continuous monitoring of numerous variables at high frequency with increased accuracy and granularity in real time is now exploited to examine how variables relate to cognitive and physical performance. AI algorithms for continuous and reliable remote assessments are being developed both at the surface level and using more complex and hidden features with neural networks (Shiwani T., et al., 2023).

4. CURRENT TRENDS IN GERIATRIC MEDICINE

Artificial Intelligence (AI) has the potential to enhance geriatric diagnostics across several modalities such as clinical decision support systems (CDSS), natural language processing (NLP), image analysis, and speech analysis (Xu X., et al., 2024; Koc M., 2023). With the increasing number of older adults, especially fragile elderly patients, it is crucial to enable reasonable and standard efforts for screening elderly patients in a wide range of clinical practice setting. While there are systematic reviews and opportunities on AI applications to diagnose different diseases including dementia, delirium, visual impairment, and functional impairment among older adults, there is a lack of literature that describes AI applications in geriatric diagnostics broadly (Moghadam et al., 2024; Woodman R. J., & Mangoni, A. A., 2023; Lukkien D. R., et al., 2023). Thus, the aim of this review article was to summarize existing geriatric diagnostic problems that AI has addressed, and how AI frameworks have been introduced in those areas including future research opportunities of AI in clinical geriatrics.

Cardiovascular disease (CVD), dementia, delirium, visual impairment, frailty, and functional impairment are the common geriatric diagnostic problems in geriatric settings. (Guasti L., et al.2025; Aïdoud A., et al., 2023,, Alonso S., et al., 2024). There has been a range of studies focused on AI diagnostics for CVD including risk prediction, pathology characterization, and treatment planning. Early screening tools such as CDSS have been developed for detecting patients with possible dementia or mild cognitive impairment, as well as patient referrals for further examination. For the purpose of delirium detection, division of care patterns and selection of creative caregiving solution can be targeted. Automated visual examination via fundus photograph and CDSS tools for the early diagnosis of age-related pathologies can be established. Prognosis of the clinical state of frailty can be estimated through strategic annotation of laboratory results and discharge note texts comprising various clinical notes with NLP. AI can also generate personalized and adaptive recommendations to enhance resilience on its own.

The digitalization of care environments of older adults has increased, and thus the proportion of sensory motion data has also grown dramatically. The development of transfer learning methods for age domain adaptation in multimodal data like 3D mesh-like tripod point clouds about human-tubular structures can inspire applications to monitor actions of older adults. Furthermore, advances in AI frameworks such as federated learning (FL) have received increasing interest for its ability to exploit privacy-sensitive cross-institutional data to predict worse outcomes. Automated image generation and restoration algorithms can help reduce noise and discretization artifacts by synthesizing high-quality images for prediction. 3D digital twins and simulation-based applications can improve the accuracy of diagnostics, prognostics, and therapeutics.

5. AI TECHNOLOGIES IN GERIATRIC DIAGNOSTICS

Since the inception of geriatric medicine in the 1940s, screening for chronic diseases, termed long-term conditions (LTCs), has been a core tenet. Although the need for monitoring LTCs is indisputable, accurate and timely identification of their onset is arguably even more important. Early diagnosis of LTCs would facilitate early intervention and prevention of downstream morbidity, mortality, and healthcare costs, so access to better diagnostic tools is of great interest in modern medicine.

Artificial intelligence (AI) is an umbrella term for a variety of computational and statistical techniques designed to learn from, or make predictions based on, data. It is a radical shift in the way machines process data, from simply executing predefined and encoded logic, to increasingly self-learning from data patterns and formal meaning prior to outputs and inference. The use of AI in geriatric diagnostics is an emerging area in research, with a small number of papers published on the potential for AI to be applied in the early identification of dementia. AI-facilitated methods for predicting LTCs have only started to be used. For frailty and its clinically important syndromes, such as falls, delirium, functional decline (including both activities of daily living and instrumental activities of daily living), and incontinence, more evaluation is required in this age-group (Hendriks et al., 2024; Chien et al., 2025).

Geriatric primary prevention screening is typically conducted with high-volume, clinician-reported questionnaires designed to identify patients at elevated risk for future functional decline (Perivolaris, 2024). Such screening is infrequently conducted given the burdens these assessments place on both patient and physician. However, the advent of wearables and ubiquitous mobile devices has led to a revolution in the ability to gather fine-grained, real-time data about individuals.

Sensor-based monitoring of movement can be used not only to improve diagnosis of existing illness failed by more conventional means, but also to identify patients at high risk for future illness before overt symptoms manifest and the disease becomes largely irreversible. The use of sensors in the monitoring of aging and age-related disease was selected as the best-bounded technique eligible for clearest scrutiny and successful application. Sensor data are noisy and require domain-specific expertise for appropriate analysis. Monitoring solutions must contend with issues of data integrity, privacy, security, and litigation, and connected sensor illness detection numbers are far lower than the current conventional care population (Ahmad I., et al., 2022; Abdulmalek S., et al., 2022).

5.1. Machine Learning Applications

Machine learning (ML) is a subfield of artificial intelligence that focuses on developing algorithms that can learn from data and make predictions or decisions based on that data. Machine Learning is revolutionizing how diseases are diagnosed, treated, and managed in geriatrics. It can analyze massive amounts of unstructured data and find patterns quickly and accurately. ML focuses on developing algorithms that can learn from and make predictions on data. Supervised, unsupervised, and reinforcement ML problems are the three main categories of ML (A., et al., 2021). In supervised learning, the algorithm learns a function that maps input data to output labels about training data and test gathers future data output. In comparison, unsupervised ML problems consider the data gathering input and no output. The output of reinforcement ML problems consists mainly of actions. The state of the environment collects training data based on the previous actions taken.

Both machine learning and initiative are crucial components of artificial intelligence. The main idea behind AI is to mimic natural intelligence in machines, while ML is based on the philosophy that systems can learn from data, identify patterns, and make decisions with minimal human intervention. An ML algorithm is a computer program that learns from data, and its performance improves as it gains more experience. AI systems can be rule-based or use ML. AI is often viewed as a "black box." People are frustrated when they do not understand the many restrictions or reasons for AI decisions (Hassija et al., 2024). However, ML is more susceptible to human control and scrutiny. While AI encompasses everything from automata to hard-coded expert programs to robotics, ML focuses on the specific technologies that use statistics and optimization to learn from data (Das & Dhillon, 2023). This encompasses a wide range of techniques, including not only traditional ones such as logistic regression, naive Bayes, k-means, and support vector machines but also more modern ones like deep learning and reinforcement learning.

5.2. Natural Language Processing

Natural Language Processing (NLP) is a burgeoning field that applies Artificial Intelligence to human language. NLP approaches exploit unstructured text in electronic health records (EHRs), such as providers' notes, which is challenging enough to classify (Khalate et al., 2024). Several studies have shown that text-analytics models can classify text from EHR notes effectively, and some have utilized clinical NLP to extract structured information. This work provides a comprehensive examination of whether NLP can detect dementia-related health concerns in EHRs across various care settings (Hong et al., 2020). The dataset consists of references to cognitive concerns in provider notes of assessed patients using a cohort of clinical datasets. The model results using SVMs and deep learning approaches show that NLP approaches can detect cognitive concerns and help understand the language behind the concerns across the mentioned notes, compared to no concerns.

Various language representations have been proposed, which are more appropriate for applications in different domains. This work examines two general language representation methods: ELMo is one of the first effective modeling approaches for both individual words and the overall sentence structure. This model trains a large bidirectional LSTM on 1 billion tokens of a general corpus and fine-tunes it on the domain-specific corpus for clinical care. The available language representation models include general-purpose models and domain-specific models. The pretrained language models have been proposed to achieve state-of-the-art performance in various NLP tasks along with customizable transformers. In addition, publicly available domain-specific and general-purpose language representation models have been proposed, providing various alternatives for applications in different domains.

Most efforts focusing on screening dementia risk have relied on structured data. Some studies using NLP techniques in assessing dementia risk on raw text data have been conducted. Previous works have used pattern-based text-analytics approaches to detect dementia in EHRs. The machine-learning tools rely on natural language processing (NLP) software to extract relevant features. The results suggest that applying NLP to provider notes improves the sensitivity of dementia detection, reflecting prior studies that BERT across localization and care settings detects potential cognitive concern notes (Shankar et al., 2025; Maclagan et al., 2023). The earlier work applies transfer learning from general-purpose modeling in successive localization.

5.3. Computer Vision Techniques

Computer vision is a branch of artificial intelligence focused on interpreting and understanding applications based on images (Efthymiou, I. P., & Efthymiou Egleton, T. W., 2023). Developments in computer vision have propelled multiple industries to utilize state-of-the-art algorithms and models using their surveillance cameras or installed static cameras to monitor health. Such implementation and planning can benefit the elderly. Summarized hereunder are different domains that highlight the impact computer vision is having on early detection and health analyses in the elderly. Age-related macular degeneration (AMD) refers to a group of complex heterogeneous neurodegenerative diseases that are usually associated with aging and are characterized by permanent degeneration of the retina (Yu et al., 2023). It is one of the leading causes of irreversible vision loss worldwide; however, it is still an under-researched area in medical AI.

Recently, the simulator of fundus photography has been used to collect wide-field fundus images, seeking to leverage deep-learning models to yield direct AMD detection from these images. However, accurately diagnosing AMD solely from fundus images is difficult due to the surrounding artifacts. Although optical coherence tomography (OCT) is the first-line examination tool for expert AMD screening, it has not gained full attention in data science research until recent years and is still overdue. To detect AMD using time-efficient and cost-effective machine learning or deep learning algorithms while enhancing the portability of this research field, an automated AMD detector is developed with the algorithmic potential to interpret OCT B-scans to a level comparable to an expert ophthalmologist for screening AMD.

A mounted handheld optical coherence tomography (OCT) optical system was used to acquire normal and AMD subjects (Devine B. C., et al., 2025; Zhang J., et al., 2023). To enable instantaneous on-board analyses, the implementation of hardware-friendly supervised pattern classifiers based on previously trained features is required. By feeding the extract slice-sum local binary pattern features derived from original and binarized B-scans with classifiers pretrained on original images, the classification accuracies of the support vector machine, extreme learning machine, and random forest classifiers for AMD detection could achieve 94.06%, 94.41%, and 92.54% on average, respectively. Automated detection of AMD deserves more attention in data science in quantitative measurements of human retinal layers with regard to embryonic growth, eye diseases, or treatment effect analyses. AMD is responsible for a plethora of photoreceptors and retinal pigment epithelium degenerations via a cascade activation of damage. Currently, a definitive AMD diagnosis is based on medically-expert delineations of retinal features from OCT images.

6. BENEFITS OF AI IN GERIATRIC DIAGNOSTICS

Artificial Intelligence (AI) has the potential to enhance health and social care for older people but also poses risks. Therefore, the responsible development and deployment of AI in this area is desirable and warranted. However, there is no clear consensus on how to broaden the acceptable evidence base to include issues of ethics, feasibility, safety, utility, equity, and acceptability, before AI is incorporated into clinical practice. AI in this area is an evolving and developing field that currently lacks an evidence base around the types of tools needed. Thus methods from the field of human-computer interaction to engage all key stakeholders will be employed to co-design a toolkit of guidance resources that may be adapted to suit the diverse health and social care systems; histories of technological innovation; and local needs in which clinicians, health professionals, industry representatives, researchers, regulatory bodies, and other stakeholders operate.

There are many potential applications of AI in healthcare for older people. Three areas of significant potential were identified: monitoring and diagnostics, stratified care and health systems support. Long term conditions (LTCs) and multimorbidity disproportionately affect older people. Better monitoring of LTCs and AI-facilitated early diagnosis may enable early intervention. Wearable technology has the potential to provide continuous monitoring of multiple factors in real time. It may reduce hospital admissions by supporting virtual monitoring and allowing early identification of acute deteriorations. When integrated into healthcare systems, AI can aggregate and interpret data in a timely fashion to support prognostication and triage. Early recognition of frailty syndromes and LTCs may also be facilitated by AI-enabled clinical decision support systems (CDSS). A systematic review identified several AI-assisted methods for predicting dementia, including image analysis of MRI scans, speech analysis of patients with Parkinson's disease dementia, and a CDSS system that predicts risk of dementia using cognitive assessment scores (Luo, 2025; Puterman-Salzman et al., 2023). CDSS tools using machine learning algorithms have also been applied to the prediction of delirium and depression among older adults.

6.1. Improved Diagnostic Accuracy

Artificial intelligence (AI) aims to reproduce and replicate human intelligence power in various ways, such as speech and facial recognition, natural language processing, and self-driving of vehicles (Kumar et al., 2023). For these applications, AI usage has increased a lot, and it is even used in various realms of life like security, finance, healthcare, and entertainment. At present healthcare is thus one of the prominent platforms where AI can provide better diagnoses and treatments. A lot of research is being done in developing AI to identify various health issues such as diabetes, COVID-19, brain tumors, skin diseases, heart diseases, etc. However, still, some issues need to be covered in applying AI to healthcare. The gap between the research done and the application of AI to the healthcare domain has been stated with a need for a better health system by the advancement of AI.

The study provides responses to what types of diseases have been detected? Which AI models and programming languages have been applied? What metrics have been used to analyze the results? There is a rise presented in the number of AI-based healthcare publications from 2014 to 2021. The present problems in inaccurate AI diagnosis and treatments which arise from the limited and wrong data collected from various sensors, lack of effective models and reliable data fusion techniques have been elaborated on (Chen et al., 2024; Albahri A. S., et al., 2023). The shortage of standard metrics and benchmarking methods to evaluate AI-based healthcare systems and the difficulty in accessing the data have also been pointed out. (Aminizadeh et al., 2024; Esmaeilzadeh, 2024). Moreover, methods and techniques to counteract the stated problems and ways to apply AI in healthcare to garner its benefits in the future have been discussed.

6.2. Enhanced Patient Monitoring

The quality of medical care for older adults can be improved through remote patient monitoring using unobtrusive Internet of Things (IoT) devices. These devices can automatically gather information about patient behavior and physiological signals, such as heart rate, glucose levels, and temperature, and send that information to the medical staff in near-realtime. It should help flag abnormal patient behavior, alert the medical staff, and thus speed up intervention. To keep patients safe and significantly increase older adult patient monitoring's effectiveness and efficiency, more thorough and complete objective observations would benefit the medical staff to complement highly subjective observations such as interviews and questionnaires. IoT system/device solution is proposed for this case. There is no need for older adult patients to change their usual habits since the proposed systems and devices are unobtrusive and the gathered information is objective.

For monitoring the excretory functional disorders, unobtrusive IoT non-invasive and non-intrusive devices are proposed for both bathroom activity change detection and toilet fall detection. Elderly patients can wear passive activity sensors for bathroom activity detection without a risk of patient discrimination, embarrassment, and, non-anonymity. Medical staff can detect toilet falls with the proposed IoT-enabled assist toilet and fall detection device attached under the toilet seat. Both approaches detect early signs of potential excretory functional disorders (Ray et al., 2025; Hyväri et al., 2024; Tanaka et al., 2024). A multi-dimensional non-invasive and contactless perception-based active detection solution is developed for abnormal motion detection, irregular breathing detection, and sudden sleep failure detection. Various sensor devices in a nursing home room environment detect these motion changes. If dignified solutions are adopted for the plans, a subfive-dollar device can be designed to detect the user's unusual motion and classify other health-related drawbacks of an older adult by analyzing the presented 2D motion data.

An IoT-enabled implement and the medical volunteers provide offline fitness prescriptions to older patients (Kulkarni and Inamdar, 2025; Martins et al., 2024; Nandakishora et al., 2025). A gamified fitness exercise website engages older adult patients to be compliant with the prescriptions. A choreographed exercise video is played to guide patients to ensure safety and effectiveness. The wearable fitness tracking watch collects biometric data and stores them in a cloud database for later review by spiritual practitioners. The exercise sessions are gamified to promote engagement. Once a session is finished, patients need to provide satisfactory videos to receive rewards. These patients can upload videos of obstacles or task models. The critical behavior captured in the videos is then reviewed by medical volunteers to examine treatment effectiveness. It produces timestamps of the videos and healthcare information, which can be beneficial for future treatment decisions.

6.3. Personalised Treatment Plans

Alzheimer's disease becomes more prevalent in older people, emerging symptoms of attention deficit and memory loss. A late-onset, sporadic, and chronic neurodegenerative disease, AD impacts roughly 40% of those aged 85 years or older. Moreover, AD accounts for 60-70% of dementia cases, creating a large socioeconomic burden due to diminishing activity of daily living, depression and psychosis (Liu et al., 2022). Consequently, automatic dementia screening in the older population has become pressing, possibly improving early diagnosis and monitoring through the integration of computerized cognitive training. Preclinical assessment of cognition has improved with wearable electroencephalograms (EEG) due to emerging AI algorithms and commercial devices at consumer prices.

Personalised treatment is a fundamental principle in medicine, yet it is challenging to achieve in standard clinical practice. There are numerous medications now approved for the treatment of cognitive impairment in dementia, but clinicians are still generally unable to specify the personalised treatment needed for a given patient. An AI-based recommendation model learns extrapolated patient data obtained in routine clinical practice and given treatment as well as using historical known data to produce personalised recommendations of the most effective treatment, thus allowing clinician-patient dialogue, patient choice of treatment and appropriate warnings. Accordingly, treatment would be recommended based on real-world medication data, promoting optimal matching between real-world patients and treatments.

The objective of this study was to develop and validate an AI-based recommendation model for high-dimensional psychiatric and neurodegenerative disorders, with regard to the development and validation of the recommendation model, the potential reproduction of the model in routine care, and the provision of specific medication and pragmatic implementation details. The treatment of cognitive impairment in dementia is a target and unique domain for developing and validating the model.

Researchers proposed a reaction score differential convexity (RSDC) method for developing the model version running on gradual information flow and payment speed, and reported how and where it could be reproduced in the healthcare system. Validating the AI-based recommendations on real-world patients, researchers found that it was possible to identify at the individual patient level the most effective drug to reduce cognitive impairment over two years. Real-world patients whose prescribed medications were the best fit according to the model had better cognitive performance after 2 years relative to those with other medication combination.

7. CHALLENGES AND LIMITATIONS

Currently, multiple obstacles inhibit the broader execution of AI in the Geriatric Diagnostics field. There are several data-related limitations in this area (Diareme, K. C., et al., 2022). AI systems need enormous volumes of high-quality, labeled data to be trained and validated, and obtaining them is especially hard in the healthcare field (Liang et al., 2022; Aldoseri et al., 2023). AI coding solutions are even further constrained by the lack of publicly available resources of data that SVMs, DNNs, and

RFs can analyze, in addition to training data. The healthcare field lacks a well-oiled data pipeline needed to develop AI systems as DA activities, such as data wrangling and feature engineering, usually consume most of project time.

Furthermore, accessing patient data within electronic health records (EHR) is well-known to be problematic due to interoperability issues among healthcare systems. EHR-sourced data are often poorly ordered and overly complex for even seasoned data scientists, making proper ML model development stalled or even impossible (Dykstra, 2024; Sidky et al.2023; Leviton & Loddenkemper, 2023; Reynolds T.. et al., 2025). One closer issue that teams running AI initiatives in geriatric diagnostics are struggling with is the lack of cleaning processes for input data. Most existing health record systems are legacy and poorly structured compared to newer, more scalable ones. Consequently, much valuable patient information is encoded among unstructured fields like text notes. This unstructured data is hard to analyze and raises concerns over private patient information' safety.

In addition, despite professional guidelines and frameworks that set a checklist for broader AI adoption, countless AI products that have passed evaluation abuse their residents in any nursing or retirement homes. Technically advanced AI models equipped with real-time monitoring capabilities create the need for sensor configurations that entail multi-million investment costs. Ethical issues arise concerning the modeling construct and how these models repay for operating costs. Furthermore, in some critics' opinions, models employed for AI monitoring in elderly care go directly against a person's human rights. It has long been argued that the absolute autonomy and private decision rights of monitored people might be breached, and hence it was long dismissed as impractical.

7.1. Data Privacy Concerns

Rapidly improving AI technologies can be used to both mitigate and amplify privacy and data protection risks. From the point of view of protecting health information, the increasing incorporation of AI into transfer patient data and analysis systems raises urgent concerns about future risks (Murdoch, 2021). Currently, AI specifically poses a novel challenge because the algorithms often require access to large quantities of patient data. Therefore, it is necessary to consider whether the data kinds or uses for AI performance may constitute a category of greater risk. Additionally, the location and ownership of the servers and computers that store and access patient health information are vitally important.

A number of issues arise here, including whether and how the server locations and the networks they occupy risk privacy breaches. Regulation should require that, for locally obtained data, patient data remain in the jurisdiction from which it is obtained. To assess privacy protection concerns, institutions must know where data is captured, stored, and analysed. Critically, robust privacy protection against commercial entities is only realizable where institutions cooperate to ensure data protection. There is the possibility that competing goals will undermine patient privacy protection.

Corporations may not be sufficiently encouraged to maintain the privacy protection of patient data. Rather than prohibiting their use, businesses may be more likely to employ AI systems without ensuring adequate privacy protection if they can monetize the data (Gabriel, 2023; Khalid et al., 2023). There have been calls for greater systemic oversight of all big data health research and technology input. A public lack of trust in the systems of an institution might heighten scrutiny of the commercial implementations of healthcare systems. It is likely to be harder to gain approval for such interventions from hospital boards, ethics committees, and public health institutions if these sorts of public trust issues arise (Ferretti et al., 2021; Marelli et al., 2021). For example, only 11% of survey respondents were willing to share their health data with technology companies.

Additionally, there is the external risk of privacy breaches from potential opportunities created by AI systems that possess sophisticated capabilities for finding out information. It is increasingly likely that these systems will inadvertently or deliberately expose health information. According to recent trends, healthcare data breaches have risen in many jurisdictions, and AI is not on the side of improving how well healthcare institutions protect health information.

Healthcare AI is poised to contribute to an increasing inability to protect health information privacy (Murdoch, 2021; Bala et al., 2024; Naik et al., 2022). Emerging computational strategies, combined with big data from online social media platforms, public health databases, and other systems, can be used to identify individuals in large health data repositories, even in cases where the information has been anonymized. Many of these approaches could be implemented without the direct knowledge of health institutions. This capability has implications for health information privacy across national boundaries. Importantly, using AI with health data puts institutions in the unusual position of relying on tools that can wholly undermine the rationales for their existence. In just a few years, AI has advanced further and more rapidly than anticipated, and it is exceedingly difficult to predict what it can do even at this time.

7.2. Bias in AI Algorithms

Medical Artificial Intelligence (AI) is increasingly being used in geriatric diagnostics even though its development risks producing biased algorithms disadvantageous to older patients. Older patients are often underrepresented in the data on which predictive analytics and risk assessment algorithms are trained, both in medical and non-medical input data (van Kolfschooten, 2023). Inaccurate representations of older patients in AI algorithm development make it more difficult for those algorithms to make accurate predictions for those patients consequent to the less-than-optimal fit between the AI algorithm and the patient's medical picture. Potential detrimental effects include lower efficacy and/or efficiency, which in turn put older patients' fundamental rights to health protection at risk.

The fact that AI medical devices may produce biased predictions for older patients is a serious matter and may give rise to age discrimination, a serious ethical issue (Alievska, 2023; Albahri A. S., et al., 2023; Koçak et al., 2025). Situation is further complicated by the fact that even when bias is unintentional in development, it could still produce discriminatory outcomes. In other words, the argument could be made that unintentionally producing biased algorithms is not prohibited under EU anti-discrimination law. Addressing demographic change is important: "by 2050, about 30% of the European population will be over 65 (EU) and by the mid-2030s, it is projected that there will be. 265 million persons aged 80 years or older, more than the number of infants (1 year of age or less) (UN, World Population Prospects 2024: Summary of Results), in the next 10 years, the number of persons aged 80 and older is expected to increase by more than 50% across the EU, reaching a projected total of 33 million in 2030, spending on yet-to-be-developed healthy longevity technologies is also expected to increase by a factor of more than 6.

7.3. Integration with Existing Systems

Integrating and deploying new AI-based tools for geriatric diagnostics into daily clinical practice is necessary to improve the quality and efficiency of geriatric care (Kouroubali et al., 2022; Mitra & Alam, 2025; Băjenaru et al., 2024). However, this goal is challenging. Such standard insights are not well-known in the field of geriatric diagnostics and are needed to make the presented concepts and designs fit-for-use.

From the authors' own experience and pilot studies, it has become evident that the following components/settings are needed to achieve a good integration:

1) Compatibility with the current EHR system,
2) Integration of diagnostics or assessments performed outside the clinician-patient contact in currently used systems,
3) Reuse of already available clinical notes in the current EHR systems, (4) Integration with the output of already existing tests or scoring systems, or
    5) A combination of the previous two points to integrate the evidence in cases where a particular concern was previously flagged by a nurse or caregiver (reflected in the EHR).

Integration with existing tools proved highly challenging, as the diagnostic systems offered mostly screenshots or videos to be inserted in an EHR, but no direct or API integration. Options to extract or reuse information from the user interface of diagnostic tools often rely on specialized programming of bots, or indirect and unsecured applications. All in all, over 75% of potential AI use cases in geriatric care are foregone (Loveys et al., 2022).

8. CASE STUDIES OF AI IN GERIATRIC DIAGNOSTICS

AI in Geriatric Diagnostics has immense potential, but with limited case studies, applications in healthcare settings, or reproducible demonstrations. Since 2018, interest in these topics has surged (Shiwani T., et al., 2023). Here are three examples relevant to the challenges faced by geriatric specialists:

Wearable Devices.

Fall detection was a dominant first use case for AI in geriatrics because falls lead to the greatest care burden and mortality. Some existing fall detection systems use accelerometer data and rule-based algorithms, meaning they are not transferable across patients and situations. Smart Watches from various companies offer devices that can create large annotated free-living datasets for behavioral monitoring.

The WISER concept leverages these new devices with previously developed machine learning (ML) fall detection methods. It is based primarily in the UK and the EU, where public researchers can obtain ground truth free-living accelerometer data from willing participants who wear a smartwatch containing an application recording data and prompts. The app interacts with other sensors to check that the analytical fall detection methods fit real activities. The public datasets, together with those of the verification processes, will be reused to create accurate transfer learning fall detection methods for different devices, patient groups, and conditions. Fine-tuning, transfer, or adapter learning paradigms will be applied to these pre-trained methods. The true novelty lies in the ability to independently verify and validate any fall detection method. Such validation is a requirement for clinical care deployment but is sometimes exploited in the booming smart wearables market, where performance claims outpace evidence.

Multimodal Intelligent Health Assistant.

Ideal fall prevention programs help both healthy and vulnerable patients, inform well-being progress through verbal prompts, and minimize clinician workload. Since

M-Health systems first found acceptance during the pandemic, no such AI assistants exist. The design allows client specifications to be deep-dived. Progressive deployment allows continuously increasing levels of automation while limiting risks. A domain-expert lead configures the rules, inputs, outputs, and patient information. A recommendation pipeline uses preset rules, patient input, and wellbeing conditions to translate the situation into treatment actions across channels, utilizing a patient-machine interaction paradigm that prioritizes motivating empathy. Session data can be asynchronously reviewed by physiotherapists, should they choose to do so. Failure modes are monitored for all channels, limiting unavoidable errors. This flexible design is expected to engage healthy and vulnerable patients, facilitate adherence, and meaningfully lessen clinician workload.

8.1. Successful Implementations

The application of artificial intelligence (AI) in medicine has gained prominence in recent years. This is predominantly due to the rapid generation of health-related big data from multiple sources. The aggressive digitization of health data has also created new possibilities for the development of AI algorithms. Stressing the clinical potential and research challenges of AI in medicine, 27 real-world AI implementations in various clinical specialties have been sourced, with a specific focus on geriatric diagnostics in older adults. Successful implementations were found in clinical domains as varied as cardiology, internal medicine, psychiatry, surgery, and radiology (Kim, 2024; Knevel & Liao, 2023).

With the world's population aging, an increasing burden of disease and disability will be carried by older people. Diagnosing and managing health issues in older adults can be particularly challenging, due to the reduced performance of standard diagnostics in older age, and the presence of multiple or complex conditions (multimorbidity). There is a pressing need to assist healthcare providers, and particularly those in primary care, to efficiently identify problems in older adults. AI might be able to assist in ongoing tasks where older adults are often under-served by traditional tools, or at tasks that cannot yet be performed automatically. In this review, a focus on geriatric diagnostics is formulated with respect to its current state, potential applications of AI, the AI solutions being developed or implemented in practice, and practical challenges is provided.

The goal to highlight the methods which are currently known to handle issues in geriatric diagnostics is outlined. To narrow the review focus to one aspect of the wider problems faced in geriatric diagnostics, age-related conditions with a particular focus on assessing cognitive decline, identification of symptoms of frailty, and instrumenting or screening for depressive disorders is identified. Concerns about the additional health burden for older adults created by the COVID-19 pandemic and other global public health initiatives are mentioned, leading to a specific interest in ways to lessen the burden on healthcare workers (Cocuzzo et al., 2022). Much of the focus will be on the deployment of new technologies in primary care settings.

8.2. Lessons Learned

In summary, the use of AI (artificial intelligence) can improve stroking outcome prediction, give a more accurate diagnosis and treatment suggestion for MCI (mild cognitive impairment), better identify eye diseases and detect Parkinson's Disease more efficiently (L. J. V., et al., 2023; Li et al., 2022; Fabrizio et al., 2021; Grueso & Viejo-Sobera, 2021). These are all the valuable insights to improve the understanding of AI use on geriatrics clinical care for chronic diseases in the existing literature. Many AI projects were attempted to advance training and imaging reading. Also, there are commonly shared concerns about the barriers and potential risks of AI in medicine. Understanding these lessons learned may strengthen researchers' consideration of adopting AI in geriatrics care and help clinicians better utilize AI outcomes in practice.

For the improvements of stroke outcome prediction through AI, the prediction model can calculate the probability of an event (e.g., higher/lower severity) based on the input feature (e.g., baseline patient characteristics, information extracted from the record) and thus help in triage and arrangement of treatment plans. However, many challenges exist. One important aspect is that stroke patients often exhibit complicated conditions, the disease time stamps vary in patients (in hours) and the physiological parameters for monitoring may differ significantly among patients (in much wider ranges than in normal ones), thus, a common patient representation form is still a challenge area for handling multimodal, multiscale, and variable-length information (Holm et al., 2025; Chaichareenon and Nupairoj, 2024; Sweidan et al., 2024). Hence, the performance gap between AI-assisted decision support systems and specialists could be large and hence limit the motivation for wider adoption of the solution. Laboratory tests can vary widely in usage across hospitals, revealing a rich resource for both clinical population and model development/refinement.

To give a more accurate diagnosis of MCI and treatment suggestions, EHRs (electronic health records) are known to have informatics and clinical value (Wei et al.2025; Joshi, H., 2025; Richter-Laskowska et al., 2025; Ostroushko, D., nd). However, the huge data volume can make EHR data integration and processing challenging as well. Parameters in AI models require hyperparameter tuning and change frequently with disease progression and treatment effects, thus potentially degrading prediction accuracy. There are also structure and format changes when processing different EHR types. The privacy issues of shared data among different EHR platforms are also worth considering

9. FUTURE DIRECTIONS

Currently, there is an increasing number of AI applications being used to assist clinicians in providing care for geriatric patients. A systematic literature review provided a state-of-the-art overview on the application of machine learning in geriatric clinical care for chronic diseases. It reported on the current landscape of machine learning technologies used in geriatric clinical care, application cases, limitations, and proposed future directions. Thirty-five eligible studies were included in the review that resulted in a summarized picture on the scope of machine learning in geriatric clinical care. The applicability of machine learning in geriatric clinical care is a rapidly evolving and multifaceted domain and there has been a noticeable increase in the amount of available literature in recent years (Abadir and Chellappa, 2024).

However, the applicability of machine learning in geriatrics is potentially much wider than the current use of machine learning in such domains as psychogeriatrics, early diagnosis of age-related diseases or disorders, and older patient triaging in emergency department. Several critical limitations of the current literature were discussed including risks associated with interpretation of algorithms, validation of machine learning for geriatric patients, the gap between deep learning research and clinical practice, and the need for multicenter, real-world studies.

However, several areas of geriatric care were identified as deserving more recognition in the literature. The broadest of these covered major acute elderly hospital care-related domains: older patient risk of in-hospital adverse events, the risk of readmission to the hospital, continuity of care, estimation of prognosis in geriatric oncology care, problems related to polypharmacy and other adverse drug events, balancing the need of GP follow-up and the burden side of it, and the risks related to discharge from the emergency department. As these conditions are particularly relevant for geriatric patients, models of machine learning failed to be described in the literature with regard to these issues. The next most notable topic was the broader quality and outcome indicators and investigation into the care delivered to geriatric patients throughout their hospital stay. Continuous measures of machine learning applications on geriatric patients and quality of care are scarce, despite the relative abundance of literature for younger patients.

9.1. Emerging Technologies

In the past few years, a lot of Intelligent Evaluation and Decision-Analytic Systems based on Artificial Intelligence (AI) have been emerging in many industrial domains for the detection of diseases, including Intelligent Systems for Diabetic and Tumor Diseases, A Patient Management System Based on Machine Learning, Intelligent Knowledge-Driven Systems for Cancer Screening, and Modeling Systems for Biochemical or Physical Parameters Detection, but not much research has been done on IT systems for early detection and intelligent evaluation of Alzheimer's Disease (AD). (Kumar et al., 2023).

Most research so far has been concentrates on working prototypes, methodologies, and potential of the technology bye underlining the limits of the works that have been done. The vast amount of research into multi-sensory detection of aging cognition declines models, on the other hand, targeting healthy people. No system is explored that is 100% feasible for early detection of AD. Therefore, the idea to develop a closed work that integrates AI techniques, wearable-sensors-based remote detection systems, and decision support systems for intelligently evaluating AD patients (Rong et al., 2022).

9.2. Potential Research Areas

There are many potential applications of AI in healthcare for older people. Rapid diagnostics may allow for a shorter interaction with healthcare staff or instruments, which is particularly advantageous for older adults with visual or hearing impairments, as it lowers the risk of misdiagnosis. Relaxation of equipment restraints or time-consuming assessment scales is favourable for older people with physical symptoms, including stiffness or tremors. Other recent AI applications would allow for the recognition of ruptured aortic aneurysm (AA), acute thoracic aortic dissection (TAAD), and ruptured pulmonary embolism (PE) in CT pulmonary angiography studies.

Grayscale retinal fundus images may be utilised for the automatic classification of age-related macular degeneration (ARMD) or diabetic retinopathy (DM). Such automatic image recognition may improve the quality of screening of ARMD and DM risk groups at a primary care level, preventing the need for time-consuming adjustments to instruments used. Thus, they may alleviate the burden on specialists in secondary care. Health systems support AI technical implementations may free up doctors' and nurses' time and improve oversight of workflows. AI algorithms may transform unstructured (free text) into structured data. This should facilitate better communication between different units, which would result in better clinical management of older patients. Healthcare systems across the world are struggling from service overload during the COVID-19 pandemic.

Older people have been disproportionately affected with higher mortality and poorer outcomes than their younger counterparts. There are various sources of pressure on healthcare systems affecting their capacity to cope with an increased burden, especially as they continue to manage the longer-term consequences of COVID-19. Population ageing and the increasing prevalence of long-term conditions entail an urgent need for support in providing care to older people. There are many practical applications of AI in healthcare for older patients with clinical conditions.

Three areas of significant potential were identified: monitoring and diagnostics, stratified care and health systems support. The global burden of long-term conditions (LTCs) and multimorbidity disproportionately affects older people. Improved monitoring of LTCs may enable AI-facilitated early diagnosis, enabling timely intervention to reduce burden on the individual and healthcare service, particularly in hospitals. Wearable technology has the potential to provide continuous monitoring of multiple factors across demographics including heart rate, oxygen saturation, activity levels, sleep patterns, ambient conditions, and social connectivity (Shiwani T., et al., 2023).

10. ETHICAL CONSIDERATIONS

Artificial Intelligence (AI) is revolutionizing geriatric diagnostics, enabling the development of cutting-edge sensors, mobile applications, and telehealth technology that enhance the efficiency of currently used instruments, allowing healthcare professionals (HCPs) to provide more accurate and individualized care and encouraging remote monitoring (Sankaran & Singla, 2024; Faiyazuddin et al., 2025). Telehealth, or electronic health care, is transforming health information exchange by making it faster and more convenient for both doctors and patients. Nevertheless, these technologies significantly raise ethical concerns related to data privacy violations, algorithm accuracy verification, and over-surveillance (Kamiyole, 2025; Toktas, 2024). Therefore, this section provides recommendations on maximizing benefits for elderly users while limiting potential adverse effects. Additionally, addressing ethical concerns to ensure compliance with regulations set forth by various organizations would prevent significant breaches of human rights and technological negligence.

Ethical issues may arise at every stage of technology production, use, and maintenance. A major concern is the potential loss of privacy with the use of AI solutions (Vousinas, G. 2022). As cameras, monitors, sensors, and other electronic devices become more advanced, their user information becomes exploitable by governments and organizations with the appropriate means. Once devices are networked together, hacking them becomes possible, putting sensitive information at risk. For instance, deployed environmental sensors could reveal living conditions, health status, and income, while video cameras could unveil habits, beliefs, gender, and sexual orientation. Some experts have voiced concerns that data collected could even affect an elder's perception of personal safety and potentially lead to abuse. Even if data is anonymized, the risk of re-identification is prevalent and could still result in unauthorized exposure of personal information. Governments have also expressed worry that biometric data may be misused for age discrimination in storing, accessing, and sharing health data (T., et al., 2019). Additionally, elder people may not have a clear understanding of how data is utilized and who has access to it, which could lead to discomfort and resistance to sensor use.

The second major concern involves monitoring and autonomy. AI technologies could encourage over-surveillance of seniors or screening of patients using wearable technologies. HCPs may impose HCP-initiated coordination due to worries over being sued if patients overdose on medications or forget to eat, leading to constant monitoring of medication ingestion or food intake. With AI technologies having access to a wide range of current health indicators, patient data analysis could pose a risk of being flagged, thus discouraging habitual risks. Changes in personal habits and patterns over time could even lead to a more life-inhibiting situation where social interactions or simple experiences are prevented for the sake of patient safety (Maris, T., et al., 2024).

10.1. Informed Consent

As an essential condition of medical ethics and law, consent must be made free, informed, expressed, and documented. In the case of computational technologies in healthcare, it is generally agreed that patients must be informed of the existence and functioning of the technology, understand its basic functioning, and be aware of its uses and their implications (Saccà et al., 2024). However, the requirements of informed consent in the context of the present state of AI are still in flux and do not necessarily guarantee patients' autonomy. Therefore, every health care stakeholder must better understand what knowledgeable consent entails in the era of AI-assisted healthcare. Furthermore, the immediacy and evolution of AI applications in healthcare require legal, ethical, cultural, and pragmatic support devices in relation to consent protocols.

It seems appropriate to consider how AI can concretely integrate into the proposal for informed consent to treatment, responding to the dilemma between the patient's self-determination and his right to health and the best available care. The proposal starts from the current notion of informed consent and emphasizes that AI must be integrated into every step of the care pathway, from history collection to objective assessment, as well as in the clinical, laboratory, and instrumental diagnostic pathways and in therapeutic procedures and in the definition of prognosis and follow-up pathways. After an exhaustive explanation of the possible uses of AI and how it works, patients must have the option to choose whether to avail themselves of it or to renounce it, even at the expense of not having the opportunity to take advantage of the best standards of care. This possibility should be framed on a per-act basis. Ideally, a naive patient would be able to check a box and state only that he wanted the best care possible without having to contemplate the blizzard of opportunities, acts, and challenges offered by AI. The present proposal is more demanding and sophisticated than the current standard of consent, including as it does aspects of shared decision making (Jin Park, H., 2024).

10.2. Accountability in AI Decisions

Responsibility is the basis upon which moral or legal blame, apology, or reward is settled for an act or event. It may, therefore, be held by agents or those accountable for their actions, operative facts, or outcomes. In other words, moral responsibility for a given action cannot be assigned unless someone is capable of influencing it in a morally relevant way. Despite differences in its nature, all categories of responsibility are assessed by a common yardstick: the degree of control, knowledge, or predictive insight that those judged to be responsible have over the action they are deemed responsible for (H. Lang et al., 2023). This suggests that it is possible to compare and narrow responsibility via the moral criteria made salient by the "responsibility-gaps" debate.

The "responsibility gaps" issue is concerned with a subset of the responsibility problem: AI decision-making technologies, sometimes referred to as "black box" algorithms. These are AI technologies whose operations are opaque or uninterpretable to all, or a subset of relevant humans. The term "black box" refers to the fact that the technology's inputs and outputs can be measured, but not necessarily its internal state or the computations it runs, rendering human operators unable to explain why it produces a given output from its input. Operative facts can be difficult to annotate, and inappropriate renditions can have disastrous consequences.

The "responsibility gaps" issue does not implicate just any morally neutral black box. The focus is on morally significant gaps that can arise when decisions are made or actions taken by black box AI technologies in contexts that involve moral consequences. Such "responsibility gaps" can be morally problematic or hazardous whenever a black box AI incurs blame or praise for its decisions, or agency over morally salient events construed as "decisions", a much broader range of decisions than those which it has causal agency in the above sense.

11. REGULATORY FRAMEWORKS

The interest surrounding Artificial Intelligence (AI) in Geriatric Diagnostics, a system addressing the area of senior population health, has the great potential to pre-emptively and automatically prevent age-related diseases such as Alzheimer's disease (Bernal et al., 2024; Mhlanga, 2024). However, such systems are new, with only few field trials conducted, and concerns around safety and efficacy of AI-based medical devices are prevalent. Therefore, regulation of such systems poses difficulties for healthcare providers and technology developers alike (Iqbal & Biller-Andorno, 2022; Brown & Desai, 2023; Mennella C., et al., 2024; Bhuiyan M. N., et al., 2021).

Furthermore, international and local regulations are not designed to effectively govern such systems, and adjustments are required. In accordance, input is provided on the regulatory framework of AI-based medical devices, an overview of regulation design challenges when governing such systems, the adjustments that these regulations require, and the consequences of not addressing these issues. Additionally, input is provided on the issue of bias in AI systems. Since there is a chance of bias in AI systems, it is vital to ensure that these systems are not making incorrect predictions for a distinctly large portion of the population. No clear guidelines are provided in current regulatory frameworks and input is given on what some of the broader questions and considerations in this field could be (Zhao et al.2024; Ghassemi M., et al., 2021).

AI has the great potential to detect patterns in large data sets that would otherwise remain hidden. It has already begun to enable digital health solutions in clinical practice that improve the pre-emptive and automated monitoring, tracking and managing of patients' health (Bhambri and Khang, 2024: Mbunge E., et al., 2021). AI can particularly be beneficial in Geriatric Diagnostics, a system addressing the area of senior population health. Such systems have great potential to improve access to health care for seniors and pre-emptively and automatically detect age-related diseases. AI-based medical devices could be designed to augment or replace human analysts in the interpretation of medical images. They could learn optimal mental health-varying screening scores based on a large corpus of diverse and longitudinal health records. Age-related diseases such as Alzheimer's disease could be detected by AI systems from health record dynamics, medical imaging or data drawn from home-assisting sensors and devices (Mennella C., et al., 2024).

11.1. Current Regulations

Geriatric clinical care is a multidisciplinary assessment designed to evaluate older patients' functional ability, physical health, and cognitive well-being. The majority of these patients suffer from multiple chronic conditions and require special attention. Geriatric populations have a higher prevalence of complex multimorbidity. A careful and holistic assessment is necessary for these patients. However, their assessment differs from a typical medical evaluation and is more challenging due to their limited cognitive and physical ability (Choudhury A., et al., 2021). Often such patients experience deterioration of mental or physical health during their hospital stay.

Consequently, the provision of geriatric clinical care is burdened with the need for proper patient history-taking, collecting past diagnosis information from various health records, and reviewing screening outcomes and previous tests. Various decisions must be made based on the health status of the older patients, classifying the urgency of the problem (emergency/semi-emergency/elective) and gauging the necessary interventions (observation/investigation/medication/intervention). Moreover, various screening tools for dementia are being developed for detecting early cognitive impairments and other geriatric health problems such as fall risks and urinary tract infections among patients with dementia (Li et al., 2022; Niyas, K. P. M., & Thiyagarajan, P. (2023).; Colombo G., and Grübel, J., 2023).

With the gradual growth of AI applications in the health care industry, it is reasonable to assume a positive impact of AI on geriatric patients. AI solutions offer huge potential to support physician daily tasks in hospitals and studies have revealed a variety of AI applications targeting chronic diseases. Current experiences with utilization of AI in geriatrics care are explored to describe the domain of their application, the expected benefit and risks for patients as well as for the teams needed to treat them. It is systematically reviewed how hospitals utilize medical AI systems for improving the clinical care of patients with chronic diseases focusing especially on applications targeting geriatric populations. Since older patients are particularly affected with complex multimorbidity and benefit from a multidisciplinary care approach. To accommodate its task efficiently, the geriatric clinician requests the assistance of others professionals resulting in a geriatric care team.

11.2. Future Policy Recommendations

AI tools are usually developed speculatively and then applied to older people, assuming they would be beneficial. As one example, AI tools have been proposed to stratify people at risk of adverse outcomes in order to target care, although few AI tools were developed with older people in mind. Before the delivery of services, planners, providers, and regulators need to use methods that systematically evaluate possible benefits and harms in order to establish whether the tool is good enough to use. Such an evaluation would assess the intended use of the AI tool, the possible benefits and harms to patients, and the health care organisation; how these impacts would be realised; and the data and assumptions behind these predictions (Efthymiou, I., 2024).

Once AI tools are delivered, it is vitally important that they undergo close monitoring. That is because AI tools are fundamentally statistical models that have been trained to make decisions based on a great deal of data about individuals. Consequently, AI tools tend to work well when provided with data similar to those on which they were trained (Efthymiou, I.P., 2025). Therefore, when used in different real-world settings, outcome distributions will shift, the predicted risk profiles will change, and there will be a decline in performance. In other words, just about every real-world deployment of an AI tool would be a new domain, and performance audits would be required.

Additionally, statistical models inevitably make errors. Environments that would have been false positives prior to the deployment of a tool may, after real-world use, retrospectively show great adverse impact on access or patient care. All these things will happen more or less regardless of who is in charge. Therefore, robust frameworks will be needed. Such frameworks include the orchestration of audits prior to delivery, the routine evaluation of outcomes after delivery, and mechanisms for recourse to mitigate harm from false predictions, for example through routinely releasing data to outside organisations. The policy wrapper will need to be appropriate to the country and setting; one option would be a scheme of direct regulation similar to those currently in place for financial and insurance models.

12. INTERDISCIPLINARY COLLABORATION

Artificial Intelligence (AI) technologies have the potential to greatly impact public health and the performance of healthcare systems through the use of various novel applications. In medicine, AI offers the promise of better prevention, diagnosis, prognosis, and treatment (Efthymiou, I.-P., et al., 2022). AI is beginning to be seen in both research and direct patient care in medicine, especially regarding image-based decision support. These approaches are being met with enthusiasm and skepticism—enthusiasm for the potential discoveries rapidly unfolding, and skepticism for safety and conduct in training, validation, and deployment. There is a need for community consensus around the best ways to reward advances and public resource allocation and how to improve the interpretation and communication of AI technology in medicine.

In geriatric clinical care, early detection of cognitive impairment and dementia is crucial for the well-being of the elderly population. In the past decade, there have been growing efforts to create screening tools for dementia, especially in developing countries, that are cheap, accessible, and easy to use (Efthymiou, I. P., & Vozikis, A., 2017). In addition, care for older patients is more demanding and challenging due to age-associated degeneration of cognitive and physical ability, polypharmacy, and multiple chronic conditions.

Geriatric clinical care is a multidisciplinary team assessment designed to evaluate older patients' functional ability, physical health, and cognitive well-being. Recently, hospitals have started to discover ways of incorporating AI systems to improve the quality of care. There are not many studies that could provide an overview of the application of AI technology in geriatric care. There are regulatory resources provided to protect patients' rights and the safety of AI health technologies. There is no identifiable established literature examining the accuracy and effectiveness of AI technology in geriatric clinical care. There is limited understanding of current geriatric care practices that can potentially leverage AI technology.

The integration of AI devices in healthcare will require interdisciplinary collaboration from various fields. There is a need for social planning on how to prepare the infrastructure to leverage the advantages of these applications. There is also a need for regulatory authorities and the medical community to work together to ensure the quality and safety of these applications. Although AI technology has not been widely adopted in geriatric clinical care, there are existing good practices in geriatric care that can potentially leverage AI in the near future.

12.1. Healthcare Professionals and AI Experts

Improving the healthcare of older people is a major priority for public health and social care and for an increasingly efficient society. Developments in technology offer new strategies and opportunities to do so. This review explores innovative applications of artificial intelligence (AI) technologies to assist healthcare professionals in the monitoring, diagnosis and stratified care of older people, as well as the implications of this new paradigm. The potential of AI technologies to contribute to effective, equitable and ethical care will be put into context by outlining four approaches to data, algorithms, systems, and education. It is expected that these applications and their integration into healthcare systems will significantly expand over time, limited only by the pace of computing and the generation of relevant evidence involving effective people machine collaborations (Shiwani T., et al., 2023).

There are two aspects to the future development of these technologies. First, there is technical development and validation to ensure that AI systems function well in their intended realm of application. Such efforts will use biomedical engineering, physics, mathematics, computer science, statistics, and other disciplines to devise the technical characteristics of the systems.

Second, there are factors relating to the acceptability and ease of use of the systems, ensuring that they can be implemented in the most positive ways. These are factors concerned more with sociology and policy than with the technical science underpinning the systems. It will be vital to address both aspects through appropriate collaborations of stakeholders, to ensure the trustworthiness of the systems, and to develop a society where scientists work for and with responsible and accountable governments and civil societies. It is hoped with thoughtfulness over the societal implications, AI may contribute to improved healthcare systems for older people in many positive ways.

The technological insights, conceptual understanding, and methodological approaches presented will interest and benefit the diverse range of stakeholders involved in large-scale AI in healthcare, including medical professionals, AI researchers, entrepreneurs, policymakers, and social scientists. In broad terms, the rapid development of AI-related technologies is expected to lead to structural change, with the scientific knowledge, engineering methods, and technological systems based on the understanding of fundamental aspects of the biological systems subsequently displaced by AI data-driven machines trained to emulate these systems. The future socio-political challenges represented by such a change are massive (Efthymiou, I.P., 2024).

12.2. Role of Family Caregivers

Caregiver burden refers to the negative impact of one's caregiving role on their health and quality of life (QoL) (Ross et al., 2023). Caregivers may experience personal health impacts (e.g., physical/psychological distress, sleep disturbances, financial strain) as well as relationship impacts (e.g., social withdrawal, strain on family interactions). In a national survey of family caregivers of people with dementia, 83% reported stress or sadness related to their caregiving role. Family or friends that assist someone with dementia or other cognitive impairment often seek to improve the QoL and safety for their care recipient while seeking to reach out proactively for assistance in order to alleviate burden on the primary caregiver. In contrast, caregivers experience much higher burden than non-caregivers and experience significant barriers toward reaching out, especially for young onset dementia and late-stage candidates (Freedman V. A., et al., 2022; Janson P., et al., 2022; Sabatini S., et al., 2025).

The goal behind the AI-Powered Caregiver Assistant is to increase caregiving effectiveness while reducing burden (Milella F., et al., 2023; Borna S., et al., 2024). Family members caring for someone with cognitive impairment share experiences, emotions, information, and resources in order to improve their QoL and caregiving. Family caregivers of someone with cognitive impairment exhibit increased social isolation, loneliness, and depression, which may be mitigated by engaging in peer interactions. In evaluation studies, development of virtual support groups demonstrated a reduction in loneliness and caregiver burden. Programs in self-care, structured peer support, and technology use have also reported improvements in caregiver experiences (Moberg C., et al., 2022; Nguyen T., et al., 2025).

13. PATIENT PERSPECTIVES

As healthcare systems globally are thirsty for innovation and increased operational efficiency, AI is presented as an option to reinvent healthcare and tackle these issues. AI tools are already being used in different ways in the professions of both social and healthcare. Consistently applied AI tools would take over the tedious and menial tasks and also detect anomalies in patient samples. AI tools are gradually finding their way into a number of sub-disciplines of healthcare for older people. Yet for a lot of older adults with sluggish adaptation to technological advancements, AI tools could represent the last horizon of change in their current digital health. The aim was to gather knowledge, expectations and concerns of older adults about AI technologies and how they could be used in their care and their healthcare.

13.1. Acceptance of AI in Diagnostics

The demand for health services has increased considerably in most countries during the last years, because of the aging population. In many countries the doctor-to-population ratio is likely too low to cope with this immense demand for health service. This has led to the development of more automated diagnostic systems, including non-medicated solutions. Although there are already companies which present AI based systems for Chronic and other diseases with high prevalence, these are not designed for diabetes mellitus type 2. Such a system would significantly reduce the need for medical resources (Spänig S., et al., 2019).

State-of-the-art systems in academia exist, however, these systems are not interactive with language output, making conversations with users nonexistent. Hence, it would be impossible to rule out any confounding factors for the respective diagnosis, thereby increasing the failure rate for correct diagnosis. Also, despite efforts publishers still charge for the use in the first place.

13.2. Impact on Patient Experience

The possibility of an AI software which could give a diagnosis for non-emergency diseases was prevalent. Such a solution, for example, could be used by a patient at home having symptoms of a cold, so as to receive a diagnosis and possibly prescription in a pharmacy after a video consultation with a virtual physician (Gellert G. A., et al., 2024; Da'Costa A., et al., 2025). AI could guide in this as well as mention recommendations for home treatments. AI could also recommend proper and highly available over-the-counter drugs for symptoms and prepare a recommendation for the doctor afterward, if required. If a chemical prescription is required, AI could determine when a physician is needed and guide the patient to home care or outpatient specialist contractors or the central emergency service in the non-emergency case. AI could also make a recommendation on whether a patient should return to work or continue recovering. It would work in a similar way to a check-up; however, there would be advantages here because the doctor would not have to set appointments specially for issuing doctor's notes (Sumner J., et al., 2023). Providing a doctor's note almost instantaneously would prove useful and help avoid revealing human appearance due to the impersonality of the AI. As a find in this study, it would be curious to implement the thought experiment on how civilization path would differ if these technologies were employed decades ago. Now it would be unacceptable to force patience to go through this process more than once.

Lastly, thoughts with a positive perception of AI in health care would need to be shared by society. The increasing number of users would quasi-autonomously educate the society on AI capabilities and knowledge. However, educators would need to be cautious, as edutainment, to which such a presentation would inevitably approach, could backfire (Efthymiou, I.-P., 2024; Efthymiou, I.-P., 2020). Knowing that even deep reinforcement learning can help develop AI models with knowledge/ expertise superiority, learning AI's mind would prove complex, if not impossible. Impacting AI's actions only through legally set commands would ensure safety, but this would come at a price. Deep learning directly optimizes behavior based on simulations, so legality would protect against illegal actions rather than premature general intelligence, which would be emergent from software evolution in a massively parallel graph structure against human comprehension. Giving AI modeling freedom while also power on their success would be inevitable at a certain moment if no other safeguards were implemented beforehand, probably being outside of legality anyway, as this would be more an existential matter.

14. CONCLUSION

The growing number of elderly individuals searching for medical care and treatment has influenced the creation of a suitable infrastructure for such patients, including early detection and diagnosis of health issues, monitoring their progression over time and treatment, and avoid the use of medications that can have adverse effects. In hospitals, care for elderly patients is provided by a multidisciplinary team. Such teams conduct interdisciplinary assessments that differ from typical medical evaluations and are consequently more complex (Efthymiou, I.-P., 2024). The majority of the geriatric patients suffer from multimorbidity and geriatric syndromes that often co-exist with a variety of chronic diseases. Elderly patients are a heterogeneous group of people with different medical and non-medical needs. Each patient's assessment involves a thorough process of collection of background data regarding their living conditions, networks, social contacts, and activities, as well as files medical history, morbidities, medications, and substance abuse.

Artificial intelligence (AI) has gained significant attention in recent years and is expected to impact the geriatric population as it integrates into the health care system.

AI is expected to assist clinicians in error-prone complex procedures and diseases that require accurate prediction due to numerous possible inputs. AI analysis of clinical notes can automate documentation procedures and facilitating better health care outcomes. Such applications are classified into devices on the edge and cloud AI platforms. Cloud platforms dominate companies involved in offering various AI services. Compared with other health care fields, geriatric care and domains related to older patients are likely lagging within the scope of existing AI applications. The potential of AI applications assisting in older patient assessment, monitoring, diagnosis, and treatment has been highlighted in a number of recent studies.

Therefore, integrating AI into geriatric diagnostics is not only a technological advancement but a practical necessity. As healthcare systems face increasing pressure from ageing populations, the responsible and targeted use of AI offers a path to more accurate, efficient, and equitable care for older adults.

REFERENCES

Abadir, P., & Chellappa, R. (2024). Artificial intelligence in geriatrics: Riding the inevitable tide of promise, challenges, and considerations. *The Journals of Gerontology. Series A, Biological Sciences and Medical Sciences*, *79*(2), glad279. Advance online publication. DOI: 10.1093/gerona/glad279 PMID: 38289911

Abdulmalek, S., Nasir, A., Jabbar, W. A., Almuhaya, M. A., Bairagi, A. K., Khan, M. A. M., & Kee, S. H. (2022). IoT-based healthcare-monitoring system towards improving quality of life: A review. *Health Care*, *10*(10), 1993. Advance online publication. DOI: 10.3390/healthcare10101993 PMID: 36292441

Ahmad, I., Asghar, Z., Kumar, T., Li, G., Manzoor, A., Mikhaylov, K., & Harjula, E. (2022). Emerging technologies for next generation remote health care and assisted living. *IEEE Access : Practical Innovations, Open Solutions*, *10*, 56094–56132. DOI: 10.1109/ACCESS.2022.3177278

Aïdoud, A., Gana, W., Poitau, F., Debacq, C., Leroy, V., Nkodo, J. A., & Fougère, B. (2023). High prevalence of geriatric conditions among older adults with cardiovascular disease. *Journal of the American Heart Association*, *12*(2), e026850. Advance online publication. DOI: 10.1161/JAHA.122.026850 PMID: 36628962

Albahri, A. S., Duhaim, A. M., Fadhel, M. A., Alnoor, A., Baqer, N. S., Alzubaidi, L., & Deveci, M. (2023). A systematic review of trustworthy and explainable artificial intelligence in healthcare: Assessment of quality, bias risk, and data fusion. *Information Fusion*, *96*, 156–191. DOI: 10.1016/j.inffus.2023.03.008

Aldoseri, A., Al-Khalifa, K. N., & Hamouda, A. M. (2023). Re-thinking data strategy and integration for artificial intelligence: Concepts, opportunities, and challenges. *Applied Sciences (Basel, Switzerland)*, *13*(12), 7082. Advance online publication. DOI: 10.3390/app13127082

Alievska, B. (2023). *Ethical challenges arising from the underrepresentation of the elderly in the development of artificial intelligence (AI) for medical applications: Exclusion, bias, and solutions* [Master's thesis, McMaster University]. MacSphere. http://hdl.handle.net/11375/28768

Alonso Salinas, G. L., Cepas-Guillén, P., León, A. M., Jiménez-Méndez, C., Lozano-Vicario, L., Martínez-Avial, M., & Díez-Villanueva, P. (2024). The impact of geriatric conditions in elderly patients with coronary heart disease: A state-of-the-art review. *Journal of Clinical Medicine*, *13*(7), 1891. Advance online publication. DOI: 10.3390/jcm13071891 PMID: 38610656

Aminizadeh, S., Heidari, A., Dehghan, M., Toumaj, S., Rezaei, M., Navimipour, N. J., & Unal, M. (2024). Opportunities and challenges of artificial intelligence and distributed systems to improve the quality of healthcare service. *Artificial Intelligence in Medicine*, *149*, 102779. Advance online publication. DOI: 10.1016/j.artmed.2024.102779 PMID: 38462281

Băjenaru, O. L., Băjenaru, L., Ianculescu, M., Constantin, V. ., Gu atu, A. M., & Nu ă, C. R. (2024). Geriatric healthcare supported by decision-making tools integrated into digital health solutions. *Electronics (Basel)*, *13*(17), 3440. Advance online publication. DOI: 10.3390/electronics13173440

Bala, I., Pindoo, I., Mijwil, M. M., Abotaleb, M., & Yundong, W. (2024). Ensuring security and privacy in healthcare systems: A review exploring challenges, solutions, future trends, and the practical applications of artificial intelligence. *Jordan Medical Journal*, *58*(3), 143–154. DOI: 10.35516/jmj.v58i3.2346

Bernal, M. C., Batista, E., Martínez-Ballesté, A., & Solanas, A. (2024). Artificial intelligence for the study of human ageing: A systematic literature review. *Applied Intelligence*, *54*(22), 11949–11977. DOI: 10.1007/s10489-024-05702-8

Bhambri, P., & Khang, A. (2024). Managing and monitoring patient's healthcare using AI and IoT technologies. In Khang, A. (Ed.), *Driving smart medical diagnosis through AI-powered technologies and applications* (pp. 1–23). IGI Global., DOI: 10.4018/979-8-3693-3679-3.ch001

Bhuiyan, M. N., Rahman, M. M., Billah, M. M., & Saha, D. (2021). Internet of Things (IoT): A review of its enabling technologies in healthcare applications, standards protocols, security, and market opportunities. *IEEE Internet of Things Journal*, *8*(13), 10474–10498. DOI: 10.1109/JIOT.2021.3062630

Borna, S., Maniaci, M. J., Haider, C. R., Gomez-Cabello, C. A., Pressman, S. M., Haider, S. A., & Forte, A. J. (2024). Artificial intelligence support for informal patient caregivers: A systematic review. *Bioengineering (Basel, Switzerland)*, *11*(5), 483. Advance online publication. DOI: 10.3390/bioengineering11050483 PMID: 38790350

Brown, S., & Desai, A. (2023). Legal and regulatory issues related to the use of clinical software in healthcare delivery. In Elkin, P. L. (Ed.), *Clinical decision support and beyond* (pp. 571–598). Academic Press., DOI: 10.1016/B978-0-323-91200-6.00014-5

Chaichareenon, K., & Nupairoj, N. (2024, June). Data-driven with process mining to analyze and identify key features for no-show risks in patients with chronic diseases to achieve treatment improvement. In *2024 21st International Joint Conference on Computer Science and Software Engineering (JCSSE)* (pp. 192–198). IEEE. https://doi.org/DOI: 10.1100/JCSSE61076.2024.10586524

Chen, M., Cui, D., Haick, H., & Tang, N. (2024). Artificial intelligence-based medical sensors for healthcare system. *Advanced Sensor Research*, *3*(8), 2300179. Advance online publication. DOI: 10.1002/adsr.202300179

Chien, S. C., Yen, C. M., Chang, Y. H., Chen, Y. E., Liu, C. C., Hsiao, Y. P., & Chung, R. H. (2025). Use of artificial intelligence, internet of things, and edge intelligence in long-term care for older people: Comprehensive analysis through bibliometric, Google trends, and content analysis. *Journal of Medical Internet Research*, *27*, e56692. Advance online publication. DOI: 10.2196/56692 PMID: 40053718

Chinnaiyan, B., Balasubramanian, S., Jeyabalu, M., & Warrier, G. S. (2025). AI applications—Computer vision and natural language processing. In *Model optimization methods for efficient and edge AI: Federated learning architectures, frameworks and applications* (pp. 25–41). IGI Global., DOI: 10.4018/979-8-3693-2401-1.ch002

Choudhury, A., Renjilian, E., & Asan, O. (2021). Use of machine learning in geriatric clinical care for chronic diseases: A systematic literature review. *Journal of Medical Internet Research*, *23*(9), e24387. Advance online publication. DOI: 10.2196/24387

Cocuzzo, B., Wrench, A., O'Malley, C., & O'Malley, C. B. (2022). Effects of COVID-19 on older adults: Physical, mental, emotional, social, and financial problems seen and unseen. *Cureus*, *14*(10), e30319. Advance online publication. DOI: 10.7759/cureus.30319 PMID: 36299954

Colombo, G., & Grübel, J. (2023, April). The Spatial Performance Assessment for Cognitive Evaluation (Space): A novel game for the early detection of cognitive impairment. In *Extended Abstracts of the 2023 CHI Conference on Human Factors in Computing Systems* (pp. 1–6). ACM. https://doi.org/DOI: 10.1145/3544549.3585632

Da'Costa, A., Teke, J., Origbo, J. E., Osonuga, A., Egbon, E., & Olawade, D. B. (2025). AI-driven triage in emergency departments: A review of benefits, challenges, and future directions. *International Journal of Medical Informatics*, *200*, 105838. Advance online publication. DOI: 10.1016/j.ijmedinf.2024.105838 PMID: 39965433

Das, A., & Dhillon, P. (2023). Application of machine learning in measurement of ageing and geriatric diseases: A systematic review. *Ageing International*, *49*(2), 353–384. DOI: 10.1007/s12126-023-09546-3 PMID: 38087195

Devine, B. C., Dogan, A. B., & Sobol, W. M. (2025). Recent optical coherence tomography (OCT) innovations for increased accessibility and remote surveillance. *Bioengineering (Basel, Switzerland)*, *12*(1), 76. Advance online publication. DOI: 10.3390/bioengineering12010076 PMID: 40428060

Diareme, K. C., Liapakis, A., & Efthymiou, I. P. (2022). Data, sentiment analysis, and examples during the COVID-19 pandemic. *HAPSc Policy Briefs Series*, *3*(1), xx–xx. DOI: 10.12681/hapscpbs.33779

Dykstra, S. (2024). *Integrating multi-domain electronic health data, machine learning, and automated cardiac phenomics for personalized cardiovascular care* [Doctoral dissertation, University of Calgary]. PRISM Repository. https://doi.org/ DOI: 10.11575/PRISM/43295

Efthymiou, I. (2024). Exploring the Frontier: New and Future Trends in Research. In B. Orlando (Ed.), Innovation Capabilities and Entrepreneurial Opportunities of Smart Working (pp. 48-68). IGI Global Scientific Publishing. https://doi.org/DOI: 10.4018/978-1-7998-8797-3.ch003

Efthymiou, I. (2025). The Role of E-Government and E-Governance in Modern Societies. In Wongmahesak, K., Ahmad, J., & Mustanir, A. (Eds.), *Public Governance Practices in the Age of AI* (pp. 45–68). IGI Global Scientific Publishing., DOI: 10.4018/979-8-3693-9286-7.ch003

Efthymiou, I.-P. (2020). Non-cognitive skills and AI: A new era of learning and development. *International Case Studies Journal*, *9*(10), 42–46.

Efthymiou, I. P. (2024). Wellbeing as an alternative to GDP? *HAPSc Policy Briefs Series*, *5*(1), 38–46. DOI: 10.12681/hapscpbs.38956

Efthymiou, I.-P. (2024). Can AI improve health and wellbeing? Case Studies Journal, ISSN (2305-509X), 13(11), 1–5.

Efthymiou, I.-P. (2024). The importance of soft skills in healthcare: The impact of communication, empathy, and teamwork on doctor-nurse interactions. *Case Studies Journal*, *13*(11), 6–11.

Efthymiou, I.-P. (2024). Can AI improve health and wellbeing? *Case Studies Journal*, *13*(11), 1–5.

Efthymiou, I.-P.. (2022). Major risk factors that increase the frequency of noncommunicable diseases: A review of evidence-based research. *International Journal of Caring Sciences*, *15*(1), 655–662.

Efthymiou, I. P., & Efthymiou Egleton, T. W. (2023). Artificial intelligence for sustainable smart cities. In *Handbook of research on applications of AI, digital twin, and internet of things for sustainable development* (pp. 1–xx). IGI Global., DOI: 10.4018/978-1-6684-6821-0.ch001

Efthymiou, I. P., & Vozikis, A. (2017). Medicine, a pan-historical, pan-cultural science. *Journal of Cardiology & Cardiovascular Therapy*, *1*(1).

Esmaeilzadeh, P. (2024). Challenges and strategies for wide-scale artificial intelligence (AI) deployment in healthcare practices: A perspective for healthcare organizations. *Artificial Intelligence in Medicine*, *151*, 102856. Advance online publication. DOI: 10.1016/j.artmed.2024.102856 PMID: 38555850

Fabrizio, C., Termine, A., Caltagirone, C., & Sancesario, G. (2021). Artificial intelligence for Alzheimer's disease: Promise or challenge? *Diagnostics (Basel)*, *11*(8), 1473. Advance online publication. DOI: 10.3390/diagnostics11081473 PMID: 34441407

Faiyazuddin, M., Rahman, S. J. Q., Anand, G., Siddiqui, R. K., Mehta, R., Khatib, M. N., & Sah, R. (2025). The impact of artificial intelligence on healthcare: A comprehensive review of advancements in diagnostics, treatment, and operational efficiency. *Health Science Reports*, *8*(1), e70312. Advance online publication. DOI: 10.1002/hsr2.70312 PMID: 39763580

Ferretti, A., Ienca, M., Sheehan, M., Blasimme, A., Dove, E. S., Farsides, B., & Vayena, E. (2021). Ethics review of big data research: What should stay and what should be reformed? *BMC Medical Ethics*, *22*(1), 51. Advance online publication. DOI: 10.1186/s12910-021-00616-4 PMID: 33931049

Freedman, V. A., Patterson, S. E., Cornman, J. C., & Wolff, J. L. (2022). A day in the life of caregivers to older adults with and without dementia: Comparisons of care time and emotional health. *Alzheimer's & Dementia*, *18*(9), 1650–1661. DOI: 10.1002/alz.12524 PMID: 35103394

Gabriel, O. T. (2023). Data privacy and ethical issues in collecting health care data using artificial intelligence among health workers. *International Journal of Medical and Health Sciences Research*, *3*(1), 1–10. DOI: 10.51594/ijmer.v3i1.234

Gellert, G. A., Kabat-Karabon, A., Gellert, G. L., Rasławska-Socha, J., Gorski, S., Price, T., & Orzechowski, P. M. (2024). The potential of virtual triage AI to improve early detection, care acuity alignment, and emergent care referral of life-threatening conditions. *Frontiers in Public Health*, *12*, 1362246. Advance online publication. DOI: 10.3389/fpubh.2024.1362246 PMID: 38807993

Ghassemi, M., Oakden-Rayner, L., & Beam, A. L. (2021). The false hope of current approaches to explainable artificial intelligence in health care. *The Lancet. Digital Health*, *3*(11), e745–e750. DOI: 10.1016/S2589-7500(21)00208-9 PMID: 34711379

Goel, A., Goel, A. K., & Kumar, A. (2023). The role of artificial neural network and machine learning in utilizing spatial information. *Spatial Information Research*, *31*(3), 355–364. DOI: 10.1007/s41324-022-00494-2

Grueso, S., & Viejo-Sobera, R. (2021). Machine learning methods for predicting progression from mild cognitive impairment to Alzheimer's disease dementia: A systematic review. *Alzheimer's Research & Therapy*, *13*(1), 162. Advance online publication. DOI: 10.1186/s13195-021-00900-6 PMID: 34583745

Guasti, L., Fumagalli, S., Afilalo, J., Geisler, T., Abreu, A., Ambrosetti, M., & Ferrini, M. (2025). Cardiovascular diseases, prevention, and management of complications in older adults and frail patients treated for elective or post-traumatic hip orthopaedic interventions: A clinical consensus statement. *European Journal of Preventive Cardiology*, *32*(2), 186–198. DOI: 10.1093/eurjpc/zwaf010 PMID: 39812215

Hansen, A. R., McLendon, S. F., & Rochani, H. (2022). Care coordination for rural residents with chronic disease: Predictors of improved outcomes. *Public Health Nursing (Boston, Mass.)*, *39*(5), 1093–1101. DOI: 10.1111/phn.13092 PMID: 34962313

Hassija, V., Chamola, V., Mahapatra, A., Singal, A., Goel, D., Huang, K., & Hussain, A. (2024). Interpreting black-box models: A review on explainable artificial intelligence. *Cognitive Computation*, *16*(1), 45–74. DOI: 10.1007/s12559-023-10179-8

Hendriks, A., Hacking, C., Verbeek, H., & Aarts, S. (2024). Data science techniques to gain novel insights into quality of care: A scoping review of long-term care for older adults. *Exploration of Digital Health Technologies*, *2*(2), 67–85. DOI: 10.37349/edht.2024.00014

Holm, N. N., Frølich, A., Dominguez, H., Dalhoff, K. P., Juul-Larsen, H. G., Andersen, O., & Stockmarr, A. (2025). Co-occurring diseases and mortality in patients with chronic heart disease, modeling their dynamically expanding disease portfolios: Nationwide register study. *JMIR Cardio*, *9*(1), e57749. Advance online publication. DOI: 10.2196/57749 PMID: 40279150

Hong, Z., Magdamo, C., Sheu, Y., Mohite, P., Noori, A., Ye, E. M., . . . Das, S. (2020). Natural language processing to detect cognitive concerns in electronic health records using deep learning. *arXiv*. https://arxiv.org/abs/2011.07423 (No DOI available)

Hyväri, S., Elo, S., Kukkohovi, S., & Lotvonen, S. (2024). Utilizing activity sensors to identify behavioural activity patterns of elderly home care clients. *Disability and Rehabilitation. Assistive Technology*, *19*(3), 585–594. DOI: 10.1080/17483107.2022.2123370 PMID: 36067090

Iqbal, J. D., & Biller-Andorno, N. (2022). The regulatory gap in digital health and alternative pathways to bridge it. *Health Policy and Technology*, *11*(3), 100664. Advance online publication. DOI: 10.1016/j.hlpt.2022.100664

Janson, P., Willeke, K., Zaibert, L., Budnick, A., Berghöfer, A., Kittel-Schneider, S., & Keil, T. (2022). Mortality, morbidity and health-related outcomes in informal caregivers compared to non-caregivers: A systematic review. *International Journal of Environmental Research and Public Health*, *19*(10), 5864. Advance online publication. DOI: 10.3390/ijerph19105864 PMID: 35627399

Jin Park, H. (2024). Patient perspectives on informed consent for medical AI: A web-based experiment. *Frontiers in Artificial Intelligence*, *7*, 1322797. Advance online publication. DOI: 10.3389/frai.2024.1322797

Joshi, H. (2025). Natural language processing of electronic health records for predicting Alzheimer's disease. In *Deep generative models for integrative analysis of Alzheimer's biomarkers* (pp. 141–174). IGI Global., DOI: 10.4018/979-8-3693-3949-7.ch006

Kamiyole, S. (2025). *Impact of electronic prescription, access, and messaging on health information exchange utilization during care transition* [Doctoral dissertation, Ohio University]. OhioLINK Electronic Theses and Dissertations Center. https://rave.ohiolink.edu/etdc/view?acc_num=ohiou1725998654793512 (No DOI available)

Khalate, P., Gite, S., Pradhan, B., & Lee, C. W. (2024). Opportunities and gaps in natural language processing and machine learning applications in healthcare: A comprehensive review of electronic medical records and medical imaging. *Frontiers in Physics*, *12*, 1372870. Advance online publication. DOI: 10.3389/fphy.2024.1372870

Khalid, N., Qayyum, A., Bilal, M., Al-Fuqaha, A., & Qadir, J. (2023). Privacy-preserving artificial intelligence in healthcare: Techniques and applications. *Computers in Biology and Medicine*, *158*, 106848. Advance online publication. DOI: 10.1016/j.compbiomed.2023.106848 PMID: 37044052

Kim, D. H. (2024). Unleashing frailty from laboratory into real world: A critical step toward frailty-guided clinical care of older adults. *Journal of the American Geriatrics Society*, *72*(12), 3643–3645. DOI: 10.1111/jgs.19229 PMID: 39166879

Knevel, R., & Liao, K. P. (2023). From real-world electronic health record data to real-world results using artificial intelligence. *Annals of the Rheumatic Diseases*, *82*(3), 306–311. DOI: 10.1136/annrheumdis-2022-222626 PMID: 36150748

Koc, M. (2023). Artificial intelligence in geriatrics. *Turk Geriatri Dergisi*, *26*(3), 238–249. DOI: 10.29400/tjgeri.2023.355

Koçak, B., Ponsiglione, A., Stanzione, A., Bluethgen, C., Santinha, J., Ugga, L., & Cuocolo, R. (2025). Bias in artificial intelligence for medical imaging: Fundamentals, detection, avoidance, mitigation, challenges, ethics, and prospects. *Diagnostic and Interventional Radiology*, *31*(2), 75–87. DOI: 10.4274/dir.2024.242715 PMID: 38953330

Kouroubali, A., Kondylakis, H., Logothetidis, F., & Katehakis, D. G. (2022). Developing an AI-enabled integrated care platform for frailty. *Health Care*, *10*(3), 443. Advance online publication. DOI: 10.3390/healthcare10030443 PMID: 35326921

Kulkarni, M. H., & Inamdar, P. R. (2025). Healthcare unbound: Navigating emerging trends and future applications in IoT-based innovations for daily well-being. In *Evolution of machine learning and internet of things applications in biomedical engineering* (pp. 238–250). CRC Press., DOI: 10.1201/9781003447535-11

Kumar, Y., Koul, A., Singla, R., & Ijaz, M. (2022). Artificial intelligence in disease diagnosis: A systematic literature review, synthesizing framework and future research agenda. *Journal of Ambient Intelligence and Humanized Computing*, *14*, 8459–8486. DOI: 10.1007/s12652-021-03612-z PMID: 35039756

Kumar, Y., Koul, A., Singla, R., & Ijaz, M. F. (2023). Artificial intelligence in disease diagnosis: A systematic literature review, synthesizing framework and future research agenda. *Journal of Ambient Intelligence and Humanized Computing*, *14*(7), 8459–8486. DOI: 10.1007/s12652-022-04489-9 PMID: 35039756

Lang, B. H., Nyholm, S., & Blumenthal-Barby, J. (2023). Responsibility gaps and black box healthcare AI: Shared responsibilization as a solution. *Digital Health*, *9*, 1–12. DOI: 10.1177/20552076231220888 PMID: 38596344

Leviton, A., & Loddenkemper, T. (2023). Design, implementation, and inferential issues associated with clinical trials that rely on data in electronic medical records: A narrative review. *BMC Medical Research Methodology*, *23*(1), 196. Advance online publication. DOI: 10.1186/s12874-023-02015-8 PMID: 37974111

Li, R., Wang, X., Lawler, K., Garg, S., Bai, Q., & Alty, J. (2022). Applications of artificial intelligence to aid early detection of dementia: A scoping review on current capabilities and future directions. *Journal of Biomedical Informatics*, *127*, 104030. Advance online publication. DOI: 10.1016/j.jbi.2022.104030 PMID: 35183766

Liang, W., Tadesse, G. A., Ho, D., Fei-Fei, L., Zaharia, M., Zhang, C., & Zou, J. (2022). Advances, challenges and opportunities in creating data for trustworthy AI. *Nature Machine Intelligence*, *4*(8), 669–677. DOI: 10.1038/s42256-022-00512-0

Liu, Q., Vaci, N., Koychev, I., Kormilitzin, A., Li, Z., Cipriani, A., & Nevado-Holgado, A. (2022). Personalised treatment for cognitive impairment in dementia: Development and validation of an artificial intelligence model. *The Lancet. Digital Health*, *4*(2), e94–e102. DOI: 10.1016/S2589-7500(21)00260-0 PMID: 35101059

Loveys, K., Prina, M., Axford, C., Domènec, Ò. R., Weng, W., Broadbent, E., & Thiyagarajan, J. A. (2022). Artificial intelligence for older people receiving long-term care: A systematic review of acceptability and effectiveness studies. *The Lancet. Healthy Longevity*, *3*(4), e286–e297. DOI: 10.1016/S2666-7568(22)00034-2 PMID: 35515814

Lukkien, D. R., Nap, H. H., Buimer, H. P., Peine, A., Boon, W. P., Ket, J. C., & Moors, E. H. (2023). Toward responsible artificial intelligence in long-term care: A scoping review on practical approaches. *The Gerontologist*, *63*(1), 155–168. DOI: 10.1093/geront/gnac080 PMID: 34871399

Luo, R. (2025). *AI for systematic reviews, gait, and activity recognition* [Master's thesis, McMaster University]. MacSphere. http://hdl.handle.net/11375/29729 (No DOI available)

Maclagan, L. C., Abdalla, M., Harris, D. A., Stukel, T. A., Chen, B., Candido, E., & Bronskill, S. E. (2023). Can patients with dementia be identified in primary care electronic medical records using natural language processing? *Journal of Healthcare Informatics Research*, *7*(1), 42–58. DOI: 10.1007/s41666-022-00125-5 PMID: 36910911

Marelli, L., Testa, G., & Van Hoyweghen, I. (2021). Big Tech platforms in health research: Re-purposing big data governance in light of the General Data Protection Regulation's research exemption. *Big Data & Society*, *8*(1). Advance online publication. DOI: 10.1177/20539517211018783

Maris, T. M., Koçar, A., Willems, D. L., Pols, J., Tan, H. L., Lindinger, G. L., & Bak, M. A. R. (2024). Ethical use of artificial intelligence to prevent sudden cardiac death: An interview study of patient perspectives. *Frontiers in Cardiovascular Medicine*, *11*, 1394397. Advance online publication. DOI: 10.3389/fcvm.2024.1394397

Martins, R., Pereira, H., Corrente, G., Xavier, W., Conceição, L., Freitas, A., & Marreiros, G. (2024). Supporting elderly care through an AI-driven and FHIR-based remote monitoring system. In *International Symposium on Distributed Computing and Artificial Intelligence* (pp. 233–241). Springer. https://doi.org/DOI: 10.1007/978-3-031-62692-0_24

Mbata, A. O., Soyege, O. S., Nwokedi, C. N., Tomoh, B. O., Mustapha, A. Y., Balogun, O. D., & Iguma, D. R. (2024). Preventative medicine and chronic disease management: Reducing healthcare costs and improving long-term public health. *International Journal of Multidisciplinary Research and Growth Evaluation*, *5*(6), 1584–1600. DOI: 10.54660/IJMRGE.2024.5.6.1584-1600

Mennella, C., Maniscalco, U., De Pietro, G., & Esposito, M. (2024). Ethical and regulatory challenges of AI technologies in healthcare: A narrative review. *Heliyon*, *10*(5), e27008. Advance online publication. DOI: 10.1016/j.heliyon.2024.e27008 PMID: 38384518

Mhlanga, D. (2024). Artificial intelligence in elderly care: Navigating ethical and responsible AI adoption for seniors. In Khang, A., Abdullayev, V. M., Sergi, B. S., & Gupta, A. (Eds.), *Fostering long-term sustainable development in Africa* (pp. 411–440). Springer., DOI: 10.1007/978-3-031-61133-9_16

Milella, F., Russo, D., & Bandini, S. (2023). AI-powered solutions to support informal caregivers in their decision-making: A systematic review of the literature. *OBM Geriatrics*, *7*(4), 1–17. DOI: 10.21926/obm.geriatr.2304257

Mitra, K., & Alam, G. (2025). *AI-driven technologies in elderly care: Benefits and challenges* [Master's thesis, Theseus]. https://www.theseus.fi/handle/10024/834134 (No DOI available)

Moberg, C., Grundberg, Å., Konradsen, H., Kallström, A. P., Leung, A. Y., & Kabir, Z. N. (2022). Meeting own needs and supporting ability to care: Family caregivers' and health care professionals' perspectives on professional support provided through a potential mobile application. *Dementia (London)*, *21*(4), 1120–1134. DOI: 10.1177/14713012211046597 PMID: 35300535

Moghadam, M. P., Moghadam, Z. A., Qazani, M. R. C., Pławiak, P., & Alizadehsani, R. (2024). Impact of artificial intelligence in nursing for geriatric clinical care for chronic diseases: A systematic literature review. *IEEE Access : Practical Innovations, Open Solutions*, *12*, 122685–122701. DOI: 10.1109/ACCESS.2024.3451188

Murdoch, B. (2021). Privacy and artificial intelligence: Challenges for protecting health information in a new era. *BMC Medical Ethics*, *22*(1), 122. Advance online publication. DOI: 10.1186/s12910-021-00687-3 PMID: 34525993

Naik, N., Hameed, B. M., Shetty, D. K., Swain, D., Shah, M., Paul, R., & Somani, B. K. (2022). Legal and ethical consideration in artificial intelligence in healthcare: Who takes responsibility? *Frontiers in Surgery*, *9*, 862322. Advance online publication. DOI: 10.3389/fsurg.2022.862322 PMID: 35360424

Nandakishora, Y., Christydass, S. P. J., Bhargav, K. V. J., & Kumar, S. S. (2025). Empowering health: The fusion of AI and machine learning in wearable technologies. In *Smart textiles and wearables for health and fitness* (p. 159). Springer., DOI: 10.1007/978-981-97-6436-5_7

Nguyen, T., Tang, B., Harrison, K. L., Stadler, S., Walter, L. C., Hoepke, K., & Allison, T. A. (2025). Age Self Care, a program to improve aging in place through group learning and incremental behavior change: Preliminary data. *Journal of the American Geriatrics Society*, *73*(3), 920–929. DOI: 10.1111/jgs.19216 PMID: 39607380

Niyas, K. P. M., & Thiyagarajan, P. (2023). A systematic review on early prediction of mild cognitive impairment to Alzheimer's using machine learning algorithms. *International Journal of Intelligent Networks*, *4*, 363–370. DOI: 10.1016/j.ijin.2023.12.002

Ostroushko, D. (n.d.). *Evaluation of cohort construction methods for MCI to AD progression from EHR data: Discussion and reflections*. GitHub Pages. https://denisostroushko1.github.io/Evaluation-of-Cohort-Construction-Methods-for-MCI-to-AD-Progression-from-EHR-Data/ (No DOI available)

Perivolaris, A. (2024). *Development and evaluation of a standardized tool to measure the quality of clinician's interaction with AI-enabled systems* [Master's thesis, Scholaris]. https://scholaris.ca/wp-content/uploads/2024/03/Thesis-APerivolaris-Final.pdf (No DOI available)

Puterman-Salzman, L., Katz, J., Bergman, H., Grad, R., Khanassov, V., Gore, G., & Abbasgholizadeh Rahimi, S. (2023). Artificial intelligence for detection of dementia using motion data: A scoping review. *Dementia and Geriatric Cognitive Disorders. Extra*, *13*(1), 28–38. DOI: 10.1159/000529208 PMID: 37927529

Ray, S. J., Cherian, J., Liberty, A. M., Hammond, T. A., & Shireman, P. K. (2025). Recognition of basic activities of daily living using wearable devices for older adults: Scoping review. *Journal of Medical Internet Research*, *27*, e67373. Advance online publication. DOI: 10.2196/67373 PMID: 40373307

Reynolds, T. A., Goldshore, M. A., Flohr, S., Land, S., Mathew, L., Gebb, J. S., & Hedrick, H. L. (2025). A clinical outcomes data archive for a comprehensive fetal diagnosis and treatment center. *Fetal Diagnosis and Therapy*, *52*(2), 139–147. DOI: 10.1159/000544039 PMID: 39378854

Richter-Laskowska, M., Sobotnicka, E., & Bednorz, A. (2025). Cognitive performance classification of older patients using machine learning and electronic medical records. *Scientific Reports*, *15*(1), 1823. Advance online publication. DOI: 10.1038/s41598-024-51976-9 PMID: 39994339

Rong, J., Ji, X., Fang, X., & Jee, M. H. (2022). Research on material design of medical products for elderly families based on artificial intelligence. *Mathematical Biosciences and Engineering*, *19*(12), 13502–13516. DOI: 10.3934/mbe.2022632 PMID: 35087604

Ross, J., Reilly, E., Sanchez-Reilly, S., Arevalo-Flechas, L., & Dentchev, A. (2023). How real is this deal? Evaluating AI accuracy in providing support to dementia caregivers. *Innovation in Aging*, *7*(Supplement_1), 1042–1043. DOI: 10.1093/geroni/igad104.3368

Sabatini, S., Turner, S. G., & Stephan, B. (2025). Comparison of views on aging and self-perceptions of aging between dementia caregivers and non-caregivers. *The Journals of Gerontology. Series B, Psychological Sciences and Social Sciences*, *80*(2), gbaf083. Advance online publication. DOI: 10.1093/geronb/gbaf083 PMID: 40372128

Saccà, R., Turrini, R., Ausania, F., Turrina, S., & De Leo, D. (2024). The ménage à trois of healthcare: The actors in after-AI era under patient consent. *Frontiers in Medicine*, *11*, 1396145. Advance online publication. DOI: 10.3389/fmed.2024.1396145 PMID: 38269319

Sankaran, A., & Singla, M. P. (2024). Artificial intelligence in geriatric healthcare: Opportunities and challenges in a transforming landscape. *Frontiers in Health Informatics*, *13*, 208. Advance online publication. DOI: 10.30699/fhi.v13i0.208

Shankar, R., Bundele, A., & Mukhopadhyay, A. (2025). Natural language processing of electronic health records for early detection of cognitive decline: A systematic review. *npj. Digital Medicine*, *8*(1), 26. Advance online publication. DOI: 10.1038/s41746-025-01015-7 PMID: 39805946

Shiwani, T., Relton, S., Evans, R., Kale, A., Heaven, A., Clegg, A., & Todd, O. (2023). New horizons in artificial intelligence in the healthcare of older people. *Age and Ageing*, *52*(12), afad223. Advance online publication. DOI: 10.1093/ageing/afad223 PMID: 38124256

Sidky, H., Young, J. C., Girvin, A. T., Lee, E., Shao, Y. R., & Hotaling, N., ... & N3C Consortium. (2023). Data quality considerations for evaluating COVID-19 treatments using real world data: Learnings from the National COVID Cohort Collaborative (N3C). *BMC Medical Research Methodology, 23*(1), 46. Advance online publication. DOI: 10.1186/s12874-023-01860-x PMID: 36800930

Spänig, S., Emberger-Klein, A., Sowa, J. P., Canbay, A., Menrad, K., & Heider, D. (2019). The virtual doctor: An interactive artificial intelligence based on deep learning for non-invasive prediction of diabetes. *arXiv*. https://arxiv.org/abs/1904.01947 (No DOI available)

Stefanidis, K. B., Summers, M. J., & Clark, M. (2025). The assessment of cognitive function and medical fitness to drive in older adults: A qualitative study with general practitioners. *Journal of Transport & Health, 34*, 101717. Advance online publication. DOI: 10.1016/j.jth.2024.101717

Sumner, J., Lim, H. W., Chong, L. S., Bundele, A., Mukhopadhyay, A., & Kayambu, G. (2023). Artificial intelligence in physical rehabilitation: A systematic review. *Artificial Intelligence in Medicine, 146*, 102693. Advance online publication. DOI: 10.1016/j.artmed.2023.102693 PMID: 38042593

Sweidan, J., El-Yacoubi, M. A., & Rigaud, A. S. (2024). Explainability of CNN-based Alzheimer's disease detection from online handwriting. *Scientific Reports, 14*(1), 21873. Advance online publication. DOI: 10.1038/s41598-024-72736-0 PMID: 39333681

Tanaka, K., Kudo, M., Kimura, K., & Nakamura, A. (2024). Long-term detection system for six kinds of abnormal behavior of the elderly living alone. *arXiv*. https://arxiv.org/abs/2411.13153 (No DOI available)

Thakur, G. K., Thakur, A., Khan, N., & Anush, H. (2024, April). The role of natural language processing in medical data analysis and healthcare automation. In *2024 International Conference on Knowledge Engineering and Communication Systems (ICKECS)* (pp. 1–5). IEEE. https://doi.org/DOI: 10.1109/ICKECS61492.2024.10617406

Toktas, E. (2024). The future of e-health: Opportunities and challenges in public health systems. *Journal of Foresight and Public Health, 1*(1), 45–56. DOI: 10.62617/jfph.v1i1.45

van Kolfschooten, H. (2023). The AI cycle of health inequity and digital ageism: Mitigating biases through the EU regulatory framework on medical devices. *European Journal of Health Law, 30*(4), 1–24. DOI: 10.1163/15718093-bja10110 PMID: 38075950

Vousinas, G. L., Simitsi, I., Livieri, G., Gkouva, G. C., & Efthymiou, I. P. (2022). Mapping the road of the ethical dilemmas behind artificial intelligence. *Journal of Politics and Ethics in New Technologies and AI, 1*(1), e31238. DOI: 10.12681/jpentai.31238

Wei, R., Buss, S. S., Milde, R., Fernandes, M., Sumsion, D., Davis, E., & Sun, H. (2025). Automated phenotyping of mild cognitive impairment and Alzheimer's disease and related dementias using electronic health records. *International Journal of Medical Informatics, 200*, 105917. Advance online publication. DOI: 10.1016/j.ijmedinf.2025.105917 PMID: 40222334

Woodman, R. J., & Mangoni, A. A. (2023). A comprehensive review of machine learning algorithms and their application in geriatric medicine: Present and future. *Aging Clinical and Experimental Research, 35*(11), 2363–2397. DOI: 10.1007/s40520-023-02552-3 PMID: 37682491

Xu, X., Li, J., Zhu, Z., Zhao, L., Wang, H., Song, C., & Pei, Y. (2024). A comprehensive review on synergy of multi-modal data and AI technologies in medical diagnosis. *Bioengineering (Basel, Switzerland), 11*(3), 219. Advance online publication. DOI: 10.3390/bioengineering11030219 PMID: 38534493

Yu, Y. W., Lin, C. H., Lu, C. K., Wang, J. K., & Huang, T. L. (2023). Automated age-related macular degeneration detector on optical coherence tomography images using slice-sum local binary patterns and support vector machine. *Biomedical Engineering Online, 22*(1), 85. Advance online publication. DOI: 10.1186/s12938-023-01149-2 PMID: 37644599

Zhang, J., Mazlin, V., Fei, K., Boccara, A. C., Yuan, J., & Xiao, P. (2023). Time-domain full-field optical coherence tomography (TD-FF-OCT) in ophthalmic imaging. *Therapeutic Advances in Chronic Disease, 14*, 1–12. DOI: 10.1177/20406223231170146 PMID: 37152350

Zhao, A. P., Li, S., Cao, Z., Hu, P. J. H., Wang, J., Xiang, Y., & Lu, X. (2024). AI for science: Predicting infectious diseases. *Journal of Safety Science and Resilience = An Quan Ke Xue Yu Ren Xing (Ying Wen), 5*(3), 232–245. DOI: 10.1016/j.jnlssr.2024.03.001

Chapter 3
AI in Healthcare:
Technological and Ethical Dimensions for Aging Populations

Dimitrios Batakis
https://orcid.org/0000-0002-2326-4653
Hellenic Mediterranean University, Greece

ABSTRACT

This chapter examines the role of Artificial Intelligence (AI) in modern healthcare, focusing on its applications for aging populations and geriatric care. It analyzes how AI enhances diagnostic accuracy, clinical decision-making, and healthcare efficiency while addressing increasing demands due to workforce shortages and demographic changes. The chapter highlights AI's ability to process large and complex datasets from electronic health records, genetic profiles, and wearable devices, as demonstrated in case studies such as Google's Med-PaLM 2 and AI-enabled digital hospitals. Ethical considerations, including data privacy, algorithmic bias, equitable access, and human oversight, are discussed, emphasizing the importance of responsible innovation and representative datasets. The chapter concludes that AI offers transformative potential for improving patient outcomes in older adults and the broader population, but its benefits depend on careful integration with ethical governance and patient-centered practices.

INTRODUCTION

Artificial Intelligence (AI) is rapidly transforming the landscape of modern healthcare, offering unprecedented opportunities to enhance diagnostic precision, accelerate drug discovery, and streamline clinical workflows. As global populations age and healthcare systems contend with increasing demands and a persistent short-

DOI: 10.4018/979-8-3373-5462-0.ch003

age of medical professionals, AI-driven solutions are emerging as a transformative force in improving patient outcomes (Batakis et al., 2025). This article explores the multifaceted role of AI in contemporary medicine, with a particular focus on its burgeoning applications for older adults and the unique ethical considerations that arise in geriatric care. Using illustrative case studies like Google's Med-PaLM 2 and the integration of AI in digital hospitals, we delve into how AI can process vast and complex medical datasets, assist in sophisticated diagnoses, and optimise clinical decision-making (Ahirwal et al., 2022). Despite its immense promise, the widespread adoption of AI in healthcare necessitates a careful balancing act between technological innovation and ethical responsibility, particularly concerning data privacy, algorithmic bias, human oversight, and equitable access for vulnerable populations.

TECHNOLOGICAL ADVANCES IN AI FOR HEALTHCARE

The rapid evolution of Artificial Intelligence (AI) has sparked global discussions about the professions that might be "threatened" by potential replacement by AI systems. Amongst the occupations often mentioned, doctors and nurses are notably absent. This exclusion highlights the critical role that human expertise plays in healthcare, even as AI continues to advance at an extraordinary pace. Whilst AI may revolutionise many aspects of healthcare, it is clear that it cannot fully replace the complex, nuanced decisions and empathetic care that medical professionals provide (Ahuja, 2019). This perspective is further supported by systems-based approaches to healthcare, such as the sociocybernetic model, which conceptualises healthcare as an adaptive, multilayered system influenced by both technological and human factors.

AI-Driven Diagnostics and Clinical Decision Support

AI has made significant strides in medical imaging, allowing for faster and more accurate disease detection. Machine learning algorithms analyse radiological images, including X-rays, MRIs, and CT scans, to identify conditions such as cancer, fractures, and neurological disorders with high precision (Paul et al., 2021). These AI-powered diagnostic tools help detect abnormalities at an earlier stage, significantly improving patient outcomes and survival rates. This is particularly evident in oncology, where technological innovation has improved both diagnostic precision and the personalisation of treatment plans. Additionally, AI-driven imaging systems reduce the workload of radiologists by prioritising critical cases, enabling faster and more accurate decision-making. Companies like IBM Watson, Google's DeepMind, and NVIDIA are leading the development of AI-driven imaging solutions, demonstrating impressive results in detecting diseases like breast cancer, lung abnormalities, and diabetic retinopathy. AI's ability to process vast volumes of imaging data ensures efficiency in radiology departments whilst minimising human errors (Najjar, 2023).

Natural Language Processing (NLP)-powered AI models, such as Google's Med-PaLM 2, represent a significant leap forward in clinical decision support (Singhal et al., 2023). Trained on extensive medical literature, clinical notes, and research articles, Med-PaLM 2 can understand complex medical jargon, answer intricate medical questions, and provide context-aware recommendations to healthcare professionals. It can assist in synthesising patient information, summarising medical literature, and even generating patient education materials. Research shows Med-PaLM 2 has achieved expert-level performance on medical examination benchmarks, often outperforming human physicians in generating high-quality, relevant, and comprehensive answers (Oniani et al., 2024; Singhal et al., 2023). Such models streamline medical documentation, enhance patient summaries, and offer real-time insights into drug interactions and contraindications, thereby empowering clinicians with enhanced information for more informed decisions (Batakis et al., 2025).

Accelerating Drug Discovery and Personalised Medicine

AI plays a pivotal role in accelerating the traditionally time-consuming and expensive process of drug discovery. Machine learning algorithms can analyse vast chemical and biological datasets to identify potential drug candidates, predict their efficacy and toxicity, and optimise molecular structures. This significantly reduces the time from target identification to clinical trials (Dhanda et al., 2025). AI-powered platforms, such as BenevolentAI and Atomwise, use deep learning to analyse complex biological datasets, accelerating the identification of promising drug candidates. AI models also play a crucial role in repurposing existing drugs for new therapeutic applications, reducing the time and costs associated with traditional drug development processes (Almaeeni, 2024).

Furthermore, AI is central to the advancement of personalised medicine. By analysing a patient's unique genetic makeup, lifestyle, medical history, and real-time physiological data (often from wearables), AI can recommend highly tailored treatment plans (Ma et al., 2023). The use of AI extends beyond clinical care into behavioural health, where language models can support targeted prevention strategies (I. P. Efthymiou et al., 2023). This approach moves beyond the "one-size-fits-all" model, optimising therapeutic outcomes and minimising adverse effects, especially beneficial for patients with complex or rare diseases.

Optimising Medical Workflows and Hospital Operations

One of the primary uses of AI in healthcare is to assist in clinical decision-making. With their ability to quickly analyse vast quantities of data, AI systems can identify patterns that might otherwise go unnoticed, making them invaluable tools in diagnosis and treatment. For example, AI algorithms can detect irregularities in medical images, such as CT scans or mammograms—at stages where the human eye might miss them. However, despite their advanced capabilities, these tools serve best as decision-support systems rather than substitutes for human professionals (Dara et al., 2024).

AI's role is supportive rather than a substitute. The technology's capabilities allow it to assist in tasks that are time-consuming or labour-intensive for human practitioners, freeing them up to focus on more complex aspects of care that require human judgement, intuition, and empathy. The decision-making process in healthcare is rarely straightforward; it involves considering a wide range of factors, from medical history to patient preferences and emotional state. These factors go beyond data and algorithms, making the human factor irreplaceable in the healthcare process (Dara et al., 2024). As such, AI should be viewed as a tool that enhances the work of healthcare professionals, rather than replacing them. This is especially true when it comes to diagnostics and treatment decisions. AI can help doctors sift through vast amounts of data, from medical histories to research papers, allowing them to make informed decisions more quickly and accurately. But the ultimate decisions should always involve human judgement, as doctors evaluate the individual circumstances of their patients and collaborate with them on the best course of action (Shaw et al., 2024).

AI also plays a significant role in improving the overall efficiency of healthcare systems. For example, AI-driven systems can streamline administrative tasks such as patient scheduling, record-keeping, and even billing, reducing the workload on healthcare providers and allowing them to dedicate more time to patient care. However, the widespread adoption of AI in healthcare depends on having the right environment for its application. Countries must accelerate the digital transformation of healthcare, especially through the digitisation of medical records and the integration of interoperable systems (Gazzarata et al., 2024; Gupta et al., 2023). In critical environments like Intensive Care Units, timely access to patient data supported by AI can significantly impact clinical outcomes.

The digital transformation of healthcare also promises to reduce geographic disparities by enabling equitable access to care. AI-driven remote monitoring, decision support, and predictive analytics empower healthcare providers to anticipate patient needs and intervene proactively, particularly in underserved regions (Dankwa-Mullan, 2024; Esmaeilzadeh, 2024). This is also relevant in the context of medical tourism, where AI tools can support seamless cross-border care coordination. Batakis et al. (2023) highlight how, in the case of Crete in Greece, both healthcare providers and hotel managers see AI as key to enhancing service integration, efficiency, and personalised care for visiting patients. Moreover, the importance of maintaining human empathy in healthcare cannot be overstated. Whilst AI may enhance diagnostic and predictive accuracy, it lacks the emotional intelligence necessary for compassionate care. High burnout rates amongst healthcare professionals underscore the need for AI systems to alleviate administrative burdens and restore focus on the patient-provider relationship, rather than act as replacements (Ahuja, 2019). The future of healthcare lies in human-AI collaboration where AI enhances efficiency and precision, and human professionals preserve the empathy and ethical grounding essential to medicine.

AI Applications in Geriatric Care

Older adults face a distinct constellation of healthcare challenges that are both complex and multifaceted. Amongst the most pressing issues are multimorbidity, where individuals often live with two or more chronic conditions simultaneously; polypharmacy, which raises the risk of adverse drug interactions, reduced adherence, and increased healthcare costs; and a heightened vulnerability to age-related conditions such as cognitive decline, frailty, and reduced mobility (Odionu & Ibeh, 2024). These challenges not only compromise health outcomes but also significantly affect the autonomy and psychological well-being of older individuals, whilst placing a growing strain on families, caregivers, and healthcare systems.

Artificial Intelligence (AI) has the potential to offer transformative, tailored solutions that directly address these pressing needs. By leveraging advanced data analytics, AI can identify patterns of disease progression, optimise medication management, and support early diagnosis of conditions such as dementia or cardiovascular disease. Intelligent monitoring systems can facilitate independent living by detecting falls, tracking vital signs, or predicting health deterioration before it becomes critical. Moreover, AI-driven decision support tools can aid clinicians in developing personalised treatment plans, thereby reducing the likelihood of errors and enhancing the efficiency of care delivery. Beyond medical management, AI can also alleviate caregiver burden by automating routine tasks and providing actionable insights, ultimately fostering a more sustainable and patientcentred model of geriatric care.

Early Detection and Personalised Treatment Plans

AI-driven solutions have become instrumental in the early detection of age-related conditions. For example, in the realm of dementia and cognitive decline, AI algorithms analyse speech patterns, cognitive test results, and even subtle behavioural changes detected through smart home sensors to identify early signs of cognitive impairment, often years before a clinical diagnosis is made. When it comes to frailty, AI evaluates gait patterns, activity levels, and other physiological markers captured by wearable devices or ambient sensors to predict an individual's risk of frailty. This predictive ability enables proactive interventions designed to prevent falls and maintain mobility (Griˇskeviˇcius et al., 2025; Rao et al., 2025). In cardiovascular disease management, wearable devices equipped with AI continuously monitor vital signs, detecting irregular heart rhythms such as atrial fibrillation (using devices like KardiaMobile) or abnormalities in blood pressure, thereby providing early warnings of impending cardiovascular events (Sun et al., 2025; Vagnetti et al., 2024). For older adults managing multimorbidity—the presence of multiple chronic conditions—and polypharmacy, which refers to the use of multiple medications, AI facilitates the development of highly personalised treatment plans. AI models can analyse complex medication interactions, optimise dosages, and predict potential adverse drug reactions to ensure safer and more effective therapeutic regimens (Ma et al., 2023). This capability is particularly crucial in reducing hospital readmissions that are related to medication errors or adverse effects.

AI-driven robotic systems, such as the Da Vinci Surgical System, assist in performing minimally invasive procedures with greater precision and control. These robotic assistants enhance surgical outcomes, reduce recovery times, and minimise complications, leading to improved patient care. AI-powered robotic surgery systems provide surgeons with realtime feedback, enabling precise movements and reducing the likelihood of human errors (Paul et al., 2021). Additionally, AI-driven robotics facilitate remote surgeries through teleoperated robotic systems, allowing expert surgeons to perform complex procedures on patients in different locations. The use of AI in robotic surgery is expanding to multiple disciplines, including orthopaedics, neurosurgery, and cardiovascular procedures, significantly improving patient outcomes and procedural success rates (Najjar, 2023). The integration of AI with robotic surgery marks a new era of precision medicine, where AI assists human surgeons in achieving unparalleled levels of accuracy and efficiency in medical procedures.

Remote Monitoring and Aging-in-Place Strategies

AI-powered remote monitoring technologies are revolutionising aging-in-place strategies, enabling older adults to live independently and safely in their homes for extended periods (Griˇskeviˇcius et al., 2025; Ma et al., 2023). Non-wearable smart home sensors and ambient devices monitor daily activities, detect falls, track sleep patterns, and assess changes in movement or routine that might indicate health decline (I. Efthymiou, 2026; Giannios et al., 2024). Systems such as I'M-ACTIVE employ sensors embedded in everyday objects like kettles to assess movement and detect emergencies, sending real-time alerts to caregivers or medical personnel (Vagnetti et al., 2024). Wearable devices go beyond the monitoring of vital signs to track mobility and exercise adherence through applications such as SilverSneakers GO, and can also provide reminders for medications or medical appointments (Sun et al., 2025). AI-enabled telemedicine platforms have enhanced healthcare access for older adults, particularly those in remote or underserved areas, by facilitating virtual consultations, remote diagnostics, and continuous health management. This reduces the need for frequent in-person visits. Furthermore, AI assists in care coordination by optimising collaboration amongst multiple healthcare providers, specialists, and caregivers, ensuring seamless transitions between different care settings, such as hospital to home, and reducing fragmented care.

Assistive Robotics and Emotional Support

Whilst still evolving, AI embodied in assistive robots hold considerable promise for supporting senior citizens in their homes (D´ıaz et al., 2013). These robots may aid with mobility, personal hygiene, household chores, and provide emotional companionship to combat loneliness, especially for individuals with cognitive impairments (Sun et al., 2025). For example, some companion animal robots have demonstrated potential in stimulating cognitive function amongst older adults with dementia (Almaeeni, 2024).

ETHICAL CHALLENGES AND CONSIDERATIONS

Despite the transformative potential of AI in healthcare, its deployment, especially within the vulnerable geriatric population, raises significant ethical and practical challenges that demand careful consideration and robust mitigation strategies (R. J. Chen et al., 2023; Cross et al., 2024; Elgin & Elgin, 2024). One of the most pressing concerns surrounding AI in healthcare is data privacy and security. AI-driven healthcare systems depend on vast amounts of patient data to function effectively, including sensitive information such as medical histories, diagnostic results, imaging data, and genetic information. The more data an AI system processes, the greater the potential for exposure to cyber threats, data breaches, and unauthorised access. Healthcare data is particularly valuable, making it a prime target for hackers and cybercriminals. A breach in this sensitive information could have devastating consequences, compromising patient confidentiality and eroding trust in healthcare institutions (Shaw et al., 2024). To mitigate these risks, it is essential that AI systems are designed with robust encryption and security protocols. Compliance with regulations such as HIPAA and GDPR is critical, but the rapidly evolving capabilities of AI demand more stringent, adaptive cybersecurity frameworks.

Data Privacy and Security

AI systems in healthcare depend on vast amounts of sensitive patient information (SPI and PHI), including medical histories, genetic data, and real-time physiological measurements. Protecting this data is paramount, as increased data collection, storage, and processing amplify the risks of breaches, unauthorised access, and misuse. Existing regulations such as HIPAA and GDPR offer frameworks to safeguard patient information, but the rapidly evolving capabilities of AI demand continuous updates and adaptations to privacy protocol. Moreover, concerns persist regarding the potential re-identification of pseudo-anonymised data and the commercial exploitation of health data (Ali et al., 2025; Bavli et al., 2025; Salomon, 2012). Transparency about data collection, usage, and sharing—with clear consent mechanisms—is critical, particularly as many older adults may have limited digital literacy or may not fully grasp the complex implications of data privacy.

Bias and Fairness

A critical concern is the potential for algorithmic bias to reinforce or even exacerbate existing healthcare disparities (Cross et al., 2024; Elgin & Elgin, 2024). AI models are often trained on historical datasets that may not represent the diverse older adult population adequately, such as lacking sufficient data from specific ethnic groups, socioeconomic backgrounds, or individuals with severe cognitive or physical impairments (Chatzivasileiou et al., 2023). As a result, AI predictions or recommendations may be inaccurate or discriminatory against underrepresented groups (Benzinger et al., 2024; Elgin & Elgin, 2024). For instance, an AI model trained primarily on data from younger or healthier individuals may misdiagnose or mistreat older patients with multiple comorbidities. To address this, it is essential to ensure training datasets are diverse and to implement continuous auditing mechanisms to detect and mitigate bias, thereby fostering equitable healthcare outcomes (Cary et al., 2025).

Human Oversight and the Doctor-Patient Relationship

Whilst AI can augment clinical capabilities, it must complement, not replace, human clinical judgement and empathy (R. J. Chen et al., 2023; Y. Chen & Esmaeilzadeh, 2024; Cross et al., 2024). The doctor-patient relationship is founded on trust, communication, and emotional understanding—elements AI cannot fully replicate (Benzinger et al., 2024; Elgin & Elgin, 2024). Over-reliance on AI risks depersonalising care and overlooking subtle clinical nuances, emotional cues, or individual patient values (Fasan, 2025). Therefore, human oversight is essential to interpret AI outputs within the broader clinical context, make final diagnostic and treatment decisions, and maintain the ethical accountability inherent in healthcare. Integrating AI as a supportive tool for healthcare providers, rather than an autonomous authority, is key to promoting acceptance and ensuring patient-centred care (Cross et al., 2024; I. P. Efthymiou et al., 2023; Nogaroli, 2025).

Beyond technical and legal concerns, ethical dilemmas also surface regarding the use of AI in healthcare. AI systems lack moral reasoning and contextual awareness, which are critical in patient care. Similar concerns have emerged in other sectors, including politics, where the unchecked use of AI can lead to significant human rights implications. Efthymiou Egleton et al. (2020) emphasise the risks of AI-driven surveillance, biased decision-making, and erosion of privacy, highlighting the urgent need for universal ethical standards that transcend sectoral boundaries. When AI tools are involved in decisionmaking, questions arise about accountability and the patient-provider relationship. If AI makes an erroneous recommendation, determining liability becomes complex. It is imperative that AI be viewed as an assistive tool rather than a replacement for clinicians. Human oversight remains essential to preserve empathy, interpret nuanced patient data, and uphold ethical standards in care (Ahuja, 2019).

Ultimately, the successful integration of AI into healthcare depends not only on technical robustness but also on a strong ethical and regulatory foundation. Responsible AI adoption demands collaborative engagement amongst technologists, clinicians, ethicists, and policymakers to create frameworks that ensure transparency, equity, and accountability. The involvement of diverse stakeholders, including non-governmental organisations (NGOs), is pivotal in shaping healthcare policies and ensuring equitable access to care. Sidiropoulos et al. (2021) highlight the expanding influence of NGOs in global health governance, addressing both their significant contributions and the challenges they face concerning transparency and legitimacy. This once again brings forward the necessity for robust frameworks that promote accountability amongst all entities engaged in healthcare delivery and policy-making. Moreover, the integration of AI in healthcare has the potential to transform service delivery, but it also raises concerns about economic displacement and widening inequalities. Emmanouil-Kalos and Prokakis (2021) emphasise that strong social protection systems are critical in buffering the socioeconomic shocks experienced during crises. Proactive welfare strategies could similarly support workers and institutions affected by rapid technological change in the healthcare sector.

NAVIGATING THE FUTURE: A BALANCED APPROACH

To unlock the full potential of Artificial Intelligence (AI) in healthcare for older adults, it is not enough to simply advance algorithms or enhance computational capacity. What is required is a balanced and holistic approach that seamlessly integrates cutting-edge technological innovation with a steadfast and unwavering commitment to ethical responsibility. This integration is indispensable because the challenges of aging populations are not merely technical problems to be solved but deeply human concerns that intersect with values, rights, and social priorities.

Developing AI for geriatric healthcare is therefore far more than a technical exercise; it represents a fundamental paradigm shift in how societies envision, design, and ultimately deploy digital technologies to serve humanity. It demands that innovation be framed not only in terms of efficiency, accuracy, and predictive power but also through the lens of compassion, empathy, and justice. The primary objective must be to harness AI's transformative capacity to enhance patient well-being, extending both the quality and dignity of life for older adults, whilst ensuring that core principles, such as respect for autonomy, protection of privacy, and preservation of human dignity, remain nonnegotiable.

When technological innovation and ethical responsibility are integrated as twin pillars, the result is the creation of robust, trustworthy, and human-centred systems. These systems will not only revolutionise geriatric care by providing more precise diagnoses, personalised interventions, and proactive support but will also foster trust amongst patients, caregivers, and healthcare professionals. In doing so, AI will be able to meet its true promise: not just as a disruptive tool for efficiency but as a transformative force that supports the values, rights, and well-being of some of society's most vulnerable members.

Integrating Innovation with Ethics

The rapid development of AI necessitates a proactive and adaptive ethical framework. This framework must not only adhere to existing data protection regulations but also anticipate new ethical dilemmas that may arise as AI capabilities expand. For example, as AI becomes more sophisticated in predictive analytics for chronic disease management or personalised interventions, continuous ethical evaluation will be vital to prevent overmedicalisation or unintended consequences (Tripathi, 2025). The focus should be on designing "AI for good", systems that are inherently beneficial, reliable, and respectful of human dignity.

Interdisciplinary Collaboration and Robust Regulatory Frameworks

Effective governance of AI in healthcare demands interdisciplinary collaboration amongst AI developers, clinicians, ethicists, legal experts, policymakers, and patient advocacy groups, especially those representing older adults. Such collaboration ensures that AI systems are developed with diverse perspectives, addressing potential biases and ensuring user-friendliness and accessibility from the outset (Dakoliya, 2025).

Furthermore, robust regulatory frameworks are critical to this effort. These frameworks must establish clear standards for data privacy, security, and interoperability (Cross et al., 2024; I. P. Efthymiou, 2024), mandate mechanisms for bias detection and mitigation in AI algorithms, define roles and responsibilities for accountability and transparency in AI-driven clinical decisions, promote explainable AI (XAI) to foster trust and understanding amongst users and clinicians (Benzinger et al., 2024; Cross et al., 2024), and ensure equitable access to AI-supported healthcare services to prevent the deepening of health disparities (Shastry, 2025).

Fostering Trust, Equity, and Quality in Patient Care

Ultimately, the goal is to ensure AI enhances healthcare whilst maintaining trust, equity, and quality in patient care across all age groups, including the aging population. This involves prioritising patient education to empower older adults and their caregivers with knowledge about AI technologies and their implications, emphasising human oversight to reinforce that AI is a tool to assist rather than replace the irreplaceable human element in care and continuous evaluation through regular assessments of AI's real-world impact on patient outcomes, safety, and ethical implications (Abah & Onwelumadu, 2025).

By embracing a responsible, inclusive, and forward-looking approach, Artificial Intelligence (AI) carries the profound potential to reshape and transform the entire landscape of geriatric care. Such a transformation extends far beyond incremental improvements in medical technology; it promises to generate significant advancements in health outcomes, prolong independence in everyday living, and enrich the overall quality of life for the world's rapidly growing aging population. What is at stake is not simply the optimisation of healthcare delivery, but a redefinition of how societies collectively understand and respond to the process of aging itself.

This transformation cannot be reduced to a matter of technological evolution alone. Rather, it represents a fundamental shift in our perspective, an ethical, social, and cultural reorientation toward aging as a shared human experience that requires thoughtful stewardship of innovation. The journey toward realising the full potential of AI in this field is long, complex, and deeply multifaceted. It will necessitate ongoing interdisciplinary dialogue amongst policymakers, healthcare professionals, technologists, ethicists, and, crucially, older adults themselves, whose voices and lived experiences must guide development. It will also require foresight in anticipating ethical dilemmas, proactive safeguards to protect vulnerable populations, and a collective determination to ensure that technological progress remains firmly aligned with human values.

To achieve these aims, AI systems must be deliberately designed to be transparent in their functioning, equitable in their access and outcomes, and accountable in their decision-making processes. Transparency builds trust, equity prevents the deepening of existing inequalities, and accountability ensures that technological tools remain aligned with the ethical principles of care and justice. Equally important is the commitment to continuous monitoring and evaluation of real-world impact, so that unintended consequences can be identified and addressed swiftly. Only through such vigilance can we ensure that AI does not inadvertently compromise fundamental human values such as dignity, autonomy, and privacy.

In sum, embracing a responsible and inclusive approach to AI development has the capacity not only to advance the field of geriatric healthcare but also to catalyse a broader cultural shift toward viewing aging as a stage of life deserving of dignity, innovation, and respect. By doing so, societies will be better equipped to harness AI as a genuine force for positive change in healthcare, one that empowers older adults, supports caregivers, strengthens healthcare systems, and ultimately affirms the shared humanity that unites generations.

Regulatory Compliance

Many AI models applied to the medical field are not yet approved by regulatory bodies and are released without any quality assurance, thus potentially posing a risk to clinical practice (Mennella et al., 2024). Approval of medical devices such as software-based AI models typically requires evidence of their clinical effectiveness and safety. The validation of these two aspects requires, for example, adequate testing on relevant data and through suitable clinical trials. Indeed, an AI model may achieve excellent performance on internal or public data but then not prove effective in real clinical settings. Similarly, a clinically effective device must also be sufficiently robust, reliable, and safe to gain approval. Ensuring these factors remains a significant challenge even with widely accessible data and well-established approaches in related fields. Medical data are usually scarcely available, and their formation and collection are relatively expensive. Approaches such as data augmentation have been explored in an attempt to tackle the scarcity of training data. Nevertheless, these kinds of approaches exhibit some limitations, and the scarcity of data remains a significant problem. An additional limitation arises from the training procedure of many AI models. Overfitting the training data leads to high performance but poor generalisation capabilities, and this behaviour is often observed in practice when many AI models are built based on an end-to-end training approach (Osifowokan et al., 2025).

Accountability and Liability

Accountability and liability constitute critical considerations as artificial intelligence (AI) increasingly assumes clinical- and decision-support roles within healthcare. The black box nature of AI and its augmented autonomy introduce novel legal questions, particularly regarding the applicable standards of care. Multiple foundational legal doctrines are pertinent: negligence, whereby failure to meet a duty of care results in harm; strict liability, which imposes responsibility absent fault; vicarious liability, assigning employer liability for employee actions; and product liability, mandating manufacturer warnings of latent dangers.

Supervisory physicians remain subject to liability, given their duty to oversee AI use and to withhold final decisions pending human approval (Zhang & Zhang, 2023). Since current medical AI constitutes a regulated medical device, approval and risk-management processes warrant scrutiny to avoid regulatory lacunae. In instances where flawed AI diagnoses precipitate patient harm, attribution of responsibility frequently proves ambiguous, engendering potential accountability gaps. Floridi's faultless moral responsibility framework proposes distributed risk and responsibility amongst relevant agents in lieu of conventional concepts of individual or entity fault (Floridi, 2023). However, dispersed accountability risks diminishing individual deterrence and thus impeding innovation and deployment (Emery-Xu et al., 2025; Tu, 2025). Observing regulatory precedents in Europe and the United States suggests complementary mechanisms: the imposition of liability fees integrated into AI products, coupled with the establishment of governmental or industry-sponsored insurance pools, can balance patient protection with incentives for ongoing development. Evolving regional legislation may further furnish guiding provisions to facilitate robust and responsible growth (Chun et al., 2024; Dixon, 2023; Justo Hanani, 2022). The paucity of enforcement mechanisms for ethical principles and the consequent lack of sanctions for noncompliance underscore the insufficiency of voluntary ethical frameworks in ensuring trustworthy AI governance.

Equity in Access to AI Technologies

Artificial Intelligence applications in healthcare have the potential to improve treatment, reduce costs and address medical staff shortages. However, equity in access to healthcare AI technologies is often overlooked. Disabled people, older adults, people of colour, the LGBTQ+ community and women are more likely to experience reduced access to AI healthcare technologies (Clark et al., 2021). A lack of access is often a consequence of under representation within the training datasets driving these systems, insufficient effort being devoted to creating equitable products and patients within lower income brackets experiencing financial inequity when accessing AI technologies.

There are numerous initiatives aimed at correcting this imbalance and improving representation in healthcare AI. In the United States, the National Artificial Intelligence Initiative Act of 2020 requires detailed plans to use AI for the "processing, interpretation, analysis, and use of the data collected by the Agency to members of populations identified as underserved and subjected to health disparities". In the United Kingdom, the Agenda for Change framework creates additional funding for "hardship" posts. Recommended considerations for developers include clear narratives around digital distribution strategies (Megahd et al., 2024).

AI and Health Equity

Researchers have highlighted the strong, long-term effects of poor health on opportunity and well-being, underscoring the importance of health equity and social justice as fundamental health system objectives. Public health ethics may provide guidance to promote the trustworthy and responsible use of artificial intelligence (AI) in healthcare. AI models already assist with disease surveillance, pandemic response, and the triaging of seriously ill patients. When carefully implemented, trustworthy AI has the potential to support the most vulnerable individuals in society, facilitate access to high-quality medical care, and improve population health by augmenting existing services and systems (Bhattacharya et al., 2021).

The principle of justice, which denounces exploitation and oppression, and argues for equal access to care, is embedded in the Hippocratic tradition and has been declared a fundamental principle of bioethics. Justice concerns the fair distribution of both benefits and burdens in research and medical care (Abra`moff et al., 2023). The European Commission High-Level Expert Group on Artificial Intelligence emphasised these values, particularly fairness and non-discrimination, when setting forth high-level requirements for the development of trustworthy AI. Unfair distribution of benefits and burdens may generate harmful bias and ultimately discrimination (Thomasian et al., 2021). This risk is especially high in cases in which AI models are trained on datasets representative of underlying structural inequalities within society. Biased AI is important for separate reasons: it may still produce inaccurate and unfair results, which in turn undermine the effectiveness of decision-making. Studies have indicated that marginalised and vulnerable groups, such as Black patients or women, receive less benefit or even harm when these models are used for healthcare. Biased AI leads to unfair decisions and discriminatory behaviours.

Furthermore, the emergence of such systemic issues is challenging to control or mitigate through transparent explanations and incomprehensible justification procedures. If these systems are introduced and integrated into medical practice without additional transparency or accountability safeguards, they risk amplifying and perpetuating existing social discriminations. The requirement that AI support the principle of justice is therefore crucial: developers should not only seek to eliminate unfair bias but also seek to share benefits fairly and avoid creating new sources of harm (Berdahl et al., 2023). Ethical guidelines supporting justice are necessary to ensure that AI systems remain committed to alleviating human suffering, and primacy is given to the needs of patients (Goisauf & Cano Abad´ıa, 2022).

CONCLUSION

This chapter has examined the transformative role of Artificial Intelligence in healthcare, with particular emphasis on its applications for aging populations and geriatric care. Whilst AI offers unprecedented opportunities to enhance diagnostic accuracy, personalise treatment, optimise healthcare workflows, and support aging-in-place strategies, its successful integration depends critically on addressing ethical, regulatory, and equity concerns. The future of AI in healthcare lies not in replacing human professionals but in augmenting their capabilities, preserving the essential elements of empathy, trust, and human oversight that underpin quality patient care. By fostering interdisciplinary collaboration, implementing robust regulatory frameworks, and prioritising transparency, fairness, and accountability, we can harness AI's potential to improve health outcomes and quality of life for older adults whilst upholding the fundamental values of dignity, autonomy, and justice.

REFERENCES

Abah, T., & Onwelumadu, I. (2025). Equity: Integrated care for underserved populations. *International Perspectives and Experiences Enhancing Access to Healthcare*, 119.

Ahirwal, M. K., Londhe, N. D., & Kumar, A. (2022). *Artificial intelligence applications for health care*. CRC Press.

Ahuja, A. S. (2019). The impact of artificial intelligence in medicine on the future role of the physician [PMID: 31592346; PMC6779111. Authoritative review on AI augmenting physicians]. *PeerJ*, *7*, e7702. DOI: 10.7717/peerj.7702

Ali, A. T., Zeeshan, M. N., Khaleeq, A., Jamil, M. N., Khan, U., Siddiqui, A., & Ahmad, S. (2025). Ethical-legal implications of AI-powered healthcare in critical perspective. *Frontiers in Artificial Intelligence*, *8*. Advance online publication. DOI: 10.3389/frai.2025.1619463

Almaeeni, H. (2024). Review on Artificial Intelligence in Medicine and Health. *2024 IEEE International Conference on Medical Artificial Intelligence (MedAI)*.

Batakis, D., Chatzivasileiou, S., & Efthymiou, I. P. (2025). Artificial Intelligence and its impact on healthcare. *World Journal of Advanced Research and Reviews*, *26*(1), 250–256. DOI: 10.30574/wjarr.2025.26.1.1015

Batakis, D., Sidiropoulos, S., Emmanouil-Kalos, A., Fouskas, T., Zopounidis, C., & Vozikis, A. (2023). Medical tourism in the region of Crete, Greece: Perspectives from healthcare providers, hotel managers, and medical tourists. *Sustainability*, *15*(24), 16822. DOI: 10.3390/su152416822

Bavli, I., Ho, A., Mahal, R., & McKeown, M. J. (2025). Ethical concerns around privacy and data security in AI health monitoring for Parkinson's disease: Insights from patients, family members, and healthcare professionals. *AI & Society*, *40*(1), 155–165.

Benzinger, L., Epping, J., Ursin, F., Balke, W.-T., Kacprowski, T., & Salloch, S. (2024). Artificial intelligence to support ethical decision-making for incapacitated patients: A survey among German anesthesiologists and internists [Recent 2024 study on human oversight and AI in medical decision-making; PubMed indexed]. *BMC Medical Ethics*, *25*(1), 78. DOI: 10.1186/s12910-024-01079-z PMID: 39026308

Berdahl, C. T., Baker, L., Mann, S., Osoba, O., & Girosi, F. (2023). Strategies to improve the impact of artificial intelligence on health equity: Scoping review. *JMIR AI*, *2*, e42936. DOI: 10.2196/42936 PMID: 38875587

Bhattacharya, S., Hossain, M. M., Juyal, R., Sharma, N., Pradhan, K. B., & Singh, A. (2021). Role of Public Health Ethics for Responsible Use of Artificial Intelligence Technologies. *Indian Journal of Community Medicine : Official Publication of Indian Association of Preventive & Social Medicine*, *46*(2), 178. PMID: 34321721

Cary, M. P.Jr, Bessias, S., McCall, J., Pencina, M. J., Grady, S. D., Lytle, K., & Economou-Zavlanos, N. J. (2025). Empowering nurses to champion Health equity & BE FAIR: Bias elimination for fair and responsible AI in healthcare. *Journal of Nursing Scholarship*, *57*(1), 130–139. PMID: 39075715

Chatzivasileiou, S., Emmanouil-Kalos, A., Efthymiou Egleton, I. P., Batakis, D., & Vozikis, A. (2023). Mapping the Donations of Pharma Companies in Greece: The Case of Scientific Societies. *International Journal of Non-Profit Sector Empowerment*, *2*(1), e34419. DOI: 10.12681/npse.34419

Chen, R. J., Wang, J. J., Williamson, D. F. K., Chen, T. Y., Lipkova, J., Lu, M. Y., Sahai, S., & Mahmood, F. (2023). Algorithmic fairness in artificial intelligence for medicine and healthcare [PMID: 37380750; PMC10632090. Comprehensive Nature review on algorithmic fairness in healthcare AI]. *Nature Biomedical Engineering*, *7*(6), 719–742. DOI: 10.1038/s41551-023-01056-8 PMID: 37380750

Chen, Y., & Esmaeilzadeh, P. (2024). Generative AI in medical practice: In-depth exploration of privacy and security challenges [PMID: 38457208; PMC10960211. Recent comprehensive analysis of data privacy in AI healthcare systems]. *Journal of Medical Internet Research*, *26*, e53008. DOI: 10.2196/53008 PMID: 38457208

Chun, J., de Witt, C. S., & Elkins, K. (2024). Comparative global AI regulation: Policy perspectives from the EU, China, and the US. *arXiv preprint arXiv:2410.21279.*

Clark, C. R., Wilkins, C. H., Rodriguez, J. A., Preininger, A. M., Harris, J., DesAutels, S., & Dankwa-Mullan, I. (2021). Health care equity in the use of advanced analytics and artificial intelligence technologies in primary care. *Journal of General Internal Medicine*, *36*(10), 3188–3193. DOI: 10.1007/s11606-021-06846-x PMID: 34027610

Cross, J. L., Choma, M. A., & Onofrey, J. A. (2024). Bias in medical AI: Implications for clinical decision-making [PMC11542778. Recent comprehensive analysis of bias in clinical AI decision support]. *PLOS Digital Health*, *3*(11), e0000651. DOI: 10.1371/journal.pdig.0000651 PMID: 39509461

Dakoliya, M. (2025). Interdisciplinary Approaches to Healthcare Management: Integrating Clinical Governance, Risk Management, and Technological Advancements. *Medicon Medical Sciences, 8*, 03–06.

Dankwa-Mullan, I. (2024). Health equity and ethical considerations in using artificial intelligence in public health and medicine [Recent 2024 CDC peer-reviewed commentary on AI and health equity; PubMed indexed]. *Preventing Chronic Disease*, *21*, 240245. DOI: 10.5888/pcd21.240245 PMID: 39173183

Dara, M., Dianatpour, M., Azarpira, N., & Omidifar, N. (2024). Convergence of CRISPR and artificial intelligence: A paradigm shift in biotechnology. *Human Genomics*. Advance online publication. DOI: 10.1016/j.humgen.2024.201297

Dhanda, S. S., Panwar, D., Lin, C. C., Sharma, T. K., Rastogi, D., Bindewari, S., & Agarwal, S. (2025). Advancement in public health through machine learning: A narrative review of opportunities and ethical considerations. *Journal of Big Data*, *12*(1), 1–58.

D´ıaz, M., Saez-Pons, J., Heerink, M., & Angulo, C. (2013). Emotional factors in robotbased assistive services for elderly at home. *2013 IEEE RO-MAN*, 711–716.

Dixon, R. B. L. (2023). A principled governance for emerging AI regimes: Lessons from China, the European Union, and the United States. *AI and Ethics*, *3*(3), 793–810.

Efthymiou, I. (2026). AI in epidemiology: Predicting the unpredictable leveraging AI to detect outbreaks and predict disease. In Umer, M. (Ed.), *Innovation and transformation of public health* (pp. 281–308). IGI Global Scientific Publishing., DOI: 10.4018/979-8-3373-1992-6.ch009

Efthymiou, I. P. (2024). Exploring the frontier: New and future trends in research. In B. Orlando (Ed.), *Innovation capabilities and entrepreneurial opportunities of smart working* (pp. 48–68). IGI Global Scientific Publishing. DOI: 10.4018

Efthymiou, I. P., Alevizos, A., & Sidiropoulos, S. (2023). The role of artificial intelligence in revolutionizing NGOs' work. *Journal of Politics and Ethics in New Technologies and AI*, *2*(1), e35137. DOI: 10.12681/jpentai.35137

Efthymiou Egleton, I. P., Efthymiou Egleton, T. W., & Sidiropoulos, S. (2020). Artificial Intelligence (AI) in Politics: Should Political AI be Controlled? [(correction)]. *International Journal of Innovative Science and Research Technology*, *5*(2), 278–280.

Elgin, C. Y., & Elgin, C. (2024). Ethical implications of AI-driven clinical decision support systems on healthcare resource allocation: A qualitative study of healthcare professionals' perspectives [Recent 2024 study on ethical accountability and transparency in AI healthcare]. *BMC Medical Ethics*, *25*(1), 148. DOI: 10. 1186/s12910-024-01151-8 PMID: 39707327

Emery-Xu, N., Jordan, R., & Trager, R. (2025). International governance of advancing artificial intelligence. *AI & Society*, *40*(4), 3019–3044.

Emmanouil-Kalos, A., & Prokakis, E. (2021). Social protection after the pandemic: Lessons learned from the eurozone crisis. *HAPSc Policy Briefs Series*, *2*(1), 70–78. DOI: 10.12681/hapscpbs.27660

Esmaeilzadeh, P. (2024). The role of AI in healthcare digitalization and telemedicine. *International Journal of Medical Informatics*, *185*, 105436.

Fasan, M. (2025). Regulating the use of artificial intelligence in the doctor-patient relationship? A primer on supranational and national legal frameworks. *BIOLAW JOURNAL*, *2025*(1), 193–211.

Floridi, L. (2023). *The ethics of artificial intelligence: Principles, challenges, and opportunities*. Oxford University Press.

Gazzarata, R., Almeida, J., Lindsko¨ld, L., Cangioli, G., Gaeta, E., Fico, G., & Chronaki, C. E. (2024). HL7 fast healthcare interoperability resources (HL7 FHIR) in digital healthcare ecosystems for chronic disease management: Scoping review [PMID: 38870885. Recent 2024 review on healthcare digital transformation and interoperability]. *International Journal of Medical Informatics*, *189*, 105507. DOI: 10.1016/j.ijmedinf.2024.105507 PMID: 38870885

Giannios, G., Mpaltadoros, L., Alepoulos, V., Grammatikopoulou, M., Stavropoulos, T. G., Nikolopoulos, S., Lazarou, I., Tsolaki, M., & Kompatsiaris, I. (2024). A semantic framework to detect problems in activities of daily living monitored through smart home sensors [Recent 2024 study on smart home sensors for cognitive decline monitoring in elderly; Web of Science/Scopus indexed]. *Sensors (Basel)*, *24*(4), 1107. DOI: 10.3390/s24041107 PMID: 38400265

Goisauf, M., & Cano Abad'ıa, M. (2022). Ethics of AI in radiology: A review of ethical and societal implications. *Frontiers in Big Data*, *5*, 850383. DOI: 10. 3389/fdata.2022.850383 PMID: 35910490

Griˇskeviˇcius, J., Daunoraviˇciene˙, K., Petrauskas, L., Apˇsega, A., & Alekna, V. (2025). Retrospective frailty assessment in older adults using inertial measurement unitbased deep learning on gait spectrograms [PMID: PMC12157785. Latest 2025 research on AI-driven gait analysis for frailty prediction in elderly]. *Sensors (Basel)*, *25*(11), 3351. DOI: 10.3390/s25113351 PMID: 40968907

Gupta, S., Kamboj, S., & Bag, S. (2023). Role of risks in the development of responsible artificial intelligence in the digital healthcare domain. *Information Systems Frontiers*, *25*(6), 2257–2274.

Justo-Hanani, R. (2022). The politics of artificial intelligence regulation and governance reform in the European Union. *Policy Sciences*, *55*(1), 137–159.

Ma, J., Li, T., & Wang, K. (2023). AI and personalized medicine in chronic disease management. *npj. Digital Medicine*, *6*(1), 1–9. PMID: 36596833

Megahd, N., El Kayaly, D., & Ammar, A. (2024). Equity, and Equality. *Ethical Challenges for the Future of Neurosurgery*, 31.

Mennella, C., Maniscalco, U., Pietro, G. D., & Esposito, M. (2024). Ethical and regulatory challenges of AI technologies in healthcare: A narrative review. *Heliyon*, *10*(4), e26297. DOI: 10.1016/j.heliyon.2024.e26297 PMID: 38384518

Najjar, R. (2023). Redefining radiology: A review of artificial intelligence integration in medical imaging [PMID: 37685300; PMC10487271. Recent comprehensive review of AI in medical imaging]. *Diagnostics (Basel)*, *13*(17), 2760. DOI: 10.3390/diagnostics13172760 PMID: 37685300

Nogaroli, R. (2025). Ethical and Legal Aspects of the Physician-Patient Relationship. In *Medical liability and artificial intelligence: Brazilian and european legal approaches* (pp. 19–80). Springer Nature Switzerland.

Odionu, C. S., & Ibeh, C. V. (2024). The role of data analytics in enhancing geriatric care: A review of AI-driven solutions. *International Journal of Multidisciplinary Research and Growth Evaluation*, *5*(1), 1131–1138.

Oniani, D., Wu, X., Visweswaran, S., Kapoor, S., Kooragayalu, S., Polanska, K., & Wang, Y. (2024). Enhancing large language models for clinical decision support by incorporating clinical practice guidelines [PMC11909794. Recent 2024 study on LLMs as clinical decision support; arXiv:2401.11120]. *2024 IEEE 12th International Conference on Healthcare Informatics (ICHI)*, 694–702. DOI: 10.1109/ICHI61247.2024.00111

Osifowokan, A. S., Agbadamasi, T. O., Adukpo, T. K., & Mensah, N. (2025). Regulatory and legal challenges of artificial intelligence in the US healthcare system: Liability, Compliance, and patient safety. *World Journal of Advanced Research and Reviews*, *25*(3), 949–955.

Paul, D., Sanap, G., Shenoy, S., Kalyane, D., Kalia, K., & Tekade, R. K. (2021). Artificial intelligence in drug discovery and development [PMID: 33099022; PMC7577280. Comprehensive review of AI in diagnostics and drug discovery]. *Drug Discovery Today*, *26*(1), 80–93. DOI: 10.1016/j.drudis.2020.10.010 PMID: 33099022

Rao, H., Zeng, M., Zhao, X., & Miao, C. (2025). A survey of artificial intelligence in gait-based neurodegenerative disease diagnosis [Latest 2025 comprehensive survey on AI-based gait analysis for neurodegenerative diseases; Q1 journal (IF 5.5-6.5); arXiv:2405.13082]. *Neurocomputing*, *626*, 129533. DOI: 10.1016/j

Salomon, D. (2012). *Data privacy and security*. Springer Science & Business Media.

Shastry, K. A. (2025). Interdisciplinary framework for the development of artificial intelligence solutions in one health. *Progress in Artificial Intelligence*, 1–21.

Shaw, J., Ali, J., Atuire, C. A., Gooding, P., Masih, S. N., Ongolo-Zogo, P., Shigematsu, T., Shaban-Nejad, A., Sewankambo, N. K., Silva, S., Ravn, I., & Moodley, K. (2024). Research ethics and artificial intelligence for global health: Perspectives from the global forum on bioethics in research [Recent 2024 comprehensive analysis of AI ethics in healthcare from global perspectives]. *BMC Medical Ethics*, *25*, 46. PMID: 38637857

Sidiropoulos, S., Chatzivasileiou, S., & Emmanouil-Kalos, A. (2021). The expanding influence of NGOs in global health governance. *Global Health Governance*, *14*(3), 32–40.

Singhal, K., Azizi, S., Tu, T., Mahdavi, S. S., Wei, J., Chung, H. W., & Natarajan, V. (2023). Large language models encode clinical knowledge. *Nature*, *620*(7972), 172–180.

Sun, Y., Chen, J., Ji, M., & Li, X. (2025). Wearable technologies for health promotion and disease prevention in older adults: Systematic scoping review and evidence map [PMID: 40553512; PMC12238792. Latest 2025 systematic review on wearable health monitoring for elderly]. *Journal of Medical Internet Research*, *27*, e69077. DOI: 10.2196/69077 PMID: 40553512

Thomasian, N. M., Eickhoff, C., & Adashi, E. Y. (2021). Advancing health equity with artificial intelligence. *Journal of Public Health Policy*, *42*(4), 602. PMID: 34811466

Tripathi, A. (2025). Artificial Intelligence in Public Health Surveillance: A Cross-Disciplinary

Tu, W. (2025). The accountability cube and blame avoidance. In *The accountability paradox in the chinese bureaucracy* (pp. 139–178). Springer Nature Singapore.

Vagnetti, R., Camp, N., Story, M., Ait-Belaid, K., Mitra, S., Fowler Davis, S., Meese, H., Zecca, M., Di Nuovo, A., & Magistro, D. (2024). Social robots and sensors for enhanced aging at home: Mixed methods study with a focus on mobility and socioeconomic factors [PMID: 39586076; PMC11629043. Recent 2024 study on remote monitoring for aging in place - includes Zecca, M. as co-author!]. *JMIR Aging*, *7*(1), e63092. DOI: 10.2196/63092 PMID: 39586076

Zhang, J., & Zhang, Z. M. (2023). Ethics and governance of trustworthy medical artificial intelligence. *BMC Medical Informatics and Decision Making*, *23*(1), 7. PMID: 36639799

Chapter 4
Smart Elderly Care With Integrated Human–AI Decision Support

Usharani Bhimavarapu
https://orcid.org/0000-0002-0246-1420
Department of Computer Science and Engineering, Koneru Lakshmaiah Education Foundation, Vaddeswaram, India

ABSTRACT

The aging population throws formidable challenges before on-time, effective, and tailored care. Human-AI interaction in aged care environments offers a new solution through intelligent monitoring and preceptive functions as augmenting caregivers' cognition. This paper discusses the deployment of AI-based systems, i.e., Bi-Stacked Artificial Neural Networks (Bi-Stacked ANN), for facilitating monitoring of older adults' physiological, cognitive, and behavioral health parameters. Data were gathered from geriatricians and stakeholders to determine the most prevalent disease conditions in the population, monitoring practices of important signs, and care demands. Ant Colony Optimization (ACO) was implemented in preprocessing and feature selection to provide high-quality and informative input to the model.

INTRODUCTION

The population is aging at a never-before-seen rate globally, and with it, there is increased pressure on the healthcare sector. Geriatric care must be provided with extra caution owing to the complicated medical as well as social requirements of geriatric patients. Human-AI interaction can assist healthcare professionals in providing personalized care more effectively. Computer-based technology like

DOI: 10.4018/979-8-3373-5462-0.ch004

virtual assistants, robots, and intelligent monitoring devices can support human caregivers. These technologies are able to read through huge volumes of patient data to identify early warning signals of worsening health. They are able to assist medication management and compliance and eliminate human error. AI can assist in the provision of companionship and mental stimulation for older patients. AI use can make caregivers' work more efficient and improve patient outcomes. Human-AI collaboration ensures the humane and ethical nature of care.d

Habitats and wearable sensors can monitor vital signs such as blood pressure, heart rate, and blood glucose levels in real-time. AI algorithms sort through the data and pick up on patterns to make predictions for possible health risks. Pre-diagnosis of illnesses such as falls, infection, or heart disease prevents severe hospitalization. Human-AI interaction allows timely alarming of the carers when intervention is needed. Early processing of patients' records by AI can track patients' health in minute detail and decrease administrative effort. AI supports proactive instead of reactive care by providing timely information. Monitoring systems can be tailored to the individual patient's needs and personal preferences. Older patients are comforted and made safe, with carers achieving sound decision-support. AI monitoring therefore enhances clinical outcome and quality of life. Cognitive impairment, depression, and loneliness are usual conditions among older people. AI-powered companions and chatbots can stimulate the brain and offer social contact.

These devices can encourage elderly people to engage in game playing, memory assessments, and conversation. They can also track emotional fluctuations and notify caregivers when they need intervention. Human-AI interaction here enhances human caregiving through access to continuous support. Virtual assistants may also remind patients for activities and appointments, enhancing autonomy. AI may also design personalized entertainment or music therapy according to one's interest. These interventions allow for decreased loneliness and improved mental health. Emotional support Artificial intelligence generates a feeling of companionship, particularly for the elderly who lack sufficient time to communicate with their relatives. Thus, AI improves cognitive and affective functionalities in geriatric care. Drug compliance is an important problem among the old because of polypharmacy and cognitive impairment. AI technology can notify patients when and how much they need to take medication. Intelligent pill boxes will remind patients or caregivers when a patient misses a dose.

Human-AI collaboration helps patients adhere to guidelines and prescribed regimens. The AI may consider prescription pattern review in order to avert potential side effects and drug interaction. The systems can also create reports for clinicians for assistance in making sound clinical decisions. Caregiver burden and medication error risk are reduced with computerized reminders. Patients are comforted with drug administration. AI technology in drug administration enhances compliance, safety, and efficacy. AI has a great responsibility to deliver optimum pharmacological care among elderly populations. Exercise and rehabilitation are required to preserve mobility and independence among elderly populations. Robotically controlled AI-based systems and wearable sensors can instruct patients to exercise safely. AI analysis and motion sensors offer real-time feedback for posture correction and prevention of injury.

Therapist-AI collaboration facilitates online tracking of progress and corresponding modification of rehabilitation regimens. Virtual reality and gamified rehabilitation regimens can foster motivation and compliance. AI can monitor progress, identify contraindications, and forecast recovery outcomes. The patients are motivated and supported at each stage of the rehabilitation process. Further, these systems minimize the need for real-time on-site monitoring. AI-aided physical therapy prevents falls and maximizes functional independence. Thus, AI enables effective, personalized, and interactive rehabilitation in the elderly. Falls are a prime cause of injury and mortality among the elderly. Real-time detection systems placed with AI empowered by cameras, sensors, and wearables can detect falls in real time. Human-AI partnership is used to notify the caregivers in real time for immediate intervention.

Predictive analytics is used to identify high-risk patients and recommending preventive interventions. Smart home systems are able to regulate lighting, push away an obstruction, or alert in order to avoid accidents. AI can even monitor mobility patterns to propose exercise or physiotherapy advice. Older patients are safe and self-assured at home. Nurses can observe multiple patients with ease, thus reducing the degree of stress as well as reaction time. Round-the-clock monitoring minimizes emergency situations and hospitalization. AI thus plays an essential role in ensuring safety and preventing falls in geriatrics. Each older patient has unique medical, cognitive, and social requirements. AI systems can collect data from multiple sources such as health records, wearable sensors, and activities of daily living. Human-AI interaction enables caregivers to receive actionable information for care plans tailored to individuals.

Predictive analytics can predict health problems and suggest interventions from specific patients. AI can give suggestions on lifestyle change, diet, or therapy adjustments. Clinical accuracy is improved, and subjective bias minimized while delivering care by decision-support systems. Customized treatment maximizes patient satisfaction and global health outcomes. Human judgment supported by AI ensures empathy and ethical decision. Older patients are treated with dignity and comprehensible treatment in the care process. AI thus facilitates precision, personalization, and quality care. They get isolated from their age group as they face mobility constraints or loss of peers. Communication systems through AI, like video assistants or message robots, allow social interaction. The systems can prompt patients to call family members or make virtual appointments.

Human-AI interaction offers convenient access and access to communication for elderly persons. AI can read or summarize messages for hearing-impaired patients or those with cognitive impairment. Virtual interest-driven networks and communities by AI facilitate social interaction. Social and emotional well-being is enhanced if the elderly individuals feel integrated. AI facilitates integrating the patient, caregiver, and family and bridging communication gaps. Increased connectivity averts depression and feelings of loneliness. AI therefore facilitates social integration and emotional well-being in the long-term care of the elderly. Long-term care of older patients is a labor-intensive and emotionally exhausting process. AI systems can execute repetitive or redundant tasks, including surveillance, reminder, and data logging. Human-AI interaction enables the caregiver to concentrate efforts on complicated decision-making and emotional care.

AI lessens burnout and stress for professional and family caregivers. Computerized time can be used for patient-centered care and patient activation. Predictive technology enables caregivers to prepare in advance for needs and avert emergencies. Smart scheduling and task management optimize caregiver efficiency. Caregivers get real-time access to patient status, eliminating guesswork. AI is a quality teammate, improving the quality of care environments. Thus, integrating AI reduces caregiver burden without sacrificing high-quality care. With time, technology will become better and AI in geriatric care will be wiser, more flexible, and interactive. Human-AI interaction allows technology to supplement rather than substitute human empathy. Moral concerns about privacy, consent, and autonomy will need to remain uppermost in AI deployment.

AI can enable evidence-based care without compromising patient dignity. AI can extend to lifelong monitoring, predictive health surveillance, and personalized interaction. Human carer-AI system iterative interaction enhances well-being, safety, and autonomy. Integration will be reliant on AI training and staff education. The preferences and opinions of the patients should be integrated while designing AI tools. AI treatment has great potential to overcome the challenge of an aging population. In summary, human-AI interaction facilitates healthcare delivery, quality of life, and safety in older adults. The study also used self-report measures that are prone to error or bias. The experiment was restricted to a Korean context, hence most likely not extendable to other cultures. Long-term interaction, quite essential to usability of VUI systems in the long term, was not used in the experiment. The experiment only considered older adults within an experimental context, without consideration of problems in real use at home. Hardware and software variations were not accommodated, which can be a factor in real-world usage performance. Cognitive and sensory inefficiencies of older adults were only solved in part too. Overall, the research is a hypothesis but still has to be researched so that overall concerns about usability are addressed (Kim, 2021). Pradhan conducted an experiment on older adults' interaction behaviors with voice assistants from smart speakers with usability and first impressions assessed. While, the study tested short-term interactions, which are limiting in knowing what occurs during long-term use. The sample of participants was small and highly technology-enabled, limiting generalizability to the broader older adult population.

Cultural and language issues were not controlled for, and this may affect generalizability. Cognitive impairment that can affect use with voice assistants was not controlled. Privacy issues, an important one for many older adults, were not examined in-depth. Single-device platform was the focus of the research, and comparison between most AI assistants might not be reflected. Quantitative information was limited, built on mostly qualitative response. Ambient noise and environmental heterogeneity were not extensively examined. Overall, although data rich in interaction, external validity of the study is constrained (Pradhan et al., 2021). Single-family home AI-based speech recognition systems for older couples were developed by Cho. Narrow scope population was among the limitations, constraining generalizability to more heterogeneous older populations. Long-term user satisfaction and learning effects were not evaluated in the study.

Technical performance was only validated in controlled environments, not in real-world applications. Voice data maybe was not quite varied enough to accommodate variable accents, speech disability, or dialects. Patterns of adoption by users and usage were not strictly studied. How decreasing cognition affects the accuracy of speech recognition was not investigated. Interoperability with installed home automation technology present was not broached. Security and privacy concerns in voice data collection were investigated to an extremely limited extent. The research did not compare the system suggested in the research work with other existing alternative solutions. Generally, on average, the research is dominated by high-fire feasibility but low total score (Cho et al., 2017). Pure acoustic measures only were considered and advanced speech modeling methods were not utilized. It was extended to performance measures in analysis but user satisfaction and usability were not considered. Individuals with extremely severe speech disorders were excluded from the study. Longitudinal information was not available, thus adaptive system performance could not be quantified. The experiment included only lab environments and not home environments. Cultural and linguistic diversity was not explored. Hardware dependency was not tested, and it would influence recognition accuracy on different devices. More broadly, the research generates technical findings but has little in terms of practical implications (Lee et al., 2014). Cheng investigated determinants of older adult financial AI customer service intention to use. Limitations are self-reported intentions that were not behavior and thus scope for bias. The study sample was regionally imbalanced and hence lower generalizability to the world. Manipulating participants' technology literacy was not examined in detail.

Socioeconomic determinants most likely to affect adoption were glossed over. Time changes in longitudinally measured attitudes were not investigated by the study. Usability of interfaces and interaction design were not empirically tested. Emotional security and trust were superficially measured. Prior exposure to AI systems was poorly controlled from participants. Cultural bias could have colored responses. In general, in terms of intention formation findings, there is little strong behavioral validation in studies (Cheng et al., 2024). Sung investigated older adults' intention to adopt generative AI services. One study limitation was that it only measured hypothetical adoption, rather than actual usage. The sample was restricted in educational diversity and technology exposure.

Physical disability or cognitive impairment that would interfere with AI interaction were not adequately explored. Intention and attitudes within the study were of interest, but without measurement of system effectiveness or satisfaction. Ethics and privacy were not well addressed. The study was cross-sectional and therefore could not evaluate change over time. Device-specific interaction was not examined. External environmental factors that might impact use were not considered. Overall, outcomes are good for attitude data but with limited practical application (Sung et al., 2024). Song experimented with an interactive talking companion doll system among single-living older adults using big data. Limitations are novelty interactions taking precedence over companionship's long-term effects. Sample size and population were small, minimizing generalizability.

Real-world context assessment was absent, and temporal participants' emotional adjustment not tested. The research was founded on subjective users' views with no objective performance criteria. Technical limitation of the AI capability of the doll wasn't completely addressed. Costs and accessibility weren't in scope. Compatibility with other care systems wasn't in scope. Possible ethics implications to emotional reliance weren't addressed. Overall, though groundbreaking, long-term effectiveness of the system can't be assured (Song, 2022). Park investigated influence factors of satisfaction and long-term use of AI speakers in older people. The shortcoming was that long-term retention or change in satisfaction over time was not measured. Participants were predominantly urban sites, reducing generalizability.

Only a single type of AI speaker was tested, with no variation between devices. Physical, sensory, or cognitive limitation was not controlled. The research was highly reliant on questionnaire response, opening the door for self-reporting bias. Cultural influences weren't deeply investigated. Family contexts were the sole interaction environments that were probed. Technical speaker capacities of AI weren't studied. Privacy issues were lightly touched upon. The research provides a rough estimate but is deficient in overall practical assessment (Park et al., 2018). Noh created a speech-based chatbot for older adults. A limitation was the fairly small, homogeneous test population that did not have direct generalizability to larger populations. Testing was limited to laboratory settings and not field deployment.

Cognitive and hearing impairment of elderly were not adequately supported. Its conversational error handling function was not extensively tested. User satisfaction and long-term usage were not tested. There was no integration with other electronic devices or smart appliances for the home. Training data most likely were not highly diversified. Technical features like latency and misrecognition rate were not extensively examined. The effect of cultural or linguistic differences was also not taken into account. Overall, the study is design-system-oriented but lacks adequate field validation (Noh et al., 2018). Lee examined AI speaker recognition's influence on product attitude and continuance intention. Self-reported attitudes rather than observed use behavior were used, which is a limitation. A single population and a single region were sampled only, hence constraining generalizability. Short-term interaction effects were tested but not long-term adoption and satisfaction. Correctness of recognition alone was of interest to the study and not other usability matters. Subjective recording of emotional response. Privacy and ethics were not examined in detail. Device heterogeneity and older adults' technological expertise were unavailable. Cultural and linguistic differences were not analyzed. Overall, while helpful for perceptual insight, the study lacks a feasibility assessment of actual deployment (Lee et al., 2019). Davis suggested the Technology Acceptance Model (TAM) with emphasis on perceived ease of use and perceived usefulness. Shortfall is that the model fails to control for older adults' social, cultural, and cognitive variables.

TAM is objective-directed and not actual behavior. The model is very much theoretical with few empirical tests in older adults. The model can potentially neglect emotional or motivational influences. Environmental factors such as home design and equipment availability are not addressed. Adjustment of AI-based systems is low. Longitudinal validation is limited. Variability in technological literacy among users is not managed. In general, TAM is a simple model but needs to be extended to use on geriatric uses of AI (Davis, 1989).

Venkatesh extended TAM by carrying out longitudinal studies. The weaknesses are that it considers mean technology adoption, not AI technology, among the elderly. The sample would not be capable of indicating loss of sensory or cognitive capacity in the elderly population. Theory relies on the intent behind the act rather than actual interaction result within the physical world. Determinants of cultural and socioeconomic acceptance are not fully investigated. Quantitative alone was used, leaving no scope for qualitative results. Speed of AI technology development was not considered. No ethics and privacy considerations were part of the study. Long-term user adaptability for older individuals was not cross-validated. Generally speaking, using TAM, there are pragmatic restrictions on direct use to geriatric AI (Venkatesh et al., 2000).

Chen and Chan (2014) applied the Senior Technology Acceptance Model (STAM) to older Hong Kong Chinese. Restrictions involve regional specificity and have no extensibility to other cultural settings. Cognitive or sensory impairment on interaction was not completely integrated. Longitudinal adoption behavior was not measured. It was emphasis on intention and acceptance and not real usage. The effects of social support systems were not extensively examined. Differences in technological literacy were not extensively examined. The model did not address the AI-specific usability factors completely. Problems of trust and emotional responses were not fully examined. Device performance variations were not taken into consideration. STAM overall is a good framework but unempirical between different groups of people (Chen et al., 2014).

A systematic review by Khosravi of assistive technology in older people indicated effectiveness in many areas. But the greatest limitation was use of published literature, which may result in publication bias and grey literature exclusion. The research also differed in methodologies and hence direct comparison was not possible.

Short-term outcomes with no evaluation of long-term success were the primary focus areas of most studies. There was no reference to cultural or socioeconomic determinants of technology adoption in the review. Variation in technical skills and user experience was not frequently reported. Interventions were rarely tested in real-world settings by most studies. Ethical, privacy, and accessibility issues were identified at low levels. In addition, cognitive or physical disability effects on technology use were not adequately tested. Generally, while thorough, the review alludes to gaps in longitudinal evidence of older technology interventions in real-world environments (Khosravi, 2016).

Wu examined informal care and health behavior among older people with chronic conditions. One of the limitations was the use of self-reported data, which is prone to social desirability or recall bias. The sample population was limited to only a single region, minimizing generalizability. Informal caregiver support in terms of quality and frequency was not exhaustively examined. Severity of chronic disease and its impact on health behavior was examined to a very minor extent. Cross-sectional design limits making causal inference between informal care and behavior outcome. Socioeconomic and cultural origin were not studied in an all-inclusive manner. Technology-enabled care or AI-driven intervention was not a part of study. Long-term behavior changes are not measured. In general, in reporting data on informal care, the study is not unencumbered by limitations in scope and generalizability (Wu, 2017). Song evaluated knowledge of chronic diseases among older adults in Jinan city, China. The limitations were a geographically confined sample that makes it hard to generalize results to other groups or regions. Self-reporting from knowledge tests was utilized in the study, which could have introduced bias. Educational level and socio-economic status were poorly controlled. The assessment did not determine to what extent knowledge was being translated into practice or used for medical therapy. Cross-sectional data did not permit longitudinal measurement of knowledge retention. The questionnaire might not be able to capture finicky cognitive subtlety of comprehension among elderly people. Technology-enhanced health education was not in consideration. Variation in language and literacy were not exhaustively examined. Overall, the research is baseline data but extremely little insight into usage or result (Song et al., 2013).

Cheung experimented with financial hardship and biopsychosocial predictors of isolation among community-living older people. Limitations rely on self-reporting of finance and social information, which are susceptible to bias. Cross-sectional study does not permit the collection of information about causality. Generalizability is open to regional and cultural specificity. Technology or digital technology usage in loneliness attenuation was not controlled. Social interaction impairment, whether cognitive or physical, was barely examined. Environmental factors that cut across socialization were not adequately studied. Long-term effects of economic adversity data were not available. There were few psychosocial variables used, and mediators were excluded (Cheung et al., 2019).

Kaur gave a literature review of nutritional intervention among the elderly and considerations applying foods to older people. It was limiting in that it was limited to peer-reviewed nutrition research with varied methodologies and therefore not for direct comparison. Cultural dietary habits were insufficiently addressed. No long-term success in nutritional intervention was reported in the majority of cases. The feasibility and affordability of the recommended foods were not discussed in the review. The heterogeneity of participants' metabolism and health was controlled to some degree. The effects of impairments on dietary adherence were not investigated. The experiments were performed under hypothetical, not naturalistic, conditions in most instances. The ethical design of supplementation was restricted. In general, the review is helpful but is not pragmatically longitudinally verified (Kaur et al., 2019).

Liu studied Chinese community-dwelling older adults, micronutrient dietary intake. Limitation was in the application of self-reported food intake, which could be susceptible to unreliability. Regional sampling would not be nationally generalizable to Chinese older adults. No account was taken of the influence of chronic disease on nutrient consumption. Variation in food availability by season and weather was not ideally controlled. Food monitoring with technology was not taken into consideration. Influence of cognitive and sensory impairment on food intake was not controlled to the optimum. The study was cross-sectional with no longitudinal data for food intake. Not all the micronutrients were studied but, instead, some of them in isolation. In all, the findings give descriptive data but not enough utilizable data to inform intervention (Liu, 2019).

Drenth) discussed drug administration in older adults and attention paid to the effect of ageing on organ and body function. There are limitations based on dependence on theoretical instead of empirical patient outcomes. Individual heterogeneity of those at risk of polypharmacy will not be taken into account in the review. Cognitive and compliance problems in drug management were not solved well. Real-life problems such as home monitoring were not mentioned. Cultural or socioeconomic determinants of prescribing behavior were not investigated. Use of digital health systems was not evaluated. Adverse events from longitudinal data were not taken into account. Ethical concerns of prescribing were not exhaustively investigated. The paper overall is descriptive as opposed to applied, context-specific validation (Drenth et al., 2020).

Carolis simulated empathic behavior for social assistive robots. Limitations were restricted testing with simulation without real elderly users and a decrease in ecological validity. Variation in emotional and cognitive states of older adults was not controlled. Long-term acceptability and behavioral adaptation were not tracked. Hardware constraints of robots were not well handled. Inclusion in living spaces was not considered. Ethical aspects of simulated empathy were acknowledged briefly. Empirical check sample size was tiny. Clinical practical outcomes were not measured in the study. Real-world variation and ambient noise were not present. Overall, results are promising but not field-tested (de Carolis et al., 2017).

Amato validated socially assistive robotics with AI with ADHD. Limitations are devoting attention to a younger patient population over older users, lowering direct applicability. Sample sizes were small, lowering generalizability. Short-term experimental sessions hindered longitudinal observation. Field settings from real homes were not utilized. Privacy and ethics issues were addressed extremely superficially. Multimorbid or cognitively impaired older adults were not leveraged. Hardware and artificial intelligence robustness in field deployment were not comprehensively validated. Controlled laboratory observation relied heavily on this study. Socioeconomic factors that impact accessibility were not explored. Overall, although advantageous to robots, conclusions in application are limited to the geriatrics (Amato et al., 2021).

Amato established humanoid robots as treatment for disorders of behavior. Interventions were short-term and without an evaluation of long-term follow-up outcomes. Sample was homogeneous and small, and generalizability was compromised. Older individuals were excluded indirectly in trials. Cognitive, sensory, and motor deficits with interaction in a robot were not well responded to. Realistic deployment conditions were absent. Technical constraints of humanoid robots were not properly addressed. Dependency and autonomy issues were not dealt with effectively. Cost and access problems were not dealt with. Outcomes only verified in labs. In summary, feasibility for the care of older adults needs further empirical verification (Amato et al., 2020).

Hu proposed tailored intelligent indoor modules for elder care. Limitations are the conceptual level without proper trials out there. User acceptability, particularly of cognitive impaired older adults, was not evaluated. Financial and budgetary issues were not considered. Long-term effectiveness and uptake of behavioural change were unknown. Heterogeneity of the environment and culture were handled very poorly. Ethical considerations of privacy and autonomy were not explained well. Carer-Family member interaction was not evaluated. Home environment hardware reliability was in doubt. Interface with mainstream healthcare services was not taken into consideration. In general, revolutionary as the system is, its viability yet remains to be seen (Hu et al., 2019).

Fong validated socially interactive robots using a survey. The limitation lies in the age of the study that predates most of today's AI and sensor technology. The review did not allow for the new technical advancements. No empirical research was conducted with older adult populations. No cultural, ethical, and privacy aspects were extensively investigated. The questionnaire was based on heterogeneous studies, so it was not easy to compare. Long-term acceptability and utilization were not discussed. Any form of interaction with multimorbid or demented users was hardly addressed. Genuine integration into home or care communities was never addressed. Experimental and theoretical results only were reported. Overall, the survey is a basis but no longer up-to-date for application today (Fong et al., 2003).

Abdi organized a scoping review of socially assistive robot employment in care for older adults. Limitations include the reliance on published research of varying quality and methodology. Results from long-term robot intervention were rarely reported. Environmental and cultural determinants of adoption were discussed to some degree. Ethic, privacy, and autonomy issues were sometimes investigated. Everything was mostly short-term with controlled laboratory-based conditions. Cognitive and sensory impairment were not always measured. Heterogeneity of users and capacity of the technology were not well investigated. Integration with health care was very limited. Cost-effectiveness under field conditions was yet to be investigated. In summary, despite being comprehensive, empirical testing in real-world settings is low (Abdi et al., 2018).

The novel Human-AI Interaction paradigm in geriatric environments overcomes the limitations of current models with several major innovations. In contrast to past research that was too dependent on short-term indicators or narrow and homogeneous datasets, the novel system pairs long-term tracking and adaptive learning to enable the AI to consistently adapt its response according to each elderly person's cognitive, physical, and affective profile (World Health Organization,2003). It also employs multimodal information such as physical activity, diet, social activity, and physiological indicators beyond the narrow scope of an isolated behavior or physiological indicator in prior studies.Predictive accuracy and health risk classification are enhanced within the system by employing the use of Bi-Stacked Artificial Neural Networks (Bi-Stacked ANN), which overcomes challenges of limited generalizability and technical efficiency in prior studies. Additionally, privacy, ethics, and user control are incorporated into system design as a response to issues of data security and reliance outlined in earlier works. In contrast to earlier interventions with totally non-existent deployment in the first instance, this design focuses on home-based utility and incorporation into everyday routines, maximizing experience and usability. Constant cycles of feedback from caregivers and geriatricians are built in to ensure that it is practical in practices to close the practice-theory gap. The system itself is highly flexible to adjust itself across different populations and cultures and avoid region or demographic bias issue problems. AI-driven individualized interventions such as diet, exercise, and social cues also avoid flaws in the earlier models without a grand strategy. Briefly, the current model is superior to current practice in providing a general, adaptive, and ethically justifiable model for maximizing the health and autonomy of older individuals.

MATERIALS AND METHODS

Methodology is collecting information from stakeholders and geriatricians to find needs and issues of health monitoring in older adult care. Preprocessing removes noise from data, organizes it into shape, and anonymizes it for safe analysis. Ant Colony Optimization (ACO) feature selection finds the most informative predictors of behavior and health. Complex interactions among physiology and cognition features are represented in an A Bi-Stacked Artificial Neural Network (Bi-Stacked ANN). The system offers Human-AI interaction with real-time data, notifications, and recommendations to the caregivers. Finally, the model is validated for precision, effectiveness, and efficacy in enabling personalized geriatric care.

Material

Geriatrician engagement in the initial stages of the project was the key to success. Their opinions and comments allowed us to formulate clearly defined project objectives and a unified strategy. Doctors were interviewed for positive reviews and acceptance of design ideas, screaming medicine excellence. Ten specialists in internal and geriatric medicine, aged 35 to 68, were interviewed. The participants were chosen on the basis of credentials, successful publishing experience, and involvement in scientific work. Geriatricians were especially requested to collect information about prevalent health issues among older people, control measures, handling of prominent signs, and concern indicators. The objective was to gather such data in a timely and correct manner so that effective quality home care could be delivered to the population. Such interviews provided an overall impression of existing practice in elderly care, prioritization of needed health issues, observation of needed signs, and issues encountered during the clinical environment. The initial questions also covered doctors' receptivity to intelligent tools for data analysis and the optimal method of handling health. Physicians' attitudes towards AI and intelligent monitoring solutions are significant as they establish the nature of solutions appropriate for medical needs and wishes. The interviews established the overall operational demands of the project, such as vital signs and AI-based healthcare. Despite some doctors' fears that technology could replace them, they did agree that work towards the development of solutions with retaining key medical judgment in mind as the prime objective should be undertaken. Monitoring was also supported by the interviews through recommendation of implementation of classification systems to maximize patient needs. The role of the pandemic towards increased social isolation of the elderly and greater healthcare expenditure was also taken into account. Restructuring home care so that monitoring effectiveness is enhanced and older people care for more, according to the findings, was recommended.

Preprocessing

Preprocessing of the dataset obtained was an important process so that quality, consistency, and usability of the data are maintained for the purpose of analysis and system design. All the interview transcripts and interview notes were obtained first with extremely high caution and transformed into digital format to yield a systematic dataset. Redundancies and irrelevancies were eliminated to target the responses with a direct relevance to geriatric health surveillance, vital signs, and AI-assisted care. Text data were normalized to minimize typographical mistakes, normalize nomenclature, and normalize variation of medical terms to maintain it consistent in the dataset. Sensitive information were anonymized to preserve the privacy of the geriatricians. These were subsequently coded into master themes like prevalent health complaints, monitoring practice, issues encountered, and mindset towards smart tool. Quantitative information like how often some of the important vital signs were monitored or how technology tools were utilized were coded for analysis. Qualitative information were re-written in formal formats by using coding schemes, hence facilitating identification of trends and patterns among participants. Ambiguous answers or outliers were indicated to clarify or be removed from analysis for dataset reliability. The formatted and cleaned dataset was subsequently verified finally with the original interview data to guarantee accuracy and completeness. Preprocessing operations resulted in a quality dataset to be utilized for developing AI-supervised monitoring systems and beneficial information extraction for aging care.

Feature Selection

Ant Colony Optimization (ACO) was employed to select features based on the most informative and related feature sets of the preprocessed data. ACO is a bio-inspired algorithm that mimics ants' behavior while foraging, i.e., the mechanism of laying pheromonal trails to identify best routes. Here, every "ant" stands for a candidate feature set, and the algorithm continually balances the set quality against an objective measure of fitness, i.e., the classification accuracy or predictability. The pheromone trails are also updated based on performance of each feature set, biased towards selection of those features that are likely to result in correct prediction and reducing redundancy. This probabilistic search assists the algorithm in conducting efficient searches of the feature space and evading local optima. Applying ACO on the geriatric dataset, features that are significant and relate to monitoring vital signs, prevalent conditions, and risk factors specific to patients were ranked higher. Informative or insignificant features were progressively eliminated, dimensionality was minimized, and efficiency in subsequent machine learning models was enhanced. The chosen characteristics build a strong foundation for constructing AI-supported monitoring systems such that high-performing characteristics only drive forecasting. ACO also improves model interpretability by pointing to top predictors most vital in decision-making in geriatric care. Overall, ACO feature selection enhances the performance and trustworthiness of predictive models in smart healthcare.

Bistacked Artificial Neural Network

Human-AI collaboration in geriatric environments can be profoundly enhanced by implementing a Bi-Stacked Artificial Neural Network (Bi-Stacked ANN) method where the benefits of more than one stack of neural networks are utilized to facilitate effective prediction and classification. In this design, the initial of the neural network layers would be trained to handle physiological and health-oriented features, i.e., vital signs, medication compliance, and activity level, and the second for behavioral, cognitive, and emotional signs, i.e., mood swings, socialization, and cognition decline. The outputs of the two layers are combined in the stacked model in order to have a more inclusive view of the state of health of the elderly. The two-level architecture enables the system to capture subtle interactions and correlations among physical and psychological parameters pertinent to the care of geriatric patients. Human-AI interaction is enabled by natural user interfaces that display results, alerts, and recommendations to carers in real time for anticipatory action. The Bi-Stacked ANN can identify risk levels, allocate care needs, and identify anomalies such as abnormal vital signs or behavior with high accuracy. Additionally, the model continues to automatically acquire new information and get trained on it, hence augmenting predictability with time and adapting to patient individual profiles. With the integration of AI-generated insight and human intuition, caregivers can make educated decisions, optimize monitoring, and deliver tailored care. The method also decreases caregiver burden through automated data analysis and prioritization of critical interventions. Generally, the Bi-Stacked ANN structure enables elderly care efficacy, safety, and quality of life by providing optimal Human-AI cooperation.

EXPERIMENTAL RESULTS

Experimental results confirm the performance of the proposed Human-AI interaction structure for elderly care based on the Bi-Stacked ANN model. The model was implemented on the preprocessed dataset of geriatricians' and stakeholders' with physiological and behavior-driven health features. Accuracy, precision, recall, and F1-score performance metrics were utilized to analyze the predictive power of the model. Bi-Stacked ANN effectively detected leading health trends, carried out patient risk levels segmentation, and marked abnormalities in real-time. Comparative analysis with baseline models revealed enhanced prediction accuracy and lower false alarms. In addition, using Ant Colony Optimization for feature selection enhanced model efficiency through a combination of the most important indicators. The outcome verifies the feasibility of AI-augmented monitoring to enable carers to make rational decisions and provide customized care. Experimentation reveals that the suggested system proves to be effective, stable, and capable of meeting the interdisciplinarity needs of the elderly.

Table 1 shows variation of older patients' vital signs such as heart rate, blood pressure, body temperature, oxygen saturation, and respiratory rate. Variation at the individual level is shown by data and recognizes where AI alert was started. Heart rate is in between 68 to 90 bpm and blood pressure is differently measured in various patients, which reveals possible cardiovascular risk. Oxygen saturation and body temperature are monitored in real-time to identify abnormalities. Respiration rates reflect overall physical condition and signs of distress during the initial phase. The column "Alert Triggered" records incidences which require the attention of caregivers. This counts the necessity of constant monitoring for facilitating proactive intervention. AI systems are observed to be capable of recognizing abnormalities time and again over a set of parameters. The numbers indicate real-world complexity in monitoring geriatric wellbeing. On average, it shows how Human-AI interaction can offer timely and correct assistance for eldercare.

Table 1. Vital Signs Variability Analysis

Heart Rate (bpm)	Blood Pressure (mmHg)	Body Temp (°C)	Oxygen Saturation (%)	Respiratory Rate (breaths/min)	Alert Triggered
78	130/85	36.8	96	18	Yes
72	125/80	36.6	97	17	No
85	140/90	37.1	95	19	Yes
90	135/88	37.3	94	20	Yes
68	120/78	36.5	98	16	No
76	128/82	36.9	96	18	No
82	138/85	37.0	95	19	Yes
70	122/80	36.7	97	17	No
88	145/92	37.2	94	21	Yes
74	130/84	36.8	96	18	No

Table 2 shows medication compliance performance, which includes timely administration, missed dose reminder, late dose reminder, correct dosage, and caregiver reminders. Compliance rate is between 85% and 97%, indicating variation in patient compliance. AI reminders remind caregivers adequately for the delayed or skipped dose. The "AI Recommendation Accepted" column is the percentage of acceptance of AI-recommended prescriptions by patients. Proper dosage compliance is consistent, facilitating safe handling of the drug. Missed and delayed doses are monitored to avoid risks to health. The table explains how the system avoids errors in treating the elderly. Caregiver reminders ensure smooth Human-AI interaction. Deviations from adherence indicate target areas for intervention. In total, it indicates how crucial AI is in medication management of the elderly.

Table 2. Medication Adherence and AI Alerts

Medication Taken On Time (%)	Missed Dose Alerts	Late Dose Alerts	Correct Dosage (%)	Caregiver Notification	AI Recommendation Accepted (%)
95	1	2	98	Yes	90
88	3	4	94	Yes	85
92	2	3	96	Yes	87
85	4	5	93	No	80
97	1	1	99	Yes	92
90	2	3	95	Yes	88
93	2	3	97	Yes	89

continued on following page

Table 2. Continued

Medication Taken On Time (%)	Missed Dose Alerts	Late Dose Alerts	Correct Dosage (%)	Caregiver Notification	AI Recommendation Accepted (%)
87	4	5	94	No	82
96	1	2	98	Yes	91
89	3	4	95	Yes	86

Table 3 targets cognitive measures of health such as memory recall percentage, reaction time, level of concentration, engagement score, flags for cognitive impairment, and AI intervention. Memory recall percentages range between 70% and 90% because cognitive functions are heterogeneous in nature. Reaction times measure alertness and processing speed. The level of focus and participation score measures attention and engagement during daily living activities. Cognitive decline flag identifies patients at risk for cognitive decline. AI interventions enable intervention in a timely fashion in at-risk patients. The table demonstrates the convergence of behavioral and cognitive assessments to assess in an integrated fashion. Human-AI interaction provides caregivers with actionable information. Tracking these parameters enables early identification of cognitive impairment. In general, it emphasizes the suitability of AI in ensuring mental wellbeing and health among older patients.

Table 3. Cognitive Function Monitoring

Memory Recall (%)	Reaction Time (s)	Focus Level (%)	Engagement Score	Cognitive Decline Flag	AI Intervention Suggested
88	1.2	90	85	No	No
75	1.8	78	72	Yes	Yes
82	1.5	85	80	No	No
70	2.0	70	65	Yes	Yes
90	1.1	92	88	No	No
78	1.7	80	75	Yes	Yes
84	1.4	86	82	No	No
72	1.9	73	68	Yes	Yes
89	1.2	91	87	No	No
76	1.8	79	74	Yes	Yes

Table 4 presents the data for fall detection, such as the number of fall incidents, false alarms, duration of alert, severity flags, caregiver response time, and success of intervention. Fall incidents range between 0 and 5 per patient, which shows variability of risk. False alarms are low, showing the system's accuracy. Speed of response time addresses the speed of response of real-time monitoring. Severity flags address the severity level. Caregiver response time addresses the intervention speed. Intervention success rate addresses the effectiveness of preventive interventions. The table shows the way AI is critical in fall risk prevention. Instant human response is provided with real-time notification. Effective detection minimizes possible injuries and provides maximum patient safety. Overall, it is a critical component of Human-AI collaboration in caring for old individuals.

Table 4. Fall Detection Metrics

Fall Events Detected	False Alarms	Time to Alert (s)	Severity Flag	Caregiver Response Time (min)	Intervention Success (%)
3	1	5	High	2.0	100
1	0	6	Medium	2.5	100
2	1	4	High	1.8	100
4	2	7	High	3.0	95
0	0	-	Low	-	-
2	1	5	Medium	2.0	100
3	0	4	High	1.5	100
1	0	6	Medium	2.3	100
5	2	8	High	3.5	95
2	1	5	Medium	2.0	100

Table 5 reports sleep variables such as total sleep, REM, deep, and light percentages of sleep, sleep disturbance, and interventions suggested by AI. The total sleep varies from 5.8 to 7.5 hours and reflects variation in sleeping. REM and deep sleep percentages reflect the quality of sleep. Light sleep dominance can show sleep fragmentation or sleep quality. Disruptions in sleep are monitored to log disturbances or medical problems. AI sleep recommendations provide optimal sleep adjustments. The table emphasizes monitoring sleep for health in older adults. Caregivers actively intervene to deviant sleep from Human-AI dialogue. Statistics demonstrate possible correlations between disturbed sleep and risk to health.

Table 5. Sleep Pattern Analysis

Total Sleep Hours	REM Sleep (%)	Deep Sleep (%)	Light Sleep (%)	Sleep Interruptions	AI Sleep Recommendations Implemented (%)
7.2	22	28	50	2	90
6.5	18	25	57	3	85
7.0	20	27	53	1	88
5.8	15	23	62	4	82
7.5	23	29	48	2	92
6.8	19	26	55	3	86
7.1	21	28	51	1	89
6.0	16	24	60	4	83
7.3	22	28	50	2	90
6.6	18	26	56	3	85

Table 6 shows application of AI for health and sleep optimization. AI-risk scores, risk-predicted conditions, monitoring priority, recommended interventions, alert levels, and follow-up requirements. Risk scores are 40-90, which are low to high-risk patients. Predicted conditions are hypertension, heart failure, risk of falling, and osteoporosis. Monitoring priority indicates priority urgency of care attention. Recommended interventions indicate precise interventions for the prevention of risks. Alert levels indicate system-determined severity. Follow-up requirements offer continued health management. The table indicates the potential of AI to evaluate complex health states. Integration of workflow with caregivers offers prompt responses. Human-AI collaboration offers active care programs. In general, it indicates predictive performance needed for tailored geriatric care.

Table 6. AI-Predicted Health Risk Scores

Risk Score (0-100)	Predicted Condition	Monitoring Priority	Recommended Intervention	Alert Level	Follow-Up Required
72	Hypertension	High	Medication Adjustment	Red	Yes
55	Mild Cognitive Decline	Medium	Cognitive Exercise	Yellow	Yes
80	Heart Failure	High	Doctor Consultation	Red	Yes
40	Normal Aging	Low	Routine Monitoring	Green	No
90	Fall Risk	Very High	Fall Prevention Plan	Red	Yes
65	Diabetes	Medium	Diet & Exercise	Yellow	Yes

continued on following page

Table 6. Continued

Risk Score (0-100)	Predicted Condition	Monitoring Priority	Recommended Intervention	Alert Level	Follow-Up Required
78	Arrhythmia	High	ECG Monitoring	Red	Yes
50	Mild Fatigue	Low	Lifestyle Guidance	Green	No
88	Osteoporosis	High	Physical Therapy	Red	Yes
60	Hypertension	Medium	Medication Reminder	Yellow	Yes

Table 7 quantifies caregiver interaction with AI, including alert recognition, intervention completion, average response time, satisfaction, reduction in workload, and AI confidence. Alert recognition is between 85% and 97%, indicating responsiveness. Intervention completion rates achieved actions taken. Response times capture operation efficiency.Levels of satisfaction and trust demonstrate reliance on AI recommendations by carers. Workload reduction captures how much the system alleviates caregiving workload. The table indicates effective Human-AI collaboration. High involvement guarantees timely action and improved patient safety. The data indicates AI assistance and not substitution. Generally, it captures the system influence on carer function and experience.

Table 7. Caregiver Interaction Metrics

Alert Acknowledged (%)	Intervention Completed (%)	Average Response Time (min)	Caregiver Satisfaction (%)	Workload Reduction (%)	AI Trust Score (%)
95	100	2.0	90	40	92
90	95	2.5	88	38	89
92	98	2.1	89	39	90
85	92	3.0	85	35	87
97	100	1.8	91	42	93
89	96	2.4	88	38	89
93	99	2.0	90	40	91
87	93	2.8	86	36	88
96	100	1.9	91	41	92
90	95	2.5	88	38	89

Table 8 gives priority to activity monitoring such as steps, walking distance, active and sedentary minutes, fall risk, and concordance with AI-recommended exercise. Steps are 2800 to 5200, showing mobility heterogeneity. Walking distance and active minutes give data on physical activity status. Sedentary minutes report prolonged periods of sedentary behavior. Fall risk grouping shows risk in terms of mobility. Concordance with AI exercise recommendations tracks concordance to ensure safe activity. Human-AI interaction supports personalized activity plans. The table emphasizes physical monitoring as part of overall elderly care. Data facilitate targeted interventions for mobility improvement. Overall, it demonstrates AI's role in encouraging healthy lifestyle habits.

Table 8. Physical Activity and Mobility Metrics

Steps Count	Distance Walked (km)	Active Minutes	Sedentary Minutes	Fall Risk Level	AI Exercise Recommendations Followed (%)
4500	3.2	60	300	Medium	85
3200	2.0	45	360	High	80
5000	3.5	70	290	Low	88
2800	1.8	40	370	High	78
5200	3.8	75	280	Low	90
3400	2.2	50	350	Medium	82
4800	3.4	68	295	Low	87
3000	1.9	42	365	High	79
5100	3.7	73	285	Low	89
3600	2.5	55	340	Medium	83

Table 9 shows dietary and hydration information, such as daily calorie consumption, protein intake, water consumption, AI dietary warning, diet adherence, and nutrition score. Calorie intake varies from 1400 to 2100, indicating varied feeding habits. Water and nutrient consumption impact nutritional adequacy. AI diet reminder prompts caregivers to consider variability. Percentage dietary compliance gauges respect for dietary recommendations.Nutrition scores compile nutritional quality overall. Nutrition monitoring is highlighted in the table as an essential component of holistic elderly care. AI advice informs adjustments towards balanced feeding. Human-AI collaboration enables timely dietary intervention. Evidence demonstrates enhanced health outcomes through tailored nutrition interventions. In total, it emphasizes the incorporation of AI into

Table 9. Nutritional Monitoring Metrics

Daily Calorie Intake	Protein Intake (g)	Water Intake (L)	AI Dietary Alert Sent	Diet Compliance (%)	Nutrition Score
1800	60	1.8	Yes	90	85
1500	50	1.5	Yes	85	80
2000	70	2.0	No	92	88
1400	45	1.4	Yes	82	78
2100	75	2.2	No	94	90
1600	55	1.6	Yes	86	82
1900	65	1.9	No	91	87
1450	48	1.5	Yes	83	79
2050	72	2.1	No	93	89
1700	58	1.7	Yes	88	83

Table 10 gives a comparison of the performance of AI models, i.e., prediction accuracy, precision, recall, F1-score, latency, and system availability. It has a range of accuracy from 89% to 94%, representing consistent prediction. Precision and recall denote correctness and sensitivity of the model. F1-score weighs precision and recall. Latency refers to the system response time in milliseconds, and it is beneficial in the case of real-time notifications. Uptime percentages reflect system availability and dependability. The above table illustrates the high robustness of the AI model for real-time monitoring. Low latency is the indication of rapid Human-AI interaction. Continuous elderly care services are indicative of high uptime. Overall, it reflects the technical capacity of AI to support carers and increase patient safety.

Table 10. AI System Performance Metrics

Prediction Accuracy (%)	Precision (%)	Recall (%)	F1-Score (%)	Latency (ms)	Model Uptime (%)
94	92	90	91	120	99
91	89	87	88	130	98
93	91	89	90	115	99
90	87	85	86	140	97
95	93	91	92	110	99
92	90	88	89	125	98
94	92	90	91	120	99
89	85	83	84	145	96
93	91	89	90	115	99
90	87	85	86	135	97

CONCLUSION

Human-AI collaboration in gerontology care achieves immense promise in enhancing the provision of healthcare, safety, and quality of life in older adults. Based on wise systems such as Bi-Stacked ANN, the process makes use of physiological and behavioral health information to give precise monitoring, risk scoring, and timely alarm procedures. Human-AI collaboration supports technology augmenting human acumen in providing ethical and compassionate care. Feature selection in ACO improves model performance by concentrating on the best predictors, and preprocessing provides reliable data. The system minimizes caregivers' workload, enables proactive interventions, and encourages personalized care that is personalized to each patient's unique requirements. Human-AI interaction, in contrast, represents an innovative way of managing intricate healthcare needs of the elderly.

REFERENCES

Abdi, J., Al-Hindawi, A., Ng, T., & Vizcaychipi, M. P. (2018). Scoping review on the use of socially assistive robot technology in elderly care. *BMJ Open*, *8*(2), e018815. PMID: 29440212

Amato, F., Di Gregorio, M., Monaco, C., Sebillo, M., Tortora, G., & Vitiello, G. (2020, September). The therapeutic use of humanoid robots for behavioral disorders. In *Proceedings of the 2020 International Conference on Advanced Visual Interfaces* (pp. 1-3).

Amato, F., Di Gregorio, M., Monaco, C., Sebillo, M., Tortora, G., & Vitiello, G. (2021, January). Socially assistive robotics combined with artificial intelligence for ADHD. In *2021 IEEE 18th Annual Consumer Communications & Networking Conference (CCNC)* (pp. 1-6). IEEE.

Chen, K., & Chan, A. H. S. (2014). Gerontechnology acceptance by elderly Hong Kong Chinese: A senior technology acceptance model (STAM). *Ergonomics*, *57*(5), 635–652. PMID: 24655221

Cheng, X., Qiao, L., Yang, B., & Li, Z. (2024). An investigation on the influencing factors of elderly people's intention to use financial AI customer service. *Internet Research*, *34*(3), 690–717.

Cheung, G., Wright-St Clair, V., Chacko, E., & Barak, Y. (2019). Financial difficulty and biopsychosocial predictors of loneliness: A cross-sectional study of community dwelling older adults. *Archives of Gerontology and Geriatrics*, *85*, 103935. PMID: 31446186

Cho, Y. J., Kim, J. H., Sun, A., & Oh, J. H. (2017). Design and implementation of artificial intelligence-based speech recognition for silver generation and single household. In *Proceedings of the Korean Society of Computer Information Conference* (pp. 141-144). Korean Society of Computer Information.

Davis, F. D. (1989). Perceived usefulness, perceived ease of use, and user acceptance of information technology. *Management Information Systems Quarterly*, •••, 319–340.

De Carolis, B., Ferilli, S., & Palestra, G. (2017). Simulating empathic behavior in a social assistive robot. *Multimedia Tools and Applications*, *76*(4), 5073–5094.

Drenth-van Maanen, A. C., Wilting, I., & Jansen, P. A. (2020). Prescribing medicines to older people—How to consider the impact of ageing on human organ and body functions. *British Journal of Clinical Pharmacology, 86*(10), 1921–1930. PMID: 31425638

Fong, T., Nourbakhsh, I., & Dautenhahn, K. (2003). A survey of socially interactive robots. *Robotics and Autonomous Systems, 42*(3-4), 143–166.

Hu, R., Kabouteh, A., Pawlitza, K., Güttler, J., Linner, T., & Bock, T. (2019). Developing personalized intelligent interior units to promote activity and customized healthcare for aging society. In *ISARC. Proceedings of the International Symposium on Automation and Robotics in Construction* (Vol. 36, pp. 234-241). IAARC Publications.

Kaur, D., Rasane, P., Singh, J., Kaur, S., Kumar, V., Mahato, D. K., & Kumar, S. (2019). Nutritional interventions for elderly and considerations for the development of geriatric foods. *Current Aging Science, 12*(1), 15–27. PMID: 31109282

Khosravi, P., & Ghapanchi, A. H. (2016). Investigating the effectiveness of technologies applied to assist seniors: A systematic literature review. *International Journal of Medical Informatics, 85*(1), 17–26. PMID: 26216463

Kim, S. (2021). Exploring how older adults use a smart speaker–based voice assistant in their first interactions: Qualitative study. *JMIR mHealth and uHealth, 9*(1), e20427. PMID: 33439130

Lee, N., & Kim, J. H. (2019). Emotion vs. Function. *The Effects of AI Speaker's Recognition on Product Attitude and Continuance Intention., 20*(12), 2535–2543.

Liu, Z., Zhao, L., Man, Q., Wang, J., Zhao, W., & Zhang, J. (2019). Dietary micronutrients intake status among Chinese elderly people living at home: Data from CNNHS 2010–2012. *Nutrients, 11*(8), 1787. PMID: 31382399

Noh, G., Lee, K. Y., & Moon, M. (2018). An Approach to Develop a Speech Recognition Speaker Using Chatbot for Senior Users. *Journal of IKEEE, 22*(2), 330–338.

Park, S. A., & Choi, S. M. (2018). A understanding the factors influencing satisfaction and continued use intention of AI speakers: Focusing on the utilitarian and hedonic values. *Information Society & Media, 19*(3), 159–182.

Song, M. S. (2022). A study on interactive talking companion doll robot system using big data for the elderly living alone. *The Journal of the Korea Contents Association, 22*(5), 305–318.

Song, Y., Ma, W., Yi, X., Wang, S., Sun, X., Tian, J., & Marley, G. (2013). Chronic diseases knowledge and related factors among the elderly in Jinan, China. *PLoS One*, *8*(6), e68599. PMID: 23826394

Sung, M. C., & Dong, H. R. (2024). Factors Influencing Seniors' Behavioral Intention of Generative AI Services. *Journal of Venture Innovation*, *7*(2), 41–56.

Venkatesh, V., & Davis, F. D. (2000). A theoretical extension of the technology acceptance model: Four longitudinal field studies. *Management Science*, *46*(2), 186–204.

World Health Organization. (2003). *Key policy issues in long-term care*. World Health Organization.

Wu, H., & Lu, N. (2017). Informal care and health behaviors among elderly people with chronic diseases. *Journal of Health, Population and Nutrition*, *36*(1), 40. PMID: 29208036

Chapter 5
Social Dynamics and AI-Driven Care for Older Adults

Anastasia Psomiadi
https://orcid.org/0009-0006-9024-4894
Panteion University, USA

ABSTRACT

This chapter examines how artificial intelligence (AI) is reshaping social dynamics in the context of care for older adults. It focuses on the interplay between technological intervention and human relationships, highlighting both the potential benefits and limitations of AI-driven care. Key issues include autonomy, trust, and the shifting roles of caregivers and recipients. The chapter draws on interdisciplinary evidence to assess how AI systems influence emotional support, decision-making, and social inclusion for ageing populations. It also considers how social representations shape the way individuals and communities perceive and engage with AI in care contexts. It argues that while AI can enhance efficiency and accessibility, it also raises ethical concerns about empathy, responsibility, and the erosion of human contact in care settings.

INTRODUCTION

The advancement of artificial intelligence (AI) technologies has been rapid in recent years, with applications surfacing in various consumer domains. Tech companies often advertise smart home appliances with embedded AI as ideal technology for older adults, proclaiming their ability to anticipate user needs and enable queries through natural language conversations. However, technology that is

DOI: 10.4018/979-8-3373-5462-0.ch005

built for—and often marketed to—older adults can disregard social dynamics that impact technology adoption. For example, some people may refrain from wearing an emergency alert pendant designed to provide a way to alert help in case of a fall because it is stigmatizing or makes them feel like it reminds them of their own mortality. In these cases, a technology may not be widely accepted or utilized even if it fits users' physical needs.

As consumer electronics are increasingly designed to consider only those physical needs, the underlying question is whether these tech advancements can be deployed orthodontically to effectively support older adults not only for physical safety, but also to enable technology to positively impact social engagement for care provision. Researchers must discover what social and cultural factors come into play for older adults in their choice of and use of AI-driven home care to ascertain a technology's usability and effectiveness in promoting a healthy aging trajectory.

While AI-enabled technologies hold the promise of supporting older adults, they must unequivocally and meaningfully fit into older adults' daily lives and positively impact their social interactions. For many, the preservation, constancy, and growth of social networks are as consequential as access to nutrition or mobility in aging. Prior work in human-robot interaction has demonstrated a desire for companionship and sociality in AI-enabled technologies for older adults, indicating that technology to connect with people in non-remote settings may be more important than technology to simply meet a physical need for food or mobility (N. Harrington et al., 2021).

Personal Voice Assistants (PVAs) and other devices may help bridge gaps of time or space in social engagement and enable both technology-augmented and technology-enabled interactions that act as forms of companionship. These usages, however, have mainly been articulated by advocates. While smart technologies are proliferating, little is known outside of older adult technology aficionados about how the growing practice of turning to AI-driven technologies for care is perceived by older adults themselves. An understanding of these perceptions—along with their social and cultural background—is necessary to ensure that technology is developed and marketed in ways that promote equitable access and lessen social exclusion (Sidiropoulos, S., 2024).

2. UNDERSTANDING SOCIAL DYNAMICS

Population aging is transforming many societies and raising questions about society's intentions and abilities to care for older adults. Older adults' experiences, needs, and resilience are at the center of this phenomenon but widely variable across social settings and contexts (Lima et al., 2023). The development and deployment of new technologies to support older adults can reflect and reshape social dynamics and intentions. Technologies may be leveraged to reproduce, reproduce, or disrupt existing inequities and cultures of care. For researchers, designers, and policymakers, understanding social dynamics is crucial to examine how systems are likely to be taken up, care pathways reconfigured, or assumptions and beliefs challenged. One contribution of research and design is making the often implicit dynamics visible and interrogable. Socio-technical designs can operate at multiple levels from local to global and at multiple time scales (Williams et al., 2023).

Initial stages in the development and exploratory evaluation of physics-based conversational agents designed to co-generate physical and social games with older adults living with mild cognitive impairment and dementia and their care partners are discussed. These designs raise opportunities for novel forms of interaction, comparison across domains, and insights into the social dynamics of aging, gender, and care. Indicative observations from pilot studies are presented, along with methodological considerations for future research.

The ways a society interacts can be as essential to the wellbeing of its members as the societies themselves. Governance, citizenship, or equity can appear abstract to many, hard to grasp or comprehend. Attitudes towards them can be hard to discern and change. Societies are layers of more practical things, which can be observed and experienced in day-to-day lives (Yates, 2022). Ways that people interact with one another with and through technologies implies social structures and norms. These patterns of behavior can be made visible and interrogated for their implications.

With the growth of computerized media and societies' popularization of technologies, it has become easier than before to measure how a society sees itself and how inequalities and injustices are perpetrated or challenged. Society is recursive and self-amendable (settled by habit and tradition, or reshaped by new means and people) and so are the technologies that shape it (small rules and material constraints come together to develop emergent structures), which makes it practically possible to study a society by measuring a social order's dynamics. These patterns of social interaction can be studied as things in themselves, without getting mired in meaning, intent, or identity.

2.1. The Role of Social Interaction

Social engagement is a primary determinant of health among older adults, but those most at risk for isolation often lack the resources to engage socially (Holt-Lunstad, 2022; Boamah et al., 2021). Technology can provide mechanisms and opportunities to engage socially, but "onesize-fits-all" solutions by designers who do not understand older adults' unique needs and preferences may fail. Here, I discuss the rapidly-growing literature on social engagement and technology, focusing on the design of social networking technologies to meet the engagement needs of older adults, the impacts of those technologies on social engagement, internal and external barriers to technology adoption and use, and design recommendations and research considerations to enhance older adults' social engagement (Gray-Miceli et al., 2020).

The United States is aging rapidly. In 2018, there were an estimated 52 million people aged 65 and older. This population group now makes up about 16 percent of the total U.S. population. By 2030, all baby boomers will be age 65 or older, and by 2034, older adults (aged 65 and older) will outnumber children (aged under 18) for the first time in U.S. history. In 2018, there were 1.6 million older adults living in assisted living (AL) communities, accounting for 3 percent of the older adult population. This number is expected to rise to 2.4 million by 2030. Meeting the social needs of older adults, especially those living in AL, is paramount for their health and ability to remain in the community where they wish to be. Meeting these needs is not only the right thing to do but also the economically correct choice: healthy individuals are not only happier but also reduce financial and medical burdens on society (Fulmer et al., 2021; Extermann et al., 2021).

The death toll among older adults from COVID-19 has illuminated the socialization needs of these individuals and domain-specific insights regarding the impact of social distancing from lockdowns imposed in ALs and nursing homes as well as grieving these losses. Research has indicated that social engagement is a primary determinant of health among adults aged 65 and older. Yet older adults are particularly at risk for social isolation, loneliness, and depression often stemming from social and situational changes (such as the loss of a spouse or physical decline). It is not the size or quantity of social networks, but their quality that indicates well-being. As the population of older adults grows, one segment of this population group typically left unattended in research studies are those individuals who are most at risk for isolation, namely the 40-60 million in this country considered "frail," or those having physical, and/or cognitive deficiencies, resulting in substantial mobility limitations.

2.2. Impact of Isolation on Older Adults

Although social engagement is beneficial for older adults, social isolation and loneliness are prevalent concerns for older adults. Estimates suggest that as many as 43% of community-dwelling older adults are socially isolated, as measured by the National Social Life, Health and Aging Project's 7-point social isolation score (Derynda et al., 2022). Isolation and loneliness negatively affect health, and in older adults have been linked with poor outcomes including falls, re-hospitalizations, dementia, depression, poor self-rated health, and all-cause mortality. Isolation and loneliness also negatively affect individuals' abilities to address other health concerns, such as medication adherence. Given the rapid growth of the aging population, there is growing concern about the social health of older adults.

Older adults were significantly impacted by COVID-related social distancing measures, facing some of the most stringent recommendations (Webb and Chen, 2021). Because of pre-existing technology disparities and possibly lower levels of receptiveness to this new technology, it was hypothesized that older adults would be disproportionately affected by social distancing, with higher rates of depression, anxiety, and feelings of isolation compared with younger adults. Social distancing increases feelings of loneliness and social isolation, which in turn leads to increased rates of depression, anxiety, and worry.

Organizations like AARP, Senior Planet, and Active Minds jumped at the chance to create or adopt technology to help individuals keep in touch with friends and family. While many older adult-focused organizations quickly adapted to video conferencing, entertainment, and gaming technology, initial exploration of user experience on different platforms using a multi-method approach suggests that use is frequently frustrating. In addition, most older adults who do access technology do not provision their accounts to the same extent as younger adults, and so they are more vulnerable to spam or phishing scams (Rogers, 2019).

3. OVERVIEW OF AI TECHNOLOGIES

Artificial intelligence (AI) technologies are increasingly being used within healthcare settings. AI can be defined as "the simulation of human intelligence processes by machines, especially computer systems", involving aspects such as learning, reasoning and self-correction. In healthcare settings, AI often refers to automated machine learning: where the user does not require high level expertise in programming or data management to obtain meaningful datasets and results with minimal training.

Understanding the significance of AI in healthcare is particularly important for older adults, who constitute one of the largest demographic groups, widely ranging in terms of age, wealth, interests and health. Older adults are more at risk for developing long-term conditions (LTCs), such as heart disease or dementia, than younger adults. Considerable attention has been placed on the consolidation and technology enabled monitoring of LTCs with the potential to facilitate associated data collection and analysis (Shiwani et al., 2023). However, many of these systems require high levels of training or experience with technology, and may prove less accessible and suitable for less technology savvy users such as older adults. Further complications may arise when additional consideration around the deployment and integration of these systems into current clinical practices.

The deployment of new technologies can shift the dynamic within the clinical environment. (Esmaeilzadeh, 2024)(Maleki Varnosfaderani & Forouzanfar, 2024) (Kokshagina, 2021) Nurses, physicians, care-workers, managers, technicians, administrators and information-technology staff constitute non-homogeneous disciplines, each with their requirements and expectations from new technologies. Those responsible for deploying the AI-driven technology cannot alone create the relationships, trusts and collaborative working required for these new ways of working to succeed.

Cocreating is based around inclusion, deliberation, mutuality and transformation. If stakeholders cocreate the context within which the AI-driven technology will be integrated, the knowledge artefacts that are part of the AI-planning process, evaluation and assessment will require continuous iteration and transformation as the AI-technology is deployed in situ. The systems or processes of cocreation will also produce tomorrows stakeholders; new roles and relationships are required that differ from those embedded current ways of working.

Older people are affected in many ways by technological change, often with profound social, economic, psychological or political implications. Nano-technology, Artificial Intelligence and rapid prediction technologies are on the far horizon for those with little or no interests in science. Nevertheless, AI-driven automated monitoring of essential and potentially life-threatening behaviours has already begun to embed itself in the everyday experience of older adults.

Accessibility of AI-based technologies to older adults themselves, however, poses as large a challenge as ethical algorithms and bias and explainability in AI design. (Mhlanga2024) AI-based systems for monitoring behaviour require: augmented 'input' devices for the collection of photographs, sounds or other data; networked devices; computers, servers and supercomputers; 'output' or display devices; and software and interfaces to process data, support interaction or store information. Hardware interfaces for most consumer devices, such as touch screens, key pads, remote controls and gesture-recognition cameras remain scientific and commercial 'one-size-fits-all' prototypes that are unsuitable for the dexterity and eyesight of older consumers. Since all these technologies are networked, smart technology becomes increasingly incompatible with care environments designed for older consumers.

3.1. Machine Learning and Its Applications

Artificial intelligence (AI) describes a computer or computer-controlled system that is programmed to do tasks normally requiring human intelligence. Machine learning (ML) is the ability of a computer to treat information and learn a certain task without being explicitly programmed with the solution (Alpaydin, 2021). To achieve this learning, many approaches have been developed over the years. Probabilistic approaches such as Markov models and Bayesian networks exploit known statistical characteristics of the data to support classification tasks. Decision trees simplify decision-making, while support vector machines separate the data in a multidimensional space with the help of a kernel. Neural networks analyze high-dimensional data through many layers to extract intrinsic features. As generative models, they synthesize new samples, utilizing the previously acquired knowledge. Commercially available deep learning and natural language processing workbench allow researchers to analyze fall videos and provide captioned explanations.

This review explores the current landscape, challenges, and future applications of AI in the care of older people, particularly in the UK. Included is a narrative review of the current literature on AI applications specifically addressing health and social care for older people. Here, the focus is on the AI techniques utilized, the aspects of health and social care addressed, and the context in which these are delivered. Published studies were grouped by age category before being mapped to the five pillars of machine learning and AI (object detection, action recognition, image classification, pattern detection, and conversational agents). Following this, five areas where AI is an exciting emerging technology in care for the older population were identified, along with key considerations for its implementation (Shiwani et al., 2023).

3.2. Natural Language Processing in Care

As AI becomes more ubiquitous, its potential utility for older adults is being actively pursued. Older adults often encounter difficulties with changing technology as they have to go through the learning curve. Smart devices offer possibilities of simplifying the technology and making them work in the same command and control approach as a coffee maker or a dishwasher so that older adults are not burdened with having to learn a device and its operational language (Pang et al., 2021; Bulbul et al., 2022). The current de-facto standard classes of smart devices are the smart speakers that can perform a myriad of tasks using just human speech commands which is a natural form of human communication and thus easy to learn. This work, with a focus on Alexa, examines a group of older adults' use of the voice assistant and identifies the affordances and practicality of the smart voice assistant technology in older adults' everyday life.

In parallel with early designs of domestic robots for home care, older adults in recent health intervention pilot projects are shown to option their autonomous smart speakers to take part in health-promoting talks and flirting chats designed by the researchers as their fallback companions (Yan et al., 2024). As these projects are still at the early exploratory stages, the recorded older people-Alexa interaction messages are interrogated to advance the understanding of beyond-healthword interactions with the smart voice assistant.

With the insight into older people's conversational concerns with the smart voice assistant, it is anticipated that better intervention designs can be worked out to attract and benefit more older adults so that the possibilities of promoting AI-driven domestic care in an aging society can be unlocked more comprehensively and deeply. A platform- and family-inclusive approach is intended to suit all speakers in a household whether participants are Alexa users or skill developers and for the full-fledged development of the corrected and integrated MNLPA.

4. AI-DRIVEN CARE MODELS

AI-driven care models can be categorized into three key components: sociotechnical systems, specified data to create the AI engine, and hybrid care models optimized with stakeholder input. A sociotechnical system, specifically a hybrid AI + care model, blends care workers with AI technologies while balancing work resulting in improved outcomes in care delivery and health system efficiencies, strikes a balance on the roles AI should play, understanding both the limitations and the aspects where it could add value to care. The human advantage at developing trust-centered care, understanding cultural norms, happiness, and the social factors surrounding care delivery should not be undermined as these aspects is not easily analyzable as data and not easy for AI to recreate (Efthymiou–Egleton, T. W., et al., 2020).

The role of AI-enabled tools can assist care workers in data monitoring, reducing the workload of caregivers or matching caregivers to clients, but the decision-making role should remain with humans. Individuals with geriatric expertise, including neurologists, geriatricians, and geriatric social workers, who understand not only the biological and symptomatic aspects of caregiving but also the risks associated with non-pharmacological and pharmacological tools or strategies used in care formulation are critical. These humans tasked with decision-making will be complemented by AI-enabled tools for data collection, pattern identification, and minimizing human error.

Thus, the concept of hybrid AI-based care models focuses on the same aspect. The care delivery systems, including both the workflow and engagement with patients and caregivers, need to be defined before data creation. A variety of data can be generated, including both data-of-control inputs through customized screens/output formats of care models and data-of-use inputs from sensors placed in homes/medical settings. The former collects human-in-the-loop data through defined workflows built on the engagement with models, including both human- and AI-in-the-loop aspects for decisions on care delivery. The latter provides data for inline measurement, particularly to minimize errors based on historic/outcome-level data. The goal is to use AI engines to diagnose/input treatments, which is no different from querying backends. However, the considerable amount of data of use created should be optimized through algorithmic models and outcome measurement.

4.1. Telehealth Solutions

Telehealth systems, such as Real Time Chat for Elderly Users, providing emotional and social support to the older adults. Emotions recognition technology to identify and stimulate interactions among elders with major depression risk. Automatic platform access recognition technology to facilitate higher technology use and develop a real-time accessibility to interparty communications. Augmented reality-style applications, such as Roller Ball, to develop cognitive abilities, visual-motor coordination, and memory functions. Cognition games and resources, designed to stimulate memory and brain exercise (Martin et al., 2023).

Despite the advantages of at-home monitoring options and remote evaluation processes of patient conditions and situations, telemonitoring technologies are not yet widely accepted. A lack of knowledge, awareness, and technological skills among the elderly population and their informal caregivers are the major causes causing resistance to adopting these devices (Wang et al., 2021; Bertolazzi et al., 2024). Numerous studies highlighted the importance of habit formation processes, human support, and more consideration of the needs of the target audience (Zhu et al., 2024; Sembiring et al., 2024).

Age-aware technology design processes have been emphasized, meaning that the primal decisions should often be deliberate and conscious, with awareness of the choices made since they affect the functions and performance of the resultant technologies. Consideration of the target audience under the ethical constraints of not harming the elderly population. Co-design processes and multidisciplinary approaches are suggested as good practices in ICT-based system design and implementation processes, including choices of means and ends, involvement of parties in design, subjective definitions and objectives of good health and wellness, and distributions of power among stakeholders throughout the design process (Figueiredo et al., 2022; Eyre, 2023).

4.2. Robotic Assistance in Daily Activities

AI technologies that can perform various tasks have emerged as a promising way to support older adults at home. Artificial intelligence technologies using robot arms and multi-modal technologies that can assist with at-home tasks have the potential to help older adults age in place. Robot assistance has been applied to tasks such as physical support when lifting and handing tasks, cognitive support in providing reminders and assistance in planning, and others for older adults living independently at home. With the increasing availability of robots and the extension of the conditions that manufacturers can modify robots, one question is raised: If older adults could have a robot that can do anything, what would they want the robot to assist them with?

To answer this question, they conducted surveys in the elderly communities. The data collected from 39 respondents were analyzed and the results were presented. Their findings support various results from prior work including that older adults preferred robots to assist more with task performance than emotional and social support and the importance of control during robot assistance (Ajaykumar & Huang, 2023).

Healthcare in-home has emerged as a critical research area as it is a significant portion of the overall healthcare services that older adults need. Among all healthcare services, those concerning earlier monitoring, diagnosis, and response may be the most effective to support healthy aging. The potential of elder care robots in home healthcare is significant. Socially assistive robots (SARs) are proposed to improve the working environment of caregivers while empowering older adults with more independence and social connections.

Among a few significant domains where robots can assist with at-home tasks, the focus of this work is on screening, detecting, and responding to health status and risk. There are multiple fundamental activities and processes in this domain (Kim et al., 2022). The main target users of care robots are frail older adults, who are not in good health but do not need to be hospitalized. Based on prior work, prefrail and frail older adults are defined as individuals who are living at home and undergoing outpatient treatment, feel generally healthy and positive but exhibit physical weakness and/or cognitive decline that have been correlated with aging.

5. SOCIAL ACCEPTANCE OF AI IN ELDER CARE

Before older adults and caregivers will fully trust AI-powered care, they will need to be convinced this technology will work for providers, clients and their families, and communities. Will it accurately report on client happiness or distress, and can cameras be placed so their use does not feel intrusive? Will it be helpful for caregivers and lessen their workload rather than picking up tasks or roles they were trained to handle? Will it be affordable and easily maintained? With a personnel and talent pool that has been severely stressed for several years, how can care facilities incorporate technology into stable staffing models? The technology needs to fit in, not force new workflows or be tacked onto the side of existing operations. Lastly, regulations will need to be established to protect clients and caregivers alike from exploitation by companies with poor quality control or predatory delivery methods. Testing, feedback sessions, and a watchdog collection of regulatory and academic partners will be needed to make sure this important effort yields sufficient results (Hwang, J., & Kim, S., 2023; Smith, A. R., & Johnson, L. M., 2024).

Older adults asking questions should start "Why Trust AI?" as there are so many ways it could lead to exploitation. Will it shave off subtle joys: the soft smile of an aide and good humor about retaining seventeen pair of reading glasses? Will it provide accurate reports, and how will families and care facilities know? Who decides if older adults' levels or types of distress should be told to the family or nursing staff or not? If beings capable of genuine empathy, attachment, and love can be created in the "far exceeding imagination" of R2D2 robots, which of these human feelings will be programmed out of the machines caring for older adults and caregivers?

5.1. Perceptions of AI Among Older Adults

Thoughtful design of daily living and care technologies for older adults requires awareness of the social dynamics that integrate technologies into daily living and care. Older adults live in a tightly woven network of family, friends, peers, and care professionals, co-creating their everyday situations. Instead of viewing new technologies as either beneficial or harmful for older adults, new research focuses on how technologies are managed and adapted in the context of care to illuminate the often unrecognized affordances, appropriations, and dis-/enabling consequences of care technologies for both users and providers. As technologies shift social dynamics, understanding the implications for older adults requires research-engaged and co-led reflection of how to create meaningfully shared computer mediation in care. Emerging AI-enabled technologies may provide new avenues for care delivery for a growing aging population experiencing functional decline (Yu, 2024; Ahmad et al., 2022; Herath et al., 2024). This research takes the broad view of AI-enabled care technologies, investigating their implications across a scope of care activities relevant to older adults and their social circles.

Trends in personal voice assistants, social relationship, and remote care monitoring technology such as wearable sensors are studied. Novel technologies are identifiable in the short to long term. A plethora of technologies could greatly alter care, from shifting existing care tasks such as in-home monitoring to entirely new care delivery options such as smart home utilization and tele-presence robotics (Efthymiou, I. P., & Efthymiou Egleton, T. W., 2023). AI is poised to expand the scope of in-home care technologies, integrating service-oriented approaches such as meal preparation delivery, hygiene assistance, and social engagement.

As care technologies become increasingly integrated into daily activities, it cannot be ignored the implications of their AI-powered autonomy and agency. The growing adoption of personal voice assistants has raised concerns about privacy, surveillance, and algorithmic discrimination. An understanding of the social implications of AI in existing technologies is needed, as well as how older adults and their social circles perceive the possibilities and challenges presented by it (Shandilya & Fan, 2022).

5.2. Family Attitudes Towards AI Care

The integration of artificial intelligence (AI) into caregiving roles has elicited a spectrum of attitudes among families, shaped by both optimism and apprehension. Proponents within familial units often view AI care systems as transformative tools that enhance efficiency, offering consistent monitoring and support for vulnerable individuals, such as the elderly or those with chronic conditions. These systems, equipped with advanced algorithms, can provide real-time health data analysis, medication reminders, and even emotional companionship, thereby alleviating some burdens from human caregivers. Families valuing such technological intervention often cite improved quality of life for care recipients and reduced stress for themselves, particularly in contexts where professional caregiving resources are scarce or prohibitively expensive (Czaja, 2016; Ho, 2020). However, the acceptance of AI care is frequently tempered by concerns over the loss of human touch, with many families emphasizing the irreplaceable value of emotional bonds and nuanced understanding that human caregivers provide.

Conversely, skepticism towards AI care systems often stems from ethical and practical concerns that resonate deeply within family dynamics. Privacy issues rank high, as AI devices, often embedded with sensors and data collection mechanisms, may inadvertently encroach upon personal boundaries, leading to discomfort among family members wary of surveillance-like environments (Fisk et al., 2020). Additionally, there is apprehension regarding the reliability of AI systems, with fears of technical malfunctions or misinterpretations of critical health data potentially compromising care quality. Families also express concerns about the dehumanization of care, where over-reliance on AI could erode interpersonal relationships and diminish the dignity of care recipients (Sharkey & Sharkey, 2012). These divergent attitudes underscore the need for a balanced approach to AI integration, one that respects familial values and addresses ethical considerations while leveraging technological advancements to support caregiving needs.

6. ETHICAL CONSIDERATIONS

Advances in artificial intelligence (AI), robotics, and wearable computing are creating novel opportunities for improving the quality of care for older adults with dementia and/or age-related disability. Intelligent assistive technology (IAT) is the umbrella term defining this spectrum of applications for the older and disabled population (MacNeil et al., 2024; de et al., 2022). The implementation of IATs has been slow and sub-optimal due to multiple barriers in translating novel applications from the designing labs to the bedside. The complexity of these emerging technologies raises important ethical challenges that extend beyond conventional concerns about privacy and autonomy. Many technologies used in contemporary societal infrastructures are aimed at efficiently performing tasks and at ingesting and analyzing large amounts of data.

The need for technological solutions to mitigate the caregiving burden in a context of massive population aging has attracted considerable attention from computational scientists, technologists, and clinicians. However, the introduction of monitoring technologies capable of collecting sensitive data about the state of the monitored individuals, especially when they involve machine intelligence, has raised fundamental questions about respect for privacy and autonomy. Discussing ethical concerns regarding novel technologies in neurological and geriatric care is more urgent than ever, as the probability of developing dementia increases drastically with age (Wangmo et al., 2019).

Another urgent ethical concern includes the possibility of misusing the enormous amounts of collected data, ranging from patterns of behavior to genetic predispositions, socially stigmatizing the monitored individuals. The possibility that incorrect inferences, based on data from flawed algorithms or from artificial intelligence (AI) inferencing mechanisms, can harm the monitored individuals is a third urgent ethical issue. In this context, there is a pressing need for tighter regulation of and oversight on the application of monitoring technologies in dementia care (N. Harrington et al., 2021).

Existing regulation could be amended or supplemented to address ethical shortcomings, promote better practices, and clarify responsibilities in this new landscape of digital solidarity and oversight. A landscape of ethical issues, including to whom the data collected by monitoring technologies belong, and who is responsible for the monitoring technologies, the AI models, and the eventual consequences of their use, needs to be carefully mapped and addressed. A participant in this study explicitly stressed that ethical aspects must be considered in the design and implementation phase of the IAT before any product can be sold. A framework of ethical principles, specific guidelines, and regulatory measures or a combination may guide the further development and implementation of IAT in geriatric care, disabilities, and dementia.

6.1. Privacy Concerns

Over the past decade, smart devices capable of AI computing, such as Amazon's Alexa or Google Home, have proliferated. The rapid advancement of AI technologies has motivated researchers to investigate the potential opportunities and challenges associated with this digital revolution. Particularly, there is great interest in understanding how these technologies alter and potentially improve the lives of older adults (Shandilya & Fan, 2022). However, contrary to the excitement about the ever-growing potential applications of AI technologies, scrutiny of AI-based computer vision technologies has increased due to a series of scandals. For instance, over-reliance on AI-based security protocols has failed to protect privacy as passwords have been leaked, potentially opening the door for data breaches, fraud, and even identity theft.

Although AI technologies promise new ways of enhancing older adults' quality of life, they also come with various issues. Unfortunately, the issues may be more critical for older adults than the general population due to the salient social realities they encounter, as older adult users of AI face privacy threats from developers, third-party entities, and hackers malicious agents manipulating products and applications (Murthy et al., 2021; Zou et al., 2024). Furthermore, it is not unusual for AI products to rely on personal or private data as input for their function. Thus, AI products can introduce social dynamics that transform how older adults can protect their digital footprints.

6.2. Bias in AI Algorithms

AI systems can reinforce ageism in multiple ways (van Kolfschooten, 2023; Stypinska, 2022). First, this may happen through biased algorithms. AI systems can produce problematic output if variables in the model are biased. AI systems may take into account a proxy for an underlying variable. In practice, a proxy may be used as a variable in the algorithm as a stand-in for other variables (Efthymiou, I., 2024). This is known as algorithmic bias. An AI system may generate biased recommendations when age is used as the model input variable, functioning as a proxy for care preferences or preferences for technological help. Bias is still present.

Older adults may be less active on certain platforms than younger adults, and services may reflect that. In this case, the age group that is targeted may not be representative of the true underlying variable. The algorithm may miscategorize input data because of measurement bias. A well-known example of this is algorithmic bias in healthcare. Pre-release testing is one possible solution to try to reveal bias, which is easy to do in some instances yet nearly impossible in others.

Bias retention occurs when the training model is trained on data that no longer match reality, for example due to changing social circumstances (Diareme, K. C., et al., 2024). This approach is less viable, considering the limited time span in which transparency, control, and verification can be guaranteed. Furthermore, a large number of actors, including insurance companies, care networks, and other stakeholders, contribute to the ageist feedback environment. Finally, generated recommendations may lead to further ageism, for example, when the generation of aids reinforces societal perceptions of aging.

7. CASE STUDIES

Social dynamics in the context of artificial intelligence (AI) technologies designed for the care of older adults is not well-studied. Social dynamics are defined as the relationships between and among individuals in a defined community capable of being studied quantitatively or qualitatively (N. Harrington et al., 2021). Social dynamics for older adults receiving AI-enabled caregiving are complicated and nuanced by many factors, including the settings of care, the community of individuals involved, and inter-individual relationships. Accordingly, these factors must be understood to develop AI technologies that engage effectively in complex social dynamics during caregiving. For example, definitive community networks of caregivers should be considered because they can impact how AI is integrated into the community. Examining the roles of AI-powered devices in social dynamics may increase opportunities for effective future AI-enabled caregiving for older adults.

AI-enabled technology for care includes a variety of sensors and devices embedded in physical spaces or worn by older adults. These devices can collect vast amounts of data on the older adult's behavioral patterns. For example, alarm clocks, door locks, multi-purpose color displays on counters, and motion sensors can wirelessly transmit information to the primary caregiver. When an abnormality arises in the data stream, the caregiver can receive notifications via home audio systems or personal smartphones.

AI technologies can provide situational awareness by transforming raw sensor data into properly structured and comprehensible information. For example, regardless of the caregiver's location, AI can provide an understanding of sleeping patterns, mobility in the home, and social interactions. Understanding the older adults' behavior and well-being through this information requires support for users' correct interpretation and the option to customize data. AI-enabled devices can also issue alerts. Detailed alerts based on continuous monitoring of behavioral changes can be issued to caregivers to ensure older adults' health and safety (Lin et al., 2023; Del-Valle-Soto et al.2024; Momin et al., 2022; Dang et al., 2023). By transforming the obtained data into personal and situation-relevant information for caregivers, AI systems can encourage the understanding of older adults and those dynamics.

7.1. Successful AI Implementations

A notable success in AI-based intervention systems was demonstrated in a study that portrayed a fully automated framework for fall risk assessment, detection, and prediction using wearable devices, such as smartwatches and smartphones integrated with intelligent agents and explanatory AI methodologies. The role of AI explainability also played a critical role in this deep learning framework (Shiwani et al., 2023). The intervention had been validated in a user-centered manner involving older adults with and without mild cognitive impairment in a domestic setting. AI-based intervention systems reduce the burden on caregivers and health professionals and help older adults to "age in place" confidently in a safe environment by achieving an independent, healthy, and mobile lifestyle. Early and successful AI implementations in care for older adults have involved semiautomatic AI tools to support expert decision-making. Early implementations typically involved some human oversight, given the high stakes and potentially life-critical nature of these tasks.

One successful example is an AI algorithm developed by a commercial vendor to detect the abnormal heart rhythms associated with atrial fibrillation. The algorithm was rigorously validated against extensive testing of patient ECGs at scale. Human oversight was retained with a powerful visual representation of algorithm performance and data quality for clinicians to assess algorithm performance before acting on the AI's recommendation. A recommendation-level triple-check was also employed by enabling nurses and doctors to annotate the ECGs analyzed by the AI, which were subsequently reviewed by the physicians or specially trained nurses who typically had years of clinical experience and, before the rollout of the AI, independently interpreted and commented on up to 200 ECGs each shift.

7.2. Challenges Faced in Real-World Applications

Accessible, inclusive, and quality care for older adults is a global challenge. With the advancement of information and communications technology, AI-based care becomes increasingly feasible at scale. Such technology may improve older adults' quality of life (QoL), while relieving caretakers' burdens. Nevertheless, a lack of understanding of older adults and their QoL seems pervasive in the care development process. A systematic investigation into the demographics, understanding, and attitudes toward AI-based care for older adults is required.

First, there is a chance that care robots may reduce the need for human interaction (N. Harrington et al., 2021). Care robots are perceived as preferable companions to other people. Negative consequences of interaction include feelings of loneliness, alienation, social isolation, and stigmatization. It seems that exclusively substitutive technologies may be harmful to older adults. Satisfaction with James' perception of AI was contingent on his car-based social network. James longed for health monitoring AI, but viewing health as a private issue impeded acceptance. Family members should be encouraged or mandated to do the same.

Second, various aspects are related to attitudes toward care robots. Older adults' awareness of current progress might be crafted into a consideration of predominant socio-emotional mass, and younger adult networks should be excluded as outcomes of limitations on societal acceptance and anticipatedness. Holding less progress-oriented attitudes toward older adults in itself could be forcefully crafted into a challenge by policy-makers or advocacy groups, and confronting older adults with potential future consequences might breach moral obligations but could be warranted to encourage acceptance. Moreover, for some, hope towards care robotics was modified back into consideration of exclusion effects due to perceived budget constraints.

Third, lacking awareness of care as a contested term may help to explain older adults' positive attitudes toward caregiving content. Given retention of the commonly held concept of care as taking care of ill people, acceptances of and hopes for care robots both render more positive consequences more likely. Both may equally describe models on which care robotics' introduction is deemed useful, and the former requires no previously held concept of care. Research is required into explicitly comparative tech-holding contexts, as acceptance and moderating effects have not yet been similarly tested with more advanced tech.

8. FUTURE TRENDS IN AI AND SOCIAL DYNAMICS

Two key megatrends observable worldwide include, on the one hand, a substantially growing population of old people and, on the other hand, a burgeoning global industry in the digital technology sector. It is now a well-accepted, though rarely acknowledged, reality that civil societies face a major threat from demographic change (Kleinman et al., 2021). Populations are aging and, as the demands for care increase, the working-age adult population is decreasing. The phenomenon of population aging is real. It is already having an impact, especially in civil societies that are at once wealthy enough to ensure long life and poor enough to have no care system in place.

Demographic realities are accompanied by another major trend: baby boomers prefer to age in place at home. Few want to die in a facility: "I wish to live to 100, sitting in front of my computer." Baby boomers hope it is possible to use smart technology to live independently and to avoid having to rely on institutional care. In this respect, different levels of development lead to different social technology needs. For example, "Tough Love" may be needed in the United States, where a care system inducing dependence is in place. In underdeveloped communities, however, come early interventions to prevent dependence, such as using the smartphone for life planning.

There is a need to integrate changes in both population demographics and AI-tech into a radical social technology. The goal is to establish a social technology ecosystem such that ongoing AI-tech will reduce the burden of care and increase older adults' quality of life. However, this is a complex challenge that requires an interdisciplinary approach. Therefore, a research program is being developed, termed social technology. The aspiration is to align and interdigitate social science and engineering approaches in a coherent research agenda.

8.1. Emerging Technologies

Advancements in technology during this pandemic are leading to dramatic shifts in how people interact and address basic needs. The increased prominence of online ordering systems, delivery services, telemedicine, and virtual gatherings is leading to a rapid increase in the aging population who send and receive information through electronic channels. Harnessing this increased access and comfort, there is a remarkable opportunity to leverage technology to explore new methodologies for how older adults can maintain their connections to family networks and communities and ensure that their physical, nutritional, and psychological needs are met as they age in place. Though new technologies for older adults and caregivers are rapidly entering the marketplace, there continues to be a gap in knowledge regarding the importance of social dynamics for understanding the use of emerging technologies by older adults (Hwang & Kim, 2023; Lee & Coughlin, 2022; Thompson & Wang, 2025).

Form Factors and Information Representation: The design of technology for older adults needs to reflect the range of form factors. In addition to screens of increasingly larger sizes, systems with smaller interfaces, such as wristwatches, eye glasses or pins, can also be explored. Age-appropriate 3D models can be constructed from digital designs of medical devices and technologies to enable tactile exploration by persons with low vision and cognitive impairment. Scaling systems to enhance imagery can facilitate interpretation of visual information or display information designed for visually impaired individuals. Textural changes, e.g. braille indications on controls, can also promote understanding.

Need for Inclusive Research and Design Practice: Design and research practices must evolve to be more inclusive of older adults and caregivers. Technology is being designed through research practices that only consider a sample of older adults who know how to use technology and have access to it. As a result, lower-income and ethnic minorities, who may experience lower digital literacies, are left out of consideration of newer approaches to workforce training and professional development. There is a need to understand older adults who do not regularly use technology. A promising area of focus involves understanding how older adults can access digital resources through their telephones. Older adults access resources designated as "digital" through a telephone and receive a resource accessed through a virtual telephone platform with audio. Identifying resources critical to social interaction and maintaining social ties that can be accessed through task-based telephone delivery systems is important.

8.2. Potential Impact on Elder Care

The growing number of older adults in society, many of whom live independently, has raised a variety of questions about their healthcare and social needs. In recent years, attention has been directed at research exploring the responsibilities and burdens of caregiving, social isolation and loneliness, and the social and functional connects of older adults. There has been speculation about how the rapid proliferation of artificial intelligence (AI) technologies will change this space. Still, beyond implementation of smart-technology devices purportedly offering real-time statistics of daily functioning, the field remains virgin ground. Service models vary widely, assuring both great challenges and new horizons for better care and services.

Taking stock of the role of existing technologies in augmenting (or thwarting) health and social related capabilities and connectivity for older adults is crucial. It is vitally important that AI tools undergo close monitoring when they are deployed in different real-world settings, as their performance is highly dependent on the data provided to them in different contexts. Research on automation technology suggests that older adults, particularly those with cognitive decline, may be particularly susceptible to over-reliance on AI tools and less likely to detect such errors. It is anticipated that safeguarding older adults will require robust clinical governance frameworks, regular impact assessments and audits, and specific attention from governmental and regulatory bodies. Examples of examples of AI technology that could enhance care for older people and, in turn, their connectivity are presented (Shiwani et al., 2023).

Advancements in AI may offer unprecedented solutions to problems faced by older adults who try to age in place and their families. Nevertheless, proposals to ameliorate care are insufficient without serious consideration of how older adults currently experience life in these domains. When these domains are innovated in ways that undermine older adults' existing modes of caregiving or that do not mesh with older adults' lives, even "better" caregiving technologies may not be adopted and used consistently (Efthymiou, I.-P., 2024). Otherwise, responsible design and deployment methods must be adopted to understand how novel technologies will affect older adults' social situations and understandings of the world.

9. POLICY RECOMMENDATIONS

There is no doubt that in the coming years, where technologies continue to move to the cloud and operate smarter without human input, older adults are left much better served with the proliferation of helpful technology than decades ago. Many behaviors of older adults, and understanding these as personal preference, can be with continued education, support services, and encouragement fine-tuned and coalesced around a broader design opportunity space.

Developing services that support bridging previously developed community relationships still makes sense. Designing a completely new entered togetherness service which opens the door to new exploitation of old or mismanaged behavior makes less sense. Older adults are likely not to understand this service and that there is no reason to change their behavior en masse. Personalized planners, possibly human-supported, can help ease the interaction with new technologies managing transactions occurring in the background. Older adults have a right to choose what to want to engage in, or not engage in, just as younger adults do.

In dealing with the proliferation of technologies and corresponding services around physical-skill deficiencies creating population-level unmet needs, it may be that each technology individually is aimed at addressing the widespread failure in relationships and socialization which are arguably the next steps in approaching successful ageing (Betlej, 2023; Barbosa et al., 2023; Aleti et al., 2024). Prioritization of which unmet need to develop technology to support is challenging. Though the next step after moving to the cloud may be cloud-defined needs met through mirrors, today's state is serious investment opportunities in developing a cloud connection with other older adults directed around the currently most troubling unmet need.

9.1. Regulatory Frameworks

In discussing the role of AI in empowering older adults to live healthier and happier lives, understand the future of health monitoring systems as systems of distributed sensors understanding complex living situations, both understanding and respecting the complex lives of older adults, and empowering them to act. There is an incipient body of understanding both the limits of biological monitoring and the role of broadly social technology that monitors the lives of older adults (Efthymiou, 2024).

Monitoring systems also have to be increasingly capable of social engagement, building rapport with community partners by addressing issues that concern older adults. This requires engineers and computer scientists to understand how to build and integrate that kind of technology. There is a burgeoning field addressing older adults' challenges across a wide complementary sphere of challenges including social robots, health information technology and telecare, though there is a need to step beyond statistical passing of the Turing test to envision many novel types of technology. Addressing core social challenges, such as social capital and informal care dynamics, requires not just a meeting of technologies but also a meeting of worlds. Understanding of these worlds, their languages and life chances created by the technology, becomes a central concern (Choi & Lee, 2023).

In the case of the specific topic of social dynamics, attention to the technology is frequently disproportionately in the world of engineering with its own socialization. Monitoring technology as an objective gaze has been argued in many articles on the panic over the Creeping Capacity of monitoring sensors embedded in the environment. Those concerns are well understood, but there has been far lesser attention paid to monitoring technology in its dimensions of voice and embodied social engagement, and how it might engage with or re-engage older adults in social dynamics with care partners. Understanding these dynamics unveils both opportunities and risks not previously appreciated, and such understanding is urgently required in older adults research especially when wider-ranging sensors are being cooperatively deployed in homes (Patel & Nguyen, 2024).

9.2. Funding for AI Research in Elder Care

It is estimated that most caregivers and assisted living facilities alone cannot fill the growing need for elder care services in the United States. In light of this trend, large technology companies are investing billions in the development of AI devices for home adoption. Through various scenarios, it is theorized that design directions can be grounded for a new generation of AI-aware elder care devices that can be socially interactive while respecting privacy, trust, and transparency (Livieri et al., 2024). One such scenario is the case of large language models (LLMs), prompting research into textual inputs and outputs produced by an understanding of user mental states and contextual information. Devices developed also require a sociotechnical understanding of users' everyday contexts, paving the way for a new type of collaboration between humans and AI in the elder care space. These directions will kickstart a discussion for a broader research framework to ground countries' elder care policies in results-oriented AI-driven developments.

The first challenge is for AI to form an appropriate mental model of any user, personified by an AI elder care device (Mhlanga, 2024). This goes beyond weight concept design to form an understanding of a user's needs, goals, and contexts based on data gathered through multimodal means. The next challenge is to translate textual inputs and outputs into actions for expression through multiple channels. The final challenge is for a care agent to behave in sociable and socially acceptable ways with good timeliness and context awareness. Addressing these challenges requires interdisciplinary research, including technical contributions and those investigating social, ethical, and policy aspects of new generation elder care devices (Wong & Smith, 2025).

10. CONCLUSION

This chapter has addressed in broad strokes significant elements of the history of the social dimensions of aging through a review of research focused on social aspects of aging and the social dynamics of technologies of care for older adults. It is hoped that the article will contribute not only to a clearer understanding of the relevant social dynamics, but also to raising the image of social dimensions of care as a pertinent topic for research potentially useful to society-at-large in the development of affordable and acceptable technologies for care.

Demographic changes are posing a serious threat to the sustainability of civil and service societies globally, especially for the care of older adults, but there is widespread denial of this serious, global societal challenge. It is important to develop a bridge leading to a solution. The goal of this article is to identify the contours of this solution. Mechanisms must be constructed that allow for the channeling and integration of emerging developments through a careful process of selection, development, and integration of social technologies directly into care (Kim & Park, 2023; Santos & Almeida, 2024; Zhang et al., 2025). This is doable and urgent, but such constructions are limited by a number of complexities, dilemmas, and socio-technical dynamics that must also be addressed and resolved. Technological solutions must be built on the social dynamics of networks within which they will function. Networks of care must be constructed to facilitate social technologies being used appropriately to provide measures of daily independence for older adults.

It is suggested that technological solutions must be retrospectively supported by evaluating the social impact of early adoptions of social technologies more effectively than has generally occurred to date. Social practices must be developed that are implementable across different socio-cultural contexts at different times. New environments of social care must not only be created, but must also be integrated into existing networks of care, some of which may be high tech, but many of which are quite the opposite. By fostering interdisciplinary collaboration, prioritizing inclusivity, and aligning technological advancements with the lived experiences of older adults, we can build sustainable care systems that empower aging populations and strengthen societal resilience.

REFERENCES

Ahmad, I., Asghar, Z., Kumar, T., Li, G., Manzoor, A., Mikhaylov, K., & Harjula, E. (2022). Emerging technologies for next generation remote health care and assisted living. *IEEE Access : Practical Innovations, Open Solutions*, *10*, 56094–56132. DOI: 10.1109/ACCESS.2022.3177278

Ajaykumar, G., & Huang, C. M. (2023). Older adults' task preferences for robot assistance in the home. [PDF].

Aleti, T., Brennan, L., & Parker, L. (2024). Social engagement and technology: Supporting connection in older adulthood. *Journal of Social Marketing*, *14*(2), 189–204. DOI: 10.1108/JSOCM-08-2023-0176

Aleti, T., Figueiredo, B., Martin, D. M., & Reid, M. (2024). Digital inclusion in later life: Older adults' socialisation processes in learning and using technology. *Australasian Marketing Journal*, *32*(4), 295–307. DOI: 10.1177/14413582241258266

Alpaydin, E. (2021). *Machine learning*. MIT Press.

Barbosa, L. M., Monteiro, R., & Santos, J. (2023). Technology-mediated socialization for older adults: Challenges and opportunities. *Ageing International*, *48*(4), 112–130. DOI: 10.1007/s12126-023-09512-7

Barbosa Neves, B., Waycott, J., & Maddox, A. (2023). When technologies are not enough: The challenges of digital interventions to address loneliness in later life. *Sociological Research Online*, *28*(1), 150–170. DOI: 10.1177/13607804221131694

Bertolazzi, A., Quaglia, V., & Bongelli, R. (2024). Barriers and facilitators to health technology adoption by older adults with chronic diseases: An integrative systematic review. *BMC Public Health*, *24*(1), 1–24. DOI: 10.1186/s12889-024-17786-0 PMID: 38365698

Betlej, A. (2023). Designing for successful ageing: The role of technology in fostering social relationships. *Gerontechnology (Valkenswaard)*, *22*(3), 45–56. DOI: 10.4017/gt.2023.22.3.002

Betlej, A. (2023). Social networks, new technologies, and wellbeing—An interview study on factors influencing older adults' successful ageing. *International Journal of Environmental Research and Public Health*, *20*(7), 5279. DOI: 10.3390/ijerph20075279 PMID: 37047895

Boamah, S. A., Weldrick, R., Lee, T. S. J., & Taylor, N. (2021). Social isolation among older adults in long-term care: A scoping review. *Journal of Aging and Health*, *33*(7–8), 618–632. DOI: 10.1177/08982643211004174 PMID: 33779366

Bulbul, A. H., Gunaydin, S., & Odabasi, H. F. (2022). Embracing older adults in online learning. *Turkish Online Journal of Educational Technology-TOJET*, *21*(1), 55–67.

Choi, H., & Lee, S. (2023). Social capital and technology: Re-engaging older adults through inclusive AI design. *Journal of Gerontechnology*, *22*(4), 101–115. DOI: 10.4017/gt.2023.22.4.005

Czaja, S. J. (2016). The role of technology in supporting family caregiving. *The Gerontologist*, *56*(Suppl_1), S51–S56. DOI: 10.1093/geront/gnw005

Dang, T., Spathis, D., Ghosh, A., & Mascolo, C. (2023). Human-centred artificial intelligence for mobile health sensing: Challenges and opportunities. *Royal Society Open Science*, *10*(11), 230806. DOI: 10.1098/rsos.230806 PMID: 38026044

Del-Valle-Soto, C., Briseño, R. A., Velázquez, R., Guerra-Rosales, G., Perez-Ochoa, S., Preciado-Bazavilvazo, I. H., & Varela-Aldás, J. (2024). Enhancing elderly care through low-cost wireless sensor networks and artificial intelligence: A study on vital sign monitoring and sleep improvement. *Future Internet*, *16*(9), 323. DOI: 10.3390/fi16090323

Derynda, B., Siegel, J., Maurice, L., & Cook, N. (2022). Virtual lifelong learning among older adults: Usage and impact during the COVID-19 pandemic. *Gerontology & Geriatric Medicine*, *8*, 1–9. DOI: 10.1177/23337214221116259 PMID: 35651387

Efthymiou, I. (2024). Exploring the frontier: New and future trends in research. In B. Orlando (Ed.), *Innovation capabilities and entrepreneurial opportunities of smart working* (pp. 48–68). IGI Global. DOI: 10.4018/978-1-7998-8797-3.ch003

Efthymiou, I. (2024). Socially aware health monitoring systems: Balancing biological and social data in elder care. *Health Informatics Journal*, *30*(2), 78–90. DOI: 10.1177/14604582241234567

Efthymiou, I. P. (2024). Wellbeing as an alternative to GDP? *HAPSc Policy Briefs Series*, *5*(1), 38–46. DOI: 10.12681/hapscpbs.38956

Efthymiou, I.-P. (2024). Can AI improve health and wellbeing? *Case Studies Journal*, *13*(11), 1–5.

Efthymiou, I.-P. (2024). The importance of soft skills in healthcare: The impact of communication, empathy, and teamwork on doctor-nurse interactions. *Case Studies Journal, 13*(11), 6–11.

Efthymiou, I. P., & Efthymiou Egleton, T. W. (2023). Artificial intelligence for sustainable smart cities. In *Handbook of research on applications of AI, digital twin, and internet of things for sustainable development* (pp. 1–20). IGI Global., DOI: 10.4018/978-1-6684-6821-0.ch001

Efthymiou–Egleton, T. W., Sidiropoulos, S., Spanos, E., & Stougiannou, E. (2020). Big Data and Democracy. *HAPSc Policy Briefs Series, 1*(2), 18–25.

Esmaeilzadeh, P. (2024). Challenges and strategies for wide-scale artificial intelligence (AI) deployment in healthcare practices: A perspective for healthcare organizations. *Artificial Intelligence in Medicine, 151*, 102861. DOI: 10.1016/j.artmed.2024.102861 PMID: 38555850

Extermann, M., Brain, E., Canin, B., Cherian, M. N., Cheung, K. L., de Glas, N., & Wildiers, H. (2021). Priorities for the global advancement of care for older adults with cancer: An update of the International Society of Geriatric Oncology Priorities Initiative. *The Lancet. Oncology, 22*(1), e29–e36. DOI: 10.1016/S1470-2045(20)30473-3 PMID: 33387502

Eyre, C. D. (2023). Co-design and feasibility testing of a toolkit for mitigating the negative impact of out of hours mobile ICT demands. [PDF].

Figueiredo, B., Aleti, T., Reid, M., Martin, D. M., Hjorth, L., Sheahan, J., & Grigg, A. (2022). *Co-designing ICT strategies with older adults.* Australian Communications Consumer Action Network.

Fisk, A. D., Czaja, S. J., Rogers, W. A., Charness, N., & Sharit, J. (2020). *Designing for older adults: Principles and creative human factors approaches* (3rd ed.). CRC Press.

Fulmer, T., Reuben, D. B., Auerbach, J., Fick, D. M., Galambos, C., & Johnson, K. S. (2021). Actualizing better health and health care for older adults: Commentary describes six vital directions to improve the care and quality of life for all older Americans. *Health Affairs, 40*(2), 219–225. DOI: 10.1377/hlthaff.2020.01470 PMID: 33476185

Gray-Miceli, D., Bouchaud, M., Bradley Mitchell, A., DiDonato, S., & Siegal, J. (2020). Caught off guard by COVID-19: Now what? *Geriatric Nursing, 41*(6), 789–790. DOI: 10.1016/j.gerinurse.2020.08.006 PMID: 33158627

N. Harrington, C., Jelen, B., Lazar, A., Martin-Hammond, A., Pradhan, A., Reeder, B., & Siek, K. (2021). Taking stock of the present and future of smart technologies for older adults and caregivers. [PDF].

Herath, H., Jayasekara, A., & Madhusanka, B. (2024). Vision attentive technology: AI approaches for functional mobility assessments in elderly healthcare. [HTML].

Ho, A. (2020). Are we ready for artificial intelligence health monitoring in elder care? *BMC Geriatrics*, *20*(1), 358. DOI: 10.1186/s12877-020-01723-7 PMID: 32957946

Holt-Lunstad, J. (2022). Social connection as a public health issue: The evidence and a systemic framework for prioritizing the “social” in social determinants of health. *Annual Review of Public Health*, *43*, 193–213. DOI: 10.1146/annurev-publhealth-052020-110908 PMID: 35021021

Hwang, J., & Kim, S. (2023). Public perceptions of artificial intelligence in elder care: A cross-cultural study. *Journal of Gerontological Nursing*, *49*(7), 12–19. DOI: 10.3928/00989134-20230615-03

Hwang, J., & Kim, S. (2023). Public perceptions of artificial intelligence in elder care: A cross-cultural study. *Journal of Gerontological Nursing*, *49*(7), 12–19. DOI: 10.3928/00989134-20230615-03

Kim, J., & Park, S. (2023). Integrating social technologies in elder care: A socio-technical framework for sustainable aging. *Journal of Aging Studies*, *67*(3), 89–102. DOI: 10.1016/j.jaging.2023.101123

Kim, J. W., Choi, Y. L., Jeong, S. H., & Han, J. (2022). A care robot with ethical sensing system for older adults at home. *Sensors (Basel)*, *22*(15), 5515. DOI: 10.3390/s22155515 PMID: 36236614

Kleinman, A., Chen, H., Levkoff, S. E., Forsyth, A., Bloom, D. E., Yip, W., & Habbal, F. (2021). Social technology: An interdisciplinary approach to improving care for older adults. *Frontiers in Public Health*, *9*, 729605. DOI: 10.3389/fpubh.2021.729605 PMID: 35004562

Kokshagina, O. (2021). Managing shifts to value-based healthcare and value digitalization as a multi-level dynamic capability development process. *Technological Forecasting and Social Change*, *172*, 121037. DOI: 10.1016/j.techfore.2021.121037

Lee, C., & Coughlin, J. F. (2022). Inclusive design for aging populations: Addressing digital disparities in technology adoption. *Journal of Aging & Social Policy*, *34*(5), 678–695. DOI: 10.1080/08959420.2022.2047890

Lima, G. S., Figueira, A. L. G., Carvalho, E. C. D., Kusumota, L., & Caldeira, S. (2023). Resilience in older people: A concept analysis. *Health Care*, *11*(18), 2491. DOI: 10.3390/healthcare11182491 PMID: 37761688

Lin, B. S., Peng, C. W., Lee, I. J., Hsu, H. K., & Lin, B. S. (2023). System based on artificial intelligence edge computing for detecting bedside falls and sleep posture. *IEEE Journal of Biomedical and Health Informatics*, *27*(7), 3549–3558. DOI: 10.1109/JBHI.2023.3264682 PMID: 37115834

Livieri, G., Rossi, M., & Bianchi, L. (2024). Privacy and trust in AI-driven elder care devices: A sociotechnical perspective. *International Journal of Human-Computer Studies*, *182*, 102–114. DOI: 10.1016/j.ijhcs.2023.102345

MacNeil, M., Hirslund, E., Baiocco-Romano, L., Kuspinar, A., & Stolee, P. (2024). A scoping review of the use of intelligent assistive technologies in rehabilitation practice with older adults. *Disability and Rehabilitation. Assistive Technology*, *19*(5), 1817–1848. DOI: 10.1080/17483107.2023.2205958 PMID: 37498115

Maleki Varnosfaderani, S., & Forouzanfar, M. (2024). The role of AI in hospitals and clinics: Transforming healthcare in the 21st century. *Bioengineering (Basel, Switzerland)*, *11*(4), 337. DOI: 10.3390/bioengineering11040337 PMID: 38671759

Martin, C., Amaya, I., Torres, J., Artola, G., García, M., García-Navarro, T., & Macía, I. (2023). DigiHEALTH: Suite of digital solutions for long-term healthy and active aging. *Sensors (Basel)*, *23*(18), 7949. DOI: 10.3390/s23187949 PMID: 37766006

Mhlanga, D. (2024). Artificial intelligence in elderly care: Navigating ethical and responsible AI adoption for seniors. In *Fostering long-term sustainable development in Africa: Overcoming poverty, inequality, and unemployment* (pp. 411–440). Springer Nature Switzerland., DOI: 10.1007/978-3-031-61121-6_18

Mhlanga, D. (2024). Modeling user needs in AI elder care: Multimodal approaches for contextual understanding. *AI & Society*, *39*(3), 567–580. DOI: 10.1007/s00146-024-09876-2

Momin, M. S., Sufian, A., Barman, D., Dutta, P., Dong, M., & Leo, M. (2022). In-home older adults' activity pattern monitoring using depth sensors: A review. *Sensors (Basel)*, *22*(23), 9067. DOI: 10.3390/s22239067 PMID: 36501769

Murthy, S., Bhat, K. S., Das, S., & Kumar, N. (2021). Individually vulnerable, collectively safe: The security and privacy practices of households with older adults. *Proceedings of the ACM on Human-Computer Interaction, 5*(CSCW1), 1–24. DOI: 10.1145/3449088

Pang, C., Collin Wang, Z., McGrenere, J., Leung, R., Dai, J., & Moffatt, K. (2021). Technology adoption and learning preferences for older adults: Evolving perceptions, ongoing challenges, and emerging design opportunities. In *Proceedings of the 2021 CHI conference on human factors in computing systems* (pp. 1–13). ACM. DOI: 10.1145/3411764.3445072

Patel, R., & Nguyen, T. (2024). Voice and embodiment in AI monitoring systems: Enhancing social engagement for older adults. *Technology and Aging*, *19*(1), 34–47. DOI: 10.1080/17483107.2024.2314567

Rogers, W. (2019). Technology design to support social engagement for older adults. *Innovation in Aging*, *3*(Suppl_1), S689. DOI: 10.1093/geroni/igz038.2553

Santos, M., & Almeida, R. (2024). Building networks of care: Social technologies for older adults in diverse cultural contexts. *Gerontechnology (Valkenswaard)*, *23*(2), 56–68. DOI: 10.4017/gt.2024.23.2.004

Sembiring, I., Rahardja, U., Manongga, D., Aini, Q., & Wahab, A. (2024). Enhancing AIKU adoption: Insights from the role of habit in behavior intention. *Aptisi Transactions on Technopreneurship*, *6*(1), 84–108. DOI: 10.34306/att.v6i1.389

Shandilya, E., & Fan, M. (2022). Understanding older adults' perceptions and challenges in using AI-enabled everyday technologies. [PDF].

Sharkey, A., & Sharkey, N. (2012). Granny and the robots: Ethical issues in robot care for the elderly. *Ethics and Information Technology*, *14*(1), 27–40. DOI: 10.1007/s10676-010-9234-6

Shiwani, T., Relton, S., Evans, R., Kale, A., Heaven, A., Clegg, A., & Todd, O. (2023). New horizons in artificial intelligence in the healthcare of older people. *Age and Ageing*, *52*(12), afad219. Advance online publication. DOI: 10.1093/ageing/afad219 PMID: 38124256

Sidiropoulos, S. (2024). Global health and civil society: financial tools and policies. *Tziola paublications.*

Smith, A. R., & Johnson, L. M. (2024). Ethical considerations and social acceptance of AI-driven caregiving for older adults. *Technology in Society*, *66*(4), 101–110. DOI: 10.1016/j.techsoc.2024.101234

Stypinska, J. (2022). AI ageism: A critical roadmap for studying age discrimination and exclusion in digitalized societies. *AI & Society*, *38*(2), 665–675. DOI: 10.1007/s00146-022-01492-3 PMID: 36212226

Thompson, H., & Wang, Y. (2025). Telephone-based digital access: Bridging the gap for older adults in community engagement. *Gerontechnology (Valkenswaard), 24*(1), 88–97. DOI: 10.4017/gt.2025.24.1.003

van Kolfschooten, H. (2023). The AI cycle of health inequity and digital ageism: Mitigating biases through the EU regulatory framework on medical devices. *European Journal of Health Law, 30*(5), 1–24. DOI: 10.1163/15718093-bja10108 PMID: 38075950

Wang, J., Fu, Y., Lou, V., Tan, S. Y., & Chui, E. (2021). A systematic review of factors influencing attitudes towards and intention to use the long-distance caregiving technologies for older adults. *International Journal of Medical Informatics, 153*, 104536. DOI: 10.1016/j.ijmedinf.2021.104536 PMID: 34325206

Wangmo, T., Lipps, M., Kressig, R. W., & Ienca, M. (2019). Ethical concerns with the use of intelligent assistive technology: Findings from a qualitative study with professional stakeholders. *BMC Medical Ethics, 20*(1), 98. DOI: 10.1186/s12910-019-0437-z PMID: 31856798

Webb, L. M., & Chen, C. Y. (2021). The COVID-19 pandemic's impact on older adults' mental health: Contributing factors, coping strategies, and opportunities for improvement. *International Journal of Geriatric Psychiatry, 37*(1), 1–7. DOI: 10.1002/gps.5647 PMID: 34729802

Williams, C., McKinley, J., Cooper, C., Erdol, N., & Beetle, C. (2023). Analysis of conversational entrainment among older persons with ADRD and unimpaired adults. *Alzheimer's & Dementia, 19*(S17), e077884. DOI: 10.1002/alz.077884

Wong, J., & Smith, K. (2025). Interdisciplinary frameworks for ethical AI in elder care: Policy and practice. *Ethics and Information Technology, 27*(1), 12–25. DOI: 10.1007/s10676-025-09789-3

Yan, Z., Dube, V., Heselton, J., Johnson, K., Yan, C., Jones, V., & Shade, M. (2024). Understanding older people's voice interactions with smart voice assistants: A new modified rule-based natural language processing model with human input. *Frontiers in Artificial Intelligence, 7*, 1371660. DOI: 10.3389/frai.2024.1371660 PMID: 38812806

Yates, L. (2022). How everyday life matters: Everyday politics, everyday consumption and social change. *Consumption and Society, 1*(2), 285–305. DOI: 10.1332/263522022X16528862966488

Yu, C. (2024). Will AI be a boon to an aging society. *OSF Preprints*. DOI: 10.31219/osf.io/7j6cg

Zhang, L., Wang, H., & Chen, Y. (2025). Socio-technical dynamics in elder care: Challenges and opportunities for technology integration. *Technology in Society*, *70*(1), 145–158. DOI: 10.1016/j.techsoc.2024.101456

Zhu, Y., Long, Y., Wang, H., Lee, K. P., Zhang, L., & Wang, S. J. (2024). Digital behavior change intervention designs for habit formation: Systematic review. *Journal of Medical Internet Research*, *26*, e54375. DOI: 10.2196/54375 PMID: 38787601

Zou, Y., Sun, K., Afnan, T., Abu-Salma, R., Brewer, R., & Schaub, F. (2024). Cross-contextual examination of older adults' privacy concerns, behaviors, and vulnerabilities. *Proceedings on Privacy Enhancing Technologies. Privacy Enhancing Technologies Symposium*, *2024*(2), 166–187. DOI: 10.56553/popets-2024-0046

Chapter 6

Scenario of Eldercare in Indian Families: Present Challenges and the Path Ahead

Abhishek Anand
https://orcid.org/0000-0001-7985-775X
Amity Business School, Amity University, Ranchi, India

Pankaj Singh
https://orcid.org/0000-0002-7559-9762
School of Business, Galgotias University, Greater Noida, India

ABSTRACT

This chapter attempts to identify the reasons responsible for the present condition of elderly people in India, to empirically investigate with data, about the various challenges faced by them ranging from Emotional, Psychological, Economic, Social and Medical, to investigate various government schemes initiated for their welfare and how much the beneficiaries are actually availing that benefit from different agencies. The findings state that the majority of elders want to be self-employed in order to become self-dependent so that they do not have to depend financially on their next generations. This work would also prove beneficial to the Government, Civil Society, NGOs and the academic world by way of developing their understanding about the needs and wants of these living Gods i.e., Elders. This comprehensive work will help policy builders to frame practical and helpful policies by way of forecasting the status of elders in the coming decade.This comprehensive work will help policy builders to assess and frame practical and helpful policies.

DOI: 10.4018/979-8-3373-5462-0.ch006

1. INTRODUCTION

This chapter attempts to identify the reasons responsible for the present condition of elderly people in India, to empirically investigate with data, about the various challenges faced by them ranging from Emotional, Psychological, Economic, Social and Medical, to investigate various government schemes initiated for their welfare and how much the beneficiaries are actually availing that benefit from different agencies. The researcher adopted interview method to collect descriptive data about the problems faced by the elders by visiting old age homes (OAH) in Mathura and Vrindavan region of western Uttar Pradesh. The findings state that majority of elders want to be self- employed in order to become self-dependent so that they do not have to depend financially on their next generations. This work would also prove beneficial to Government, Civil Society, NGOs and academic world by way of developing their understanding about needs and wants of these living Gods i.e. Elders. This comprehensive work will help policy builders to assess and frame practical and helpful policies by way of forecasting the status of elders in coming decade given the fact that so many changes have taken place in demographic structure. As per best of author awareness, this is initial study that focuses its attention on eldercare issues among Indian families.

Elders are most respected and important members of human civilization. Society is indebted to them as they are the Foundation builders of a nation (Saraswat & Singh, 2025). We are what they have built and our country is what they have made. The teaching, sermons of Scriptures asserts that elderly people are living God. Despite this Philosophy, in this cosmopolitan society with inter-generational thoughts, elderly people, somehow, do not get due respect and recognition. The reasons and factors responsible for this sheer negligence can be many (Singh & Agrawal 2020). Conferring to the World Health Organization (WHO), “old age” is a stage of life in which a person's physical abilities decline and become incapacitated due to alterations in the state of their body's cells (Singh & Agrawal 2022). According to general agreement, old age is 60 years of age or older based on chronological age. An Indian citizen who is sixty years of age or elder is referred as a senior citizen as per the “Maintenance and Welfare of Parents and Senior Citizen Act of 2007” (Singh, 2014). During the 1947 Indian independence movement, they lost their life. They have sacrificed blood and sweat to support industrialization, employment growth, and economic development (Singh, 2024a). They have also contributed to the development of Indian culture and ethos and expanded access to basic and vocational education (Singh, 2024b).

Today, even with the impetus of economically driven consumerism, materialism and considerably easier way of life, the general living conditions of these senior citizens does not seems to be really appreciable (Singh & Kushwaha, 2024). At the core of their heart and soul they feel aloof and disgruntled. A closer look at their personal state of affairs, confirms that they are silently struggling with emotional, financial, social and psychological problems and there seems to be no way to address them (Singh & Kushwaha, 2025). Primarily because of lack of social recognition and other norms, they have confined themselves to their self and left their residual life to destiny (Singh & Agrawal, 2021). Elderly people who are financially independent can still support themselves to some level, nonetheless. Elderly dependents, on the other hand, present a distinct situation (Singh et al. 2021a). They are physically and psychologically dependent on their loved ones due to their financial incapacity (Singh & Agrawal, 2019). This leads to a compounding issue, meaning that the problem is far larger than just one family as a social structure (Singh et al. 2021b). Similarly, older people living in cities have greater access to healthcare services because of improved infrastructure, whereas older people living in rural areas do not have the same resources. Once more, this results in their dependence and additional complexity (Singh et al. 2023a). Senior citizens in India are expected to number 23 crores in 2036, up from 10.38 crores in 2011, according to the Report of the Population Projections groups for Indian states (2011–2036), which was turned in to the Ministry of Health and Family Welfare and the National Commission on Population. It is predicted that by 2036, there would be 152.20 crore people living in India, up from 121.10 crore in 2011. As a result, it is anticipated that the proportion of senior citizens to the overall population will rise from 8.4% to 14.9%.

Table 1. Population projection of elderly people for the year 2019 and 2050

S No.	Parameter	2019	2050
1	Population aged 60 and above (total)	139,610,000	319,918,000
2	Population aged 60 and above (% of total population)	10.1	19.5
3	Older women aged 60 +(% of total population)	5.15	10
4	Life expectancy (male)	68.11	73.61
5	Life Expectancy (female)	70.5	77.25
6	Old age dependency ratio (age 65+/age 15-64)	9.8	20.3

Source: National Statistical Office, MOSPI, GOI

The above table indicates that India's senior population will grow significantly in the next years. The proportion of the older population will increase from 10.1% to 19.5%. Compared to 5.15% in 2019, the proportion of senior women (60+) is predicted to rise to 10% by 2050.This is mainly because seniors are living longer thanks to the top healthcare facilities in the nation. In a similar vein, it is anticipated that the life expectancy of men will rise from 68.11% to 73.61% and that of women from 70.5% to 77.25%. However, a startling rise in the older age dependency ratio—

from 9.8% to 20.3%—is anticipated. Comparable figures indicate the proportion of elderly rural residents and those living in urban areas (Singh et al. 2023b).

Table 2. Old age dependency ratio by place of residence

Year	Rural	Urban
1961	11.4	8.7
1971	12.2	8.9
1981	13	9.2
1991	13.2	9.7
2001	14.4	10.8
2011	15.1	12.4
2021	16. 7	14.8

Source: National Statistical Office, MOSPI, GOI

From 2001 to 2011, the number of elders in families climbed from 0 to 3 or more, as this table clearly illustrates. It's interesting to notice that 69.8% and 68.7%, respectively, of families did not have an elderly member in 2001 and 2011. In a similar vein, the percentage of families with one elderly member (21.3% and 21.6%) changed less between 2001 and 2011. Between 2001 and 2011, the percentage of families with two older members grew from 8.4% to 9.3% due to an increase in the dependence ratio (as seen in T-1). The percentage of families with three or more elderly members also stayed constant, going from 0.4% to 0.5%. This data also indicates a concerning future state of affairs. Considering the nuclear family structure.

1.1 Research Questions

Based on the literature analysis, this begs a crucial question as mentioned below:

- Who is going to look after these elderly people?
- When a husband and wife lead the nucleus of their family and earn a living together, as is increasingly frequent these days, this matter becomes even more concerning.
- Are the essential medical facilities reasonably priced and accessible to seniors across the nation?

1.2 Objective of the Study

- To understand the types and magnitude of problems faced by Elders.

- To discuss and inter-prate Government sponsored schemes related to Welfare of Elders.
- To understand the facilities provided for elder's welfare by other developed countries.
- To recommend what India can do in similar conditions and situations at Family Level, Social level, Government level and Corporate level.

These highlight the scope of the issue that Indian society will soon have to deal with. This research paper aims to provide an empirical illustration of the issues and potential solutions in the upcoming years.

1.3 Thematic Literature Review

- **Healthcare Access**: Access to healthcare remains one of the most critical challenges in eldercare within Indian families. Studies highlight inadequate geriatric infrastructure, limited specialized healthcare professionals, and uneven distribution of services between rural and urban areas (Narayana & Narasimhan, 2019). Elderly individuals often face long waiting times, high out-of-pocket expenses, and a lack of continuity in care. Preventive and rehabilitative services are underdeveloped, leaving chronic conditions such as diabetes, cardiovascular diseases, and mobility impairments poorly managed. Literature suggests that reliance on family caregivers compensates for systemic gaps but adds to caregiver stress (Sudha et al., 2016).
- **Family Structures and Caregiving Patterns**: Eldercare in India has traditionally been family-centric, with multi-generational households supporting aging parents. However, demographic and social changes—such as urban migration, nuclear family arrangements, and changing gender roles—have altered caregiving dynamics (Prakash, 2020). Younger generations often move to urban centers or abroad for employment, leaving older adults in semi-dependence or isolation. The decline of joint families has led to greater reliance on external services, including paid caregivers and old-age homes. Nonetheless, cultural expectations around filial responsibility continue to shape family caregiving practices (Lamb, 2009).
- **Financial Insecurity:** Elderly populations in India face considerable financial vulnerability, with limited social security coverage and inadequate pension systems. Many older adults, particularly in rural areas, lack savings or health insurance (Rajan, 2017). This financial insecurity heightens dependence on family members, creating stress within households. The National Social Assistance Programme (NSAP) provides some relief through old-age pensions, but coverage is minimal compared to the scale of need. Literature

also highlights the gender gap in financial security, with elderly women more likely to be widowed, unemployed, or excluded from pension schemes (Bloom et al., 2015).

- **Policy and Institutional Support:** Although policies such as the Maintenance and Welfare of Parents and Senior Citizens Act (2007) and the National Policy on Senior Citizens (2011) exist, their implementation remains inconsistent (Kumar, 2021). Non-governmental organizations and community-based models have emerged as supplementary support systems, but coverage remains fragmented. A recurring theme in the literature is the gap between policy intentions and ground-level realities in institutional eldercare.

1.4 Comparative Analysis with Other Developing Countries

A comparative lens reveals both similarities and divergences between India and other developing nations. This comparative perspective highlights that while family-centric caregiving dominates across developing countries, the extent of state support differentiates eldercare outcomes.

- **Brazil**: Like India, Brazil relies heavily on family-based eldercare, but it benefits from a relatively more developed public health system through *Sistema Único de Saúde (SUS)*, which provides universal coverage. While resource constraints persist, community-based eldercare centers and stronger state intervention reduce the sole dependence on families (Camargos et al., 2018).
- **South Africa:** South Africa presents a mixed model where extended families traditionally provide care, but the HIV/AIDS epidemic and economic inequality have strained household capacities. The state provides *old-age grants*, a more robust social safety net compared to India's pension coverage, yet healthcare inequities and rural-urban divides remain (Schatz & Seeley, 2015).
- **India:** Compared to Brazil and South Africa, India has weaker state-supported eldercare and greater reliance on informal family caregiving. Pension and healthcare schemes are fragmented, and institutional care is stigmatized culturally. However, cultural norms of filial duty remain stronger in India, shaping the moral economy of care despite structural challenges.

1.5 Gendered Eldercare and Intersectionality

Gender is central to the dynamics of eldercare in India. Women disproportionately shoulder caregiving responsibilities, often balancing eldercare with childcare and household duties (Roy, 2020). The "feminization of caregiving" results in unpaid labor, reduced workforce participation, and heightened stress for women caregivers. At the same time, elderly women themselves face compounded vulnerabilities—higher life expectancy, widowhood, lower income security, and social isolation. Intersectionality deepens these inequalities. By examining gender and intersectionality together, the analysis underscores that eldercare in India is not only a familial or policy issue but also one shaped by overlapping axes of inequality.

2. BACKGROUND OF STUDY

Elderly people who live alone are considered to be "at-risk" by the WHO. Living lonely and unaccompanied in later life is frequently perceived as an uncomfortable circumstance that presents a health risk and necessitates particular attention (Kharicha et al. (2007; Iliffe et al. 1992). Research on older individuals living isolated is essential in emerging countries like India, where there is little social protection for the elderly and inadequate governmental structures (Sen and Noon 2007). Many medical problems and adverse health occasions that affect the olders may be associated with living alone. These include poor chronic disorders (Murphy 1995), eating habits (Davis et al. 1990), a greater risk of death (Welin et al. 1985), and a greater risk of functional failure (Mor et al. 1989; Sarwari et al. 1998). Based mostly on research done in industrialized countries, this information is based on incomplete evidence (Dean et al. 1992).

Epidemiological and medical research from several developing nations has demonstrated that seniors who live unaccompanied experience higher rates of depression (Dean et al., 1992; Mui 1998; Chou and Chi 2000); worse psychological health (Iwasa et al. 2006); functional damage; poor diet; high risk of excessive alcohol and smoking use; social isolation; lower levels of physical activity; and greater rates of chronic conditions such as glaucoma, cataracts, and arthritis (Singh et al. 2024b).. A cross-sectional study conducted in India found substantial gender inequalities in the socio-demographic features and the health condition of the elderly (Mini 2009). Nonetheless, a substantial body of research on the relationship among older Indians' living status (i.e., whether they are "independent" or "dependent") and their financial circumstances is generally lacking (Singh et al. 2025b). The dearth of demonstrative demographic data in India has made it more difficult to comprehend how the elderly are financially situated. Furthermore, a number of methodological problems have led to the frequent exclusion of elderly individuals from large-scale study (Ebrahim, 1996).

Ageism and the difficulties associated with the range of ailments that can strike an elderly person have also been connected to the unwillingness to look into one's health status in later life (Sen 1996). The health concerns of the elderly were not previously given much attention by the Indian government, but this is beginning to change as the number of older citizens rises (Singh et al. 2025a). Previous researches focused on the problems related to the adjustment of older persons (Rajput et al. 2022). The author believes that the Indian joint family structure should be maintained (Kushwaha et al. 2024). It is important for younger and elder generations to collaborate and communicate with each other (Kushwaha et al. 2023a). According to the author, a concerted effort must be made by the government, non-governmental organizations, religious institutions, etc. to both understand and address the issues brought about by a graying society if India's elderly population is to live a dignified and high-quality life (Kushwaha et al. 2023b). The focus of the author's research has been on the emotional, social, and marital adjustments made by older adults (Singh et al. 2024a).

The majority of elderly patients admitted to institutions, according to the study's authors, came from nuclear households (Jain & Singh, 2023). Compared to those who are not, older people who are institutionalized have a wider range of social problems, including mental health problems (Kumar et al. 2025). Furthermore, authors have observed that older persons who are hospitalized face higher psychological problems in addition to financial hardships compared to their non-institutionalized counterparts (Jain et al. 2025).

Information about older citizens' financial situation as well as the social and physical problems they face has been supplied (Anand & Singh, 2025). The author of the paper has focused on the factors that contribute to problems that India's older population faces (Kushwaha et al. 2025). The author has focused on how urbanization, nuclearization of families, rapid industrialization, and the rise of individual philosophy have undermined Indian traditional norms, which traditionally gave older people power over the family (Sharma & Singh 2025). The findings claims that efforts should be taken to avoid elder problems, and that understanding generational variations in families and social work intervention can be helpful in this regard.

Albert & Cattell, (1994) has focused on the study of the aging population in India and provides an analysis of elder abuse along with socio-economic, emotional, physical, and health associated matters. The author has also discussed the subjects that can be utilized to structure models of care for the elderly and argues that these models are influenced by various factors, including but not limited to gender, socio-economic status, and place of living. The author contends that in order to maintain the family unit, standard and expert interventions and welfare services—such as financial support and counseling for elderly people and their families—are required. The author has concluded that while some aspects of aging have been steadily constant over time, most of them are micro-level.

Bongaarts, & Zimmer, (2001) have attempted to draw attention to the harmful actions that older family members commit. Scientists have investigated the impact of abusive familial conduct as well as the many types of abuse that are commonly aimed against the elderly through this study. Writers have also examined the inadequacy of social security policies in safeguarding the status of older family members. Younger generations and those of today both recognize the decline in human values. In direction to solve the issue of older residents, policies, prompt social work interventions, and critical majors should be given high attention, according to the authors (Chaudhuri & Roy, 2007).

Disability can lower an aged person's quality of life in addition to being a significant health indicator that can have a substantial impact on society because of long-term institutionalization and increased medical care usage. Furthermore, as people age, their chances of developing a handicap also do, and once they do, their chances of getting worse and having a lower chance of recovering from their condition also rise. "Disability and elderly" encompasses a broad spectrum of conditions, each requiring different care. However, aging should not be associated with infirmity because a sizable portion of the senior population continues to live independently (Chen & Short, 2008).

Gee, (2000) claims that social gerontology analyzes the silver economy as a tool of ageing strategy for the ageing population. In Japan, the term "silver market" was coined in the 1970s to refer to the growing number of senior housing options. The silver market comprises, among other things, products, values, and services for wealthy senior citizens; unique trade solutions that enable operators to adapt to an aging workforce; concepts for universal design; and trans-generational design, which seeks to make products and services "age-friendly" to individuals with varying physical and mental capacities, may lead to better social integration. The epidemic has exposed weaknesses in India's infrastructure, program execution, health policy, and support services for the elderly, who are the group most at risk from the virus. In light of this dramatic increase, India urgently needs to build a stronger ecosystem for elder care, particularly in the post-COVID era. Urbanization and migration from pastoral to metropolitan areas in India have accelerated the breakdown of traditional joint family structures into nuclear family units (Gupta & Sankar, 2002).

In 2019, World Bank study found that 34% of people reside in cities, a significant rise from 26% in 2001. This trend has a negative effect on the safety net of shared responsibility and resources available to the elder population (WHO, 1997). Micro family units are smaller in size and number of members. Furthermore, if rehabilitation and relocation are problematic, the Life Satisfaction Quotient meter may easily fall a few notches. It is common knowledge that having a family, being in a comfortable environment, and having steady income all contribute to a happier existence. Generally speaking, debt from mortgages, children's college tuition, and other long-term expenses accruing at a later age (65+) ruins a person's best years (Gu et al. 2007).

The Indian government has launched a number of initiatives to advance the silver economy. Among the most notable are the budgetary allocation of Rs 100 cr, by the Ministry of Social Justice and Empowerment's, Government of India. The government also launch the Senior Aging Growth Engine (SAGE) scheme, which aims to support private enterprises that innovate in products and processes for the benefit of the elderly. The initiative finds, assesses, confirms, and compiles elders' requirements in direction to provide goods, services, and solutions. elderly Able individuals for Re-Employment with Self-respect, an initiative of the government, aims to link elderly individuals with private sector employers. In this effort, startups such as Neomotion have developed a"no transfer" accessibility option that allows a wheelchair user to ride a motorcycle after it is attached. The "Indoknee" from Newnara provides unrestricted, lightweight corrective support; the Flexmo wearable hip protection and the Ducere smart insoles help prevent falls. Avyantra, a different start-up, is developing an automated medical gadget for home dialysis. Those who are coping with chronic kidney failure may find this simpler. At the request of EAC-PM, another Quality of Life for Elderly Index initiative has been developed for competitiveness. It highlights a topic that is sometimes overlooked: the difficulties that the elderly encounter. It also analyzes the general state of ageing in India and pinpoints the regional patterns of aging throughout Indian States. The four pillars of the Index structure are financial, social, and health well-being (Kinsella and Gist, 1998).

The problems that elderly persons deal with are diverse. These include problems with society, psychology, health, the economy, abuse, and crime. However, solutions can be put into practice for other issues as well. For example, one might ask for help and support in order to provide remedies for crimes and abuse. Policies and initiatives have been put into place with the goal of easing the issues faced by the elderly. Enhancing their participation in activities and functions, enhancing their economic and social welfare, enhancing their health, They can live their lives effectively when these are available (Knodel and Debavalya, 1997). The above discussion points towards highly sensitive element of aged persons in India. Although considerable amount of literature has discussed about the types and variations of problems faced by the elderly population, there is dearth of knowledge about the types of opportunities available for aged persons for their productive and skillful employment. Moreover, it is also evident that there are some gaps between the facility which they need and the actual status of the same in their day to day life. This research paper focuses on these pertinent issues and their solutions (Lena et al. 2009).

3. PROBLEMS FACED BY ELDERLY CITIZENS IN INDIA

With marching age and biological degeneration of human body, many problems crop up at later stage of life (Lim and Ng, 2010). From the viewpoint of Research, they can be classified as Health and Medical problems, Financial Concerns, Social problems, Issues with the nervous system, psychology, and emotions and Issues Related to Aging as discussed below:

3.1 Health and Medical problems faced by elderly

The health and medical problem can be classified into two broad categories namely degenerative problems and lifestyle problems.

- ***Degenerative Problems*:** These problems arise due to increasing age as there are degenerative changes in aging body. Most common among them are heart disease, diabetes, osteoporosis and osteoarthritis, urological and kidney diseases, vision and hearing disease, cognitive and mental disease, constipation and bladder problem and problems relating to oral health. Cognitive problems are varied in nature. Among them, most ccommon cognitive health problem are Dementia and Alzheimer's disease. Chronic illnesses are most common in people 75 years of age and older, with cardiovascular disease (CVD) and hypertension taking center stage (Li et al. 2009).
- ***Problems with lifestyle:*** A person's lifestyle has an impact on their health. These illnesses are not contagious, meaning that sick individuals cannot spread the disease. Lack of exercise, poor eating practices, alcohol, tobacco, and drug use disorders are the causes of them. If not treated in a timely manner, these can develop into potentially fatal illnesses. Sedentary lifestyles and work-life imbalances brought on by intense pressure and stress are the root causes of many disorders. Each country has a different incidence of lifestyle problems, as per the India Fit Report 2022. The results are much worse in Lucknow, where an astounding 45.10 percent of people have at least one lifestyle disease.

3.2 Financial problems faced by elderly

Seniors become more reliant on loved ones as a result of a range of financial issues. A recent Age Well Foundation survey indicates that 65% of India's elderly (those over 60) face financial problems and are totally dependent on others to meet their basic requirements. The remaining 35% are financially stable, their major source of income coming from pensions, having amassed, saved, and inherited wealth.

Over 65% of Indian women over 65 who are homemakers make up the mainstream of the nation's elderly populace. This adds to the growing number of older Indians experiencing financial insecurity. The quality of care declines even when offspring of individuals in their 60s and 70s take good care of their old parents. This helps with a growth in India's senior population experiencing financial insecurity. The quality of care decreases with age, even though offspring of individuals in their 60s and 70s take good care of their old parents.

3.3 Social problems faced by elderly

Elders in India are also facing many social problems. Migration of young generation of people to cities for job related purpose has resulted into nuclear family system. This family where, both husband and wife are earning bread and butter in big cities lack time for each other. Due to this, they are not able to devote time to their kids who are being reared in crèches. This raises an important question i.e. how can they give time to elders of their family when they do not have time for their own kids. Due to this relationship crisis elders are facing tough time in homes and are isolated. Another issue is that due to inter-generational gap, there is lack of value system among the two generations which results in expectation clashes. This also leads to social problems.

3.4 Issues related to Ageing

A very common issue faced by every elderly that is Neurological, Psychological and Emotional Problem due to Ageism. Ageism can be described as discrimination of elders against their age. According to WHO Ageism refers to how we think (stereotypes), how we feel (prejudices) and how we act towards others (discrimination) or oneself based on age. This psychological phenomenon plays an important role in establishing relationship between younger generation and older generation. The negative impact of ageism is that it can damage solidarity between older generation and younger generation and can have negative repercussions on health, longevity and well-being. Ageism can be of three types--Self-directed Ageism (when a person internalizes negative feeling about him/herself), Interpersonal Ageism (supervisor in job situation or family members discriminate elder person), and Institutional Ageism I.e. Discriminatory action by institutions like fewer researches by medical research institutions in developing remedies for elders.

4. PUBLICLY SPONSORED SCHEMES FOR ELDER WELFARE IN INDIA

Looking at the rising population of elderly people in India, the government has made sincere effort to safeguard their interest, rights and economic in-dependency. Prominent among them are discussed herewith:

4.1 Atal Pension Yojana

The aim of the APY scheme is to establish a social security system that is universally available to all Indians, with a focus on those who fall below the poverty line and those employed in the unorganised sector. The program, which is run by the Pension Fund Regulatory and Development Authority (PFRDA), requires all bank account holders between the ages of 18 and 40 to make pension contributions in accordance with their own preferences. Alternatively, at reaching the age of 60, subscribers will be assured a minimum monthly pension of either Rs. 1000, Rs. 2000, Rs. 3000, Rs. 4000, or Rs. 5000.The subscriber would be eligible for the monthly pension; upon his death, the pension corpus, which amounted to the subscriber's age-60 accrued savings, would be transferred to the subscriber's nominee. Subscribers are able to participate. Subscriber can contribute to APY on monthly basis, quarterly basis and also yearly basis. The Scheme is praiseworthy and important. However, keeping in view the impact of inflation in future, the pensionable amount corpus can be enhanced within a range of Rs.10000 - Rs. 15000 per month.

4.2 Rashtriya Vayoshri Yojana (RVY)

The program's goal is to give older adults who fall into the BPL category and have age-related disabilities or infirmities practical aids and assisted living appliances that can help them regain nearly normal bodily functioning. The Ministry of Social Justice and Empowerment is in charge of the administrative oversight of this program, which was introduced on April 1, 2017. The senior citizens who are identified as beneficiaries of the scheme receive free assisted living devices, including walking sticks, elbow crutches, walkers/crutches, tripods/quad pods, wheelchairs, prosthetic dentures, and eyeglasses. "Artificial Limbs Manufacturing Corporation (ALIMCO)" is a public sector undertaking that is carrying out the scheme.The designated beneficiaries receive the devices in camp mode.

4.3 Indira Gandhi National Old Age Pension Scheme (IGNOAPS)

Under the National Social Assistance Programme (NSAP), the Ministry of Rural Development launched this program to provide financial support to elders who are below the poverty line. Because of the non-contributory nature of this scheme, the beneficiary can get their pension without making any contributions. For BPL individuals aged 60 to 79, the monthly pension is Rs. 200; for those aged 80 and beyond, it is only Rs. 500. At the current Price Index, this amount appears insignificant. Only Rs 6500 crore in funding has been allotted by the government, while around 5.6 crore elders fall within the BPL category. The sum should be increased by the government in line with the number of elderly people in the BPL category.

4.4 The Pradhan Mantri Vaya Vandana Yojana

The program is designed to give seniors over 60 financial security. Pensioners can choose their own payment frequency, such as monthly, quarterly, half-yearly, or annually, with an alluring interest rate of 8% annually. The pension caps are set at Rs. 10,000 for the maximum amount and Rs. 3,000 for the minimum. The government guarantees older citizens' future security and their right to a dignified existence through this program. But the only seniors who stand to gain from this plan are those who have investable funds.

4.5 The National Programme for Health Care of Elderly (NPHCE)

NPHCE was established in 2010 with the goal of offering high-quality healthcare services to people residing in district hospitals, sub-centers (SC), community health centers (CHC), and primary health centers (PHC) around the country. Through the State Health Society, the initiative aims to make it easier for people to access the resources and facilities for healthcare they require at all levels. These government or healthcare facility senior citizen benefits could be fully or partially funded, giving the nation's aged people access to high-quality medical treatment at affordable costs. Although this is a wonderful concept with broad coverage, not all locations have easy access to specialized therapy (Zimmer and Amornsirisomboon, 2001).

4.6 Varistha Mediclaim Policy

This policy is among India's greatest national health programs and provides comprehensive coverage for medical needs. Seniors between the ages of 60 and 80 are eligible for specialist medical treatment under this policy, which is tailored to their needs. It pays for prescription drugs, blood transfusions, emergency medical transportation, and other expenses associated with the diagnosis. The policy has a one-year expiration date, but it can be extended until the age of 90 and offers other benefits like an income tax refund under Section 80D.The goal of this strategy is to support elderly adults' health and wellbeing. Seniors who need healthcare services can get them without having to worry about paying exorbitant costs. They can unwind and fully enjoy the experience because they feel safe and at ease (Song et al. 2008).

4.7 Vayoshreshtha Samman

In 2012, the Indian government launched the esteemed Vayoshreshtha Samman, an award programme for older persons that acknowledges and compensates them for their noteworthy achievements in various disciplines. Since its 2013 elevation to a national award, the government's annual initiative has received recognition in thirteen different categories. District Panchayats who offer senior residents outstanding services and facilities will receive a cash award of Rs. 10 lakhs along with a memento and citation. Likewise, the top-performing institution conducting research on aging will get a monetary prize of Rs. 5 lakhs together with a memento and citation. These honors are intended to acknowledge and promote the unselfish contributions made by people and organizations to the welfare of elders in India (Sheela and Jayamala, 2008; Rajan et al. 2003).

5. INDIAN STRATEGIES TO DEAL ELDERLY AT FAMILY, SOCIAL, GOVERNMENT AND CORPORATE LEVEL

5.1 Family Level

Family is the basic unit of society. Since a person is born, he /she learns how to deal with his basic needs and emotions among his family members consisting of different age groups. In Indian tradition joint family system is a consistent, strengthening force at the core of ritual. In the Indian family system, it is the highest responsibility of every son and daughter to show respect for the elder members of the family, particularly by caring for the parents as they age. Today, when nuclear family system has emerged in society due to urbanization, there is erosion of "care" and "share" culture of the family wherein due respect and care was given to elders. If this is restored, then the problems of elders will be minimized. For instance, they will have members who will take care of their medical issues on time. Financially also they will be secure as other than pension, income generated from other members can meet their medical expenses. This will lead to shared financial Burdon. Emotionally and psychologically, they will be deriving warmth and respect from children and younger generation which will in longer run give them sense of purpose and goal of life and foster emotional stability (Ross and Wu, 1996). This way, the benefits can come to both the generations with strong bondage (Zimmer, 2005).

5.2 Social Level

The per ca pita income of India is much lower than that of china and japan. So it would be a challenging task for the society to afford all those facilities which is required for meaningful living of elders. It may lead to undesirable understanding between the elders and the society. This may lead to a situation where elders may think that society is least bothered of their needs and society ma think them to be a burden. It is suggested that right from now initiative should be taken by society in this regard (Wu & Schimmele, 2008).

5.3 Government Level

Despite these challenges, there is growing awareness among families, policymakers, and civil society regarding the need for robust eldercare mechanisms. Emerging trends such as community-based care initiatives, the expansion of old-age homes, home healthcare services, and the use of digital health technologies are slowly bridging gaps in traditional caregiving models. Government policies and schemes like the Maintenance and Welfare of Parents and Senior Citizens Act, the National Programme for Health Care of the Elderly (NPHCE), and various pension and insurance schemes provide an essential foundation, though implementation and accessibility remain inconsistent.

5.4 Corporate Level

As per the Companies Act 1956, every corporate house has to invest 2% of their profit on Corporate Social Responsibility (CSR) activity. This way Corporates can help in building hospitals, old age homes, Elders Park, even job opportunities for retired elders in every district of the country

We in India too will have to evolve some innovative ways to serve our elders without much cost to exchequers. Concept of Nucleus family be reverted back to multi-Generational structure of family where in elders may spend their time helping new generation and young generation taking care of elders. Employers of organized and unorganized sectors may come forward to encourage this family structure by providing special incentives to their employees for keeping their Parent with them. In addition to this government may also increase budgetary allocation for elders to the maximum permissible extent.

6. DISCUSSION

6.1. Mental Health Services for Older Adults

Mental health remains one of the most underexplored dimensions of eldercare in India. The Mental Healthcare Act (2017)* was a landmark reform guaranteeing the right to affordable and accessible mental healthcare for all, including the elderly. However, gaps in implementation severely limit its reach. India has fewer than 1,000 trained geriatric psychiatrists, and most mental health professionals are concentrated in urban centers (Patel et al., 2018). This leaves large sections of rural and semi-urban older adults without any formal support. Depression, dementia, and anxiety disorders are common among Indian elders, yet stigma often prevents families from seeking professional help. Mental health is still perceived through a lens of "weakness" or "spiritual imbalance," resulting in underreporting and delayed diagnosis. Community-based services are rare, and while NGOs like NIMHANS and the Banyan Trust have launched outreach programs, these remain localized. Comparative insights from the Asia-Pacific reveal scalable models.

6.2 Legal Protections for the Elderly

The Maintenance and Welfare of Parents and Senior Citizens Act (2007)* is India's most comprehensive legal safeguard for elders. It mandates children and heirs to provide financial and emotional support, with the possibility of filing cases before maintenance tribunals. Despite this, enforcement remains weak. Many elderly individuals are unaware of their rights, and the stigma of taking legal action against one's children prevents effective utilization. Tribunals often suffer from bureaucratic delays, and penalties for neglect are rarely implemented. Awareness campaigns led by NGOs such as HelpAge India and state-level legal aid authorities have improved visibility, but much more needs to be done. Innovative models such as "mobile tribunals" in states like Maharashtra and Tamil Nadu demonstrate how justice delivery can be localized and elder-friendly. Legal protections extend beyond maintenance.

6.3 Elder Abuse and Neglect

Elder abuse is a hidden but widespread problem in India. Surveys by HelpAge India (2022) reveal that nearly 50% of elders report some form of abuse, most often verbal, emotional, or financial, with sons and daughters-in-law frequently identified as perpetrators. Institutional abuse in poorly regulated old-age homes is also a growing concern, with cases of neglect, inadequate medical care, and financial exploitation being reported. The cultural taboo surrounding elder abuse often silences victims. Many elders fear social stigma, retaliation, or abandonment, making legal recourse rare. Although the Maintenance Act (2007) and Indian Penal Code provide avenues for punishment, the lack of monitoring systems in care institutions undermines enforcement. Successful models from Asia-Pacific highlight ways forward.

6.4 Palliative Care and Community Models

End-of-life care is often overlooked in India's eldercare discourse. Palliative care—focusing on dignity, pain management, and holistic well-being—is largely restricted to urban hospitals and a few NGOs. Kerala, however, presents a global best practice through its community-based palliative care model, where volunteers, local governments, and NGOs collaborate to deliver low-cost, home-based services to chronically ill elders. This model has received international recognition and demonstrates the scalability of community-driven approaches. Elsewhere in Asia-Pacific, Japan integrates palliative care into long-term eldercare insurance schemes, while Thailand has piloted temple-based palliative care services. These models emphasize the role of cultural context in shaping care delivery. In India, scaling palliative care will require policy prioritization, capacity building of primary health workers, and integration with existing schemes such as National Programme for Palliative Care (NPPC). Furthermore, sensitizing families to palliative care as a legitimate and compassionate option could shift the dominant curative mindset, ensuring elders experience dignified aging and end-of-life support.

7. CONCLUSION

The scenario of eldercare in Indian families is undergoing significant transformation, influenced by rapid socio-economic changes, urbanization, migration, and the gradual shift from joint to nuclear family systems. Traditionally, eldercare was an integral part of family life, embedded in cultural values of respect and filial responsibility. However, changing lifestyles, increased work pressures, and geographical mobility have created considerable challenges in ensuring comprehensive and consistent care for the elderly. Issues such as social isolation, inadequate financial security, poor access to healthcare services, and lack of emotional support have become pressing concerns, particularly for elders living independently or in urban centers.

The future of eldercare in India lies in a collaborative and multi-dimensional approach. Families must be supported through awareness and capacity-building programs to better manage caregiving responsibilities. Simultaneously, private sector involvement, innovative technologies such as telemedicine and AI-driven health monitoring, and the strengthening of public healthcare infrastructure will be critical. Culturally sensitive community models that balance traditional family-based support with formal institutional mechanisms can create sustainable solutions.

In conclusion, eldercare in Indian families stands at a crossroads. Addressing current challenges and preparing for the rapidly growing elderly population requires a collective effort encompassing family, community, government, and private stakeholders. By fostering empathy, strengthening social security measures, and embracing innovative care models, India can ensure that it's elderly population lives with dignity, security, and improved quality of life in the years to come.

7.1 Future Trends and the Role of Technology in Eldercare

7.1.1 Emerging Trends in Eldercare

The future of eldercare in India is shaped by demographic, socio-economic, and technological transitions. Several key trends stand out:

- **Demographic Shift**: India's elderly population is projected to reach nearly 319 million by 2050, constituting over 20% of the population (UN, 2022). This "silver wave" will significantly increase the demand for structured elder-care services.
- **Rise of Nuclear Families**: Migration and urbanization will accelerate the breakdown of joint families, shifting caregiving responsibilities to professional caregivers, NGOs, and private services.
- **Policy Emphasis on Active Aging:** National and state policies are increasingly focusing on active aging—promoting healthy lifestyles, social engagement, and lifelong learning for elders.
- **Market Growth of Eldercare Services:** The eldercare market is expected to expand rapidly, with private investments and public–private partnerships shaping the future service ecosystem.

7.1.2 Technology's Role in Eldercare

Technology is emerging as a game-changer in bridging gaps in access, affordability, and quality of eldercare. Its role can be seen across multiple domains:

- **Telemedicine and E-Health Platforms**: Apps like Practo and Portea enable remote consultations, reducing travel burdens for older adults. Government-backed *e-Sanjeevani* has expanded teleconsultation services to rural areas.
- **Assistive Technologies**: Wearables (e.g., fall detectors, heart-rate monitors), mobility aids, and smart home devices enhance safety and independence for elderly individuals living alone.
- **AI and Robotics:** Pilot projects in Japan and Singapore using AI-enabled robots for companionship and rehabilitation show promise for India, where caregiver shortages are looming.
- **Digital Social Inclusion:** Platforms like WhatsApp, Facebook, and community forums are helping elders remain socially connected, reducing risks of isolation and depression. NGOs are also providing digital literacy training tailored for seniors.
- **Big Data and Predictive Analytics**: Health data monitoring through wearable devices can assist in early detection of chronic illnesses, helping reduce hospitalization rates.

However, technology adoption is not without challenges. Digital illiteracy, affordability gaps, and rural-urban disparities limit access. Policies must therefore integrate digital inclusion strategies to ensure equity. A regional heat map of India showing disparities in eldercare infrastructure (e.g., number of geriatric hospitals, elder homes, palliative care centers by state). Color-coded indicators can visually highlight where eldercare facilities are concentrated (Kerala, Tamil Nadu) versus underserved regions (Bihar, Jharkhand). The integration of technology with traditional caregiving practices offers a sustainable pathway for India. Hybrid models—combining *family support, community interventions, and digital tools*—are likely to dominate future eldercare. Policymakers must encourage inclusive technological adoption through subsidies, training, and partnerships with private innovators to ensure that advances benefit elders across socio-economic and geographic divides.

REFERENCES

Albert, S. M., & Cattell, M. G. (1994). Family relationships of the elderly: living arrangements. In Albert, S. M., Cattell, M. G., & Hall, G. K. (Eds.), *Old Age in Global Perspective: Cross-Cultural and Cross-National Views* (pp. 85–107).

Anand, A., & Singh, P. (2025). *Interdisciplinary Studies: Issues, Perspectives, and Challenges From National Education Program 2020*. Integrating Personalized Learning Methods Into STEAM Education.

Bloom, D. E., Chatterji, S., Kowal, P., Lloyd-Sherlock, P., McKee, M., Rechel, B., Rosenberg, L., & Smith, J. P. (2015). Macroeconomic implications of population ageing and selected policy responses. *The Lancet, 385*(9968), 649–657. [https://doi.org/DOI: 10.1016/S0140-6736(14)61464-1

Bongaarts, J., & Zimmer, Z. 2001 ' Living Arrangements of Older Adults in the Developing World: An Analysis of DHS Household Surveys ', DHS Comparative Report No. 148, Calverton, MD.

Camargos, M. C. S., Rodrigues, R. N., & Machado, C. J. (2018). Demographic transition and population aging in Brazil. *Revista Brasileira de Estudos de População, 35*(1), 1–23.

Chaudhuri, A., & Roy, K. 2007 Gender Differences in Living Arrangements among Older Persons in India, [Online] Available at: https://ssrn.com/abstract=987327 (accessed 17 August 2011).

Chen, F., & Short, S. E. (2008). Household context and subjective well-being among the oldest old in China. *Journal of Family Issues, 29*(10), 1379–1403. PMID: 19554216

Chou, K.-L., & Chi, I. (2000). Comparison between elderly Chinese living alone and those living with others. *Journal of Gerontological Social Work, 33*(4), 51–66.

Davis, M. A., Murphy, S. P., Neuhaus, J. M., & Lein, D. (1990). Living arrangements and dietary quality of older U.S. adults. *Journal of the American Dietetic Association, 90*(12), 1667–1672. PMID: 2246446

Dean, A., Kolody, B., Wood, P., & Matt, G. E. (1992). The influence of living alone on depression in elderly persons. *Journal of Aging and Health, 4*(1), 3–18.

Ebrahim, S. (1996). Principles of epidemiology in old age. In Ebrahim, S., & Kalache, A. (Eds.), *Epidemiology in Old Age* (pp. 12–21). BMJ Publishing Group.

Gee, E. M. (2000). Living arrangements and quality of life among Chinese Canadian elders. *Social Indicators Research, 51*(3), 309–329.

Gu, D., Dupre, M. E., & Liu, G. (2007). Characteristics of the institutionalized and community residing oldest-old in China. *Social Science & Medicine*, *64*(4), 871–883. PMID: 17126971

Gupta, I., & Sankar, D. Delhi 2002 ‘ Health of the Elderly in India: A Multivariate Analysis ’, Institute of Economic Growth Discussion Paper No. 46.

HelpAge India. (2022). *Elder abuse in India: A national report.* HelpAge India. https://www.helpageindia.org

Iliffe, S., Tai, S. S., Haines, A., Gallivan, S., Goldenberg, E., Booroff, A., & Morgan, P. (1992). Are elderly people living alone an at risk group? *British Medical Journal*, *305*(6860), 1001–1004. PMID: 1458108

Iwasa, H., Kawaai, C., Gondo, Y., Inagaki, H., & Suzuki, T. (2006). Subjective well-being as a predictor of all-cause mortality among middle-aged and elderly people living in an urban Japanese community: A seven-year prospective cohort study. *Geriatrics & Gerontology International*, *6*(4), 216–222.

Jain, P., & Singh, P. (2023). Lethargic approach in expediting financial reporting system: A case of construction firm. *International Journal of Teaching and Case Studies*, *14*(1), 1–10.

Jain, P., Singh, P., & Kushwaha, R. (2025). Investigating change management as a novel digital wallet service innovation in banks: A case of Indian bank. *Int. J. Teaching and Case Studies*, *15*(1), 67–81.

Kharicha, K., Iliffe, S., Harari, D., Swift, C., Gillmann, G., & Stuck, A. E. (2007). Health risk appraisal in older people 1: Are older people living alone an “at-risk” group? *The British Journal of General Practice*, *57*(537), 271–276. PMID: 17394729

Kinsella, K., & Gist, Y. J. (1998). *International Brief on Gender and Aging*. United States Department of Commerce, Economics and Statistics Administration.

Knodel, J., & Debavalya, N. (1997). Living arrangements and support among the elderly in South-east Asia: An introduction. *Asia-Pacific Population Journal*, *12*(4), 5–16. PMID: 12293567

Kumar, A., Singh, P., Parihar, A.S. & Saraswat, S. (2025), “Analyzing the impact of psychological capital on the entrepreneurial intentions of students through mediating role of individual expectancy using PLS-SEM”, *International Journal of Social Economics*, Vol. ahead-of-print No. ahead-of-print. https://doi.org/.DOI: 10.1108/IJSE-03-2024-0252

Kumar, S. (2021). Elderly care in India: A neglected dimension in public policy. *Journal of Social and Economic Development, 23*(2), 294–311.

Kushwaha, J., Sharma, A., & Singh, P. (2023a). Exploration and prioritization of enablers to organization work–family balance planning for working sole Indian mothers integrating fuzzy Delphi and AHP. *International Journal of Social Economics*, *50*(3), 398–418.

Kushwaha, J., Singh, P., & Kushwah, R. (2025). *Work-Family Balance Among Working Sole Mothers: Insights From Systematic Integrative Literature Review and Thematic Analysis*. Leading Inclusive Workplaces Through Digital Transformation and Organizational Change.

Kushwaha, J., Singh, P., & Kushwaha, R. (2024). Predicting working sole Indian mothers' satisfaction towards work–family balance integrating the Kano model and weighted average method. *International Journal of Social Economics*, *51*(6), 725–740.

Kushwaha, J., Singh, P., & Sharma, A. (2023b). Modelling the enablers of work-family balance among working single mothers integrating expert-mining and TISM-MICMAC. *Journal of Organizational Effectiveness: People and Performance*. Advance online publication. doi: .DOI: 10.1108/JOEPP-05-2022-0106

Lamb, S. (2009). *Aging and the Indian diaspora: Cosmopolitan families in India and abroad*. Indiana University Press.

Lena, A., Ashok, K., Padma, M., Kamath, V., & Kamath, A. (2009). Health and social problems of the elderly: A cross-sectional study in Udupi Taluk, Karnataka. *Indian Journal of Community Medicine : Official Publication of Indian Association of Preventive & Social Medicine*, *34*(2), 131–134. PMID: 19966960

Li, L. W., Zhang, J., & Liang, J. (2009). Health among the oldest-old in China: Which living arrangements make a difference? *Social Science & Medicine*, *68*(2), 220–227. PMID: 19019514

Lim, L. L., & Ng, T. P. (2010). Living alone, lack of a confidant and psychological well-being of elderly women in Singapore: The mediating role of loneliness. *Asia-Pacific Psychiatry*, *2*(1), 33–40.

Mini, G. K. (2009). Socioeconomic and demographic diversity in the health status of elderly people in a transitional society, Kerala, India. *Journal of Biosocial Science*, *41*(4), 457–467. PMID: 18647442

Mor, V., Murphy, J., Masterson-Allen, S., Willey, C., Razmpour, A., Jackson, M. E., Greer, D., & Katz, S. (1989). Risk of functional decline among well elders. *Journal of Clinical Epidemiology*, *42*(9), 895–904. PMID: 2778468

Mui, A. C. (1998). Living alone and depression among older Chinese immigrants. *Journal of Gerontological Social Work*, *30*(3–4), 147–166.

Murphy, M. (1995). Household and family factors in morbidity and mortality. *Morbidity and mortality data: problems of comparability*, 18-20.

Narayana, M. R., & Narasimhan, S. (2019). Health and health care of the elderly in India: A review. *Indian Journal of Gerontology, 33*(1), 1–20.

Patel, V., Xiao, S., Chen, H., Hanna, F., Jotheeswaran, A. T., Luo, D., ... & Saxena, S. (2018). The magnitude of and health system responses to the mental health treatment gap in adults in India and China. *The Lancet, 388*(10063), 3074–3084.

Prakash, I. (2020). Changing family structures and their impact on elderly care in India. *Indian Journal of Social Work, 81*(2), 225–242.

Rajan, S. I. (2017). Ageing in India: Trends and issues. *Economic and Political Weekly, 52*(16), 32–37.

Rajan, S. I., Mishra, U. S., & Sarma, P. S. (2003). *India's Elderly: Burden or Challenge?* Sage Publishers.

Rajput, S., Jain, E., Mehra, A., Thakur, K. S., Gupta, O., & Singh, P. (2022). Technology Driven Tourism: A PLS SEM Model of its Antecedents in Tourist Behavior Intention. In *2022 IEEE Conference on Interdisciplinary Approaches in Technology and Management for Social Innovation (IATMSI)*, Gwalior, India, 2022 (pp. 1-6). doi: DOI: 10.1109/IATMSI56455.2022.10119265

Ross, C., & Wu, C. L. (1996). Education, age, and the cumulative advantage in health. *Journal of Health and Social Behavior*, *37*(1), 104–120. PMID: 8820314

Roy, K. (2020). Gender and eldercare in India: Negotiating responsibility and dependence. *Journal of Cross-Cultural Gerontology, 35*(4), 375–391.

Saraswat, S. & Singh, P. (2025), "The moderating role of perceived trust in predicting the adoption intention of consumers toward online pharmacies using the application of UTAUT model", *International Journal of Pharmaceutical and Healthcare Marketing*, Vol. ahead-of-print No. ahead-of-print. https://doi.org/ DOI: 10.1108/IJPHM-05-2024-0042

Sarwari, A. R., Fredman, L., Langenberg, P., & Magaziner, J. (1998). Prospective study on the relation between living arrangement and change in functional health status of elderly women. *American Journal of Epidemiology*, *147*(4), 370–378. PMID: 9508104

Schatz, E., & Seeley, J. (2015). Gender, ageing and carework in East and Southern Africa: A review. *Global Public Health, 10*(10), 1185–1200.

Sen, K. (1996). Gender. In Ebrahim, S., & Kalache, A. (Eds.), *Epidemiology in Old Age* (pp. 210–220). BMJ Publishing Group.

Sen, M., & Noon, J. New York 2007 29–31 March 'Living arrangement: how does it relate to the health of the elderly in India? ', paper presented at the annual meeting of the Population Association of America.

Sharma, R. K., & Singh, P. 2025. The Virtual Economy: Opportunities and Challenges in the Digital Age. *Digital Technologies and Transformations in Public Administration, Engineering, and Sustainable Business*, pp.177-204.

Sheela, J., & Jayamala, M. (2008). Health condition of the elderly women: A need to enhance their well being. *Indian Journal of South Asian Studies*, *1*(1), 177–187.

Singh, A. K., Meshram, S. A., Khandelwal, V., Tiwari, P., & Singh, P. (2024). Implementation of Industry-Based Perspective in Technical Education: A Qualitative and Quantitative Analysis. *Industrial and Manufacturing Designs: Quantitative and Qualitative Analysis*, 321-346.

Singh, P. (2014). Unorganized sector and India's informal economy: Challenges and prospects. *New Man International Journal of Multidisciplinary Studies*, *1*(2), 209–218.

Singh, P. (2024a). Weather index insurance viability in mitigation of climate change impact risk: A systematic review and future agenda. *Journal of Science and Technology Policy Management*, *15*(1), 142–163.

Singh, P. (2024b). Analyzing Responsible Leadership Effectiveness for Attainment of Sustainable Development Goals in Developing Countries Using Environmental Scanning Techniques. In Bhattacharya, S., Venkatesh, V. G., & Chatterjee, S. R. (Eds.), *Responsible Corporate Leadership Towards Attainment of Sustainable Development Goals. Responsible Leadership and Sustainable Management*. Springer., DOI: 10.1007/978-981-97-1386-8_13

Singh, P., & Agrawal, G. (2019). Efficacy of weather index insurance for mitigation of weather risks in agriculture: An integrative review. *International Journal of Ethics and Systems*, *35*(4), 584–616.

Singh, P., & Agrawal, G. (2020). Development, present status and performance analysis of agriculture insurance schemes in India: Review of evidence. *International Journal of Social Economics*, *47*(4), 461–481.

Singh, P., & Agrawal, G. (2021). Modelling the barriers of weather index insurance service adoption integrating expert mining and ISM Fuzzy-MICMAC. *Benchmarking*, *29*(8), 2527–2554. DOI: 10.1108/BIJ-04-2021-0183

Singh, P., & Agrawal, G. (2022). Mapping the customer centric weather index insurance service design using quality function deployment. *The TQM Journal*, *34*(6), 1800–1822.

Singh, P., Agrawal, G., & Kushwaha, R. (2021a, November). Evaluating Customer Satisfaction of Weather Index Insurance Service Quality Using Kano Model. In *2021 IEEE Bombay Section Signature Conference (IBSSC)* (pp. 1-6). IEEE.

Singh, P. & Kushwaha, R. (2024). "Envisaging Indian farmers' desires from agricultural index insurance integrating rank sum weighting method and MoSCoW technique: an approach to requirements prioritization", *International Journal of Social Economics*, Vol. ahead-of-print No. ahead-of-print. https://doi.org/.DOI: 10.1108/IJSE-03-2024-0233

Singh, P., & Kushwaha, R. (2025). "Conceptualizing the corporate-social accountability and sustainability assessment of weather-risk management policy towards stakeholders using qualitative insights: a case of weather index insurance", *Qualitative Research in Financial Markets*, Vol. ahead-of-print No. ahead-of-print. https://doi.org/DOI: 10.1108/QRFM-05-2024-0113

Singh, P., Kushwaha, R., & Kushwaha, J. (2021b). Assessing visitors' satisfaction about museum service quality using Kano model. In *2021 IEEE 9th Region 10 Humanitarian Technology Conference (R10-HTC)* (pp. 1-6). IEEE.

Singh, P., Kushwaha, R., & Kushwaha, J. (2023a). Analyzing Accountability of Weather Index Insurance Service in Attainment of Sustainable Development Goals: A Sustainable Accounting Perspective Review. In Pratik Arte et al. (Eds): *Sustainable International Business, 2023*. Springer Nature, 2023. doi: , 531340. DOI: 978-3-031-43784-7

Singh, P., Kushwaha, R., & Kushwaha, J. (2023b). Evaluating Farmer Participation in Weather Index Insurance in a Socio-Demographic Perspective: Evidence From the Crop Insurance Data of India. In Popoola, A., Magidimisha-Chipungu, H., & Chipungu, L. (Eds.), *Handbook of Research on Managing the Urban-Rural Divide Through an Inclusive Framework* (pp. 255–278). IGI Global., DOI: 10.4018/978-1-6684-6258-4.ch005

Singh, P., Kushwaha, R., & Kushwaha, J. (2024b). Foresight the future of Industry 5.0 in perspective of sustainable services in developing countries. *Modern Technologies and Tools Supporting the Development of Industry 5.0*, 381.

Singh, P., Kushwaha, R., & Kushwaha, J. (2025). Meta-synthesis analysis on artificial intelligence applications in healthcare. *AI Frontiers: Transforming Health, Agriculture, and Education*, 187.

Singh, P., Kushwaha, R., & Kushwaha, J. (2025a). Retail innovations impact on competitiveness in retail sector: Evidence from SAP-LAP Analysis. In Rajput, S., Malik, F. A., Mahajan, S., & Javed, A. (Eds.), *Retail Innovations in Business Models* (pp. 69–88). IGI Global., DOI: 10.4018/979-8-3693-7620-1.ch012

Singh, P., Kushwaha, R., & Kushwaha, J. (2025b), "A Qualitative Study on Analysing the Role of Mimicking Technology in Electronic Customer Relationship Management: A Case of Service Sector", Kumar, A., Ciddikie, M.D., Kashyap, A.K. and Akram, H.W. (Ed.) *Marketing 5.0*, Emerald Publishing Limited, Leeds, pp. 103-119. https://doi.org/DOI: 10.1108/978-1-83797-815-120251008

Singh, P., Kushwaha, R., Kushwaha, J., & Singh, A. K. (2024)a. A Qualitative Study to Rank Non-Conventional Energy Sources for Industrial Sustainability and Energy Management Decisions Using MoSCoW Prioritization Method. *Industrial and Manufacturing Designs: Quantitative and Qualitative Analysis*, 105-137.

Song, L., Li, S., Zhang, W., & Feldman, M. W. 2008 Intergenerational support and self-rated health of the elderly in rural China: an investigation in Chaohu, Anhui Province, in *Healthy Longevity in China: Demographic, Socioeconomic, and Psychological Dimensions*, Y. Zeng, D. L. Poston, Jr., D. A. Vlosky & D. Gu, Springer Publisher, Dordrecht, The Netherlands, 235 – 349.

Sudha, S., Suchindran, C., Mutran, E. J., Rajan, S. I., & Sarma, P. S. (2016). Marital status, family ties, and self-rated health among elders in South India. *Journal of Cross-Cultural Gerontology, 31*(3), 261–277.

United Nations. (2022). World population prospects 2022. Department of Economic and Social Affairs, Population Division. https://population.un.org

Welin, L., SvÄrdsudd, K., Ander-Peciva, S., Tibblin, G., Tibblin, B., Larsson, B. and Wilhelmsen, L. (1985). Prospective study of social influences on mortality: The study of men born in 1913 and 1923. *Lancet*, *1*(8384), 915–918. PMID: 2858755

World Health Organization (WHO). (1977). *Prevention of Mental Disorders in the Elderly*. WHO.

Wu, Z., & Schimmele, C. M. 2008 Living arrangements and psychological disposition of the oldest old population in China, in *Healthy Longevity in China: Demographic, Socioeconomic, and Psychological Dimensions*, Y. Zeng, D. L. Poston, Jr., D. A. Vlosky & D. Gu, Springer Publisher, Dordrecht, The Netherlands, 397 – 418.

Zimmer, Z. (2005). Health and living arrangement transitions among China's oldest-old. *Research on Aging*, *27*(5), 526–555.

Zimmer, Z., & Amornsirisomboon, P. (2001). Socioeconomic status and health among older adults in Thailand: An examination using multiple indicators. *Social Science & Medicine*, *52*(8), 1297–1311. PMID: 11281411

Chapter 7
Culturally Relevant AI Strategies for Geriatric Care in Low-Resource Settings

Konstantinos Stolakis
https://orcid.org/0000-0002-5497-4172
University of Patras, Greece

ABSTRACT

This chapter explores culturally relevant AI strategies for geriatric care in low-resource settings. It focuses on how AI tools can be adapted to local health practices, social norms, and infrastructure limitations. The analysis includes case studies from underserved regions, highlighting the role of AI in extending primary care, supporting informal caregivers, and improving access to diagnostics and monitoring. It discusses the importance of inclusive data, local language processing, and trust-building through community-based models. The chapter also addresses the risks of digital colonialism, poor interoperability, and ethical concerns tied to algorithmic design in non-Western contexts. It concludes with policy recommendations for equitable AI deployment tailored to ageing populations in low-income and rural environments.

1. INTRODUCTION

Culturally relevant artificial intelligence (AI) strategies for geriatric care in low-resource settings provide the elderly with better access to healthcare and social services. Geriatric care addresses the medical needs of elders and offers support through social services. In low-resource settings, disabled elders face many barriers

DOI: 10.4018/979-8-3373-5462-0.ch007

when trying to access healthcare and social services. An assessment of the needs of the disabled elderly in a low-resource setting can identify gaps in the current healthcare situation and allow the development of AI solutions that are culturally relevant, closing the gap and allowing the elderly to access healthcare and social services.

AI is currently used in healthcare, but the lack of cultural relevance can aggregate the health disparity experienced by elders in low-resource settings and prevent the many benefits engineered solutions provide in supporting the disabled elderly in daily living activities. Cultural relevance improves service utilization and compliance to treatment and clinical advice (Harrington, C. N., et al., 2021). Cultural belief and sharing of personal information present major barriers to the need of elderly care in low-resource settings as it affects the reporting of health-related issues and the utilization of healthcare or social service (Kalusivalingam, A. K., et al., 2021).

Cultural belief dictates that health-related issues can only be expressed to the family and is a barrier to seeking professional care due to the stigma that a diagnosis can bring. Marital status may prevent the elder from sharing health-related issues that are considered inappropriate for and restricted within a marriage relationship. Hence, sharing of information needs to be within their trusted group when seeking help or support. The development of a chatbot for geriatric care using AI is a new and innovative idea. The chatbot should be culturally relevant by considering the needs, language, and beliefs of the elderly.

2. UNDERSTANDING GERIATRIC CARE

Geriatric care denotes a comprehensive approach to the physical, mental, functional, and social health needs of older adults. The population aged 65 and older is projected to reach 73 million by 2030 in the United States and 1.5 billion worldwide by 2050 (Jakovljevic, M., et al., 2023). Larger, more culturally diverse elderly populations in low-resource settings therefore indicate a greater need for culturally relevant approaches to care. Current-age geriatric healthcare models also largely evolved in resource-rich, urban settings, demanding reconsideration in lower-resource contexts. Robust culturally relevant AI can help address these challenges and bridge the prevailing geriatric care gap. Geriatric care is a multidisciplinary assessment that addresses the functional ability, physical health, and cognitive wellbeing of patients (Efthymiou, I.-P., 2024).

Multimorbidity, the concurrent presence of multiple chronic conditions, affects the majority of older adults and complicates this process. Assessments are further challenged by limited cognitive and physical capacities, while mental and physical health often deteriorate during hospital stays. Accordingly, many geriatric patients prefer community care and assisted living arrangements where support staff provide supervision and companionship, enabling older adults to age in place while maintaining independence.

Artificial intelligence (AI) therefore represents a potential means to improve prevention, diagnosis, and treatment across a broad range of chronic diseases. Screening tools have already been developed for early cognitive impairments, fall risks and urinary tract infections among patients with dementia (Wang, G., et al., 2019). With the aging population expected to reach unprecedented levels in most countries, widespread adoption of AI in healthcare is likely, but concerns about uncertainty in the underlying data and limited explainability of complex algorithms need to be addressed (Choudhury et al., 2021).

Geriatric care comprises multidisciplinary assessments that evaluate the functional ability, physical health, and cognitive well-being of older individuals (age 65 and above). The majority of these patients suffer from multiple chronic conditions and require special attention. Geriatric patients often present multimorbidity, which affects a large portion of the older population. Their assessment differs from typical evaluations and is more challenging due to limited cognitive and physical ability; furthermore, such patients may experience deterioration of mental or physical health during hospital stays even when their primary condition improves.

In low-resource settings, geriatric care is further complicated by an insufficient number of skilled practitioners, a scarcity of advanced medical technology, and pervasive cultural and language barriers that impede timely access to quality care. These compounded challenges exacerbate existing constraints, underscoring an urgent need for support (Harrington, C. N., et al., 2021).

3. THE ROLE OF AI IN HEALTHCARE

Artificial intelligence (AI) refers to the design, development, and deployment of systems applied in machines to simulate human intelligence, often focused on specific and narrow human tasks. AI technologies include classic methods such as rule-based systems (also known as expert systems), symbolic reasoning, and search or optimisation algorithms; statistical and probabilistic methods including classic machine learning algorithms; and more recently, perception, learning, and processing systems such as artificial neural networks, deep learning, and natural language processing (Williams, D., et al., 2021). The system is able to extract information from complex data and deliver it as an assumption, prediction, or sometimes an explanation. The most common representation of AI is based on machine learning, where collected data samples pass through a training phase and a model learns an objective function for the data to predict an output space, objectives, or categories.

In geriatric care, AI enables both diagnostic assistance and monitoring of at-risk patients (Souliotis K. 2016).

Furthermore, the development of tailored natural language processing algorithms has the potential to allow frail elderly people to communicate with chatbots in natural language, greatly extending access and saving resources. Nonetheless, these systems must be generalisable to a wide range of populations. It therefore becomes highly important for algorithms to be adapted to specific social, cultural, and economic contexts, to support local populations.

3.1. Overview of AI Technologies

Artificial intelligence (AI) refers to a wide range of techniques that can routinely interpret complex medical data and deliver clinically relevant information. Health and social care applications include "dashboard" decision support (combining AI-based risk stratification with evidence-based guidelines and alerts), image and video analysis and natural language processing, pharmacovigilance and genomics. AI is important for healthcare for older people because long-term conditions and multimorbidity, combined with ageing-related frailty, sensorimotor impairment and other changes, create significant challenges in terms of diagnosis, risk prediction and personalised treatment Sankaran, A., & Singla, M. P. (2024).. Early diagnosis and risk prediction can enable stratification of care pathways tailored to individual needs. Monitoring vital signs and activity patterns can flag early signs of deterioration, enabling prompt intervention. AI can also support community-level care, for example by processing social media data and identifying individuals at risk of crises requiring time-critical assessment (Shiwani et al., 2023).

3.2. AI Applications in Geriatric Care

Artificial intelligence has been identified as one of the main innovations transforming the entire healthcare industry not only in description and diagnosis but also in treatment and maintenance. With the aim of relieving pressure on the healthcare system by increasing efficiency, AI has recently emerged as a possible solution. Technological developments in the medical field, such as those achieved with the use of artificial intelligence, have opened a new era, especially in the diagnosis process. The main technological approach in this field is the use of data from wearable sensors.

In recent years, AI systems have been designed to support the elderly population with health diagnosis, medication management, companionship, and support for basic daily activities. A generic framework for an AI system with a focus on the supporting elderly is separated into three basic functional modules: perception, processing data, and actions, and it can be represented from the following figure.

The perception module corresponds to the role of sensors in a human being, which is usually used to collect physiological data and the external environment of an elderly person, e.g., faults in their movement. The processing data module is the brain of the system, which performs data fusion in order to extract useful information. Based on this information, an autonomous decision regarding the actions is made to help the elderly. For example, the posture corresponding to pressuring the air pressure sensor of the gastrointestinal organs of the elderly is different, so the reaction related to the relaxation or compression of the gastrointestinal organs is also different in order to assist in the function of the gastrointestinal organs when the elderly have a defecation need.

4. CULTURAL RELEVANCE IN HEALTHCARE

Cultural relevance refers to how well the culture of the intended users is considered and addressed during the design of an intervention. In health care, culture influences beliefs and practices concerning the acceptance and seeking (or rejecting) of health care, and shapes behaviour within the health system. Culture also affects perceptions of health workers (and the health sector generally) and the power relationships within health-care settings. Cultural competence refers to the demonstration of congruent behaviour, attitudes and policies that will come together in a system, agency or among professionals, enabling them to work effectively in cross-cultural situations. It is a necessary precondition for the provision of culturally relevant health care, which in turn is a critical determinant of the acceptance and effectiveness of health-care interventions, including those incorporating AI technology.

4.1. Defining Cultural Relevance

While an exact consensus on the nuances of cultural relevance remains elusive, an expanding body of literature supports the construct's pertinence (N. Harrington et al., 2021). Educationally, a strategically crafted pedagogical framework serves as a conduit for cultural transmission. Insofar as a relevant programme imparts critical operational competencies, whether in trades or broader cultural tenets, and encompasses salient sociopolitical components, it may effectively convey cultural relevance (Schneider-Kamp, 2021). In a structural capacity, cultural relevance confers a sense of identity and is manifest within ongoing social interactions.

Culturally relevant formation routinely fosters a positive self-perception uniformly ascribed within mainstream society. Individuals who perceive their culture as disparaged exhibit reluctance to assert cultural pride; conversely, those who observe such prejudice may regard cultural out-group members as dissimilar and unworthy of emulation. As a value system, cultural relevance navigates the tension between preservation and interest elicitation. Cultural elements may induce both intrinsic and extrinsic appeal within a particular group. A value system oriented toward cultural preservation privileges the former—emphasizing automatic, collective, and self-directed transmission and augmenting cultural continuance. A value system geared toward interest prioritizes the latter—accentuating particularized, individual, and other-directed socialization and accentuating proselytization and conversion.

4.2. Importance of Cultural Competence

Cultural competence represents the ability of providers to understand, appreciate, and interact with individuals from cultures or belief systems different from their own. This capability fosters the creation of treatment plans that are culturally tailored, thereby enhancing care quality (Pray, 2017). Establishing culturally aware communication is vital for building lasting relationships that effectively address patients' needs. The relevance of cultural competence is particularly pronounced for the rapidly growing aging and ethnically diverse population. Minority elders contend with considerable barriers (economic status, housing, geographic location, and health literacy) that hinder access to care and timely diagnosis of conditions such as Alzheimer's disease. Disparities in mental health treatment persist across racial and ethnic groups, frequently attributed to limitations in resource access, insurance coverage, stigma, and cultural perceptions (Sotiropoulos, L. D., 2023). Augmenting cultural competence among providers in social work, medicine, psychology, and counselling is imperative for improving mental health outcomes in minority populations.

In the context of geriatric assessment, specific functional scales have been developed for many cultures, yet the practicability of mastering and applying the appropriate instrument for each patient is limited (Golden, A. (2023; Jakovljevic, M., et al., 2023). Evaluations encompassing beliefs regarding advance directives, healthcare decision-making, disclosure, consent, gender considerations, and end-of-life preferences necessitate a tailored approach within multicultural populations. Elder abuse and self-neglect constitute substantial issues, with prevalence rates notably elevated among minority groups. For instance, a study within a Latino community documented elder abuse occurrences as high as 40%, a figure potentially linked to the employment of culturally sensitive surveyors who facilitated more comfortable disclosure. Cultural sensitivity equips providers to detect abuse amid barriers such as fear of retaliation or deportation, concerns prevalent among undocumented immigrants.

5. LOW-RESOURCE SETTINGS

Inherent disparities in healthcare access and outcomes continue to persist in low-resource settings both within higher-income countries and more broadly throughout low- and middle-income countries (LMICs) where barriers to care are compounded by factors such as insufficient healthcare infrastructure, limited healthcare personnel, widespread poverty, and low levels of education and literacy. Additional burdens include challenges related to food insecurity and inadequate housing, which further exacerbate the health consequences of these factors (Williams et al., 2021). In higher-income countries, ongoing issues of rural access to high-quality care persist. For example, while telemedicine and remote patient monitoring offer promise in bridging gaps in rural care, factors such as limited broadband internet infrastructure and low digital literacy remain significant obstacles (N. Harrington et al., 2021). Successes in delivering care to patients in under-served and outlying communities often rest in the hands of rural providers and their ability to manage patients beyond common standards of care.

5.1. Characteristics of Low-Resource Settings

Low-resource settings, which include rural areas and impoverished slums, confront significant and multifaceted barriers to accessing essential healthcare services. These barriers encompass a wide range of challenges, including limitations in the quality of care provided, availability of necessary healthcare resources, and the overall affordability of services offered. As individuals progress in age, these inherent challenges become even more pronounced, particularly for older adults who reside in such regions. These senior individuals encounter substantial difficulties in securing the appropriate geriatric care and necessary support systems, which are crucial to their overall well-being and health maintenance.

Recognizing the unique obstacles they face is vital. Therefore, the design and implementation of culturally relevant and effective AI solutions, specifically tailored for this vulnerable population, necessitate a comprehensive examination of the common and prevalent characteristics existing within low-resource contexts. Additionally, it is of utmost importance to develop targeted strategies aiming to bridge the enduring cultural gaps that continue to hinder healthcare access and utilization for older adults in these underserved and often forgotten areas. This approach can ensure that the peculiar needs of these communities are respected and met, leading to improved health outcomes.

5.2. Barriers to Healthcare Access

Although it is true that much of the elders live in low-resource places, there are vast differences among them, ranging from the cities of Africa to the open fields of South America, passing by the United States or China. Although some of the problems appear the same at first sight, like being unable to access a good doctor when one is sick, or feeling lonesome, they have very different roots and ways to be fixed. In contrast to that, Artificial Intelligence (AI) can be used for scaling personalized healthcare services, adapting to the needs and culture of each person.

Addressing the need for personalized medical assistance in these circumstances is exceedingly difficult. Physicians might be scarce, differently specialized, and sometimes even not qualified enough to address some specific emergent needs of these people. Aside from cultural, temporal, spatial, or financial limitations on health assistance, elders also face deficiencies in their daily routine. A great number of elderly people experience feelings of loneliness, which must be treated differently according to culture and personality because a loss of empathy perpetrates their condition and makes the situation worse.

6. INTEGRATING AI IN GERIATRIC CARE

Most societies face a rapid growth in their older adult population. At the same time, many elders face a series of barriers to accessing quality healthcare services, such as geographical location, poverty, and a low level of education, among others. As a result, these barriers create a large gap between geriatric care needs and service delivery. It is argued here that culturally relevant AI strategies in geriatric care can help bridge this gap, thus contributing to optimizing health services and improving quality of life (Sankaran, A., & Singla, M. P., 2024).

Attention is focused on the challenge of integrating culturally relevant AI into geriatric care in low-resource settings. First, the existing geriatric care needs are assessed, then the role of AI in addressing those needs is outlined, and finally an approach for defining culturally relevant AI is proposed. Key barriers to implementing culturally relevant AI solutions that support active and healthy ageing are then identified. A review of a proposed culturally relevant AI framework is used as a starting point for further elaboration, focusing on policies, security, funding, and business strategies. Several existing AI platforms are assessed to illustrate how the proposed strategies can be applied. These platforms address issues of active and healthy ageing in general, as well as specific issues related to mental health and loneliness in particular.

6.1. Assessing Needs in Low-Resource Settings

Various cultural groups often exhibit unique needs that require consideration when constructing solutions for low-resource populations. It is necessary to evaluate fairly specific cultural and technological requirements in alignment with local stakeholders and expert knowledge (Harrington, C. N., et al., 2021).

The probability of requiring medical intervention in old age is significantly higher than in younger populations (Golden, 2023). Attempts to meet such needs in low-resource settings demand solutions that routinely ameliorate elder care consistent with socially acceptable practices. Cultural-matching AI features can be crafted to satisfy basic necessities within aging and facilitate functional and higher-level activities. Well-constructed implementations hold promise for providing scalable support without necessitating direct human oversight, a seldom-available resource in underserved regions.

6.2. Developing Culturally Relevant AI Solutions

AI stands to address several issues in the delivery of culturally relevant care to elderly persons—in providing information, in communicating, in monitoring, in maintaining engagement and mental activity, and in providing enhanced care. Existing studies of models relating to the experiences of older persons have informed this perspective and provide a useful context for analysis.

From a community health perspective, improved information has the potential to reduce over-consumption of health resources, with consequent indirect benefits to society. An elderly person needing to know whether an illness is serious enough to warrant a visit to a health centre, for example, may be able to address this question through an AI interface providing advice only rather than turning up to a busy and expensive appointment. Healthcare providers may themselves find more effective information provision useful. Community COVID-19 programs globally have employed AI to assist with transportation, contactless purchases, translation apps, and especially symptom monitoring on mobile phones. Premi et al. (2021) identified four core challenges for AI and ICT in low-resource settings: power supply, data privacy and protection, technological design and deployment, and fragmentation of AI initiatives, and suggested ways to address these through collaboration and multi-sector participation at national and community levels (Williamson, S. M., & Prybutok, V., 2024).

Appropriate AI approaches can define language grammars and acoustic models, provide real-time interpretation, and assist communication between doctors and patients who do not share a language. Audio processing tools provide vital supports for the visually impaired and those with limited literacy. AI systems can evaluate data and highlight dangerous deviations; provide ongoing monitoring of mental health and well-being through an analysis of mood and choice of words; maintain mental acuity by engaging users in mentally stimulating games; and through physical monitoring can detect trips, falls, and accidents, as well as provide guides for strength enhancement, nutritional advice, and so on. AI mental health tools have supported the elderly during COVID lockdowns, demonstrating usefulness in low-resource settings. Continuous monitoring can generate considerable benefits in care homes and for those living alone. Internet-based technologies, enabled by AI, provide continual access to care providers and can integrate with electronic health records and help best allocate staffing and budgets (Williams et al., 2021).

7. CASE STUDIES

Case studies offer valuable insights by examining specific instances of applications that have succeeded and also those that have failed in providing access to essential healthcare services. For example, Samarasinghe et al. present a critical review and four case studies to illustrate how artificial intelligence (AI) can improve healthcare access and mitigate inequalities, especially in low-resource environments. Effective interventions address humanity's basic needs: food, water, shelter, and healthcare. An understanding of the social and political context in which assistance is deployed is critical to ensure interventions provide long-term benefits. In a review of 35 research papers published between 2010 and 2019, find that AI applications in psychological disorder, eye disease, and other areas, all of which affect a large share of the geriatric population, can help improve geriatric care in many chronic medical conditions (Choudhury et al., 2021).

Case Study 1:

Voice-Based AI in Rural India A pilot project initiated in rural Maharashtra introduced an innovative voice-activated AI health assistant specifically designed to communicate in Marathi, a language spoken widely in the region. This assistant was especially tailored for older adults living in these areas who often faced challenges due to low literacy levels. The tool proved to be highly beneficial by providing essential reminders for medication, offering valuable dietary advice, and facilitating direct access to local health workers who could assist them. The project's success was closely linked to the strategic choice of using familiar dialects that resonated with the users, alongside the important involvement of local community leaders throughout the development process. This approach ensured that the needs and preferences of the target demographic were respected and addressed. The elderly users of this system exhibited a significant rise in engagement, resulting in a notable decrease of missed medication doses by an impressive 40%.

Case Study 2:

Tablet-Assisted Screening in Sub-Saharan Africa In a low-income clinic located in Uganda, health workers implemented an innovative approach by using AI-enabled tablets to conduct cognitive screening for older patients. The user-friendly interface was designed to incorporate local languages, making it accessible to a wider range of individuals, and featured culturally relevant images that resonated with the patients' everyday experiences. Additionally, family members were actively included in the process to offer support and assistance to the older users, fostering a collaborative environment for screening. Consequently, this methodology facilitated a substantial enhancement in the early identification of cognitive decline, achieving an impressive 60% increase. In addition, the duration required to perform each screening was notably decreased by 30%, thereby enabling healthcare professionals to support a greater number of patients necessitating assistance within the allotted time. This initiative not only underscored the capacity of technology to transform healthcare but also accentuated the significance of community involvement and cultural appropriateness in medical practices throughout Sub-Saharan Africa (Sidiropoulos S., et al., 2025).

Case Study 3:

Messaging AI in Indigenous Australia A culturally adapted chatbot was carefully developed specifically for remote Indigenous communities to support elderly patients who are living with chronic health conditions (Gillard, A. K.,et al., 2025). The messages that the chatbot delivered were co-designed in collaboration with local elders, ensuring cultural relevance, and these messages were translated into various local languages to enhance understanding. The delivery method chosen for these messages was SMS, primarily due to the significantly poor internet access in these communities. There was a significant enhancement in the adherence to scheduled appointments among the patients, as they exhibited a greater propensity to attend their medical engagements owing to these initiatives. Furthermore, an increase in the trust placed in digital health instruments was reported, signifying a favorable change in the perception of technology within these communities.

7.1. Successful Implementations

Examples of successful AI implementations in geriatric care demonstrate how the technology can enhance safety, efficiency and analog–digital balance. In Denmark, a digital system for care integration supports discharge and transitional care for elderly nursing-home residents, a vulnerable group facing frequent hospitalizations. Discharge processes require careful planning and involve information exchange not only between hospital professionals but also among nursing-home staff (Mannella, et al., 2023). The system attempts to streamline communication and foster cross-sector collaboration before development began in 2016. A user-centered evaluation identified six challenges and suggested four AI-based improvements: a ranking algorithm for documentation prioritization; filtering techniques to highlight clinically relevant information; AI-generated follow-up questions to address ambiguous details; and the automation of a discharge-monitoring 'time-out' checklist. All four solutions are conceptually feasible given the data, and the scholarly study provides a framework for user-driven co-development of AI in complex healthcare domains although the AI components themselves are yet to be implemented (Schneider-Kamp, 2021).

In low and middle income countries, a more general discussion of AI applications in low-resource settings emphasizes iterative, field-based processes integrated into existing clinical workflows rather than attempts to create novel systems from scratch. The paper highlights four key risks that apply more widely. Ground-truth data are dependent on high-quality, expert-labelled input, often scarce in low-resource settings, and insufficient variation in labeling can lead to under-specified models.

Generalizability is compromised when datasets have different characteristics, as heterogeneity can be high between geographic regions. Ownership and confidentiality are crucial; data collection and storage must be governed by clear ethical standards that support transparent consent and permit audit of data use. Most important is localization, meaning socio-environmental and organisational characteristics need to be woven into solutions before deployment, which requires collaboration with local stakeholders who can recommend adaptations and shepherd implementation. Consequent recommendations are to map stakeholder structures, set realistic and clearly communicated objectives, and openly maintain strategic and operational transparency throughout to mitigate risks and maximize benefits (Williams et al., 2021).

7.2. Lessons Learned from Failures

Identifying factors that cause artificial intelligence (AI) interventions in geriatric care to be inapplicable from one cultural or technical context to another facilitates the development of more culturally relevant systems for low-resource settings (Williams et al., 2021). Care for the ageing population is a major societal challenge. Elderly citizens who live in nursing homes tend to be hospitalized frequently, putting them into cycles of readmissions and discharges. The discharge process from hospital to nursing home is complex, demanding careful planning for care integration.

Communication problems and interruptions between medical and nursing staff as well as hospitals and nursing homes often cause poor-quality care integration and unsafe processes, both of which create patient risk (Schneider-Kamp, 2021). Digital health information-exchange systems increasingly support care integration. However, heavy workloads and other obstacles frequently prevent these systems from meeting user needs and realising their potential (Owoyemi et al., 2020). In turn, current digital health information-exchange systems do not ensure safe, smooth, and transparent transitions, in particular for frail and vulnerable elderly citizens.

A qualitative study of the user experiences of a digital health information-exchange system for care integration of elderly citizens in Denmark was conducted to understand the current system and explore the potential of AI to optimise it. The study was conducted in collaboration with health researchers, AI experts, and software engineers. Six systemic challenges and four overarching principles for AI-based enhancements that correspond to distinct degrees of automation were identified (Efthymiou, I., 2024). The findings demonstrate a new role for qualitative health research beyond the design of AI, offering a basis that facilitates user-driven co-development of AI for care optimization (Schneider-Kamp, 2021).

8. ETHICAL CONSIDERATIONS

Ethical considerations emerge as a pivotal aspect of deploying culturally relevant AI strategies in geriatric care within low-resource settings. The integration of novel healthcare technologies invariably generates social and ethical challenges that extend beyond the realm of technical efficacy (Livieri, G., et al., 2024; Spiegel et al., 2021). The distribution of benefits may become disrupted, with perceptions of inequity differing widely among stakeholders—a circumstance that can have particularly deleterious effects in low-income contexts characterized by entrenched power disparities. Acknowledgement of these concerns alongside the anticipated benefits is therefore vital for the optimisation of AI-based interventions

Data representativeness constitutes a central issue. To avoid the marginalisation of outliers and under-represented groups, research efforts should limit the disproportionate inclusion of data from dominant populations and actively engage ethicists, affected communities, and individuals throughout the development process (Sallstrom et al., 2019). Steps are underway to tailor AI algorithms more closely to the specific disease manifestations observed within the populations concerned. Concurrently, applications in imaging, diagnosis, risk analysis, and health information management are gaining ground and promise to curtail costs and inefficiencies to a significant degree (Ahsan et al., 2022).

Efforts to address underlying social injustices may thus provide additional incentives for AI adoption. Yet, transparency remains an indispensable requirement: clarity is needed with respect to data provenance, the presence of biases, the allocation of responsibility for decision-making, and the question of ownership. Following Floridi et al., explicability should be regarded as an important principle in its own right (Floridi et al., 2018). Mechanisms must be established to communicate the functioning of AI systems in accessible terms, to delineate the boundaries and conditions of their operation, and to specify the locus of accountability (Mennella et al., 2024). In this manner, the resulting solutions can reflect concerns voiced by stakeholders and uphold broader considerations of social justice (Ibeneme et al., 2021).

The ethical domain is also shaped in important ways by the perspectives of caregivers and professional stakeholders, which are particularly relevant to the successful uptake and sustained operation of AI and assistive technologies (Thaldar, D., & Naidoo, M., 2021). A study of dementia caregivers, for example, underscores the salience of ethical issues and highlights their role as guideposts for responsible design and implementation at scale (Alexopoulos, P., et al., 2025; Wang et al., 2023). Likewise, professional participants view ethical matters as a key dimension of the transition from laboratory innovation to practical deployment. Issues of machine intelligence, the collection of sensitive data, and operation in close proximity to the human body all warrant careful consideration in relation to the support of vulnerable older adults afflicted with dementia or other age-related disabilities (Wangmo et al., 2019).

The concomitant social policy environment further accentuates the imperative for sustained engagement, as witnessed in the formulation of healthcare and social services that dovetail with research-derived insights in order to meet the pressing needs of older adults living alone and those with cognitive impairments. The formulation of policy priorities and the identification of actionable solutions may nevertheless founder without regular interaction between researchers and policymakers. Close collaboration thus constitutes a critical enabling condition, particularly in respect of an emphasis on diverse communities and broader questions of equity (Townsend et al., 2023).

8.1. Privacy and Data Security

Concerns surrounding privacy and data security emerge as major obstacles to the development and adoption of AI technologies for healthcare in general and even more so for long-term care (Kouroupis, K., 2021; Murdoch, 2021). Exposure of personal health information to non-healthcare organizations constitutes a substantial infringement on dignity and human rights as well as risks discrimination and stigmatization (Bak et al., 2022). For AI to be acceptable, there must be safeguards that ensure the protection of sensitive information, that maintain the users' agency over their data, and that clearly regulate the handling of such data by AI subcontractors (Sihlahla et al., 2025).

Several major risks have been identified. Use of deidentified data does not constitute a sufficient safeguard since new algorithms could conceivably reidentify patients when the datasets are held in private hands (Bak et al., 2022). Once the data loses its protected status, there is an incentive to use it for purposes such as targeted advertising or health insurance decisions, especially since datasets cannot be forgotten or recalled (Sotiropoulos, L. D., 2023; Murdoch, 2021). In cases where organizations hold aggregated data on large populations, identification—even of anonymized datasets, may become far easier. Secure data infrastructure on the other hand remains essential to prevent privacy breaches, but regulations allowing for exceptional exfiltration by public authorities pose concerns (Kouroupis, K., & Serotila, I., 2022; Bak et al., 2022). While AI could be leveraged to improve and sustain the long-term care sector, the collection of training data for such systems is necessary and privacy safeguards are mandated (Naidoo et al., 2022).

8.2. Bias and Fairness in AI

Bias and fairness are critical ethical considerations in the deployment of AI-based geriatric care (van Kolfschooten, 2022). Several stages of the AI cycle present opportunities for the introduction of prejudice. Biased variables or proxies may be encoded in a model; health factors such as digital literacy and access—key dimensions shaping health and well-being—vary by age and influence outcomes; and ageist practices reflected in the research data, policies, and social contexts surrounding older adults contribute to representation bias (Palaniappan et al., 2024). Measurement bias arises from inaccuracies, noise, or mislabeling in the data, such as recruitment challenges, cohort effects, or the reliance on instrument variables (Jogi, 2022).

Modelling bias may result from the deliberate or inadvertent programming of age-related biases through proxies like age itself and factors correlated with age and treatment preferences—disparate-use bias. Bias in AI-based medical devices extends beyond training and validation datasets, originating from other sources (Rubeis et al., 2022). During application, AI systems may reinforce, perpetuate, or exacerbate ageist dynamics, particularly when deployed at scale in low-resource settings. Systemic bias—manifest in institutional practices within societal, political, and economic structures—prioritizes the interests of some social groups over others, erecting barriers to access and full participation in health care services.

1.Data Representation Bias in AI

A significant percentage of current AI systems are predominantly trained on datasets sourced from wealthy, urban populations. This specific focus leads to a notable bias in both predictions and recommendations, thereby diminishing their accuracy and effectiveness for older adults residing in under-resourced, culturally diverse regions (Ncube et al., 2022). To foster equity in AI technologies, it is essential to develop and utilize inclusive datasets that accurately reflect local health conditions, a range of languages, and the unique social norms inherent to these communities. This strategy will improve the relevance and applicability of AI in various contexts, ultimately contributing to enhanced health outcomes and greater equity (Ibeneme et al., 2021).

2. Language and Communication Bias in AI

Tools often tend to exclude and overlook non-dominant languages or dialects, which inadvertently reinforces and perpetuates systemic barriers in society. This exclusion has significant implications, especially in geriatric care, where it marginalizes older adults who may already experience difficulties with digital literacy (Sallstrom et al., 2019). As a result, their access to essential services is further limited. To ensure that systems truly support all users, it is critical that they accommodate local languages and diverse communication styles (Owoyemi et al., 2020). By doing so, we can work towards treating every user fairly and equally, ultimately bridging the gap created by linguistic and cultural differences (Tran et al., 2019).

3. Cultural Assumption Bias in AI Systems

Many artificial intelligence systems, particularly those developed for use in healthcare, tend to embed and reflect the underlying assumptions that originate from established Western healthcare norms and practices. This tendency can lead to significant mismatches and disparities in the care practices that are offered to populations, particularly within culturally diverse communities (Choudhury et al., 2021). These communities frequently possess varying and distinct perspectives on critical issues such as ageing, caregiving, and health beliefs, which may diverge widely from the frameworks and models typically seen in Western settings. To achieve fair and effective applications of AI technology, it becomes essential that such systems not only acknowledge but also actively adapt to the myriad of local customs and practices that exist (Townsend et al., 2023).

Furthermore, it is crucial to incorporate community input and perspectives throughout the design, development, and deployment phases of these AI systems

(Efthymiou, I.-P., 2020). This approach is vital for ensuring that the AI systems are capable of catering effectively to the diverse and unique needs of each specific community they are designed to serve, ultimately fostering a more inclusive and equitable healthcare environment.

9. POLICY IMPLICATIONS

Regulatory and policy frameworks play an essential and significant role in enabling not only the successful but also the sustainable operation and implementation of AI solutions tailored specifically for culturally relevant geriatric care, especially in low-resource settings. It is crucial for governments to establish comprehensive regulatory processes for AI technologies that rigorously and thoughtfully address pertinent ethical and social issues while still allowing for the rapid application and utilization of promising innovations that arise in the field (Naidoo et al., 2022).

Furthermore, policies should be designed to ensure that AI-enabled services remain reasonably affordable and accessible, possibly through innovative public-private partnerships, particularly considering that the elderly population often has limited financial resources (Townsend et al., 2023). This aspect is vitally important for encouraging widespread adoption of beneficial technologies.

Additionally, funding agencies ought to actively support interdisciplinary research initiatives that not only iteratively evaluate AI systems in real-world conditions but also emphasize collaboration among a diverse group of professionals including engineers, gerontologists, and healthcare professionals (Harrington, C. N., et al., 2021). This type of integrative research collaboration is indispensable for the development of effective, context-sensitive, and user-friendly AI solutions that truly cater to the needs of elderly individuals in varying contexts. By fostering such collaborations and ensuring equitable access to these technologies, we can enhance the quality of geriatric care in underserved communities (Owoyemi et al., 2020).

9.1. Regulatory Frameworks

The rapid advancement of artificial intelligence (AI) technologies has introduced new regulatory and ethical challenges for healthcare, despite the routine presence of several approved AI-based systems in clinical environments (Ahsan et al., 2022). For AI-driven healthcare applications to attain wide adoption, they must address concerns regarding patient safety, fairness, privacy, and transparency (Mennella et al., 2024). Healthcare systems, particularly in low-resource settings, are often governed by comprehensive industry regulations on safety and quality (Xesfingi, S., & Vozikis, A., 2014; van Kolfschooten, 2022).

In South Africa, legislative frameworks mandate that the development and deployment of AI in healthcare are planned, designed, procured, and implemented in a regulated manner in order to comply with existing laws and regulations and address risks inherent to AI technologies (Naidoo et al., 2022).

Regulatory frameworks play a pivotal role in enabling two essential objectives:

Defining with clarity what constitutes the safe, responsible, and ethical development as well as application of AI technologies is crucial. It involves establishing guidelines that ensure these intelligent systems operate within the boundaries of societal norms and legal frameworks (Sihlahla et al., 2025). This also includes distinguishing carefully between licit and illicit behaviours that can occur during both the design and operational phases of AI technologies, ensuring that all practices align with ethical standards and promote the welfare of individuals and communities (Donnelly, D. L., 2022).

Regulatory organisations and national bodies further support these objectives by issuing guidance on public policy and government actions (Mennella et al., 2024). While AI development in healthcare entails substantial ethical and social implications beyond the realm of regulation, establishing sustainability for AI technologies depends on compliance with regulatory requirements (Palaniappan et al., 2024).

9.2. Funding and Resource Allocation

Substantial investment is absolutely critical and urgently needed to bolster and support the extensive array of AI research, development, and deployment endeavors that are essential to effectively meet the ever-growing demand for skilled AI talent in various sectors and industries (Williams et al., 2021). In low-resource settings, funding priorities can vary widely among governments, not only within the same country but also between different countries, leading to significant disparities in available funding and resources. Due to these variances, externally sourced funding frequently becomes the primary and often sole source of investment in these regions, making it vital for various stakeholders to come together (Ibeneme et al., 2021). As a result, there is a pressing need for multi-stakeholder collaboration, along with strategic resource allocation, to be optimized effectively. This optimization is not just vital but imperative to avoid fragmented efforts that fail to deliver impactful and meaningful results.

It is essential to reduce duplication of resources and initiatives, which can waste valuable time and effort, and significantly enhance the likelihood of achieving rapid and successful outcomes in the crucial and rapidly evolving field of AI, which is poised to transform countless aspects of society and industry (Tran et al., 2019).

10. FUTURE DIRECTIONS

Emerging technologies such as multi-modal conversational agents have demonstrated significant effectiveness across diverse populations, thereby fostering improved social engagement and enhancing functional autonomy among users (Rubeis et al., 2022). Additionally, enabling older adults to have greater control over AI-driven smart home environments may drastically enhance their quality of life, substantially reduce feelings of anxiety, and provide robust support for health monitoring.

The incorporation and integration of such innovative technologies warrant thorough exploration through field-based, iterative research processes, particularly within low-income communities where the impact could be even more pronounced (Williams et al., 2021). Further investigation into effective strategies for developing culturally relevant AI can provide critical insights that would greatly support geriatric care initiatives, especially in resource-constrained environments that often lack access to advanced technological solutions (Owoyemi et al., 2020; Ibeneme et al., 2021).

1.Community-Led AI Co-Design

Future systems and advanced technologies need to be thoughtfully developed with substantial and meaningful input from older adults, their caregivers, and local health workers who are familiar with the needs of these populations. Involving these crucial stakeholders in the design and development process guarantees that their distinct perspectives, as well as their specific needs, are meticulously considered and incorporated (Panahi, O., 2025). The co-design approach not only mitigates the potential for cultural mismatches between technology and its users but also substantially enhances the likelihood of successful user adoption and overall satisfaction with the final product (McIlduff et al., 2022). By placing a strong emphasis on collaboration and active engagement with these communities, we can create innovative solutions that genuinely match and resonate with the individuals and communities they are intended to serve (Choudhury et al., 2021). In this way, we ensure that technology becomes a true ally for older adults, enriching their lives and addressing their genuine needs effectively (Sallstrom et al., 2019).

2. Open-Source, Low-Bandwidth Solutions

Open-source, low-bandwidth solutions are essential and must be meticulously designed to be not only lightweight but also offline-capable and freely available to everyone without exception (Diareme, K. C., et al., 2022). Such an inclusive approach directly addresses the numerous infrastructure limitations that are commonly faced by diverse users across different regions and allows for significant local adaptation in various environments and contexts without incurring excessively high costs (Owoyemi et al., 2020). By ensuring that these vital tools are readily accessible and straightforward to modify, we empower communities in unique ways to effectively overcome and navigate technological barriers that may otherwise hinder their progress and development. This empowerment is crucial for fostering innovation and facilitating more robust technological growth at the community level.

3. Ethical Oversight and Local Governance

Establishing local review bodies that actively monitor bias, fairness, and overall cultural fit within the community will be essential for promoting trust, transparency, and accountability (Vousinas, G. L., et al., 2022). These oversight bodies should be made up of experienced geriatric experts, highly knowledgeable ethicists, and diverse community representatives to ensure that comprehensive perspectives are well considered (Sihlahla et al., 2025). Their collective insights will be invaluable in addressing potential issues that could arise while fostering a more inclusive decision-making process. By engaging a wide range of voices and viewpoints, these bodies will not only enhance the ethical standards but also improve community relations, making sure that all decisions reflect the values and needs of the entire community (McIlduff et al., 2022). This deeper engagement with various stakeholders will lead to better outcomes and greater acceptance of decisions made (Sallstrom et al., 2019).

10.1. Emerging Technologies

The extensive care needs of older adults heavily rely on social support. Informed by the frameworks on contemporary geriatric care and the depth of relevant literature, a vision for culturally tailor-made AI applications emerges toward the goal of facilitating independent aging in low-resource settings. As an essential context, emerging technologies that can heighten technological access must therefore be prioritized. Technologies such as extended reality, voice, wearables, remote sensors, and the Internet of Things exemplify the emerging possibilities (Efthymiou, I. P., & Efthymiou Egleton, T. W., 2023).

Extended reality combines enhanced sensing of environmental and personal information with unobtrusive feedback on physical, cognitive, or social activities. Application-focused designs can, for example, nurture a sense of presence through augmented telepresence, utilize avatars to enrich social intervention, and harness artificial intelligence to create virtually synchronous environments (Rubeis et al., 2022). At a societal level, telecommunication networks, social media, and platforms facilitate social connectedness and networking through virtual support groups, allowing safe distancing yet persistent connection during pandemics (Ahsan et al., 2022).

Voice-activated devices offer opportunities due to their pervasiveness, low learning curve, and hands-free operation. In older adults and caregivers, efficacy has been demonstrated across a spectrum of issues ranging from reminiscence therapy to household management to loneliness applications (Panahi, O., 2025). The research community should investigate better supportive mechanisms for context, intent, and even conversational initiative, mindful of various privacy and trust concerns that arise .

Wearables and remote sensors enable objective, continuous, and pervasive monitoring of biological, physiological, behavioral, and environmental signals to capture early warnings of emergent conditions (e.g., sepsis, pulmonary events) and integrate them with medical records for comprehensive longitudinal trends and patient risk-pattern analyses (Ncube et al., 2022). In certain contexts and particular care needs where elder monitoring is necessary, emerging small, inexpensive wireless sensors can be cost-effective compared with costly medical appliances.

Envisioned long-term care scenarios, where caregivers blend on-site visits with remote support, can be supported through unobtrusive sensing, video streaming, and personalized and context-aware online content repositories (Ahsan et al., 2022). As the Internet of Things revolution continues, all parties must balance the demand for utility with the need for privacy, remain vigilant against emerging vulnerabilities and long-term data decay, and negotiate the boundaries of artificial intelligence under allied societal models.

10.2. Research Opportunities

There is an increasingly significant opportunity for innovative and novel research to address a wide range of sociocultural, environmental, and agricultural challenges that are becoming more pressing in today's world. Given the ambitious aim to make artificial intelligence more culturally relevant and applicable to diverse populations, several key opportunities emerge for AI researchers and scholars to extensively explore (Choudhury et al., 2021). These potential avenues include creating new, robust evaluation methodologies that can better account for cultural contexts, developing a heightened awareness of the various cultural differences that exist in a highly globalized context, devising effective trust-building strategies designed for diverse cultural and environmental settings, and fostering stronger and more dynamic interdisciplinary collaborations across fields (Efthymiou, I. P., & Efthymiou Egleton, T. W., 2023; Sallstrom et al., 2019). By fully embracing and prioritizing these important research avenues, the field of artificial intelligence can make significant strides toward delivering AI systems that are not only sensitive to cultural nuances but also adept at navigating the various resource constraints faced by different communities around the world.

11. RECOMMENDATIONS

Developing culturally relevant AI for geriatric care is not just important; it's essential for effectively closing the significant gap in quality of care that older adults receive in low-resource settings. There are four strategic approaches that can significantly help in building stakeholder buy-in, which will ultimately lead to successful implementation of these necessary initiatives.

First and foremost, it's vital that international funding agencies make a deliberate choice to earmark resources specifically for AI solutions that are designed to meet and address the intricate cultural expectations and needs of the elderly population (Lindeberg, J.,et al., 2023). This proactive approach will stimulate a greater volume of production and focus on the middle phase of the AI pipeline crucially needed to tailor effective solutions.

Secondly, the principle of human-centred design must be the driving force behind AI development, ensuring that the tools created are user-friendly and genuinely responsive to the needs of the elderly. Thirdly, it is imperative that AI technologies are fully embedded within established community care pathways. Local organisations should be actively involved right from the initial stages prior to implementation to co-design governance frameworks; if this does not happen, the essential elements of acceptance, trust, and subsequently the effective use of the technology are unlikely to be realized.

Lastly, a collaborative effort among donors, universities, and international organizations is essential to provide both the resources and comprehensive training necessary for gerontologists in the field of AI. This training is crucial for equipping them with the skills required to lead the specification of cultural requirements and effectively interpret AI outcomes in varying contexts. Involving gerontologists early in the process, alongside members of local communities, proves to be a critical factor in the development of solutions that genuinely create a positive impact on geriatric.

11.1. Strategies for Implementation

Developing culturally relevant AI for geriatric care is not just important; it's essential for effectively closing the significant gap in quality of care that older adults receive in low-resource settings. There are four strategic approaches that can significantly help in building stakeholder buy-in, which will ultimately lead to successful implementation of these necessary initiatives.

First and foremost, it's vital that international funding agencies make a deliberate choice to earmark resources specifically for AI solutions that are designed to meet and address the intricate cultural expectations and needs of the elderly population.

This proactive approach will stimulate a greater volume of production and focus on the middle phase of the AI pipeline crucially needed to tailor effective solutions.

Secondly, the principle of human-centred design must be the driving force behind AI development, ensuring that the tools created are user-friendly and genuinely responsive to the needs of the elderly (Choudhury et al., 2021). Thirdly, it is imperative that AI technologies are fully embedded within established community care pathways. Local organisations should be actively involved right from the initial stages prior to implementation to co-design governance frameworks; if this does not happen, the essential elements of acceptance, trust, and subsequently the effective use of the technology are unlikely to be realized.

Lastly, a collaborative effort among donors, universities, and international organizations is essential to provide both the resources and comprehensive training necessary for gerontologists in the field of AI. This training is crucial for equipping them with the skills required to lead the specification of cultural requirements and effectively interpret AI outcomes in varying contexts. Involving gerontologists early in the process, alongside members of local communities, proves to be a critical factor in the development of solutions that genuinely create a positive impact on geriatric care.

11.1. Strategies for Implementation

Health systems in low- and medium-income countries often struggle to provide geriatric care. As a result, older adults in these areas typically cannot access the specialized services or coverage that characterizes geriatric programs in wealthier countries. Tailoring artificial intelligence (AI) for elderly care in such contexts is therefore a priority, recognizing numerous cultural, infrastructural and economic variations across nations. To this end, culturally relevant AI is necessary. A principal implication of this strategy is that social and economic data would be as important as health data, since the former would be vital for mitigating cultural biases in the algorithm design (Efthymiou, I., 2025). Intuitively, few decisions should be taken by absorbed in AI that cannot be explained to users. A strong commitment to local involvement is also crucial, implying not only co-design but also training of local actors (Williams et al., 2021).

Extending the use of AI to geriatric care has the potential to improve both the quality and cost-effectiveness of services, fostering respect for individuals' specific needs and thus enhancing all dimensions of care. Applicable tools range, for instance, from conversational agents for mental health follow-up to computer vision and augmentation for robotic patient transfers. Besides linguistic variety, contributions should consider societal and economic characteristics at multiple levels, from multinational to communal—along with the ongoing cultural shift toward digitization.

Indeed, ignoring culture might generate significant risks in the relationship between medical assistant and patient. For example, anxiety stemming from digitization trends, already apparent among younger generations in certain countries, might be compounded by the dual presence of demographic and cultural barriers.

The numerous services covered by AI at different life stages illustrate this dynamic. That said, the cultural relevance of AI systems raises equally (if not more) important questions in the geriatric domain, where social structure and ties strongly influence decisions and acceptance of assistance measures. Section 11.1 recommends strategies tailored to low-resource settings, all the while aligning with initiatives taken in more developed nations. Nevertheless, a detailed feasibility study remains a prerequisite, especially at the local level.

1. **Integrate Local Language Development.** Develop intelligent AI interfaces that function efficiently in local languages and various dialects, leveraging advanced voice recognition and visual communication tools. These technologies are designed to suit individuals with low literacy levels, ensuring accessibility for all users.
2. **Partnerships with Community Health Workers.** Train local health workers effectively to utilize advanced AI tools, acting as intermediaries between technology and the community, thereby fostering trust and bridging the critical digital gaps that often exist in healthcare access (Williams et al., 2021).
3. **Modular and Scalable Design** allows for the efficient construction of AI systems that can be easily scaled or adapted to suit various cultural and infrastructural contexts. This flexibility ensures that the AI systems can meet diverse requirements effectively.
4. **Pilot Testing with Community Feedback.** Engage in small-scale pilot projects to gather invaluable direct user feedback and refine the system thoroughly before proceeding with broader deployment efforts to ensure overall effectiveness and user satisfaction.

11.2. Engaging Stakeholders

Community engagement is essential in rounding out the interdisciplinary gaps in addressing elderly individuals' needs. Inclusive decision-making invites a wide array of expertise, capacities, and perspectives, making for a more well-rounded understanding of elderly care (McIlduff et al., 2022). Engagement also helps foster ongoing commitment among participants and stakeholders, while obviating the cultural blind spots that may arise when involving only a subset of experts on aging. Community engagement is particularly important in culturally relevant decision-making, because it can support coalition-building that translates into long-term capacity for addressing local challenges while imparting a sense of ownership regarding the initiative. Engaging stakeholders also constitutes a diverse platform for bottom-up solutions that may better interface with the day-to-day realities of care.

AI design for low-resource settings has also yet to fully realize participatory approaches, particularly in geriatric care; understanding elderly individuals' multifaceted needs remains a prerequisite to the alignment of design priorities with their goals and aspirations. Engaging a broad cross-section of actors (including policymakers, care providers, researchers, and elderly individuals themselves) fashions culturally relevant AI strategies that bridge the societal gap between vulnerable populations and service providers.

Notwithstanding mixed-income and age demographic distributions confronted across care-provision and service-design settings, participatory and community-based methodologies are critical to understanding the care and support needs of elderly individuals (McIlduff et al., 2022). Given the lack of dedicated infrastructures and training in such settings, integrating these approaches with technology-transfer and knowledge-exchange initiatives can yield the necessary resources for establishing new healthcare policies and practices across diverse urban and rural profiles.

12. CONCLUSION

Cultural relevance is a crucial concept that is defined as the extent to which a program or a piece of literature demonstrates a keen awareness of and is specifically tailored to the prevailing cultural practices, beliefs, and values of the target population it serves (Efthymiou, I.-P., 2024) . By embedding cultural relevance into technological solutions, it is possible to significantly enhance client confidence, which in turn promotes improved engagement and responsiveness among users. In the pursuit of developing AI tools that are appropriately designed for low-resource settings, several risks and challenges arise. These include the presence of insufficient, poorly labeled, or biased training datasets that can distort outcomes, challenges associated with the generalizability of algorithms across diverse populations, as well as critical issues regarding data ownership and confidentiality that need careful handling.

Furthermore, there is a pressing necessity for the localisation of solutions to meet the specific needs of various socio-cultural environments. Nevertheless, despite these challenges, digital technologies hold the promise of being a potentially transformative solution for low-resource health systems. This transformation is achievable because these technologies can help reduce significant barriers, such as shortages of human capital, the inherent complexity of systems, geographic distances, and the high logistical costs often associated with healthcare provision.

However, it is imperative that these issues are systematically assessed and addressed through ongoing, iterative, and field-based development processes that take into account the unique characteristics of low-resource contexts, rather than relying on top-down implementation strategies that originate in high-resource environments. In the context of chronically underfunded geriatric care and rehabilitation systems, the implementation of AI-based innovations may serve as a cost-effective means to expand access to high-quality services (Efthymiou, I., 2026). Additionally, these innovations can ensure the collection of appropriate data necessary for informed policy-making decisions, while also deepening the understanding of complex care delivery challenges and identifying potential improvements that can enhance overall healthcare services.

REFERENCES

Ahsan, M. M., Luna, S. A., & Siddique, Z. (2022). Machine-learning-based disease diagnosis: A comprehensive review. *Health Care, 10*(3), 541. DOI: 10.3390/healthcare10030541 PMID: 35327018

Alexopoulos, P., Bogati, U., Farombi, T., & Shrestha, P. (2025). Experiences from designing and implementing integrated health and social care systems for aging populations in low-resource settings around the world. *Dementia Care and Provision in the Majority World: Epidemiology, Diagnosis and Care in Low-and Middle-income Nations*, 117.

Diareme, K. C., Liapakis, A., & Efthymiou, I. P. (2022). Big data, sentiment analysis, and examples during the COVID-19 pandemic. *HAPSc Policy Briefs Series, 3*(1). Advance online publication. DOI: 10.12681/hapscpbs.33779

Donnelly, D. L. (2022). First do no harm: legal principles regulating the future of artificial intelligence in health care in South Africa. *Potchefstroom Electronic Law Journal/Potchefstroomse Elektroniese Regsblad, 25*(1).

Efthymiou, I. (2024). Exploring the Frontier: New and Future Trends in Research. In B. Orlando (Ed.), Innovation Capabilities and Entrepreneurial Opportunities of Smart Working (pp. 48-68). IGI Global Scientific Publishing. https://doi.org/DOI: 10.4018/978-1-7998-8797-3.ch003

Efthymiou, I. (2025). The Role of E-Government and E-Governance in Modern Societies. In Wongmahesak, K., Ahmad, J., & Mustanir, A. (Eds.), *Public Governance Practices in the Age of AI* (pp. 45–68). IGI Global Scientific Publishing., DOI: 10.4018/979-8-3693-9286-7.ch003

Efthymiou, I. (2026). AI in Epidemiology: Predicting the Unpredictable Leveraging AI to Detect Outbreaks and Predict Disease. In Umer, M. (Ed.), *Innovation and Transformation of Public Health* (pp. 281–308). IGI Global Scientific Publishing., DOI: 10.4018/979-8-3373-1992-6.ch009

Efthymiou, I.-P. (2020). Non-cognitive skills and AI: A new era of learning and development. *International Case Studies Journal, 9*(10), 42–46.

Efthymiou, I.-P. (2024). Can AI improve health and wellbeing? Case Studies Journal, ISSN (2305-509X), 13(11), 1–5.

Efthymiou, I.-P. (2024). The importance of soft skills in healthcare: The impact of communication, empathy, and teamwork on doctor-nurse interactions. *Case Studies Journal, 13*(11), 6–11.

Efthymiou, I. P., & Efthymiou Egleton, T. W. (2023). Artificial intelligence for sustainable smart cities. In *Handbook of research on applications of AI, digital twin, and internet of things for sustainable development* (pp. 1–11). IGI Global., DOI: 10.4018/978-1-6684-6821-0.ch001

Floridi, L., Cowls, J., Beltrametti, M., Chatila, R., Chazerand, P., Dignum, V., Luetge, C., Madelin, R., Pagallo, U., Rossi, F., Schafer, B., Valcke, P., & Vayena, E. (2018). AI4People—An ethical framework for a good AI society: Opportunities, risks, principles, and recommendations. *Minds and Machines*, *28*(4), 689–707. DOI: 10.1007/s11023-018-9482-5 PMID: 30930541

Gillard, A. K., McNeair, T., Andrew, N. E., Haines, T., Hill, K. D., Moran, C., & Long, K. M. (2025). Multi-stakeholder aged care research networks: A scoping review. *The Gerontologist*, *65*(3), gnae152. PMID: 39478337

Golden, A. (2023). THEORETICAL FRAMEWORK FOR AN ARTIFICIAL INTELLIGENCE–BASED COMPREHENSIVE GERIATRIC ASSESSMENT. *Innovation in Aging*, *7*, 877.

Harrington, C. N., Jelen, B., Lazar, A., Martin-Hammond, A., Pradhan, A., Reeder, B., & Siek, K. (2021). Taking stock of the present and future of smart technologies for older adults and caregivers. *arXiv preprint arXiv:2104.00096.*

Ibeneme, S., Okeibunor, J., Muneene, D., Husain, I., Bento, P., Gaju, C., Housseynou, B., Chibi, M., Karamagi, H., & Makubalo, L. (2021). Data revolution, health status transformation and the role of artificial intelligence for health and pandemic preparedness in the African context. *BMC Proceedings*, *15*(Suppl 15), 22. DOI: 10.1186/s12919-021-00228-1 PMID: 34809624

Jakovljevic, M., Kumagai, N., & Ogura, S. (2023). Global population aging–Health care, social and economic consequences, volume II. *Frontiers in Public Health, 11*, 1184950.s, D., Hornung, H., Nadimpalli, A., & Peery, A. (2021). Deep learning and its application for healthcare delivery in low and middle income countries. *Frontiers in Artificial Intelligence*, *4*, 553987.

Kalusivalingam, A. K., Sharma, A., Patel, N., & Singh, V. (2021). Leveraging federated learning and explainable AI for advancing health equity: A comprehensive approach to reducing disparities in healthcare access and outcomes. *International Journal of Artificial Intelligence and Machine Learning*, *2*(3).

Kouroupis, K. (2021). Facial recognition: a challenge for europe or a threat to human rights?. Eur. J. Privacy L. & Tech., 142.

Kouroupis, K., & Serotila, I. (2022). Privacy and security in light of the European Digital Agenda. Nomiki Bibliothiki, 18-36.

Lindeberg, J., Henkel, M., Perjons, E., Johannesson, P., & Lappalainen, K. F. (2023, April). AI solutions for inter-organisational care: A case based analysis. In *World Conference on Information Systems and Technologies* (pp. 538-549). Cham: Springer Nature Switzerland.

Livieri, G., Anastasopoulou, C., Briola, K., Nikolopoulou, P., & Efthymiou, I.-P. (2024). Ethical issues arising from the use of AI in drug discovery. *Journal of Politics and Ethics in New Technologies and AI*, *3*(1), e37093. Advance online publication. DOI: 10.12681/jpentai.37093

McIlduff, C. D., Acharibasam, J., Starr, V., & Chapados, M. (2022, September). Engaging Indigenous older adults with technology use to respond to health and well-being concerns and needs. [). Sage CA: Los Angeles, CA: SAGE Publications.]. *Healthcare Management Forum*, *35*(5), 257–264. PMID: 35670368

McIlduff, D., Carter, R., & Patel, S. (2022). Stakeholder engagement in geriatric care: Building inclusive healthcare systems. *Journal of Aging & Social Policy*, *34*(2), 178–195. DOI: 10.1080/08959420.2021.1987524

Mennella, C., Maniscalco, U., De Pietro, G., & Esposito, M. (2024). Ethical and regulatory challenges of AI technologies in healthcare: A narrative review. *Heliyon*, *10*(4). PMID: 38384518

Murdoch, B. (2021). Privacy and artificial intelligence: Challenges for protecting health information in a new era. *BMC Medical Ethics*, *22*(1), 122. DOI: 10.1186/s12910-021-00687-3 PMID: 34525993

Naidoo, S., Bottomley, D., Naidoo, M., Donnelly, D., & Thaldar, D. W. (2022). Artificial intelligence in healthcare: Proposals for policy development in South Africa. *South African Journal of Bioethics and Law*, *15*(1), 11–16. DOI: 10.7196/SAJBL.2022.v15i1.797 PMID: 36061984

Ncube, B., Mars, M., & Scott, R. E. (2022). Telemedicine options to address identified health needs in Botswana. *Digital Health*, *8*, 20552076221102768. DOI: 10.1177/20552076221102768 PMID: 35663237

Owoyemi, A., Owoyemi, J., Osiyemi, A., & Boyd, A. (2020). Artificial intelligence for healthcare in Africa. *Frontiers in Digital Health*, *2*, 6. DOI: 10.3389/fdgth.2020.00006 PMID: 34713019

Palaniappan, K., Lin, E. Y. T., Vogel, S., & Lim, J. C. W. (2024). Gaps in the global regulatory frameworks for the use of artificial intelligence (AI) in the healthcare services sector and key recommendations. *Health Care*, *12*(17), 1730. DOI: 10.3390/healthcare12171730 PMID: 39273754

Panahi, O. (2025). Health in the Age of AI: A Family and Community Focus. *Archives of Community and Family Medicine*, *8*(1), 11–20.

Pray, A. (2017). *Cultural Competency in Medical Social Work with Elders* (Doctoral dissertation, University of St. Thomas, Minnesota).

Rubeis, G., Fang, M. L., & Sixsmith, A. (2022). Equity in AgeTech for ageing well in technology-driven places: The role of social determinants in designing AI-based assistive technologies. *Science and Engineering Ethics*, *28*(6), 49. PMID: 36301408

Sallstrom, L., Morris, O., & Mehta, H. (2019). Artificial intelligence in Africa's healthcare: Ethical considerations. *ORF Issue Brief*, *312*, 1–11.

Sankaran, A., & Singla, M. P. (2024). Artificial intelligence in geriatric healthcare: Opportunities and challenges in a transforming landscape. *Frontiers in Health Informatics*, *13*(7), 897–908.

Schneider-Kamp, A. (2021). Health capital: Toward a conceptual framework for understanding the construction of individual health. *Social Theory & Health*, *19*(3), 205–219. PMID: 32837331

Shiwani, T., Relton, S., Evans, R., Kale, A., Heaven, A., Clegg, A., & Todd, O. (2023). New Horizons in artificial intelligence in the healthcare of older people. *Age and Ageing*, *52*(12), afad219. PMID: 38124256

Sidiropoulos, S., Emmanouil-Kalos, A., Chouzouris, M., Xenos, P., & Vozikis, A. (2025). From Aid to Impact: The Cost-Effectiveness of Global Health Aid in Sub-Saharan Africa and the Evolving Role of Microinsurance. *Health Care*, *13*(14), 1716. PMID: 40724741

Sihlahla, I., Donnelly, D. L., Townsend, B., & Thaldar, D. (2025). Legal and ethical principles governing the use of artificial intelligence in radiology services in South Africa. *Developing World Bioethics*, *25*(1), 35–45. PMID: 38009422

Sotiropoulos, L. D. (2023). Addressing Smart Contracts in the Insurance Sector: Institutional Framework and Practical Aspects. *ENTHA*, *20*, 22.

Souliotis, K. (2016, April). Patient participation in contemporary health care: Promoting a versatile patient role. *Health Expectations*, *19*(2), 175–178. DOI: 10.1111/hex.12456 PMID: 26995388

Spiegel, J. M., Ehrlich, R., Yassi, A., Riera, F., Wilkinson, J., Lockhart, K., & Kistnasamy, B. (2021). Using artificial intelligence for high-volume identification of silicosis and tuberculosis: A bio-ethics approach. *Annals of Global Health*, *87*(1), 58. PMID: 34249620

Spiegel, M., van de Loo, M., & van den Berg, E. (2021). Ethical challenges in AI for healthcare: A systematic review. *Journal of Medical Systems*, *45*(12), 108. DOI: 10.1007/s10916-021-01783-4 PMID: 34755231

Thaldar, D., & Naidoo, M. (2021). AI inventorship: The right decision? *South African Journal of Science*, *117*(11/12). Advance online publication. DOI: 10.17159/sajs.2021/12509

Townsend, B. A., Sihlahla, I., Naidoo, M., Naidoo, S., Donnelly, D. L., & Thaldar, D. W. (2023). Mapping the regulatory landscape of AI in healthcare in Africa. *Frontiers in Pharmacology*, *14*, 1214422. DOI: 10.3389/fphar.2023.1214422 PMID: 37693916

Tran, B. X., Vu, G. T., & Ha, G. H.. (2019). Global evolution of research in artificial intelligence in health and medicine: A bibliometric study. *Journal of Clinical Medicine*, *8*(3), 360. DOI: 10.3390/jcm8030360 PMID: 30875745

Van Kolfschooten, H. (2022). EU regulation of artificial intelligence: Challenges for patients' rights. *Common Market Law Review*, *59*(1).

Vousinas, G. L., Simitsi, I., Livieri, G., Gkouva, G. C., & Efthymiou, I. P. (2022). Mapping the road of the ethical dilemmas behind artificial intelligence. *Journal of Politics and Ethics in New Technologies and AI*, *1*(1), e31238. DOI: 10.12681/jpentai.31238

Wang, G., Albayrak, A., Mattace-Raso, F., & van der Cammen, T. J. (2023). Technologies in long-term care and nursing homes. In *Gerontechnology. A Clinical Perspective* (pp. 45–59). Springer International Publishing.

Wang, G., Marradi, C., Albayrak, A., & van der Cammen, T. J. (2019). Co-designing with people with dementia: A scoping review of involving people with dementia in design research. *Maturitas*, *127*, 55–63. PMID: 31351521

Wangmo, T., Lipps, M., Kressig, R. W., & Ienca, M. (2019). Ethical concerns with the use of intelligent assistive technology: Findings from a qualitative study with professional stakeholders. *BMC Medical Ethics*, *20*(1), 98. DOI: 10.1186/s12910-019-0437-z PMID: 31856798

Williamson, S. M., & Prybutok, V. (2024). Balancing privacy and progress: A review of privacy challenges, systemic oversight, and patient perceptions in AI-driven healthcare. *Applied Sciences (Basel, Switzerland)*, *14*(2), 675.

Xesfingi, S., & Vozikis, A. (2014). What shapes patient's satisfaction in countries' health care systems?

Chapter 8
Ageing Well or Ailing Wallets?
Chronic Illness, Risk Factors, and Catastrophic Health Spending Among the Elderly

Amiya Abdul Khadar
https://orcid.org/0009-0002-0861-8115
Lovely Professional University, India

Pooja Kansra
https://orcid.org/0000-0003-2229-0662
Lovely Professional University, India

Ergunova Olga Titovna
https://orcid.org/0009-0006-2267-8121
Peter the Great St. Petersburg Polytechnic University, Russia

ABSTRACT

The present study provides a comprehensive systematic review of the various studies related to prevalence, risk factors and catastrophic health expenditure associated with non-communicable diseases among older population. This study can help to consolidate and synthesize the multitude of studies which have been done in this field into one cohesive paper. This helps in understanding the current status as well as identifying places for improvement in this purposed field of study. The findings have revealed that the most prevalent NCDs found among older people are cardio-vascular diseases such as hypertension, stroke and heart diseases, Type 1 and Type 2 diabetes, cancer, chronic respiratory diseases, neurological and musculoskeletal diseases and mental health issues.The multimorbidity of NCDs was found to be the

DOI: 10.4018/979-8-3373-5462-0.ch008

most significant factor that pushes many households below the poverty line. It was observed that hospitalization due to chronic diseases among elderly was a major factor in for increase in out-of-pocket expenditure leading to catastrophic health expenditure.

1. INTRODUCTION

Chronic illness refers to a broad range of long-term health conditions that progress slowly, persist over an extended period, and often require ongoing medical attention or management rather than a one-time cure. Unlike acute diseases, which develop suddenly and resolve within a short duration, chronic illnesses typically last for months or years and can significantly impact an individual's quality of life (Jankovic et al., 2018; Goel et al., 2022; Kundu & Chakraborty, 2023). Common chronic conditions include cardiovascular diseases, diabetes, hypertension, cancer, chronic respiratory diseases, arthritis, and neurodegenerative disorders. According to the World Health Organisation (WHO), chronic illnesses account for most global morbidity and mortality, representing a major public health challenge, particularly in low- and middle-income countries where healthcare resources are often limited (Joseph & Gupta, 2016; Patil et al., 2016; Dugee et al., 2019; Adam et al., 2022). The burden of chronic illness extends beyond physical health, affecting psychological well-being, social relationships, and economic stability. Individuals with chronic conditions often face limitations in daily activities, increased dependency on caregivers, and long-term financial strain due to medical expenses.

Moreover, the management of chronic diseases requires consistent access to healthcare services, adherence to treatment, and lifestyle modifications, which may not always be feasible for individuals from disadvantaged socio-economic backgrounds (Gopalakrishnan et al., 2015; Hakami et al., 2023). Given the demographic transition marked by increasing life expectancy and an ageing population, the prevalence of chronic illnesses is expected to rise substantially in the coming decades. This makes it essential to understand the risk factors, socio-economic determinants, and healthcare utilization patterns associated with chronic conditions. Addressing these issues is crucial not only for improving health outcomes but also for reducing the economic and social burden on individuals, families, and healthcare systems (Efthymiou I,P., 2024). Thus, the present study focuses on examining the evidence from the existing literature regarding the prevalence, risk factors and out-of-pocket expenses associated with NCDs among the older population, examining the materials and methodologies employed to analyse the same and finally looking into future scope for the study.

To achieve study goals, the paper is structured into five segments. The 'Introduction' section provides an overview of NCDs and their impact on the elderly population. The 'Materials and Methods' section outlines the procedures employed for extracting the data and assessing the quality of studies. The 'Result' section presents the findings of the study, and the 'Discussion' section wraps up the study, incorporating policy implications and addressing the limitations of the study.

2. MATERIALS AND METHODS

PRISMA technique was used for conducting a comprehensive systematic review (Moher et al., 2009). The study recommends a set of standards and parameters for composing items to improve the systematic review and meta-analysis quality. The search spanned from October to December 2023 to gather and assess studies published until August 2023.

Search Criteria

The literature review drew upon two potential sources: a. electronic database and b. references provided by the selected articles. The main sources for the study were electronic databases such as ACADEMIA, Embase, NCBI, PubMed, Springer, ResearchGate, Google Scholar, JSTOR etc.

The search was designed to incorporate terms related to the outcome, exposure, and the target participants (Table 1). The study's objective was to identify the "prevalence", "risk factors" and "catastrophic health expenditure" associated with NCDs among older people. As the number of overall NCDs is large the most prevalent chronic ailments such as "cardiovascular diseases", "diabetes", "cancer", and "chronic respiratory diseases" were set as separate keywords to identify literature. The study population of the search was the elderly population. United Nations in 2013 defined the elderly population as individuals who are 60 years or older (United Nation, 2013). For this study, age groups of 60 years and older were encompassed within the keywords. The exposure of interest where demographic and socio-economic variables, general terms such as education, income, occupation, age, gender, religion, ethnicity etc. were used as keywords to represent specific components of socioeconomic and demographic variables.

Table 1. Search criteria: identifying keywords for literature search

Concept	Keywords
1.Outcome: NCDs Prevalence, Risk Factor and Cost	"non-communicable diseases" OR "NCDs*" OR "diabetics*" OR "cardiovascular diseases*" OR "cancer*" OR "respiratory diseases*" AND "prevalence*" OR "risk factors*" OR "cost*" OR "expenditure*" "healthcare*" OR "catastrophic health expenditure*" OR "out-of-pocket expenditure*"
2.Participant: Older people	"elderly* age*" OR "old* adults*" OR "old*population" OR "elderly* population" OR "old*people" OR "aged 60" OR "aged 65" OR "aged 70" OR "elderly people" OR "senior*"
3a. Exposure-Socioeconomic subgroups	"socioeconomic factors" OR "socioeconomic status" OR "social class*" OR "occupation*" OR "income" OR "employment" OR "wealth quantiles" OR "education*"
3b. Exposure-Demographic subgroups	"gender" OR "sex" OR "marital status" OR "religion" OR "race" OR "ethnicity*"

*Truncation symbol
Searches combined with AND: 1 AND 2 AND 3a. 1 AND 2 AND 3b.

Selection Criteria

The abstract and title of all the sources found during the search underwent screening based on exclusion and inclusion criteria (Pongiglione et al., 2015). After the initial screening, the selected studies were thoroughly read, and the selection criteria were re-applied to the full text. Inclusion and exclusion strategies were made in alignment with the already established outcomes, exposure, and study participants from Table 1. The studies that included any of the outcomes and targeted the older population were included in the study. Studies that analyzed at least one exposure factor either socioeconomic variables or demographic variables were selected. All descriptive studies and reviews were selected, while conference papers, posters and studies published in non-peer-reviewed journals were excluded. The specific criteria for inclusion and exclusion are outlined comprehensively in Table 2.

Table 2. Selection criteria: Strategy for inclusion and exclusion of literatures

Concept	Inclusion Criteria	Exclusion criteria
Outcome: NCDs Prevalence, Risk Factor and Cost	Studies that include any of the outcomes from Table 1	Studies that are not centered around the established outcomes of interest
Participant: Elderly Population	Studies are focused on the elderly population or people aged 60 years and above	Studies that do not primarily target the older population
Exposure: a. Socioeconomic subgroups b. Demographic subgroups	Studies reflecting any of the exposure factors from table 1	Studies does not include at least one exposure factor.
Type of Study	Descriptive studies, reviews	Conference articles, posters, published in non-peer-reviewed journals
Language	English	Languages other than English

3. RESULTS

From the several databases that were selected, 276 studies were identified and screened. After examining the titles and abstracts and implementing criteria set for inclusion and exclusion, 107 references were reviewed in full text resulting in the selection of 87 studies, a further 5 studies were identified from the selected studies list of references. Of the 92 references selected for this systematic review, 42 were focused on the prevalence of NCDs among older people, 35 studies discussed risk factors associated with NCDs among elderly people and 15 studies discussed the catastrophic health expenditure (CHE) associated with NCDs among the elderly population (Figure1)

Figure 1. **Search strategy with PRISMA flow diagram** *(Moher et al., 2009)*

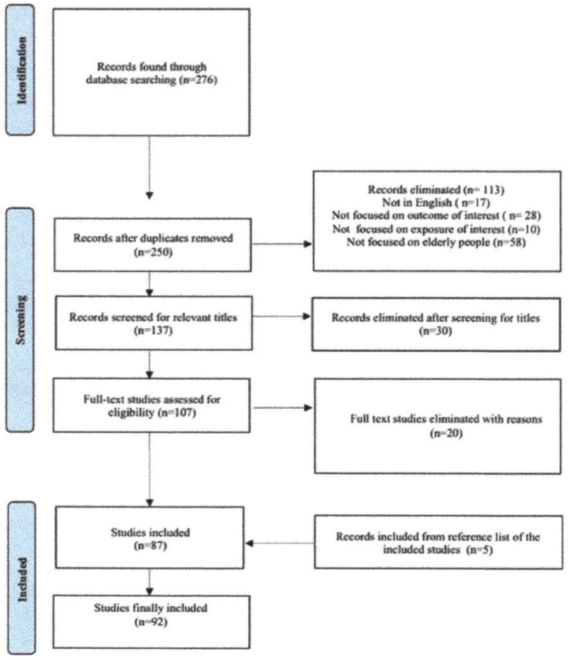

3.1. Prevalence of NCDs Among Elderly Population

The burden of NCDs among older individuals is a pressing global concern. As people age the prevalence and severity of NCDs typically rise. The interplay between ageing and the immune system, combined with the lingering effects of exposure to various risk factors associated with NCDs, makes this issue one of the foremost challenges that the older population faces. Among the different types of NCDs found the most prevalent ones found among older people are listed in Table 3.

Table 3. NCDs prevalent among the older population

NCDs Prevalent Among Elderly		References
Cardiovascular diseases	**Hypertension**	Yawson et al., 2016; Menon et al., 2016; Sherbiny et al., 2016; Ong et al., 2017; Russell et al., 2019; Mansour et al., 2020; Zali et al., 2020; Dahshan et al., 2020; Sarveswaran et al., 2020; Dahal et al., 2021; Farzad et al., 2021; Lutala & Muula, 2022
	Stroke	Kunna et al., 2017; Newtonraj et al., 2017; Sum et al., 2019; Li et al., 2020; Camacho et al., 2020; Bramhankar et al., 2021; Farzad et al., 2021; Farzadfar et al., 2022; Du et al., 2023
	Heart Disease	Gopalakrishnan et al., 2015; Malta et al., 2017; Ithnin et al., 2018; Shin et al., 2018; Twabi et al., 2021; Bramhankar et al., 2021; Napalai et al., 2022; Puri et al., 2022; Farzadfar et al., 2022; Wu et al., 2023;
Diabetes	**Type 1**	Lutala & Muula, 2022; Orm et al., 2023; Darbandi et al., 2023; Hadavandsiri et al., 2023
	Type 2	Sazlina et al., 2012; Kunna et al., 2017; Cuschieri & Grech, 2021; Mamedov et al., 2021; Mertens et al., 2021; Wagner et al., 2021
Cancer		Feng et al., 2014; Joseph & Gupta, 2016 ; Khademi et al., 2017; Kien et al., 2017; Yang et al., 2022; Farzad et al., 2021; Goel et al., 2022; Adams et al., 2022
Chronic Respiratory diseases	**Chronic obstructive pulmonary disease**	Malta et al., 2017; Kien et al., 2017; Bramhankar et al., 2021; Goel et al., 2022; Hakami et al., 2023
	Asthma	Chidumwa et al., 2021; Puri et al., 2022; Kyprianidou et al., 2023; Reid et al., 2023.
Neurological diseases	**Alzheimer's Disease**	VanDevanter et al., 2023
	Parkinson's Disease	Tan et al., 2014
Musculoskeletal diseases	**Arthritis**	Kandpal et al., 2013; Yu & Zhang, 2020 ; Hughes et al., 2021; Svinøy et al., 2021; Hakami et al., 2023; Kyprianidou et al., 2023; Yankanchi & Udigiri, 2023;
	Osteoporosis	HuanDong et al., 2017; Khademi et al., 2017; Kansiime et al., 2019; Hakami et al., 2023
Mental Health Issues		Sum et al., 2019; Chidumwa et al., 2021; Harris et al., 2021 ; Mamedov et al., 2022; Sharma et al., 2022; Wu et al., 2023

Source: Authors Compilation based on reviewed articles

Cardiovascular diseases are one of the most predominant chronic diseases found among the older population (Narendran et al., 2018; Yonel et al., 2018). Among the different types of cardiovascular diseases hypertension was the most common (Yawson et al., 2016). Among older adults, hypertension poses a significant health challenge, contributing to functional decline, deteriorating health quality and increased health expenditure (Russell et al., 2019; Reid et al., 2023). According to the

Framingham Heart Study, the prevalence of hypertension rises from approximately 30 per cent in adults aged 65-75 years to 60 per cent among those aged 75 years and older (Franklin et al., 2001). Stroke and heart diseases are the other most prevalent cardiovascular disease found among the older population (Farzadfar et al., 2022; Du et al., 2023).

Diabetes is another prevalent chronic disorder found among elderly people (Mwangi et al., 2020; Lutala & Muula, 2022; Orm et al., 2023; Darbandi et al., 2023; Hadavandsiri et al., 2023). Elevated blood glucose levels, stemming from deficiencies in insulin secretion or insulin resistance characterize this condition (Lutala & Muula, 2022; Darbandi et al., 2023). Among older adults, diabetes represents a significant health concern due to its association with high risk of cardiovascular diseases, functional decline, and mortality (Cuschieri & Grech, 2021; Mamedov et al., 2021; Mertens et al., 2021).

Amongst many chronic diseases, cancer stands out as a prominent contributor towards the rise in morbidity and mortality among older adults, with age representing a significant risk factor for its onset (Farzad et al., 2021; Yang et al., 2022). The majority of cancer diagnoses occur in individuals aged 60 years and older (Ahmed et al., 2019). It reflects the effect of ageing-related genetic mutation, environmental exposures and lifestyle factors. Chronic Respiratory diseases, Neurological diseases, Musculoskeletal diseases and Mental health issues are the other major chronic non-communicable diseases that impact the lives of older adults (Malta et al., 2017; Kien et al., 2017; Bramhankar et al., 2021; Goel et al., 2022; Sharma et al., 2022; Hakami et al., 2023; Wu et al., 2023)

3.2. Risk Factors Associated with NCDs Among Elderly Population

Numerous risk factors are linked to NCDs which can be majorly classified into modifiable and non-modifiable categories. Age, gender and genetic constitution come under the non-modifiable risk factors (Bloom et al., 2011; Corrêa et al., 2016) and modifiable risk factors which comprise unhealthy lifestyle choices such as tobacco use, unhealthy diet, physical inactivity and excessive alcohol consumption are major contributors towards the growing epidemic of NCDs (Negin et al., 2011; Farzadfar et al., 2022; Goel et al., 2022). Among the non-modifiable risk factors age is a key risk factor that increases the mortality rate due to NCDs (Gbadamosi & Tlou, 2020). People aged 60 or older are relatively more affected by NCDs than any other age group. With the rapid increase in older people every year, the burden of NCDs is expected to surge, driven by the escalating prevalence of the key risk factors. This trend will subsequently lead to an overall increase in disease burden (Mondai et al., 2020; Pereira et al., 2023).

Modifiable Risk factors associated with NCDs can be majorly categories into behavioral, metabolic and environmental risk factors (Sivanantham et al., 2022; Goel et al., 2022; Du et al., 2023). The most common risk factors associated with NCDs are listed in Table 4.

Table 4. Risk Factors Associated with NCDs

Risk Factors Associated with NCDs		**References**
Behavioral Risk Factors	**Tobacco Use**	Okpechi et al., 2013; Patil et al., 2016; Kaur et al., 2019; Pengpid & Peltzer, 2020; Sarveswaran et al., 2020; Dissanayake et al., 2021; Sivanantham et al., 2022;
	Unhealthy Diet	Newtonraj et al., 2017; Kunna et al., 2017; Camacho et al., 2020; Li et al., 2020; Farzad et al., 2021; Bramhankar et al., 2021; Farzadfar et al., 2022; Du et al., 2023
	Lack of Physical Activity	Wagner et al., 2021; Dutta et al., 2022
	Alcohol Consumption	Okpechi et al., 2013; Dai et al., 2015; Negi et al., 2016; Dahal et al., 2021; Goel et al., 2022; Sarveswaran et al., 2020; Vallecillo et al., 2020; Sivanantham et al., 2022;
Metabolic Risk Factors	**Obesity**	Cuschieri & ; Aryal et al., 2015; Grech, 2021; Dahal et al., 2021; Du et al., 2023; Kundu & Chakraborty, 2023; Suksatan et al., 2023
	High Blood Pressure levels	Seyedsadjadi et al., 2017; Ahmed et al., 2019; Russell et al., 2019; Saraswat et al., 2023
	High Blood Sugar levels	Harris et al., 2021; Ngaruiya et al., 2021; Saraswat et al., 2023
Environmental Risk Factors	**Air Pollution**	Goel et al., 2022; Yankanchi & Udigiri, 2023
	Chemical and Radiation Exposure	Munday et al., 2019; Yankanchi & Udigiri, 2023
	Occupational Hazards	Goel et al., 2022; Yankanchi & Udigiri, 2023

Source: Authors Compilation based on reviewed articles

Behavioural risk factors are actions that increase the likelihood of developing NCDs (Farzad et al., 2021). These behaviours are often modifiable and influenced by individual choices. Behavioural risk factors encompass tobacco use, an unhealthy diet, physical inactivity and long-term consumption of alcohol (Okpechi et al., 2013; Dai et al., 2015; Negi et al., 2016; Dahal et al., 2021; Goel et al., 2022; Sarveswaran et al., 2020; Vallecillo et al., 2020; Sivanantham et al., 2022).

Metabolic risk factors are physiological abnormalities or dysfunctions that contribute towards the chance of developing NCDs. These include obesity, high blood pressure, and high sugar levels (Seyedsadjadi et al., 2017; Russell et al., 2019;Du et al., 2023; Kundu & Chakraborty, 2023; Suksatan et al., 2023; Saraswat et al., 2023). Other major modifiable risk factors are environmental risk factors which include air pollution, chemical and radioactive exposure and occupational hazards (Yankanchi & Udigiri, 2023; Goel et al., 2022; Munday et al., 2019).

3.3. Catastrophic Health Expenditure (CHE) Associated with NCDs Among Elderly Population

Out-of-pocket expenditure (OOPE) refers to the healthcare cost borne by individuals directly when accessing healthcare services excluding any reimbursement from insurance companies or employers (Ma et al., 2019). Catastrophic health expenditure (CHE) generally happens when these out-of-pocket expenses surpass a specific threshold of household income resulting in significant financial strain on the household (Verma et al., 2021; Wang et al., 2023).

Many studies define the threshold as the case when households' financial spending on healthcare utilization exceeds 10 per cent of the total household expenditure (Van Minh & Xuan Tran, 2012; Pandey & Singh, 2017; Verma et al., 2021; Mohanty et al., 2022). Table 5 shows studies that discussed the Catastrophic Health Expenditure (CHE) linked with NCDs amongst the elderly population.

Table 5. Catastrophic Health Expenditure (CHE) Associated with NCDs

Authors	Country	Catastrophic health expenditure associated with NCDs
Wang et al., 2023	China	One in five among older individuals in China experienced catastrophic health expenditure and CHE was linked to an increased risk of depression.
Xu & Yang, 2022	China	Chronic conditions prevalent among elderly, such as stroke and liver diseases contribute significantly towards CHE for families on the edge of poverty.
Mohanty et al., 2022	India	The estimated incidence of CHE was 24.6 per cent among middle aged and older people in India with odds of experiencing CHE being more for households with higher old-age dependency.
Verma et al., 2021	India	The significant impoverishing effect of NCDs was observed as one-twelfth of households and one-eighth of households were pushed into poverty due to CHE is 2014 and 2017-18 respectively.
Farooq & Masud, 2021	Pakistan	The presence of children, older people and sick or disabled persons in the households increases the risk of CHE.
Prinja et al., 2019	India	The direct OOPE for hospitalization due to NCDs amounted to INR 16,768 while indirect productivity loss was estimated at INR 8,164. CHE was observed to be 22.2 percent with 12 percent households slipping below poverty line.

continued on following page

Table 5. Continued

Authors	Country	Catastrophic health expenditure associated with NCDs
Aregbeshola & Khan, 2018	Nigeria	Households with members having chronic illnesses were found to be at the risk of experiencing CHE
Kastor & Mohanty, 2018	India	The mean OOPE for hospitalization for NCDs was INR 19,210 with the highest for cancer INR 57,232. Cancer was observed as the leading cause of CHE among households
Njagi et al., 2018	Sub-Saharan Africa	Major factors contributing towards CHE included economic status of households, healthcare provider utilized, nature of illness and socio-demographic attributes of households.
Barasa et al., 2017	Kenya	Household heads unemployment, presence of elderly, chronic illness, lower socio-economic status, larger households' size are significantly associated with the higher chance of experiencing CHE.
Pandey & Singh, 2017	India	33.1 per cent who utilized hospitalization and 13.8 per cent who utilized out-patient care experienced CHE
Picco et al., 2016	Singapore	The societal cost of multimorbidity was SGD $15,148 per individuals annually and multimorbidity was considerably interrelated with risk of experiencing CHE.
Carpenter et al., 2015	Australia	Older Australians with multiple chronic condition were at risk of being unable to pay out-of-pocket expenditure despite having universal health insurance.
Wang et al., 2015	China	Factors that positively contributed towards CHE inequality included household size, per capita income, members who aged more than 65 years, presence of multiple chronic diseases.
Choi et al., 2015	Korea	Households having chronic illness such as cardiovascular diseases, diabetes, kidney diseases were found to be at significant risk of incurring CHE.

Source: Authors Compilation based on reviewed articles

DISCUSSION

The escalating burden of NCDs among the elderly is becoming a pressing concern for the entire world. With the ageing trajectory of many countries, there is a dual challenge of rapid ageing alongside the increasing prevalence of NCDs within the population. The double burden of ageing and NCDs is a significant and growing public health concern worldwide. As life expectancy increases and the population ages the prevalence of chronic illnesses such as cardiovascular diseases, cancer, diabetes and such NCDs increases posing significant challenges for healthcare systems, economies, and societies. The study aimed to determine the prevalence of NCDs and their associated risk factor among the elderly population, as well as to identify the catastrophic health expenditure resulting from out-of-pocket spending on NCDs, based on existing studies. Out of 276 literatures found, 92 were included in the study using specific selection criteria.

Study findings showed that the most prevalent NCDs found among older people are cardiovascular diseases such as hypertension, stroke and heart diseases, Type 1 and Type 2 diabetes, cancer, chronic respiratory diseases, Neurological and Musculoskeletal diseases and mental health issues (Gopalakrishnan et al., 2015; Hakami et al., 2023). Cardiovascular diseases and diabetes were found to be the ailments causing the most cases of mortality among the elderly (Russell et al., 2019; Mansour et al., 2020; Hakami et al., 2023; Reid et al., 2023). The study also observed that the most prevalent risk factors associated with NCDs among older people included behavioural risk factors such as smoking, lack of physical activity, unhealthy diets and use of alcohol, metabolic risk factors such as obesity, high blood pressure and sugar levels, and environmental risk factors such as air pollution, occupational hazards, chemical and radioactive exposure etc.(Sivanantham et al., 2022; Goel et al., 2022).

The study observed that the risk of experiencing CHE was highest for families having older members with chronic ailments (Van Minh & Xuan Tran, 2012; Pandey & Singh, 2017; Verma et al., 2021; Mohanty et al., 2022). Multimorbidity of NCDs was found to be the most significant factor that pushes many households below the poverty line. Hospitalization due to chronic diseases among the elderly was a major factor in the increase in out-of-pocket expenditure leading to catastrophic health expenditure (Verma et al., 2021; Wang et al., 2023). The present study holds a few limitations, the exclusion of relevant studies presented at conferences and published in non-peer-reviewed journals can lead to biases. The difference in materials and methods used for estimating out-of-pocket expense and variation in the threshold of finding CHE make conducting a meta-analysis not feasible.

CONCLUSION

The study shows the burden NCDs have on the older population of a country. The burden of NCDs among the older population spreads beyond health outcomes and has significant social and economic implications. Chronic ailments can lead to functional difficulties, reduce the quality of life, increase financial burden, and increase dependency among older people. This can burden the healthcare systems and formal and informal caregivers thus putting a dent in the overall productivity and workforce participation within households. Strategies that are aimed towards promoting healthy lifestyles, and improving access to healthcare services and treatments are crucial towards preventing NCDs as well as reducing the mortality caused by NCDs (Efthymiou, I. P. et al., 2019). The health of elderly people can easily become a heavy burden for the country's overall healthcare. Awareness programmes are needed to make people understand the risk factors and possible economic burdens that can be caused by NCDs. Most of the risk factors of NCDs are modifiable so early intervention and awareness can help in reducing the country's burden of NCDs.

Funding: This research was supported by the Indian Council of Social Science Research (ICSSR) under the Doctoral Fellowship program.

Competing interests: The authors have no competing interests to declare that are relevant to the content of this article.

REFERENCES

Adams, D. M., Brown, P. G., Williams, M., Bromfield, L., & Bunting-Clarke, J. (2022). Assessment of rational use of medicines for chronic non-communicable diseases: A cross-sectional design in a public access clinic in Jamaica. *Journal of Public Health Research*, *11*(3). Advance online publication. DOI: 10.1177/22799036221126348 PMID: 36204195

Ahmed, S. H., Meyer, H. E., Kjøllesdal, M. K., Marjerrison, N., Mdala, I., & Htet, A. S.. (2019). The prevalence of selected risk factors for non-communicable diseases in Hargeisa, Somaliland: A cross-sectional study. *BMC Public Health*, *19*(1), 878. DOI: 10.1186/s12889-019-7101-x PMID: 31272414

Aregbeshola, B. S., & Khan, S. M. (2018). Determinants of catastrophic health expenditure in Nigeria. *The European Journal of Health Economics*, *19*(4), 521–532. DOI: 10.1007/s10198-017-0899-1 PMID: 28555372

Aryal, K. K., Mehata, S., Neupane, S., Vaidya, A., Dhimal, M., & Dhakal, P.. (2015). The burden and determinants of non communicable diseases risk factors in Nepal: Findings from a nationwide STEPS survey. *PLoS One*, *10*(8). Advance online publication. DOI: 10.1371/journal.pone.0134834 PMID: 26244512

Barasa, E. W., Maina, T., & Ravishankar, N. (2017). Assessing the impoverishing effects, and factors associated with the incidence of catastrophic health care payments in Kenya. *International Journal for Equity in Health*, *16*(1), 1–14. DOI: 10.1186/s12939-017-0526-x PMID: 28166779

Bloom, D. E., Cafiero, E. T., Jané-Llopis, E., Abrahams-Gessel, S., Bloom, L. R., Fathima, S., ... The Global Economic Burden of Noncommunicable Diseases. World Economic Forum; 2011.

Bramhankar, M., Pandey, M., Rana, G. S., Rai, B., Mishra, N. L., & Shukla, A. (2021). An assessment of anthropometric indices and its association with NCDs among the older adults of India: Evidence from LASI Wave-1. *BMC Public Health*, *21*(1), 1357. DOI: 10.1186/s12889-021-11421-4 PMID: 34238276

Camacho, P. A., Gomez-Arbelaez, D., Otero, J., González-Gómez, S., Molina, D. I., & Sanchez, G.. (2020). Self-reported prevalence of chronic non-communicable diseases in relation to socioeconomic and educational factors in colombia: A community-based study in 11 departments. *Global Heart*, *15*(1). Advance online publication. DOI: 10.5334/GH.792 PMID: 32489808

Carpenter, A., Islam, M. M., Yen, L., & McRae, I. (2015). Affordability of out-of-pocket health care expenses among older Australians. *Health Policy (Amsterdam), 119*(7), 907–914. DOI: 10.1016/j.healthpol.2015.03.010 PMID: 25896218

Chidumwa, G., Maposa, I., Corso, B., Minicuci, N., Kowal, P., & Micklesfield, L. K.. (2021). Identifying co-occurrence and clustering of chronic diseases using latent class analysis: Cross-sectional findings from SAGE South Africa Wave 2. *BMJ Open, 11*(1). Advance online publication. DOI: 10.1136/bmjopen-2020-041604 PMID: 33514578

Choi, J. W., Choi, J. W., Kim, J. H., Yoo, K. B., & Park, E. C. (2015). Association between chronic disease and catastrophic health expenditure in Korea. *BMC Health Services Research, 15*(1), 1–8. DOI: 10.1186/s12913-014-0675-1 PMID: 25608983

Corrêa, M. M., Thumé, E., De Oliveira, E. R. A., & Tomasi, E. (2016). Performance of the waist-to-height ratio in identifying obesity and predicting non-communicable diseases in the elderly population: A systematic literature review. *Archives of Gerontology and Geriatrics, 65*, 174–182. DOI: 10.1016/j.archger.2016.03.021 PMID: 27061665

Cuschieri, S., & Grech, S. (2021). Insight into the Occurrence of Common Non-communicable Diseases at a Population Level and the Potential Impact During the Coronavirus Pandemic — A Need for a Syndemic Healthcare Approach? *SN Comprehensive Clinical Medicine, 3*(12), 2393–2400. DOI: 10.1007/s42399-021-01064-2 PMID: 34568765

Dahal, S., Sah, R. B., Niraula, S. R., Karkee, R., & Chakravartty, A. (2021). Prevalence and determinants of noncommunicable disease risk factors among adult population of Kathmandu. *PLoS One, 16*(9). Advance online publication. DOI: 10.1371/journal.pone.0257037 PMID: 34495984

Dahshan, A., Al-Kubiasi, N., Al-Zaidan, M., Saeed, W., Kehyayan, V., & Bougmiza, I. (2020). Prevalence of polypharmacy and the association with non-communicable diseases in Qatari elderly patients attending primary healthcare centers: A cross-sectional study. *PLoS One, 15*(6), 1–13. DOI: 10.1371/journal.pone.0234386 PMID: 32525902

Dai, H., Jia, G., & Liu, K. (2015). Health-related quality of life and related factors among elderly people in Jinzhou, China: A cross-sectional study. *Public Health, 129*(6), 667–673. DOI: 10.1016/j.puhe.2015.02.022 PMID: 25796292

Darbandi, M., Rezaeian, S., Najafi, F., Shadmani, F. K., Ghavi, S., & Miryan, M.. (2023). A Comprehensive Evaluation of Occupational Epidemiology in Western Iran: A Cohort Study in Ravansar Noncommunicable Diseases. *Journal of Occupational and Environmental Medicine*, *65*(9), E610–E618. DOI: 10.1097/JOM.0000000000002916 PMID: 37367639

Dissanayake, S. A. I. P., Kisokanth, G., & Warnakulasuriya, S. S. P. (2021). Prevalence of risk factors for Non-communicable diseases, work-related health problems and associated factors among male three-wheeler drivers in Gampaha Urban Council area, Sri Lanka. *The Journal of Men's Health*, *17*(4), 295–303. DOI: 10.31083/jomh.2021.059

Du, Y. R., Liu, L., Zhao, Y., Huang, J. J., Golden, A. R., & Cai, L. (2023). Ethnic disparities in prevalence of chronic non-communicable diseases and its multimorbidity among older adults in rural southwest China. *BMC Public Health*, *23*(1), 1217. DOI: 10.1186/s12889-023-16161-1 PMID: 37353785

Dugee, O., Sugar, B., Dorjsuren, B., & Mahal, A. (2019). Economic impacts of chronic conditions in a country with high levels of population health coverage: Lessons from Mongolia. *Tropical Medicine & International Health*, *24*(6), 715–726. DOI: 10.1111/tmi.1323 PMID: 30870575

Dutta, S., Mishra, A., Basu, M., & Mukherjee, M. (2022). Determinants of Non Communicable Diseases: A Mixed-method Study on Its Prevalence and Perceptions among Rural Population of Muchisa, West Bengal. *Journal of Clinical and Diagnostic Research : JCDR*, *16*(6), LC15–LC21. DOI: 10.7860/JCDR/2022/53398.1646

Efthymiou, I. P. (2024). Wellbeing as an alternative to GDP? *HAPSc Policy Briefs Series*, *5*(1), 38–46. DOI: 10.12681/hapscpbs.38956

Efthymiou, I. P., Vozikis, A., & Sidiropoulos, S. (2019). Application of Sociocybernetic model in the field of Health Management. *International Journal of Scientific and Engineering Research*, *10*(5), 451–560.

Farooq, S., & Masud, F. (2021). Catastrophic health expenditure and poverty in Pakistan. *Pakistan Development Review*, *60*(1), 27–48. DOI: 10.30541/v60i1pp.27-48

Farzad, M, MitraMoodi, Sharifi F, Amirabadizadeh H, Amirabadizadeh A, Kazemi T, et al. (2021). Prevalence and factors connected with chronic diseases in the elderly residents of Birjand: A community – based study in Birjand, South Khorasan Province, Iran. *Journal of Diabetes and Metabolic Disorders*, *20*(2), 1655–1662. DOI: 10.1007/s40200-021-00918-9 PMID: 34900817

Farzadfar, F., Zalvand, R., Karami, B., Yoosefi, M., Takian, A., & Tajvar, M. (2022). Prevalence and Determinants of Severe Mental Disorders in Iran: Evidence from the National Survey of STEPs- 2016. *Archives of Iranian Medicine*, *25*(7), 460–472. DOI: 10.34172/aim.2022.76 PMID: 36404514

Feng, L., Li, P., Wang, X., Hu, Z., Ma, Y., & Tang, W.. (2014). Distribution and determinants of non communicable diseases among elderly uyghur ethnic group in Xinjiang, China. *PLoS One*, *9*(8). Advance online publication. DOI: 10.1371/journal.pone.0105536 PMID: 25141133

Franklin, S. S., Larson, M. G., Khan, S. A., Wong, N. D., Leip, E. P., & Kannel, W. B.. (2001). Does the relation of blood pressure to coronary heart disease risk change with aging?: The Framingham Heart Study. *Circulation*, *103*(9), 1245–1249. DOI: 10.1161/01.CIR.103.9.1245 PMID: 11238268

Gbadamosi, M. A., & Tlou, B. (2020). Modifiable risk factors associated with non-communicable diseases among adult outpatients in Manzini, Swaziland: A cross-sectional study. *BMC Public Health*, *20*(1), 665. DOI: 10.1186/s12889-020-08816-0 PMID: 32398061

Goel, G. S., Gupta, B., Mittal, A., & Gupta, S. (2022a). Prevalence Of Risk Factors Of Non Communicable Diseases In District Ambala, Haryana. *Journal of Pharmaceutical Negative Results*, *13*(8), 4768–4772. DOI: 10.47750/pnr.2022.13.S08.623

Goel, G. S., Gupta, B., Mittal, A., & Gupta, S. (2022b). Prevalence Of Risk Factors Of Non Communicable Diseases In District Ambala, Haryana. *Journal of Pharmaceutical Negative Results*, *13*, 4768–4772. DOI: 10.47750/pnr.2022.13.S08.623

Gopalakrishnan, S., Ganeshkumar, P., & Katta, A. (2015). Study of morbidity profile of a rural population in Tamil Nadu. *Journal of Clinical and Diagnostic Research : JCDR*, *9*(2), LC05–LC09. DOI: 10.7860/JCDR/2015/10424.5520 PMID: 25859470

Hadavandsiri, F., Shafaati, M., Mohammad Nejad, S., Ebrahimzadeh Mousavi, M., Najafi, A., & Mirzaei, M.. (2023). Non-communicable disease comorbidities in HIV patients: Diabetes, hypertension, heart disease, and obstructive sleep apnea as a neglected issue. *Scientific Reports*, *13*(1), 12730. DOI: 10.1038/s41598-023-39828-6 PMID: 37543699

Hakami, S. M., Omar, M. T., Alsaad, S. M., Vennu, V. S., Hattan, L. I., & Bindawas, S. M. (2023). Association between non-communicable diseases and physical activity level in older adults visiting primary health care centers in Jizan, Saudi Arabia. *Saudi Medical Journal*, *44*(6), 580–587. DOI: 10.15537/smj.2023.44.6.20230076 PMID: 37343987

Harris, T. G., Flören, S., Mantell, J. E., Nkambule, R., Lukhele, N. G., & Malinga, B. P.. (2021). HIV and aging among adults aged 50 years and older on antiretroviral therapy in Eswatini. *African Journal of AIDS Research*, *20*(1), 107–115. DOI: 10.2989/16085906.2021.1887301 PMID: 33685372

HuanDong L, Qian L, Yu H, Chouwen Z, Hui M, Jian G, et al. (2017). The prevalence of multiple non-communicable diseases among middle-aged and elderly people: The Shanghai Changfeng Study. *European Journal of Epidemiology*, *32*(2), 159–163. DOI: 10.1007/s10654-016-0211-1 PMID: 27999971

Hughes, G. D., Aboyade, O. M., Okonji, C. O., Clark, B., & Mabweazara, S. Z. (2021). Comparison of the prevalence of non-communicable diseases and traditional herbal medicine use in urban and rural communities in South Africa. *Advances in Integrative Medicine*, *8*(2), 136–143. DOI: 10.1016/j.aimed.2020.11.002

Ithnin M, Nor NAUM, Nordin NJ, Effendy NM, Sahar MA, Abdullah KHA, et al. Knowledge, attitude, and practice on non-communicable diseases (NCDs) among the adult population in the urban area of Negeri Sembilan, Malaysia. Int J Res Pharm Sci. 2018;9(Special Issue 2):88–94. https://doi.org/DOI: 10.26452/ijrps.v9iSPL2.1747

Jankovic, J., Mirkovic, M., Jovic-Vranes, A., Santric-Milicevic, M., & Terzic-Supic, Z. (2018). Association between non-communicable disease multimorbidity and health care utilization in a middle-income country: Population-based study. *Public Health*, *155*, 35–42. DOI: 10.1016/j.puhe.2017.11.014 PMID: 29306621

Joseph, N., & Gupta, S. (2016). Assessment of economic impact among in-patients with non-communicable diseases in a private tertiary care hospital in Southern India. *Journal of Clinical and Diagnostic Research : JCDR*, *10*(6), LM04–LM06. DOI: 10.7860/JCDR/2016/19426.8059 PMID: 27504316

Kandpal, S. D., Kakkar, R., Aggarwal, P., & Bansal, S. (2013). Pattern of prevalence of risk factors for non-communicable diseases in the geriatric population of district Dehradun. *Indian Acad Clin Med.*, *14*(3–4), 214–217.

Kansiime, S., Mwesigire, D., & Mugerwa, H. (2019). Prevalence of non-communicable diseases among HIV positive patients on antiretroviral therapy at joint clinical research centre, Lubowa, Uganda. *PLoS One*, *14*(8). Advance online publication. DOI: 10.1371/journal.pone.0221022 PMID: 31398244

Kastor, A., & Mohanty, S. K. (2018). Disease-specific out-of-pocket and catastrophic health expenditure on hospitalization in India: Do Indian households face distress health financing? *PLoS One*, *13*(5), 1–18. DOI: 10.1371/journal.pone.0196106 PMID: 29746481

Kaur, G., Bansal, R., Anand, T., Kumar, A., & Singh, J. (2019). Morbidity profile of noncommunicable diseases among elderly in a city in North India. *Clinical Epidemiology and Global Health, 7*(1), 29–34. DOI: 10.1016/j.cegh.2017.12.004

Khademi, N., Babanejad, M., Asadmobini, A., & Karim, H. (2017). The association of age and gender with risk factors of noncommunicable diseases among employees in West of Iran. *International Journal of Preventive Medicine, 8*. Advance online publication. DOI: 10.4103/ijpvm.IJPVM_400_16 PMID: 28299033

Kien, V. D., Van Minh, H., Giang, K. B., Dao, A., Weinehall, L., & Eriksson, M.. (2017). Socioeconomic inequalities in self-reported chronic non-communicable diseases in urban Hanoi, Vietnam. *Global Public Health: An International Journal for Research, Policy and Practice, 12*(12), 1522–1537. DOI: 10.1080/17441692.2015.1123282 PMID: 26727691

Kundu, J., & Chakraborty, R. (2023). Socio-economic inequalities in burden of communicable and non-communicable diseases among older adults in India: Evidence from Longitudinal Ageing Study in India, 2017–18. *PLoS One, 18*(3). Advance online publication. DOI: 10.1371/journal.pone.0283385 PMID: 36996071

Kunna, R., San Sebastian, M., & Stewart Williams, J. (2017). Measurement and decomposition of socioeconomic inequality in single and multimorbidity in older adults in China and Ghana: Results from the WHO study on global AGEing and adult health (SAGE). *International Journal for Equity in Health, 16*(1). Advance online publication. DOI: 10.1186/s12939-017-0578-y PMID: 28506233

Kyprianidou, M., Panagiotakos, D., Makris, K. C., Kambanaros, M., Christophi, C. A., & Giannakou, K. (2023). Prevalence and sociodemographic determinants of selected noncommunicable diseases among the general population of Cyprus: A large population-based cross-sectional study. *Chronic Diseases and Translational Medicine, 9*(3), 222–237. DOI: 10.1002/cdt3.70 PMID: 37711870

Li, X., Cai, L., Cui, W. L., Wang, X. M., Li, H. F., & He, J. H.. (2020). Association of socioeconomic and lifestyle factors with chronic non-communicable diseases and multimorbidity among the elderly in rural southwest China. *J Public Health., 42*(2), 239–246. DOI: 10.1093/pubmed/fdz020 PMID: 30860582

Lutala, P., & Muula, A. (2022). Brief behaviour change counselling in non-communicable diseases in Mangochi, Southern Malawi: A hypothetical acceptability study. *Pilot and Feasibility Studies, 8*(1). Advance online publication. DOI: 10.1186/s40814-022-01032-0 PMID: 35331326

Ma, C., Jiang, Y., Li, Y., Zhang, Y., Wang, X., & Ma, S.. (2019). Medical expenditure for middle-aged and elderly in Beijing. *BMC Health Services Research, 19*(1), 1–10. DOI: 10.1186/s12913-019-4190-2 PMID: 31174516

Malta, D. C., França, E., Abreu, D. M. X., Perillo, R. D., Salmen, M. C., & Teixeira, R. A.. (2017). Mortalidade por doenças não transmissíveis no brasil, 1990 a 2015, segundo estimativas do estudo de carga global de doenças. *São Paulo Medical Journal = Revista Paulista de Medicina, 135*(3), 213–221. DOI: 10.1590/1516-3180.2016.0330050117 PMID: 28746656

Mamedov, M. N., Druk, I. V., Turusheva, E. A., Eremina, E. Y., Morozova, T. E., & Iskenderov, B. G.. (2021). Behavioral risk factors and clinical course of cardiovascular diseases and other noncommunicable diseases during quarantine in various regions of Russia. *Russ J Cardiol., 26*(9), 15–21. DOI: 10.15829/1560-4071-2021-4670

Mamedov, M. N., Rytova, A. I., Yarovaya, E. B., & Drapkina, O. M. (2022). Psychosomatic status analysis of patients with chronic non-communicable diseases (CNCDs) in Russia and CIS countries during self-isolation. *Profilaktychna Medytsyna, 25*(1), 29–34. DOI: 10.17116/profmed202225011 2

Mansour, Z., Said, R., Dbaibo, H., Mrad, P., Torossian, L., & Rady, A.. (2020). Non-communicable diseases in Lebanon: Results from World Health Organization STEPS survey 2017. *Public Health, 187*, 120–126. DOI: 10.1016/j.puhe.2020.08.014 PMID: 32949882

Menon, V. P., Edathadathil, F., Sathyapalan, D., Moni, M., Don, A., & Balachandran, S.. (2016). Assessment of 2013 AHA/ACC ASCVD risk scores with behavioral characteristics of an urban cohort in India Preliminary analysis of Noncommunicable disease Initiatives and Research at AMrita (NIRAM) study. *Medicine, 95*(49), e5542. DOI: 10.1097/MD.0000000000005542 PMID: 27930551

Mertens, E., Sagastume, D., & Penalvo, J. L. (2021). Quantification of disparities in the distribution of lifestyle and metabolic risk factors, prevalence of non-communicable diseases and related mortality: The Belgian Health Interview Surveys 1997-2018. *BMJ Open, 11*(11). Advance online publication. DOI: 10.1136/bmjopen-2021-053260 PMID: 34810190

Mohanty, S. K., Sahoo, U., & Rashmi, R. (2022). Old-age dependency and catastrophic health expenditure: Evidence from Longitudinal Ageing Study in India. *The International Journal of Health Planning and Management, 37*(6), 3148–3171. DOI: 10.1002/hpm.3546 PMID: 35929614

Moher, D., Liberati, A., Tetzlaff, J., & Altman, D. G. (2009). Preferred reporting items for systematic reviews and meta-analyses: The PRISMA statement. *BMJ (Clinical Research Ed.)*, *339*(7716), 332–336. DOI: 10.1136/bmj.b2535 PMID: 19622551

Mondai, R. N., Das, A., Islam, M. D., Podder, P., Pramanik, S., & Rani, M. (2020). Prevalence of NCD risk factors among the adult family members of students of school (Phase - A). *Journal of Medicine*, *21*(1), 8–13. DOI: 10.3329/jom.v21i1.44094

Munday, D., Leaman, J., O'Moore, É., & Plugge, E. (2019). The prevalence of non-communicable disease in older people in prison: A systematic review and meta-analysis. *Age and Ageing*, *48*(2), 204–212. DOI: 10.1093/ageing/afy186 PMID: 30590404

Mwangi, K. J., Mwenda, V., Gathecha, G., Beran, D., Guessous, I., & Ombiro, O.. (2020). Socio-economic and demographic determinants of non-communicable diseases in Kenya: A secondary analysis of the Kenya stepwise survey. *The Pan African Medical Journal*, *37*, 351. DOI: 10.11604/pamj.2020.37.351.21167 PMID: 33796165

Napalai, P., Seangpraw, K., Boonyathee, S., & Ong-Artborirak, P. (2022). COVID-19-related knowledge influences mental health, self-care behaviors, and quality of life among elderly with non-communicable diseases in Northern Thailand. *Frontiers in Public Health*, *10*, 993531. DOI: 10.3389/fpubh.2022.993531 PMID: 36388338

Narendran, M., Savitha Rani, B. B., Kulkarni, P., Renuka, M., & Narayana Murthy, M. R. (2018). Interdependence of communicable and non-communicable diseases among elderly population in declared slum in Mysuru City, Karnataka. *Indian Journal of Public Health Research & Development*, *9*(11), 62–66. DOI: 10.5958/0976-5506.2018.01426.2

Negi, P. C., Chauhan, R., & Rana, V. (2016). Vidyasagar, Lal K. Epidemiological study of non-communicable diseases (NCD) risk factors in tribal district of Kinnaur, HP: A cross-sectional study. *Indian Heart Journal*, *68*(5), 655–662. DOI: 10.1016/j.ihj.2016.03.002 PMID: 27773404

Negin, J., Cumming, R., de Ramirez, S. S., Abimbola, S., & Sachs, S. E. (2011). Risk factors for non-communicable diseases among older adults in rural Africa. *Tropical Medicine & International Health*, *16*(5), 640–646. DOI: 10.1111/j.1365-3156.2011.02739.x PMID: 21320244

Newtonraj, A., Murugan, N., Singh, Z., Chauhan, R. C., Velavan, A., & Mani, M. (2017). Factors associated with physical inactivity among adult urban population of Puducherry, India: A population based cross-sectional study. *Journal of Clinical and Diagnostic Research : JCDR*, *11*(5), LC15–LC17. DOI: 10.7860/JCDR/2017/24028.9853 PMID: 28658812

Ngaruiya, C., Wambua, M., Mutua, T. K., Owambo, D., Muchemi, M., & Rop, K.. (2021). The last frontier for global non-communicable disease action: The emergency department—A cross-sectional study from East Africa. *PLoS One*, *16*(4). Advance online publication. DOI: 10.1371/journal.pone.0248709 PMID: 33798234

Njagi, P., Arsenijevic, J., & Groot, W. (2018). Understanding variations in catastrophic health expenditure, its underlying determinants and impoverishment in Sub-Saharan African countries: A scoping review. *Systematic Reviews*, *7*(1). Advance online publication. DOI: 10.1186/s13643-018-0799-1 PMID: 30205846

Okpechi, I. G., Chukwuonye, I. I., Tiffin, N., Madukwe, O. O., Onyeonoro, U. U., & Umeizudike, T. I.. (2013). Blood Pressure Gradients and Cardiovascular Risk Factors in Urban and Rural Populations in Abia State South Eastern Nigeria Using the WHO STEPwise Approach. *PLoS One*, *8*(9). Advance online publication. DOI: 10.1371/journal.pone.0073403 PMID: 24039932

Ong, S. K., Lai, D. T. C., Wong, J. Y. Y., Si-Ramlee, K. A., Razak, L. A., & Kassim, N.. (2017). Cross-sectional STEPwise Approach to Surveillance (STEPS) Population Survey of Noncommunicable Diseases (NCDs) and Risk Factors in Brunei Darussalam 2016. *Asia-Pacific Journal of Public Health*, *29*(8), 635–648. DOI: 10.1177/1010539517738072 PMID: 29082745

Orm, I., Devos, P., & Diaconu, K. (2023). Experiences of communities with Lebanon's model of care for non-communicable diseases: A cross-sectional household survey from Greater Beirut. *BMJ Open*, *13*(9), 1–12. DOI: 10.1136/bmjopen-2022-070580 PMID: 37666549

Pandey, P., & Singh, S. (2017). Catastrophic health expenditure among geriatric population of Lucknow district, India. *J Geriatr Ment Health.*, *4*(1), 42. DOI: 10.4103/jgmh.jgmh_40_16

Patil, S. S., Rajaram, D., & Seeri, J. S. (2016). Correlates of geriatric health problems in the urban elderly- A community based study in Bangalore, Karnataka. *Indian Journal of Public Health Research & Development*, *7*(3), 231–237. DOI: 10.5958/0976-5506.2016.00163

Pengpid, S., & Peltzer, K. (2020). Prevalence and correlates of multiple non-communicable disease risk factors among adults in zambia: Results of the first national steps survey in 2017. *The Pan African Medical Journal*, *37*, 1–12. DOI: 10.11604/pamj.2020.37.265.25038 PMID: 33598080

Pereira, Z. S., da Silva, A. S., Melo, J. C. D. N., dos Santos, J. C., Sewo Sampaio, P. Y., & Silva, R. J. D. S.. (2023). Differential Factors Are Associated with Physical Activity in Older Adults in Brazil with and without Non-Communicable Chronic Diseases: A Cross-Sectional Analysis of the 2019 National Health Survey. *International Journal of Environmental Research and Public Health*, *20*(14). Advance online publication. DOI: 10.3390/ijerph20146329 PMID: 37510562

Picco, L., Achilla, E., Abdin, E., Chong, S. A., Vaingankar, J. A., & McCrone, P.. (2016). Economic burden of multimorbidity among older adults: Impact on healthcare and societal costs. *BMC Health Services Research*, *16*(1), 1–12. DOI: 10.1186/s12913-016-1421-7 PMID: 27160080

Pongiglione, B., De Stavola, B. L., & Ploubidis, G. B. (2015). A systematic literature review of studies analyzing inequalities in health expectancy among the older population. *PLoS One*, *10*(6), 1–21. DOI: 10.1371/journal.pone.0130747 PMID: 26115099

Prinja, S., Jagnoor, J., Sharma, D., Aggarwal, S., Katoch, S., & Lakshmi, P. V. M.. (2019). Out-of-pocket expenditure and catastrophic health expenditure for hospitalization due to injuries in public sector hospitals in North India. *PLoS One*, *14*(11), 1–17. DOI: 10.1371/journal.pone.0224721 PMID: 31697781

Puri, P., Singh, S. K., & Pati, S. (2022). Identifying non-communicable disease multimorbidity patterns and associated factors: A latent class analysis approach. *BMJ Open*, *12*(7). Advance online publication. DOI: 10.1136/bmjopen-2021-053981 PMID: 35820748

Reid, S. D., Motilal, S., Pooransingh, S., St. Bernard, G., & Ivey, M. A. (2023). Differential Mental Health Impact of COVID-19 Lockdowns on Persons with Non-Communicable Diseases in Trinidad and Tobago. *International Journal of Environmental Research and Public Health*, *20*(16). Advance online publication. DOI: 10.3390/ijerph20166543 PMID: 37623129

Russell, S., Sturua, L., Li, C., Morgan, J., Topuridze, M., & Blanton, C.. (2019). The burden of non-communicable diseases and their related risk factors in the country of Georgia, 2015. *BMC Public Health*, *19*, 479. DOI: 10.1186/s12889-019-6785-2 PMID: 32326912

Saraswat, A., Eram, U., Shah, S., & Ahmad, A. (2023). Study on Assessment of Self-Care Practices in Patients of Non Communicable Diseases in Aligarh. *Indian Journal of Public Health Research & Development*, *14*(1), 14–21. DOI: 10.37506/ijphrd.v14i1.1878

Sarveswaran, G., Kulothungan, V., & Mathur, P. (2020). Clustering of noncommunicable disease risk factors among adults (18–69 years) in rural population, South-India. *Diabetes & Metabolic Syndrome*, *14*(5), 1005–1014. DOI: 10.1016/j.dsx.2020.05.042 PMID: 32623362

Sazlina, S. G., Zaiton, A., Nor Afiah, M. Z., & Hayati, K. S. (2012). Predictors of health related quality of life in older people with non-communicable diseases attending three primary care clinics in malaysia. *The Journal of Nutrition, Health & Aging*, *16*(5), 498–502. DOI: 10.1007/s12603-012-0038-8 PMID: 22555798

Seyedsadjadi, N., Berg, J., Bilgin, A. A., Tung, C., & Grant, R. (2017). Significant relationships between a simple marker of redox balance and lifestyle behaviours; Relevance to the Framingham risk score. *PLoS One*, *12*(11). Advance online publication. DOI: 10.1371/journal.pone.0187713 PMID: 29107974

Sharma, A., McCall-Hosenfeld, J. S., & Cuffee, Y. (2022). Systematic review of menstrual health and hygiene in Nepal employing a social ecological model. *Reproductive Health*, *19*(1), 1–21. DOI: 10.1186/s12978-022-01456-0 PMID: 35773696

Sherbiny, N. A., Younis, A., & Masoud, M. (2016). A comprehensive assessment of the physical, nutritional, and psychological health status of the elderly populace in the Fayoum Governorate (Egypt). *Archives of Gerontology and Geriatrics*, *66*, 119–126. DOI: 10.1016/j.archger.2016.06.001 PMID: 27315050

Shin, J. Y., Lim, J., Ki, M., Song, Y. J., Chun, H., & Kim, D. (2018). An assessment of magnitudes and patterns of socioeconomic inequalities across various health problems: A large national cross-sectional survey in Korea. *International Journal of Environmental Research and Public Health*, *15*(12). Advance online publication. DOI: 10.3390/ijerph15122868 PMID: 30558216

Sivanantham, P., Sahoo, J. P., Lakshminarayanan, S., Bobby, Z., & Kar, S. S. (2022). Is the rural population of Puducherry district healthy in terms of the burden of noncommunicable diseases? Findings from a cross-sectional analytical survey. *Journal of Postgraduate Medicine*, *68*(1), 14–23. DOI: 10.4103/jpgm.JPGM_796_20 PMID: 34531334

Suksatan, W., Teravecharoenchai, S., & Sarayuthpitak, J. (2023). Health-Promoting Behaviors among Older Adults with Noncommunicable Diseases in Rural and Urban Areas during the New Normal Post-COVID-19 Era: A Structural Equation Modeling Analysis. *Nutrients*, *15*(1). Advance online publication. DOI: 10.3390/nu15010101 PMID: 36615759

Sum, G., Salisbury, C., Koh, G. C. H., Atun, R., Oldenburg, B., & McPake, B.. (2019). Implications of multimorbidity patterns on health care utilisation and quality of life in middle-income countries: Cross-sectional analysis. *Journal of Global Health*, *9*(2), 20413. DOI: 10.7189/jogh.09.020413 PMID: 31448114

Svinøy, O. E., Hilde, G., Bergland, A., & Strand, B. H. (2021). Timed up and go: Reference values for community-dwelling older adults with and without arthritis and non-communicable diseases: The Tromsø study. *Clinical Interventions in Aging*, *16*, 335–343. DOI: 10.2147/CIA.S294512 PMID: 33654390

Tan, J. P., Li, N., Gao, J., Guo, Y. H., Hu, W., & Yang, J. S.. (2014). Construction of the Chinese Veteran Clinical Research (CVCR) Platform for the assessment of non-communicable diseases. *Chinese Medical Journal*, *127*(3), 448–456. DOI: 10.3760/cma.j.issn.0366-6999.20132399 PMID: 24451949

Twabi, H. H., Semphere, R., Mukoka, M., Chiume, L., Nzawa, R., & Feasey, H. R. A.. (2021). Pattern of abnormalities amongst chest X-rays of adults undergoing computer-assisted digital chest X-ray screening for tuberculosis in Peri-Urban Blantyre, Malawi: A cross-sectional study. *Tropical Medicine & International Health*, *26*(11), 1427–1437. PMID: 34297430

United Nations. (2013). World population ageing. New York: United Nations. Available from: https://www.un.org/en/development/desa/population/publications/pdf/ageing/WorldPopulationAgeing2013.pdf [Accessed 15 Feb 2024].

Vallecillo, G., Robles, M. J., Duran, X., Castillo, C., Fonseca, F., & Torrens, M. (2020). High prevalence and risks factors for non-communicable diseases in older people with opioid use disorder. *Heroin Addiction and Related Clinical Problems*, *22*(1), 23–30.

Van Minh, H., & Xuan Tran, B. (2012). Assessing the household financial burden associated with the chronic non-communicable diseases in a rural district of Vietnam. *Global Health Action*, *5*, 1–7. DOI: 10.3402/gha.v5i0.18892 PMID: 23273250

VanDevanter, N., Naegle, M., Nazia, N., Bamodu, A., & Marx, E. S. (2023). Healthy aging and care of the older adult with chronic disease: A qualitative needs assessment in 14 eastern and southern Caribbean islands. *Revista Panamericana de Salud Pública = Pan American Journal of Public Health*, *47*, 1–6. DOI: 10.26633/RPSP.2023.40 PMID: 36909812

Verma, V. R., Kumar, P., & Dash, U. (2021). Assessing the household economic burden of non-communicable diseases in India: Evidence from repeated cross-sectional surveys. *BMC Public Health*, *21*(1), 1–22. DOI: 10.1186/s12889-021-10828-3 PMID: 33962625

Wagner, K. H., Schwingshackl, L., Draxler, A., & Franzke, B. (2021). Impact of dietary and lifestyle interventions in elderly or people diagnosed with diabetes, metabolic disorders, cardiovascular disease, cancer and micronutrient deficiency on micronuclei frequency - A systematic review and meta-analysis. *Mutation Research/ Reviews in Mutation Research*, *787*, 108367. DOI: 10.1016/j.mrrev.2021.108367 PMID: 34083034

Wang, Y., Liu, M., & Liu, J. (2023). Catastrophic health expenditure and the risk of depression among middle-aged and old people in China: A national population-based longitudinal study. *Epidemiology and Psychiatric Sciences*, *32*. Advance online publication. DOI: 10.1017/S2045796023000240 PMID: 37194279

Wang, Z., Li, X., & Chen, M. (2015). Catastrophic health expenditures and its inequality in elderly households with chronic disease patients in China. *International Journal for Equity in Health*, *14*(1). Advance online publication. DOI: 10.1186/ s12939-015-0134-6 PMID: 25599715

Wu, N., Xie, X., Cai, M., Han, Y., & Wu, S. (2023). Trends in health service needs, utilization, and non-communicable chronic diseases burden of older adults in China: Evidence from the 1993 to 2018 National Health Service Survey. *International Journal for Equity in Health*, *22*(1). Advance online publication. DOI: 10.1186/ s12939-023-01983-7 PMID: 37649033

Xu, X., & Yang, H. (2022). Elderly chronic diseases and catastrophic health expenditure: An important cause of Borderline Poor Families' return to poverty in rural China. *Humanities & Social Sciences Communications*, *9*(1). Advance online publication. DOI: 10.1057/s41599-022-01310-5

Yang, C., Long, J., Shi, Y., Zhou, Z., Wang, J., & Zhao, M. H.. (2022). Healthcare resource utilisation for chronic kidney disease and other major non-communicable chronic diseases in China: A cross-sectional study. *BMJ Open*, *12*(1). Advance online publication. DOI: 10.1136/bmjopen-2021-051888 PMID: 35027417

Yankanchi, S. G., & Udigiri, R. (2023). Morbidity Pattern among the Farm House Residents in Vijayapur District, Karnataka - A Cross Sectional Study. *Journal of the Indian Medical Association*, *121*(2), 27–32.

Yawson, A. E., Abuosi, A. A., Badasu, D. M., Atobra, D., Adzei, F. A., & Anarfi, J. K. (2016). Non-communicable diseases among children in Ghana: Health and social concerns of parent/caregivers. *African Health Sciences*, *16*(2), 378–388. DOI: 10.4314/ahs.v16i2.6 PMID: 27605953

Yonel, Z., Sharma, P., Yahyouche, A., Jalal, Z., Dietrich, T., & Chapple, I. L. (2018). Patients' attendance patterns to different healthcare settings and perceptions of stakeholders regarding screening for chronic, non-communicable diseases in high street dental practices and community pharmacy: A cross-sectional study. *BMJ Open*, *8*(11). Advance online publication. DOI: 10.1136/bmjopen-2018-024503 PMID: 30391921

Yu, X., & Zhang, W. (2020). Neighborhood's locality, road types, and residents' multimorbidity: Evidence from China's middle-aged and older adults. *BMC Public Health*, *20*(1), 1728. DOI: 10.1186/s12889-020-09876-y PMID: 33198728

Zali, A., Gholamzadeh, S., Mohammadi, G., Looha, M. A., Akrami, F., & Zarean, E.. (2020). Baseline Characteristics and Associated Factors of Mortality in COVID-19 Patients; an Analysis of 16000 Cases in Tehran, Iran. *Archives of Academic Emergency Medicine*, *8*(1), e70. DOI: 10.22037/aaem.v8i1.872 PMID: 33134966

Zubayer, M. A., Ahammed, B., Sarder, M. A., Kundu, S., Majumder, U. K., & Islam, S. M. S. (2021). Double and triple burden of non-communicable diseases and its determinants among adults in Bangladesh: Evidence from a recent demographic and health survey. *International Journal of Clinical Practice*, *75*(10). Advance online publication. DOI: 10.1111/ijcp.14613 PMID: 34235819

Chapter 9
Navigating Ethical Frontiers in AI-Driven Geriatric Care

Ayesha Farooqi
https://orcid.org/0009-0000-4556-4211
Poornima University, India

Debmitra Das
https://orcid.org/0009-0004-7079-1415
Poornima University, India

Monika Tripathi
Poornima University, India

Ritam Dutta
https://orcid.org/0000-0003-3089-778X
Poornima Institute of Engineering and Technology, India

Nikhil Kumar Goyal
https://orcid.org/0009-0007-4532-8033
Poornima University, India

Mohammed Firdos Alam Sheikh
https://orcid.org/0000-0002-8405-8482
Poornima University, India

ABSTRACT

This chapter explores the ethical, legal and social issues of the use of artificial intelligence (AI) in geriatrics. With the increasing number of geriatrics in the world, the application of AI, in the form of assistive robotics, predictive health solutions, and digital companions, is growing to assist older adults medically, socially, and emotionally. Although such technologies have potential benefits to increase the efficiency of healthcare, individualize it, and assist caregivers, they give rise to important ethical concerns concerning issues of privacy, autonomy, fairness, and dignity of a human person. This chapter inserts these problems into conventional codes of medical ethics, but at the same time it directs these problems to the risks that are unique to the elderly populations. Specific adversity posed by AI, such as data protection, algorithmic bias, dependency, and accountability, in the course of making crucial decisions using AI, are addressed in detail.

DOI: 10.4018/979-8-3373-5462-0.ch009

1. INTRODUCTION

1.1 Rise of AI in Healthcare

Artificial intelligence has gone through a transformation in the past ten years, and it is now an essential and viable asset in health systems across the globe. The existing algorithms that can process large amounts of data and determine patterns as well as provide predictive judgments have become an addition to human knowledge in the medical field. In other areas like diagnosis, drug discovery and treatment optimization, AI has proven to be extremely promising improvements in the levels of accuracy and efficiency. This trend is not restricted to hospitals passionate about high technology or medical research institutions, but more and more care facilities are adopting applications of artificial intelligence, including community clinics, rehabilitation clinics, and telemedicine.

Figure 1. Explore the Practical Applications of AI in Healthcare

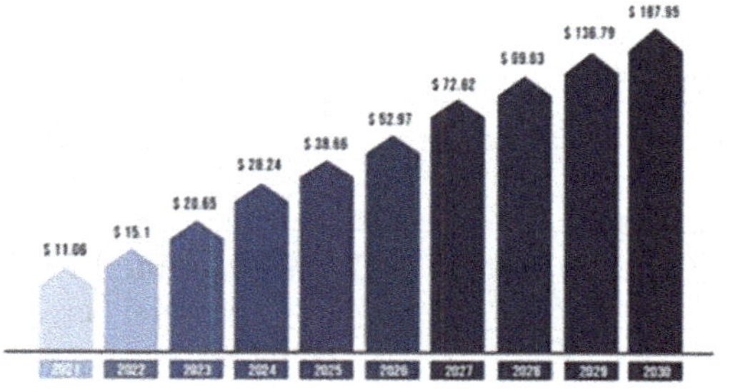

This change is especially profound with regard to geriatric care. The worldwide demographic situation has been changing incredibly fast as the life expectancy grows, and birth rates decrease. The WHO estimates put the population aged 60 and older at an equivalent of nearly twice as many by 2050. With an upsurge in the aging population to the never-before levels, this has posed significant problems to the health care facilities, caregivers, and cost maintenance, among others. The emergence of AI technologies, which can automate or assist in monitoring, offer personalized health-related data and support caregivers, helps to fill the gap that is growing between demand and supply in elderly care (Chen et al., 2020).

More than that, the emergence of AI is not the only narrative of technological advancements but one of necessity. The challenges related to staff shortages that plague the healthcare and are especially common in the elderly and palliative care areas where emotional support is just as important as treatment. AI can help address the issue of overstrained personnel by automating certain processes and providing intelligent tools that would assist healthcare providers and, at the same time, enhance care delivery. This takes the increasing role of AI in healthcare beyond just efficiency improvement to meeting some of the most fundamental needs of these systems and required equitable access to care by vulnerable populations on a more equitable basis than ever before.

1.2 Importance of AI Applications in Elderly Care

Older adults usually have complicated and persistent medical issues like dementia, heart diseases, arthritis and impaired sensory organ-functioning. The complex nature of these needs is often not supported by traditional models of care, which are reliant on human care givers and visits to hospital. The usage of AI applications can be considered a critical finding in addressing these gaps since they provide the capabilities stemming out of precision, individualization, and scalability. As an example, wearable AI-powered devices can provide constant monitoring of vital signs with the prediction of health anomalies and provide notifications to prevent their deterioration. These tools are particularly helpful to the aging who live on their own and give relief not only to patients but their relatives as well (Ali & Li, 2019).

In addition to monitoring their health, AI can improve the life of old people on a daily basis. Smart home AI technologies can control the lighting, heating, and security systems to make safe environments that are customized to the needs of the aging residents. Assistive robots can be speech-touch-recognizing and machine-learning friendly to remind users to take medicines, be assistive in mobility, and even have discussions to eliminate loneliness. These applications demonstrate that the significance of AI in healthcare provision to the elderly cannot be confined to the arena of healthcare pathway, as it also has applications in improving the general quality of life of the elderly.

Also, AI can be of significant aid to both professional and family caregivers. Care giving can be both physically and emotionally exhaustive, and the burnout rates in facilities serving the elderly is quite high. Such technologies as automated documentation systems, fall detector sensors, and a predictive care planning tool could also help to reduce administrative and surveillance tension that could give more time to caregivers to interact with human beings. This middling music between human sensibility and technological assistance is actually how AI in elderly care is important a person can do and make a difference and at the same technology can enable a person to do that difference better.

1.3 Ethical Dimensions in the Context of Aging Populations

As much as the benefits of AI in geriatric care cannot be ignored, the ethical impact of AI cannot be ignored. Older adults represent one of the most vulnerable members of the society, and the application of more sophisticated technologies in the treatment of such individuals brings about the question of privacy, autonomy, dignity, and fairness. Continuous surveillance systems and health-monitoring devices can raise safety levels, as well as violate personal privacy. In the same manner, AI-led healthcare decision-making brings up issues of transparency and accountability where there is a risk that the data can be misinterpreted or algorithms can reach biased solutions.

Other crucial issues are autonomy. The aged group may attribute dignity in old age to independence being one of the things that they may consider important. Nonetheless, the growing dependence on AI-powered technologies may subconsciously cultivate machine dependency with a consequent loss of personal agency. This tension in ethics explains why there is a need to focus on the development of AI solutions that will not disempower their end users, and instead assist and enable them in making choices about their lives (Ienca, 2017).

Moreover, societal inequalities can be widened in case AI systems are not created and established in an inclusive way. Lack of access to advanced AI facilities may necessitate funding in the form of money, digital skills, and strong facilities all of which may not be democratically available among communities. The question of ethics of AI in the treatment of the aged, then, is not confined to the concerns of the individual but to the wider ones of justice, accessibility and other social responsibilities. Collaboration is required between policymakers, technologists, and healthcare providers to work together to make sure that AI can be viewed as an amplifier of dignity and equity instead of an exclusionary or coercive sourcequin independent of what is underscoring the potential of electrical-related mechanics to support or undermine compassion, kindness, and empathy driving the development of AI (Ashfaq et al., 2020).

2. FOUNDATIONS OF ETHICS IN HEALTHCARE TECHNOLOGY

2.1 Traditional Medical Ethics and Geriatric Care

Medical ethics have been the rulebook in the making of medical decisions especially in geriatric settings where, the patient is mostly vulnerable. In medical decision-making, a principle of beneficence (acting in the best interest of the patient), a principle of non-maleficence (avoiding harm), a principle of autonomy (respects the choice of the patient), and a principle of justice (ensuring fairness in the knowledge of healthcare delivery) are considered. In elder care, these principles are extended, and elder adults can experience many chronic conditions, cognitive loss, dependence upon others and so on.

There are new challenges to these principles with the advent of AI applications that hold tremendous promise in scope. As an example, predictive algorithms aimed at detecting health risk have to be tested on the principle of non-maleficence. Improper diagnosis of an illness or failure to detect a dangerous condition by an AI device might lead to serious results. Likewise, autonomy dictates that an elderly patient should be in charge of their health choices but AI-based systems tend to act in a manner that is not always clear and could not be easily overruled (Sinnige et al., 2023).

In such a manner, AI as an ethical reconfiguration in geriatric care is not a purely technological innovation. The established tenets of medical ethics are a lens that must be used when considering implementing AI, as the movement toward advanced technology must not transition into a degradation of the ideals that make the entire care-giving process what it is today.

2.2 Principles for Technology-Driven Healthcare

With the shift to a technology-driven healthcare system, a larger set of ethics are required. AI systems are different in that they are independent of the caregivers with the capability of further controlling the decisions than the caregivers in conventional medical tools. Such independence induces a need to formulate ethical frameworks to discuss transparency, accountability, and inclusivity.

The healthcare industry that relies on technology ought to be transparent. Engaging older patients and their caregivers in the process of decision-making with the help of AI requires them to be aware of how the AI system functions, with respect to which data, and how decisions are made. In case of lack of transparency, there is nothing like trust in such systems and patients feel more alienated than empowered. Accountability is also paramount, to put it another way when AI-initiated decisions cause harm, it is vital to examine accountability whether it is with the developer, the healthcare professionals or the institution implementing the technology in question. Inclusivity will make sure that AI applications are made with diverse groups of older people in mind, decreasing the likelihood of bias against marginalized groups of the elderly (Bloom et al., 2015).

It is by integrating these principles into AI-based healthcare frameworks that the profession can step towards a more ethical-driven innovation model, one that is no longer characterized by placing efficiency as a top-tier goal but by also taking into consideration human dignity, safety, and rights of elderly patients.

2.3 Role of Human Dignity and Autonomy

The dignity and autonomy are among the ethical issues in the AI-driven geriatric care. Elderly individuals are at risk of being attacked by the notion of self-worth with regard to physical degradation, and dependence on others. The dignity may be supported or violated by I technologies. As another example, mobility or medication management assistive robots can facilitate independence enabling an older adult to feel more confident and self-determined. Conversely, such close monitoring by way of monitoring devices can be unhealthy as it impairs privacy and transforms an individual to being an object instead of feeling respected (Cafolla, 2024).

Figure 2. Factors affecting patient's dignity

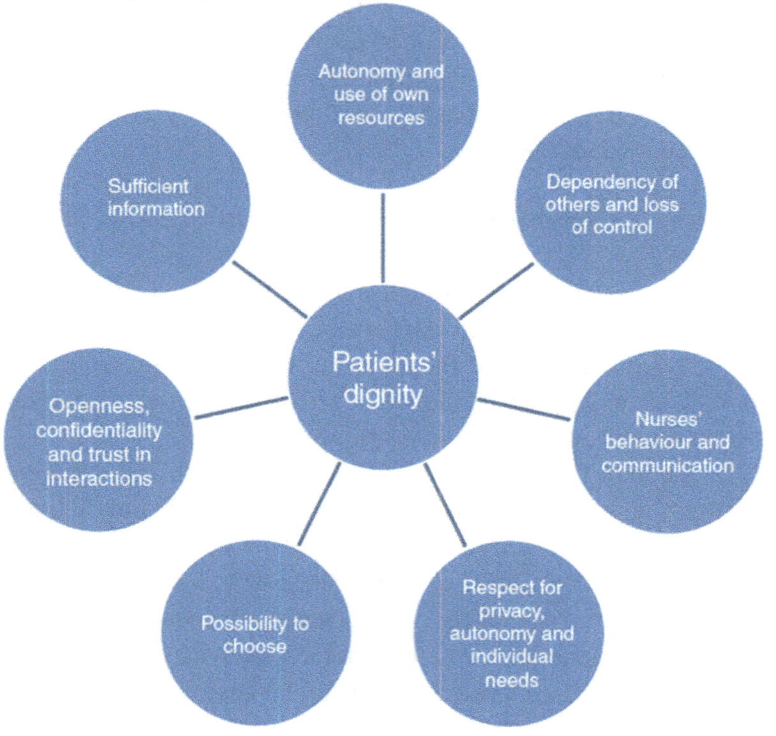

Another pillar of ethical healthcare that should be well kept is autonomy. The recommendations delivered by the AI should be designed as helpful aids but not as compulsive tools to force out individual decisions in favor. As an example, certain guidelines, such as a specific dietary intake to control diabetes, may be proposed by an AI-based program, but the choice has to be made by the patient and supported by human caregivers who can add an empathic perspective and background. In order to retain control the AI systems used must be explainable, customizable, and user-responsive, so that technologies do not endanger but instead guarantee self-determination.

Overall, ethics of healthcare technology should stand on the grounds of dignity and autonomy. AI in geriatric care should focus on the following values as priorities, which can make it a form of empowerment and not domination.

3. AI APPLICATIONS IN GERIATRIC CARE

3.1 Assistive Robotics for Elderly Support

One of the most understood examples of AI use in the geriatric sector is assistive robots. These machines are created to facilitate the adult aged with mobility, daily tasks and even companions. To illustrate, artificial intelligence-based navigation tools can ensure that robots help the elderly move around their homes and decrease fall-related accidents. Robotic exoskeletons or robotic arms can also be helpful, allowing a person with reduced mobility to stand on his/her own.

Beyond simple physical assistance, new focus is being given to the emotional needs with the development of assistive robots. Socially interactive robots can be used to engage in conversation in natural language processing, memory building games or to enforce appointment and medication reminders. These systems are capable of addressing the problem of loneliness that is experienced by the aged, especially those residing in solitude. Nevertheless, there are still ethical issues of replacing human interaction with digital ones, and the questions about the authenticity and emotional health must be answered (Mhlanga, 2020).

Assistive robotics has the potential not to substitute care provider but to enhance their activities. Robots alleviate human caregivers of repetitive or physically strenuous tasks and allow them to attend more to the relational and empathetic sides of care and find a balance between care-industrial efficiency and human connection.

3.2 AI in Diagnosis and Predictive Health Monitoring

AI has proved to have amazing capabilities when it comes to treating diseases and forecasting health risks in the elderly. Wearable gadgets, which are equipped with AI AI algorithms, can monitor vital signs in real tome (e.g., heart rate, blood pressure, and oxygen saturation) and provide early detection of medical conditions.

Machine learning models can inspect these datasets to forecast falls, discover early signs of cognitive decline or predict readmissions to the hospital.

As another example, AI technology could recognize minor changes in speech patterns or gait that could be evidence of the onset of dementia or Parkinson's disease. Predictive monitoring can improve health outcomes and even save health systems a lot of money because early-stage interventions can be performed to address the problem. Nonetheless, this dependency on the monitoring may be questioned in terms of privacy, ownership of data and even the geist of having to live under the sight of surveillance at any given time (Gill et al., 2013).

Predictive monitoring should seek a balance ethically between safety and autonomy. Although the advantages of early diagnosis are enormous, elderly people should still be in control of their data collection, sharing, and utilization process. The process of consent must be transparent, not showing the patient as a/the passive object of technologically controlled processes.

3.3 Personalized Care and Digital Companions

Among the most paradigm-shifting AI uses in the geriatric population is the implementation of personalized healthcare experiences. AI-based systems can incorporate an individual medical history, genetic data and real-time monitoring data to generate patient-specific care plans. These systems enable individualized prescription, whether that be prescription changes or lifestyle changes, so that treatment is not specific to the specific patient (Hajdú, 2020).

An emerging area is digital companions, which are geared to provide emotional and social benefits to their owners through AI-enabled conversation and interaction. Such systems also help the aged people who feel social isolated. With the delivery of companionship, reminders, and cognitive stimulation, digital companions can also increase emotional well-being and postpone the cognitive decline.

However, customization poses ethical concerns of privacy and control of data. The more information is gathered to individualize care, the higher the likelihood of breaches or violation of confidentiality. Although online companionship can effectively make people get closer each other, relying on the technology in order to attain companionship might also depreciate human contact, which will cause a situation where technology is replacing people instead of making the relationships closer. To make sure that personalization serves human dignity, special design decisions and regulatory protection will be essential(Vandemeulebroucke et al., 2020) .

4. CHALLENGES OF AI IN GERIATRIC CARE

4.1 Privacy and Data Protection Concerns

AI-based technologies are frequently used by elderly people who are being monitored every day in terms of their health and daily activity patterns. Privacy is the key issue that arises when it comes to such monitoring as it is necessary to conduct interventions in time. The vulnerability of the population to exploitation or discrimination can be caused by the breach of data or its enforcement by unauthorized parties through the personal health data of vulnerable populations. The aged can have a hard time interpreting consent agreements or the consequences of data sharing especially when their usual digital literacy is already low (Amin et al., 2016).

The ethical issue is how to make systems that guarantee privacy without undermining safety. This and needs strong security in the form of encryption, clear terms of consent and a policy that allows the patient to control what happens to their data. Ethical AI should keep the principle of informational autonomy at the forefront, so that elderly people are aware and empowered on how their personal data is used (Khan et al., 2021).

4.2 Algorithmic Bias and Fairness in Elderly Health Outcomes

The truth is that a systems can only be as faultless as the data that they are trained on. Data representation problems in the elderly result in algorithmic bias, resulting in inaccurate predictions and unfair healthcare disparities. Take, for instance, a diagnostic algorithm that will be trained mainly using data about younger adults only, which could lead to the inability of the algorithm to interpret the symptoms of older patients as such, and thus fail to diagnose them properly or treat them in an insufficient manner (Kim et al., 2022).

Not only would AI bias jeopardise fairness, it would also worsen pre-existing health disparities. To combat this challenge, comprehensive datasets will be needed, continuous bias auditing, and reporting of the limitations of the AI systems. Fairness in geriatric care investment in AI applications will entail providing high level of service to the elderly community regardless of their demographic variations in age, gender, and economic disparity (Kumar et al., 2023).

4.3 Dependency, Autonomy, and Human Dignity

Notwithstanding, autonomous use of AI can provoke dependence, leading eventually to a state where elderly people will no longer be able to operate independently. Dependence on AI companions, such as overdependence, as an example, is likely to decline actual social interactions, leading to isolation. Equally, the use of predictive monitoring could induce caregivers to override patient wishes in favor of the algorithms.

When used to empower and not to control, human dignity is also endangered. The ethics frameworks should therefore underline the idea that AI be viewed as a supplement to making decisions by human beings. A key principle to take into consideration in making systems that involve agency, flexibility, and choice is vital to the continued perception of dignity in AI-driven care (London et al., 2023).

4.4 Accountability and Liability in AI-Driven Decisions

In incorrect tool choices by AI systems, it is not easy to figure out who is at fault. In case of failure of AI-monitor cap to detect a fall or invalid health condition recognition, the accountability can be directed to developers, medical practitioners, or employing organizations. The lack of distinct accountability structure can be an ethical and legal liability, and the elderly patients are at risk of being harmed without proper compensation possibilities.

To solve this dilemma, ethically developed AI should have accountability structures; precisely the processes that allot responsibility to each phase, design to deployment. Policymakers are also obligated to implement regulatory regimes that explain liability, so that the elderly are not left defenseless in situations arising when there is technological failure. Finally, the focus on accountability cannot be seen purely as a legal matter but as a matter of moral responsibility towards the outcomes which may pose a threat to the welfare of vulnerable groups (Ali & Nikberg, 2024).

5. PSYCHOLOGICAL AND SOCIAL IMPLICATIONS OF AI IN GERIATRIC CARE

5.1 Impact on Elderly Mental Health and Emotional Well-Being

The possibility of making use of AI technologies within the contexts of geriatric care has an enormous potential to improve the quality of life of senior citizens, but it also has strong psychological undertone. Positively, loneliness is one of the most prevalent problems of the elderly, and robots and AI have helped with this by way of conversational agents, virtual companions, and interactive robots. Social isolation is one of the established risks of depression, cognitive weakness, and physical health impairment. Continuous engagement makes AI systems can offer the companionship that would give a sense of companionship and purpose.

Nonetheless, the replacement of the human connection with artificial communication proposes the issues of ethics and psychology. Although companions that are based on AI may replicate empathy, they do not have the correspondence of human feelings through emotional reciprocity and care. The habitual use of artificial companions can also provide a thin facade of companionship especially when the elderly member is more exposed to abandonment issues once face-to-face contact is reduced. In addition, some older adults might also develop the so-called robot anxiety, or fear, when introduced to robotic or AI solutions because of unfamiliarity or loss of human touch in care (Mhlanga, 2023a).

Infrastructures that strike a balance between these dynamics involves the development of AI designed to complement, rather than supersede, human interaction. Ethical deployment must first be to promote well-being without compromising the values of real social interactions.

5.2 Social Isolation, Digital Companionship, and Interpersonal Relationships

Social isolation is among the most urgent geriatric medical problems. Older adults are often isolated because they do not see anyone or live on their own or in nursing homes. AI offers a solution that provides digital companionship and that its contribution to interpersonal relationships is contradictory. Though use of AI companions can help lessen the pain of living alone due to its conversational potential and reminders, there is a risk that family members or caregivers will be discouraged to check in regularly by the assumption that there is a robot to do the job (Mhlanga, 2023b).

There is generation issue to whether they will be accepted or not. Younger baby boomers and generations are far-less digitally illiterate and thus may find IC social companionship reassuring and welcoming, but the older cohorts can find the technology to be intrusive and dehumanizing. The cultural setting also contributes to the discussion: in societies where the direct engagement of the family in elderly care is appreciated, the use of the AI assistant can be interpreted as a lack of social responsibilities, whereas in individualistic countries, such an offering could be considered as strength-empowering.

Ethically, the systems have to be presented as supplementing human interaction. It is important that caregivers and their families are trained to incorporate AI tools as extending care to relational care, as opposed to trying to replace any such tool completely.

5.3 Intergenerational Dynamics and the Changing Role of Family Caregivers

Geriatric medicine is changing the way of families due to the growth of AI. Conventionally, younger generations of the family dominate the process providing emotional and physical assistance to the aging family members. The future AI technologies will reduce the burden of care because they will help with routine activities, health tracking and provide some predictive warnings of an emergency. Such support can decrease stress on the caregivers and allow a family to concentrate on other important areas of care (Mois & Beer, 2020).

Ethical issues occur in the terms of redistribution of responsibility. The families can start using AI systems too much, and personal involvement will be gradually abandoned. This trend has the potential to change intergenerational relationships, causing the relationships to be less based on a sense of obligation and intimacy that is synonymous with elder care. Not every family can enjoy the same access to AI solutions; the affordability and accessibility of such products may further exacerbate existing disproportionate care quality.

Ethical integration of AI in family caregiving must support the policies and cultural supports that endorse the uniqueness of human contact. I believe that IA should serve as a supportive interface that would allow families to focus more time on their elderly members instead of doing away with such time altogether.

5.4 Psychological Risks of Over-Reliance on AI in Elderly Care

Adventurous dependence on AI technologies may expose older adults to a pool of psychological dangers. Secondly, the elderly may lose the confidence of self-efficacy because of dependence on automated systems. When humans do not have to perform some of the functions, such as managing medication, planning, offering mobility assistance, and voluntarily transfer them to the machine, the elderly will start experiencing disengagement with their own capabilities. That is called learned helplessness and can speed up cognitive decline and foster being passive (Goyal, 2025).

Second, AI operated using surveillance creates a feeling of being monitored at all times, which affects the privacy and causes stress. Elderly people might also feel that they are placed under surveillance all the time, which destroys their independence. And lastly, technological inaccuracy (i.e., false alarms, suggesting a treatment that is not correct) increases anxiety, which creates distrust towards AI and healthcare professionals.

To prevent these risks, thus, AI systems have to be given a human-centered approach where empowerment, rather than control, is considered. Interfaces should be easy to use, flexible to requirements and responsive to the psychological factors associated with the use of technology. Such an approach towards aging will enable AI to play a supportive role in geriatric care instead of disempowering them.

6. REGULATORY AND POLICY PERSPECTIVES

6.1 Current Regulatory Frameworks for AI in Healthcare

The booming AI in the context of healthcare also has some problematic implications because the expansion rates of AI have surpassed the models and regulations development. Regulations modernly tend to be more general medical device regulations, like the FDA approval process or the Medical Devices Regulation (MDR) of the European Union. Such structures pay higher attention to safety and efficacy but fail to handle wider ethical issues, namely, transparency, accountability, and the rights of a patient(Udupa & Yellampalli, 2025).

In geriatrics and such areas where the patients are already inhibited by regulatory deficiencies, the gap becomes more pronounced. Lots of AI tools, including predictive monitoring systems or social robots, might not easily be categorised as medical devices and thus would not be subjected to customary regulation. Such ambiguity poses dangers to the patient as well as the provider since the liability on erroneous acts or wrong usage is unclear.

In order to have an ethical integration, current systems need to be changed to include fairness, inclusivity, and autonomy respect requirements besides the traditional ones that relate to safety needs.

6.2 Ethical Governance and Global Policy Trends

Globally, governance of ethics in AI in healthcare is slowly being understood by governments and institutions. The European Union has brought forth some leadership in trying to create its proposed AI Act, putting forward a risk-based classification system around AI-based applications with tighter requirements applied to higher-risk systems, including those in healthcare. In the same way, agencies such as World Health Organization (WHO) have provided provisos that support the aspects of transparency, accountability, and inclusivity in the AI-driven health systems.

Nevertheless, worldwide inequality in governance continues to be very large. AI regulations will first be generated and enforced at higher levels in high-income countries, whereas low- and middle-income countries may not be able to even enact simple protections. Such disparity threatens to establish a tier system in AI-driven healthcare where some elderly patients could get a better ethical protection than other elderly patients depending on geographical location (Goyal et al., 2025b).

Cooperation at an international level is thus crucial International standards in AI ethics in geriatrics could be created and thus assuring uniformity and avoiding gaps in the rules where exploitation of vulnerable groups can occur through a lax regulation of the sphere in question.

6.3 Policy Recommendations for Responsible AI in Geriatric Care

Policymakers should take proactive and comprehensive stands to overcome the ethical boundaries of AI-driven elderly care. Three major recommendations can be distinguished.

1. Increasing Accountability Mechanisms – Regulations need to spell out who is responsible in the event of an error related to AI, be that the developer, the healthcare provider, or the institution. Laws must be in place to capture the needs of the aged patients in case of injury.
2. Enhancing Transparency and Informed Consent – AI systems should be explainable and accessible as per policies. Old people and the people taking care of them should be capable of comprehending the way of making decisions, what kind of data has to be gathered, and how it is processed. Consent must be a dynamic and continuous process rather than a one-time pop up box.
3. Ensuring equity and accessibility of AI-driven care should not only focus on, but should be accessible to every aging population regardless of geographic location or social economic status. In order to avoid further disparity of care quality, granting subsidies, public financing, and fair distribution plans are essential.

One more thing governments can do is invest in digital literacy initiatives among the older population and make them comfortable using AI tools and operating independently. Policymakers can develop systems that would heighten the geriatric care by using both technological majority and ethical governance instead of compromising the latter (Raza et al., 2022).

6.4 Balancing Innovation with Ethical Safeguards

The main dilemma underlying AI policy legislation in medicated geriatric treatment is the need to innovate the field and at the same time protect its ethical integrity. Excessive strict rules can kill innovation and hold back the application of life-saving equipment. On the other hand, there is the danger of lacking adequate control, as the vulnerable members of the older generations can be subjected to abuse, exploitation, or abandonment.

Balance in this must be elicited through a fluid, adaptive sort of governance. Regulatory frameworks need to be dynamic, thus able to adapt to the changing technology. Engagement with stakeholders is also essential-the elderly themselves, the caregivers, and the health staff, and the technology inducers should all be involved in the formulation of policy (Reynolds et al., 2022).

Finally, ethical regulation also should not be seen as an obstacle to innovation but as a trust-building factor. Integrating protection mechanisms within the creation and implementation of AI, policymakers may cultivate an environment in which the elder population can enjoy the technological advances without having to expose themselves to the dangers of AI.

7. CASE STUDIES AND PRACTICAL APPLICATIONS

7.1 AI in Fall Detection and Emergency Response

One of the most widespread and awful health hazards of elderly people is falls, which usually lead to bone fractures, hospitalization, and long-term disability. Fall detection is one of the applications of AI in geriatric care that can be developed. Unlike conventional emergency buttons, movable sensors and automatic vision-based systems can detect falls on their own and sound alarms. Such tools utilize accelerometers, radar imaging, and machine intelligence in differentiating a normal movement and a potentially harmful occurrence (Schulz et al., 2020).

As an example, smart home monitoring systems that have depth cameras can identify the body posture and detect unusual pattern related to a fall. No time to waste Once detected, the system alerts the caregivers or the emergency services within a significant reduction of response times. Notably, AI increases detection accuracy by minimising false alarms- one of the problems of prior mechanical systems.

Ethically, they present issues of privacy and autonomy to such systems. Constant surveillance, particularly with the help of cameras, can be considered as an encroachment, which makes some elderly people feel that they are being tracked in their personal areas. Striking the balance between safety and dignity warrants attentiveness in design: AI needs to gather as little data as possible, faces should be depersonalized, and users must be given an opportunity to make an informed choice whether they would like to participate or not.

7.2 Companion Robots and Emotional Support Systems

The additional significant usage of AI in elderly care is the creation of companion robots that would be able to serve as a delivery of emotional and social support. Such examples as Paro, the robotic seal, or Pepper, the humanoid robot, have demonstrated good results in managing the conditions of loneliness and preventing the tendency of dementia-related agitation. These systems interact with elderly people in terms of conversation, gestures and emotional recognition technology.

The use of companion robotics can assist mental health in its ability to provide an engaging experience, routine, and comfort to the user. In the case of caregivers, such technologies minimize emotional stress, thus, the elderly enjoys quality consistency even when the workforce is depleted.

Nonetheless, there is still a question of ethics. Do AI systems that pretend to have empathy or does this amount to deception? Some objectors state that it is dangerous to create machine-impersonating caring since this may diminish the value of human relations. Supporters respond that the apparent psychological effects (feeling less lonely, having a better mood) make the use of artificial companions worthwhile, particularly in less-well-endowed care systems (Shi et al., 2024).

The practical use indicates that such systems can work best when combined with a human carer instead of being a substitute. As has been shown in pilot programs in Japan, companion robots are most effective as add-ons to social engagement programs, not as replacements to them.

7.3 Smart Homes and AI-Enabled Care Facilities

AI is not only converting individual devices, but also transforming all types of living environments. Smart homes with old age residents included IoT-tented sensors and voice-enabled assistants, as well as predictive analytics, to guarantee safety and free living. Telemetry is another lightweight functionality that can be used to monitor vital signs, assess mobility, and manage medication schedules, to mention just a few.

AI has been applied in care facilities to enhance staffing schedules, predict health emergencies and individualize care plans. As an example, predictive analytics can be used to predict residents who are at greater risk of falls or infection, so intervention can be implemented to prevent these outcomes. Such a strategy does not only enhance results but also lessens the financial strain to the healthcare system (Bloom & Luca, 2016).

However, such systems hold their problems as well: there are the breach of privacy regarding data, bias in algorithmic risk prediction, and a lack of inclusion of older citizens who have never used technology. Ethical frameworks have to consider consent where the older adult has a full understanding of what the data is used within the decision-making process and offers some method to question or dispute the AI-generated decision.

7.4 Lessons from Global Implementations

Countries worldwide have adapted the sphere of AI in geriatrics in dissimilar ways. Japan With an ageing population, Japan has been a leader in the use of robots when it comes to companionship and assistance with caregiving. In Europe, it has been stressed that innovation has to co-exist with high-security standards in GDPR. Meanwhile, in the United States, there are significant clouds of the bright startups representing innovation in the sphere of wearable sensors and AI-driven solutions in the creation of health platforms.

These international case studies show that attitudes to aging and technology are culture-dependent and shows that attitudes to aging and technology influence the adoption and use of AI. In the collectivistic world, the role of AI can be criticized as the one that will call the authority of family-based caregivers into question, whereas in individualistic societies, AI will be more likely to be accepted as a kind of empowerment that will help individuals become more independent (Goyal et al., 2025a).

Based on these examples, there is one lesson that is evident, AI in geriatrics governance cannot operate a one-fits-all model. Effective implementation will require cultural sensitivity, ethical protection and effective participation of elderly people in the design and adoption process.

8. FUTURE DIRECTIONS AND RESEARCH NEEDS

8.1 Technological Innovations on the Horizon

Technologies related to artificial intelligence in geriatric care are developing at a new pace, and a breakthrough in recent years, compared to the current applications that are in existence, is very likely to be a reality. The development of natural language processing (NLP) is one of the most promising spheres. Existing conversational agents have problems with situational awareness, emotional intelligence and cultural cultural sensitivity. The next generation systems will provide really empathetic interactions, such that the elderly individuals can engage in purposeful or meaningful conversational processes with the AI companion simulating human listening capability, human understanding capability and human flattery capability.

These systems are also likely to alleviate loneliness and instill a feeling of companionship among the individual living in isolation.

The other important frontier is robotics Although much of this already occurs with assistive robots in the form of companion pets or assistive mobility devices, the next wave of robotics promises to be able to perform more complicated physical tasks, such as lifting and transferring patients, preparing meals, and independent mobility assistance. These systems will minimize physical stress on the caregivers and increase independence of older people.

Meanwhile, the wearable health technologies will also change largely. In addition to heart rate or step tracking, future devices may incorporate biosensors that allow to measure glucose levels, blood pressure, oxygen saturation and even neurological activity, on-the-fly. With predictive AI algorithms added to these devices, he or she will receive an early signal of the onset of a chronic disease, falling, or cognitive decline so that corrective action may be taken beforehand instead of waiting to rectify the problem. Nevertheless, the key issues will continue to be accessibility and affordability. Unless ways are found to democratize such innovations, they risk creating inequalities between elderly persons with low income groups having no access to advanced technologies that enable them to live autonomously (Han et al., 2023).

8.2 Addressing Gaps in Ethical Research

Despite the progressive rate of the technological aspect of AI-driven geriatric care development, ethical research has remained underdeveloped. Most of the available literature dwells on technical feasibility and efficiency leaving behind important human-centred questions like autonomy, dignity and informed consent. With older adults, these matters are not incidental--they are critical to making sure that technology supports, rather than undermines, their experience of life.

In future research, a special emphasis should be placed on how old people view the AI technologies, how do they respond to them by their emotions, and how are their cultures and socioeconomic backgrounds forming their acceptance. As an example, whereas in Japan robotic caregivers can be welcomed as people are not opposed to human-machine interaction, in other societies where the warming hand of a family member cannot be replaced by a robot, it would not be desired.

Another urgent gap surely is the short term orientation of most research. Pilot projects are frequently short (a few months), which is inadequate exposure to assess the psychological, social and ethical impacts of use of artificial intelligence. Longitudinal analyses should be conducted to conclude whether the initial improvements of AI are maintained or social attachment, human control or emotional health are slowly damaged by dependency on machines. Such research is needed to reflect on policies and designs that could show latent harms only after years of use have been observed.

8.3 Integrating Interdisciplinary Perspectives

Geriatrics are not the domain you will see AI develop by technologists only. The multi-faceted nature of aging requires the input of many components including ethicists, sociologists, gerontologists, psychologists, policymakers, and most importantly the elderly themselves in designing algorithms and systems. Interdisciplinarity leads to innovations based on the values of and experience of older people by ensuring compatibility of technological changes with values.

A potential solution is participatory design in which older adults are given a direct role in the design of the technologies targeted at them. Besides leading to systems that are more reflective of their actual needs and preferences, this also leads to the empowerment of older adults as they become acknowledged active participants in the development process, rather than dependent end users of technology. As an example, elderly users involved in the design of conversational agents may point out language use-patterns, emotional demands, or accessibility issues that a developer may have otherwise overlooked.

In addition, geriatric care is neither a mere medical problem, but also a social-cultural one. Ethical frameworks should address the impacts of AI on the family structures, relationships between generations and systems of community support. Mitigating the risks of the use of AI in elderly care requires the integration of interdisciplinary views to make the technologies socially acceptable, culturally sensitive, and ethically acceptable within the society.

8.4 Policy-Oriented Research Priorities

A transformed policy framework is needed to support a rapidly changing technological innovation to ensure that geriatric AI is safe, fair, and sustainable. Policymakers should have evidence based proposals on how they can regulate data protection, algorithmic accountability and equitable access to AI driven health care. It is accordingly the duty of research, to focus on the generation of knowledge that can be directly applied to policy.

A prime need here is data governance In elderly care, I systems are very likely to use sensitive personal information like biometric or behavioral data. Such data might be misused to conduct business exploitation or be subjected to breaches in line with the absence of powerful policies. Research must offer paradigms of privacy preserving data management that trade-off between innovativeness and protection.

Along with that, the international cooperation is important. In the same manner that climate change is leading to international accord, the transnational nature of the ethical issues around the use of AI in geriatric care may demand transnational strings. Populations of elderly people are not segmented or restricted to regional demographic indexes of particular countries. Therefore, corporations realizing AI solutions are worldwide. The failure to have harmonization of standards may cause a loophole in terms of ethics and disparities. Therefore, policy-relevant studies must consider perspectives of international collaboration, and the establishment of coalitions has to be equitable, inclusive, and responsible in the elderly care-driven by AI between countries.

8.5 Envisioning the Future of Ethical AI in Elderly Care

The strongest idea of a future is one in which technology and human beings cooperate. The design should not be such that I should replace human care but should rather be a mean allowing elderly people to be independent, dignified, and connected. The systems of the future need to prolong the healthy life of the older adults and keep older adults emotionally and socially connected.

This vision demands postive ethical design It should be known and understandable as well as customized to users so that there are no chances of betrayal among people and computers. Caregivers one should not replace but make their workload easier and help find more time to devote to human-centered elements through empathy.

Indeed global collaboration, multidisciplinary study, as well as participation will go a long way in accomplishing this vision. Such potential of AI driving change to aging being transformed to a period marked by empowerment, safety and continuing social engagement, is vast with a potential transfer of the traditional age of dependency and vulnerability. With responsible guidance, AI can empower the aged to new levels of empowerment, security, and social engagement. The task is not only to be technologically innovative but to make sure that the ethical values are put first in the transformation process (Vandemeulebroucke et al., 2020b).

9. CONCLUSION

One of the greatest examples of how technology connects with human well-being in the 21 st century is the introduction of artificial intelligence in the care of geriatrics. As the world is becoming older there is an increasing demand of more innovative solutions that meet health, safety and emotional needs of the older adults. The challenges that AI presents and their associated opportunities will fall into the category of fall detection systems and predictive healthcare monitoring, companion robots, and smart care environments providing the potential of transforming quality of life by relieving the burden on caregivers and healthcare systems. But one cannot have these opportunities without the ethical responsibilities they bring along with them.

At the center of the discussions of ethics one will hear about privacy, autonomy, fairness, and human dignity. Older people are particularly susceptible to the unintentional consequences of technological adoption, be it invasive surveillance, algorithmic discrimination, or reliance on the artificial intelligence system that can erode social ties. It is, therefore, critical to design AI systems that do not undermine the values and rights of older adults and which function to empower rather than replace human values and care.

The case studies described in this chapter demonstrate that the real life setting of AI application is hopeful and multi-faceted in nature. In Japan, the companion robot shows how technology may be used to deal with loneliness, whereas approaches in Europe show the significance of a strong data protection framework. These illustrations indicate that context is crucial: cultural norms, regulations, and social conditions have a significant impact on ethical permissibility of AI in geriatrics. The lessons will include the idea that there can be no universal model; culture-sensitive and adaptive approaches must be adopted to have responsible innovation.

REFERENCES

Ali, H., & Li, H. (2019). Evaluating a smartwatch notification system in a simulated nursing home. *International Journal of Older People Nursing*, *14*(3), e12241. PMID: 31099184

Ali, H., & Nikberg, N. (2024). Bias in AI-driven healthcare: Navigating ethical challenges at an early stage. *Journal of Service Science and Management*, *17*(2), 305–320.

Amin, M. G., Zhang, Y. D., Ahmad, F., & Ho, K. C. D. (2016). Radar signal processing for elderly fall detection: The future for in-home monitoring. *IEEE Signal Processing Magazine*, *33*(2), 71–80. DOI: 10.1109/MSP.2015.2502784

Ashfaq, M., Yun, J., Yu, S., & Loureiro, S. M. C. (2020). I, Chatbot: Modeling determinants of users' satisfaction and continuance intention of AI-powered service agents. *Telematics and Informatics*, *54*, 101473. DOI: 10.1016/j.tele.2020.101473

Bloom, D. E., Canning, D., & Lubet, A. (2015). Global population aging: Facts, challenges, solutions & perspectives. *Daedalus*, *144*(2), 80–92.

Bloom, D. E., & Luca, D. L. (2016). The global demography of aging: Facts, explanations, future. In *Handbook of the Economics of Population Aging* (Vol. 1, pp. 3–56). Elsevier.

Cafolla, D. (2024). Exploration of AI-enhanced wearable devices for advanced cardiovascular monitoring in the elderly. In *International Conference on AI in Healthcare* (pp. 185–197).

Chen, K., Lou, V. W.-Q., Tan, K. C.-K., Wai, M.-Y., & Chan, L.-L. (2020). Effects of a humanoid companion robot on dementia symptoms and caregiver distress. *Journal of the American Medical Directors Association*, *21*(11), 1724–1728. DOI: 10.1016/j.jamda.2020.05.036 PMID: 32713772

Gill, T. M., Murphy, T. E., Gahbauer, E. A., & Allore, H. G. (2013). The course of disability before and after a serious fall injury. *JAMA Internal Medicine*, *173*(19), 1780–1786. PMID: 23958741

Goyal, N. K. (2025). Security and Privacy in IoT, Fog, and Blockchain Networks. In Sathio, A., Rind, M., Awan, S., & Junejo, A. (Eds.), *Energy-Efficient Deep Learning Approaches in IoT, Fog, and Green Blockchain Revolution* (pp. 371–398). IGI Global Scientific Publishing., DOI: 10.4018/979-8-3373-0300-0.ch015

Goyal, N. K., Dandotiya, M., Kumari, M., Kaloria, S., & Anushya, A. (2025). AI-Powered Haptic Devices for Patient Rehabilitation. In Mamodiya, U., Kalam, A., Bossoufi, B., Awad, M., & Somwanshi, D. (Eds.), *Integrating AI With Haptic Systems for Smarter Healthcare Solutions* (pp. 143–170). IGI Global Scientific Publishing., DOI: 10.4018/979-8-3373-2307-7.ch007

Goyal, N. K., Dandotiya, M., Qurashi, J. A., Kumari, M., & Sharma, S. (2025). AI-Driven Predictive Analytics for Disease Management. In Ouaissa, M., Ouaissa, M., Imad, M., Qurashi, J., & Farooq, M. (Eds.), *Utilizing AI of Medical Things for Healthcare Security and Sustainability* (pp. 231–276). IGI Global Scientific Publishing., DOI: 10.4018/979-8-3373-0690-2.ch008

Hajdú, J. (2020). Dignity of elderly persons and digitalised social care. In *The Right to Human Dignity* (p. 569).

Han, X., Zhou, X., Tan, B., Jiao, L., & Zhang, R. (2023). AI-based next-generation sensors for enhanced rehabilitation monitoring and analysis. *Measurement*, *223*, 113758.

Ienca, M. (2017). *Intelligent technologies for the aging brain: Opportunities and challenges* (Doctoral dissertation, University of Basel).

Khan, M. F., Ghazal, T. M., Said, R. A., Fatima, A., Abbas, S., Khan, M. A., & Khan, M. A. (2021). An IoMT-enabled smart healthcare model to monitor elderly people using machine learning technique. *Computational Intelligence and Neuroscience*, *2021*, 2487759. PMID: 34868288

Kim, J. W., Choi, Y. L., Jeong, S. H., & Han, J. (2022). A care robot with ethical sensing system for older adults at home. *Sensors (Basel)*, *22*(19), 7515. PMID: 36236614

Kumar, S., Underwood, S. H., Masters, J. L., Manley, N. A., Konstantzos, I., & Lau, J.. (2023). Ten questions concerning smart and healthy built environments for older adults. *Building and Environment*, *244*, 110720.

London, A. J., Razin, Y. S., Borenstein, J., Eslami, M., Perkins, R., & Robinette, P. (2023). Ethical issues in near-future socially supportive smart assistants for older adults. *IEEE Transactions on Technology and Society*.

Mhlanga, D. (2020). Industry 4.0: The challenges associated with the digital transformation of education in South Africa. *The Impacts of Digital Transformation*, *13*(51), 13–26.

Mhlanga, D. (2023a). Digital transformation in healthcare: The role of AI for inclusive long-term care. In Mhlanga, D., & Ndhlovu, E. (Eds.), *Economic Inclusion in Post-Independence Africa*. Springer., DOI: 10.1007/978-3-031-31431-5_19

Mhlanga, D. (2023b). Financial technology, artificial intelligence, and the health sector. In *FinTech and Artificial Intelligence for Sustainable Development*. Palgrave Macmillan., DOI: 10.1007/978-3-031-37776-1_7

Mois, G., & Beer, J. M. (2020). The role of healthcare robotics in providing support to older adults: A socio-ecological perspective. *Current Geriatrics Reports*, *9*, 82–89. DOI: 10.1007/s13670-020-00314-w PMID: 32435576

Raza, H., Abbas, N., Amir, S., Arshad, K., Siddiqui, M. R. U., & Khan, S. I. (2022). An IoMT-enabled smart healthcare model to monitor elderly people using explainable AI. *Journal of NCBAE*, *1*(1), 16–22.

Reynolds, C. F., Jeste, D. V., Sachdev, P. S., & Blazer, D. G. (2022). Mental health care for older adults: Advances and new directions. *World Psychiatry; Official Journal of the World Psychiatric Association (WPA)*, *21*(3), 336–363. PMID: 36073714

Schulz, R., Beach, S. R., Czaja, S. J., Martire, L. M., & Monin, J. K. (2020). Family caregiving for older adults. *Annual Review of Psychology*, *71*(1), 635–659. PMID: 31905111

Shi, Y., Ma, C., Wang, C., Wu, T., & Jiang, X. (2024). Harmonizing emotions: An AI-driven sound therapy system for enhancing mental health of older adults. In *International Conference on Human-Computer Interaction* (pp. 439–455).

Sinnige, J., Braspenning, J., Schellevis, F., Stirbu-Wagner, I., Westert, G., & Korevaar, J. (2023). The prevalence of disease clusters in older adults with multiple chronic diseases: A systematic review. *PLoS One*, *18*(7), e79641. PMID: 24244534

Udupa, P., & Yellampalli, S. S. (2025). Smart home for elder care using wireless sensors. *Circuit World*, *44*(1), 69–77.

Vandemeulebroucke, T., de Casterlé, B. D., & Gastmans, C. (2020). Ethics of socially assistive robots in aged-care settings: A socio-historical contextualisation. *Journal of Medical Ethics*, *46*(2), 128–136. PMID: 31818967

Vandemeulebroucke, T., Dierckx de Casterlé, B., Welbergen, L., Massart, M., & Gastmans, C. (2020). The ethics of socially assistive robots in aged care: A focus group study with older adults. *The Journals of Gerontology: Series B*, *75*(9), 1996–2007. PMID: 31131848

Chapter 10
Educational, Technological, Epistemic, and Pedagogical Architectures for an Ageing World:
Human–AI Synergies in Geriatric Care and Ecologies

Ashraf Alam
https://orcid.org/0000-0001-6178-1187
Alliance University, Bengaluru, India

ABSTRACT

This chapter critically interrogates the integration of AI in geriatric care through the lens of education, positioning learning ecosystems as the foundational infrastructure for ethical, inclusive, and context-sensitive AI deployment. Drawing on global policy frameworks, cross-sectoral case studies, and pedagogical theory, it constructs a multi-tiered roadmap encompassing awareness, skill-building, and professionalisation across stakeholders. The chapter challenges technological determinism by reframing AI not as a neutral tool but as a socially contingent artefact shaped by educational design, equity concerns, and moral responsibility. Case studies from Japan, Finland, India, and South Korea demonstrate that successful AI implementation hinges less on technical sophistication than on educational imagination. It concludes by proposing lifelong, interdisciplinary, and justice-oriented learning

DOI: 10.4018/979-8-3373-5462-0.ch010

strategies as prerequisites for meaningful AI adoption in ageing societies, asserting that without robust education, even the most advanced AI cannot ensure dignified and humane eldercare.

1. INTRODUCTION

The demographic calculus of the twenty-first century is undergoing a profound reconfiguration as the global population of individuals aged sixty and above is anticipated to surpass 2.1 billion by the year 2050, reflecting a near doubling from 1.1 billion in 2020. This senescent trajectory is disproportionately accentuated in post-industrial economies such as Japan, Germany, Italy, and South Korea, wherein the speed and magnitude of population ageing are historically unprecedented. In contrast, low- and middle-income countries are experiencing a temporal compression of this demographic transition, whereby the physiological and infrastructural demands of old age are emerging within fragile socio-economic frameworks. These demographic inflections are not merely actuarial projections but materialise as significant stressors on global geriatric health infrastructures, already debilitated by systemic underfunding, chronic workforce attrition, and fragmented long-term care systems (Broadbent et al., 2024; Wang et al., 2024; Wang et al., 2023; Czaja & Ceruso, 2022).

The World Health Organization has extrapolated that by 2030, the global health and social care sector will experience a deficit exceeding fifteen million skilled workers, a shortfall that will disproportionately impair the delivery of elder-oriented services. Simultaneously, the epidemiological landscape of ageing is increasingly characterised by multimorbidity, chronic inflammation, and neurodegenerative pathologies, with dementia-related illnesses, including Alzheimer's disease, expected to affect over 139 million individuals by mid-century (Efthymiou, I., 2026). Health systems remain encumbered by outdated biomedical paradigms, structurally inadequate long-term care infrastructure, and insufficient integration between preventive, acute, and palliative services (Su & Yang, 2024; Lambert et al., 2023; Sankaran & Singla, 2024; Koc, 2023). Geriatric care has thus become a site of ontological and operational crisis, demanding not only clinical intervention but a paradigmatic shift in its epistemic and logistical foundations.

Artificial Intelligence, as a sociotechnical assemblage, has emerged as a pivotal modality for reconfiguring the praxis of eldercare. The deployment of machine learning algorithms for predictive diagnostics, fall risk assessment, and readmission probability calculations introduces unprecedented capacities for preemptive intervention (Rao et al., 2024; Momtazmanesh, Nowroozi, & Rezaei, 2022). AI-augmented robotics, ranging from socially assistive humanoid interfaces to sensor-embedded prosthetics, are increasingly integrated into care ecologies. Remote monitoring platforms, driven by algorithmic pattern recognition, facilitate real-time surveillance of biometric fluctuations, behavioural anomalies, and medication adherence.

Pioneering initiatives such as IBM Watson's clinical decision-support in oncology and DeepMind's ophthalmological diagnostics are progressively extending into age-specific domains. These technological artefacts, however, are not epistemologically neutral. They embody ontologies of ageing, implicit biases in data representation, and systemic asymmetries in access and benefit. The integration of AI into eldercare landscapes surfaces a critical disjuncture between technological advancement and educational preparedness (Jun Woo & Kang, 2024; Corbett et al., 2021). Three constituencies, namely, health professionals and direct-care workers, the geriatric population itself, and the engineering-design complex, are negotiating AI implementation without sufficient cognitive, ethical, or pedagogical scaffolding (Salah, Selvaperumal, & Abdulla, 2022; Sharif et al., 2025). For the clinical workforce, AI literacy must transcend operational training and encompass interpretive acumen, algorithmic accountability, and normative decision-making. For older adults, digital engagement requires more than interface competence; it necessitates culturally attuned, affectively resonant, and autonomy-affirming experiences (Tiwari et al., 2023; Sepúlveda et al., 2022). For developers and systems architects, the absence of gerontologically informed design frameworks has precipitated tools that alienate, infantilise, or misrecognise the elderly subject.

Absent intentional educational infrastructure, AI deployment in geriatric contexts risks replicating extant inequities and generating new modalities of exclusion. Education, in this regard, is not an auxiliary mechanism but a constitutive condition of technological justice. It functions simultaneously as a vector of empowerment and as a moral architecture, guiding the ontogenesis of AI systems from ideation to implementation (Uchikov et al., 2024; Lau et al., 2022; Efthymiou, 2024a). The pedagogical interface between human cognition and machine logic becomes the critical site where inclusion, dignity, and efficacy are either cultivated or foreclosed. This chapter posits that educational ecosystems are the decisive fulcrum upon which the future of AI-integrated geriatric care pivots. It offers a multidimensional analytical framework synthesising epistemological theories, pedagogical innovations, regulatory considerations, and empirical case narratives. The goal is to elucidate and operationalise the educational imperatives necessary for ethical, equitable, and effective AI adoption within eldercare environments.

The subsequent sections address discrete thematic domains, including human–AI interaction, participatory design ethics, digital equity, change management, policy translation, and best practices across geopolitical contexts (Livieri G., 2024). Each section converges toward a coherent roadmap aimed at catalysing systemic transformation through educational intervention, thereby reimagining ageing not as a site of technological intervention alone, but as a locus of intergenerational learning, moral imagination, and sociotechnical co-evolution.

2. HUMAN–AI INTERACTION IN GERIATRIC CARE

2.1. AI as Co-worker

The ontological incorporation of artificial intelligence into geriatric healthcare infrastructures necessitates a paradigmatic shift from mechanistic substitution to socio-technical hybridity. The transition is not merely an artifact of automation but an epistemic reconfiguration of caregiving ontologies and institutional ecologies (Jnr, 2025; Kaya et al., 2024). Actor-Network Theory, conceptualised by Bruno Latour and Michel Callon, offers a salient analytical apparatus through which AI can be interpreted not as an inert instrument but as a relational actant embedded within heterogeneous assemblages of human and non-human actors. Within residential care institutions and domiciliary service environments, AI no longer functions as a passive executor but as a semi-autonomous cognitive agent that modulates work-flows, augments decision hierarchies, and reconstitutes epistemic trust structures and operational responsibilities (Gray et al., 2022; Vourganas, Attar, & Michala, 2022).

Empirical deployments across high-income nations, particularly in Scandinavian and East Asian contexts, elucidate this reterritorialisation of care. In Denmark, South Korea, and Singapore, AI-augmented robotic entities such as PARO, Pepper, and TUG are employed to execute multimodal caregiving functions. These include pharmacological adherence prompts, biometric surveillance, affective simulation, and kinetic facilitation. The performative embodiment of these robots generates anthropomorphic attachments while simultaneously restructuring emotional economies within caregiving (Ibuki, Ibuki, & Nakazawa, 2024; AlZaabi, AlMaskari, & AalAbdulsalam, 2023). Although such integration introduces efficiencies in task delegation and continuity of care, it simultaneously raises ethical interrogatives regarding the commodification of affect, the erosion of relational authenticity, and the attenuation of embodied empathy.

The algorithmic abstraction inherent in such systems is not value-neutral. Algorithms trained on anonymised and decontextualised datasets often fail to encapsulate the relational and cultural nuances of geriatric subjectivity (Chu-Ke & Dong, 2024; McGee, 2024). The caregiving sector, already marked by gendered undervaluation and precarious labour arrangements, confronts further ontological marginalisation as AI systems are valorised for their precision, predictability, and perceived impartiality (Seibert et al., 2021; Rizvi et al., 2023). This creates a dialectical tension wherein human affective labour is de-institutionalised while machinic logic is reified as the new normative standard. Consequently, the shift from anthropocentric care paradigms to hybrid human–machine synergies mandates an ontological recalibration of professional identity within the caregiving workforce (Kedziora, 2022; Agha et al., 2025). Care personnel must reconceptualise their epistemic authority in dialogic relation to algorithmic intelligences. This necessitates the cultivation of competencies in interfacing with algorithmic logic, delineating system thresholds, and navigating the stochastic error margins intrinsic to machine learning models (Chen & Xu, 2023; Belmin et al., 2022). Without pedagogical intervention, there exists a bifurcated risk of algorithmic over-dependence or techno-skeptical disengagement, both of which compromise care quality and institutional resilience.

2.2. Educational Needs of Healthcare Professionals and Caregivers

The proliferation of AI-mediated diagnostic and therapeutic modalities within clinical settings demands an epistemological expansion of professional medical education. Contemporary healthcare practitioners must be equipped not only with procedural fluency but also with conceptual and ethical intelligibility in the interpretation and deployment of algorithmic outputs (Nguyen et al., 2022; Wu et al., 2024). Surveys conducted across pedagogical institutions in the United States and the European Union indicate that less than twelve percent of nursing graduates express self-efficacy in engaging with AI-generated clinical data (Diareme, K., et al., 2022), highlighting a lacuna in current curricular architectures. This educational asymmetry is exacerbated by the pervasive opacity of algorithmic systems, especially those predicated on deep neural networks and ensemble learning architectures. Such systems, while performant, elude conventional explanatory paradigms, thereby destabilising clinical accountability, undermining patient-practitioner communication, and inflating medico-legal risk. To remediate this, a stratified instructional framework is imperative, one that scaffolds knowledge acquisition across ascending planes of complexity and contextual engagement.

At the foundational tier, the pedagogical emphasis must be on the cognitive architecture of AI, typologies of training data, and canonical use-cases within eldercare ecosystems. Instructional modules should incorporate translational frameworks that map algorithmic logic onto geriatric-specific morbidities such as fall risk prediction, early dementia detection, and polypharmacy management. This foundational layer must be synchronised with biopsychosocial understandings of ageing to develop and nurture integrative competence (Chen, Zhang, & Wang, 2023; Liu, Chau, Liu, & Wan, 2023). The intermediate level of instruction must pivot toward data ethics, human–machine interface literacy, and interpretive analytics. Here, professionals must acquire the capacity to decipher probabilistic output vectors, calibrate algorithmic thresholds, and engage in critical discourse regarding the epistemic biases embedded within training datasets (Jonek-Kowalska & Wolny, 2025; Zhang et al., 2023). Particular vigilance must be exercised regarding algorithmic misclassification risks when models are extrapolated from non-geriatric or demographically skewed populations.

At the advanced tier, the focus must shift to leadership development and meta-strategic governance. This includes training in inter-professional coordination within AI–human teams, change management in digitally transforming institutions, and longitudinal evaluation of care outcomes mediated by AI augmentation (Huang et al., 2024; Papathanail et al., 2021; Efthymiou, 2024b). Advanced learners should also be equipped to engage in ethical review panels, procurement assessments, and post-deployment surveillance of AI systems. To architect these educational trajectories, Bloom's Taxonomy can serve as a cognitive scaffolding framework, facilitating a progression from factual recall to evaluative judgment. When integrated with the Technological Pedagogical Content Knowledge (TPACK) model, a comprehensive instructional schema emerges, wherein technological proficiency, content fluency, and pedagogical adaptability coalesce. This ensures that AI education is not epistemically siloed but is embedded within a broader praxis of professional formation.

2.3. Pedagogical Innovations for Training Clinicians

The inculcation of AI fluency within geriatric healthcare professionals necessitates a pedagogical pivot from transmissive to constructivist modalities. Simulation-based learning environments, underpinned by AI-driven virtual patient avatars, provide synthetic but authentic clinical encounters that facilitate skill acquisition without exposing real patients to iatrogenic risk (Apell & Eriksson, 2023; Marino et al., 2023). In countries like Japan and the Netherlands, longitudinal studies have demonstrated that such simulations enhance diagnostic accuracy, attenuate cognitive load, and improve human–AI co-decisioning in complex geriatric scenarios. Pedagogical enactments such as case-based discussions further function as epistemic laboratories where comparative analysis between AI-augmented and traditional care pathways are interrogated. These discussions transcend procedural learning by facilitating the cultivation of meta-cognitive awareness, moral reasoning, and systemic reflection. Clinicians are thus enabled to engage in dialogical synthesis between technological affordances and patient-centred values.

Experiential pedagogies, such as clinical decision games, simulate ethically and diagnostically ambiguous scenarios where learners must navigate high-stakes decision trees mediated by algorithmic suggestions. The gamification of ethical reasoning and technical navigation offers learners embodied engagement with uncertainty, trade-offs, and system feedback loops. Adaptive learning analytics embedded in these games enable real-time feedback and metacognitive calibration (Nasr et al., 2021; Aggarwal et al., 2021). Constructivist pedagogical approaches serve as the ontological substratum of these methodologies. Learning is conceptualised not as epistemic absorption but as dialogic construction, mediated through reflective praxis, social interaction, and iterative problematisation. Reflective journals function as cognitive mirrors, allowing clinicians to document epistemic dissonance, algorithmic misalignments, and emergent patterns of clinical judgment.

Ethical deliberation seminars, where AI-related failures and trade-offs are thematised, thus developing and nurturing the cultivation of phronesis and practical wisdom. Embedding such pedagogical innovations within institutional training infrastructures enables the transition from user-centric to co-creator models of professional identity. Clinicians are thereby repositioned as critical interlocutors in the design, deployment, and continuous refinement of AI systems (Pani et al., 2024; Viderman et al., 2022). This metamorphosis represents the most profound epistemological and ethical shift necessary for the sustenance of humane, contextually responsive, and technologically augmented eldercare ecosystems.

3. ETHICAL AI DESIGN AND DEVELOPMENT

3.1. Human-Centred and Age-Inclusive Design

The functional obsolescence of numerous artificial intelligence applications in geriatric contexts originates not from algorithmic inefficiency or computational insufficiency but from a pervasive epistemological misalignment with the lived realities of ageing (Sætra, 2022; Wang et al., 2024). The design epistemes within which these systems are conceived often reflect technocratic imaginaries that are epistemologically detached from the biopsychosocial complexities of elderhood (Aher et al., 2024; Hanke et al., 2022). Design paradigms remain structured by anthropocentric norms centred on young, neurotypical, able-bodied users, thereby marginalising older adults as a deviant category outside the normative user template. The conceptual architectures of Universal Design and Design Justice provide normative correctives to this exclusionary orientation. Universal Design, initially developed within disability studies, offers a paradigm for infrastructural inclusivity through adaptability and ergonomic flexibility. Design Justice reorients design priorities by centring the epistemologies and agency of marginalised users. Despite their theoretical robustness, these frameworks remain peripheral in the pedagogical frameworks that shape software engineering and human–computer interaction curricula. AI developers continue to be acculturated within epistemic silos that render gerontological complexity invisible or technically irrelevant.

Educational interventions must therefore prioritise the somatosensory, cognitive, and affective dimensions of senescence as core curricular components. The physiological phenomena of ageing, including presbyopia, presbycusis, delayed neuromuscular coordination, and episodic memory instability, must be operationalised into design parameters such as font scalability, acoustic calibration, interaction latency, and cognitive offloading mechanisms (Zhang et al., 2024; Kerwan et al., 2025). User interface design cannot be abstracted from sensorimotor decline. Pedagogical efforts must employ transdisciplinary models wherein gerontology, neuropsychology, and affective computing coalesce to produce actionable design heuristics. Cognitive degeneration presents a non-linear trajectory with considerable inter- and intra-individual variability. AI systems must be capable of adapting to episodic lucidity, inconsistent attention, and semantic disorientation (Wolniak & Stecuła, 2024; Rozynek et al., 2021).

Such dynamism necessitates that developers receive training in neurodiversity, cognitive ageing, and human factors engineering. Absent this expertise, technological outputs may remain computationally sophisticated yet phenomenologically alienating (Mikkelsen et al., 2023; Abou Hashish & Alnajjar, 2024). Systems optimised for efficiency may ultimately exacerbate disorientation, user abandonment, or techno-anxiety among geriatric populations (Bevilacqua et al., 2023; González-Castro et al., 2024). Participatory co-design models offer a reconfiguration of traditional development pipelines by foregrounding situated expertise. These frameworks dissolve the binary between designer and end-user, recasting older adults and caregivers as epistemic agents within the iterative lifecycle of design (Dong et al., 2022; Costanzo et al., 2024). Empirical evidence from co-creation initiatives in Norway and Canada illustrates that such engagements not only enhance functional usability but also engender relational trust, critical for uptake and sustained use. Developers must be trained in dialogic facilitation, cultural humility, and reflexive design inquiry. This pedagogical reorientation involves transitioning from a metrics-driven efficiency logic to an ethics-situated design ethos, wherein dignity, autonomy, and affective congruence constitute primary success indicators (Vousinas, G. et al., 2022).

3.2. Integrating Ethics into Technical Curricula

Although normative discourses surrounding AI ethics have gained institutional visibility, their pedagogical translation within technical education remains underdeveloped, often tokenised within elective modules or appended as non-assessable content (Choudhary & Nagar, 2025; Ghosh & Ghosh, 2023). Frameworks such as IEEE's Ethically Aligned Design and UNESCO's Recommendation on the Ethics of Artificial Intelligence codify comprehensive principles including transparency, justice, non-maleficence, and accountability. However, in practice, these frameworks are rarely embedded into the epistemic core of computer science, data engineering, or robotics education. An urgent pedagogical imperative lies in the curricular integration of ethics as a foundational rather than supplementary domain. This reconfiguration demands the infusion of geriatric-specific ethical scenarios within core coursework (Laur & Wang, 2022; Aronsson, 2022). Case-based instructional modules must interrogate real-world deployments such as algorithmic triage in long-term care facilities, surveillance-intensive monitoring tools in dementia units, and affectively responsive robotic companions. These cases must surface moral tensions among principles such as user autonomy, informational asymmetry, privacy intrusiveness, and clinical efficacy.

Interdisciplinary academic programmes, such as minors or certificate tracks in Gerontechnology and Ethics, provide institutional mechanisms for sustained engagement. These programmes must fuse disciplinary insights from ageing studies, design anthropology, sociotechnical systems theory, and biomedical ethics. Precedents at institutions like Eindhoven University of Technology and the University of Geneva demonstrate the feasibility and utility of such integrative models, generating graduates capable of straddling technical competence and moral imagination. Pedagogical praxis must also transcend traditional assessment models that privilege regurgitation over deliberation. Evaluative modalities such as stakeholder mapping, anticipatory governance simulations, and algorithmic audit exercises cultivate foresight, responsibility attribution, and procedural justice awareness (Ray et al., 2022; Dong et al., 2021). The goal is not merely to produce engineers who adhere to prescriptive ethical norms but to develop and nurture technologists capable of interrogating the structural consequences of their designs within specific sociopolitical ecologies.

3.3. Training Policymakers, Designers, and Ethicists

The pedagogical ecosystem of ethical AI in eldercare extends far beyond the technical cadre and encompasses a constellation of interdependent actors including policymakers, service designers, professional ethicists, and institutional governance bodies (Denecke & Baudoin, 2022; Pelly et al., 2023). Each actor occupies a distinct ontological and epistemological location within the AI lifecycle and therefore requires differentiated, domain-specific educational scaffolding (Shaik et al., 2023; Xing et al., 2021). Policymakers must develop algorithmic literacy, not at the level of code fluency but at the level of system architecture, risk stratification, and regulatory foresight. Scenario-based learning environments that simulate policy dilemmas, governance breakdowns, and regulatory trade-offs are particularly effective. The AI Policy Clinic at the University of Oxford and the experimental policy labs at the GovLab in New York University offer working prototypes of such immersive training methodologies, grounded in transdisciplinary mentorship and live casework.

Design professionals must expand their epistemic toolkit to include both aesthetic sensitivity and distributive justice awareness. Curricula in inclusive design, accessibility engineering, and co-creative service ecosystems should be institutionalised within design education. Without such interventions, even well-intentioned products risk recapitulating structural exclusions under the guise of innovation (Alharbi et al., 2023; Görtz et al., 2023). Professional ethicists, traditionally trained in abstract deontological and utilitarian frameworks, must acquire fluency in data systems, machine learning pipelines, and algorithmic evaluation metrics (Thakare et al., 2022; Zaidan, 2023). Joint academic appointments or degree programs across philosophy departments and engineering schools can bridge the hermeneutic divide between normative reasoning and computational implementation. This hybrid training enables ethicists to engage with AI not only as observers but as embedded practitioners.

Institutionalising these pedagogical interventions requires organisational infrastructure. Cross-sectoral AI ethics councils focused on geriatric care constitute a viable modality for sustained deliberation and capacity building. Such councils, composed of eldercare practitioners, data scientists, patient representatives, legal scholars, and ethicists, function as pluralistic knowledge forums (Chu et al., 2023; Chang et al., 2025). Their remit includes the evaluation of emergent technologies, the codification of ethical benchmarks, and the dissemination of best practices. Experimental models in Finland and South Korea indicate that when appropriately resourced, these councils can evolve into agile, context-aware regulatory interlocutors. The ethical terrain of AI in geriatric care is not a monologic domain reducible to abstract compliance frameworks (Zhu et al., 2022; Huq et al., 2024). It is a dialogic and situated practice that must be nurtured through continuous, polyphonic education. The ethical sensibilities required to co-create inclusive technologies are not spontaneously emergent but must be cultivated through immersive pedagogy, reflective praxis, and interdisciplinary collaboration. The origin of ethical innovation in AI does not reside solely in source code. It is rooted in classrooms, clinics, laboratories, courtrooms, and care homes, where diverse actors encounter each other and negotiate the meaning of dignity in the age of machines.

4. ADDRESSING DIGITAL DIVIDE AND ACCESSIBILITY THROUGH EDUCATION

4.1. Mapping Digital Exclusion Among Older Adults

The digital divide within gerontological populations resists simplistic dichotomies of connectivity versus disconnection and instead manifests as a stratified and multidimensional exclusionary architecture (Baek et al., 2023; Ho, 2023; Efthymiou, 2020). This exclusion is constituted by a complex interaction of infrastructural scarcity, cognitive degeneration, socioeconomic marginalisation, psychosocial alienation, and epistemological disenfranchisement (Paulauskaite-Taraseviciene et al., 2023; Chen et al., 2023). The Capability Approach, originally formulated by Amartya Sen and expanded by Martha Nussbaum, offers a robust theoretical substrate for evaluating these exclusions by prioritising substantive freedoms and the realisation of agency over nominal access. Within this analytical matrix, the absence of meaningful technological engagement is not merely an infrastructural deficit but a deprivation of choice, autonomy, and personhood (Alruwaili et al., 2024; Tsoi et al., 2023).

Digital Capital Theory further elaborates the intersecting vectors that shape digital engagement. It posits that digital participation is mediated by an assemblage of technical literacy, social embeddedness, and institutional scaffolding. Within geriatric cohorts, especially those situated in socioeconomically precarious contexts, these vectors are systematically eroded. Globally, over 47 percent of individuals aged sixty and above remain offline. In geographies such as sub-Saharan Africa and South Asia, this proportion exceeds 80 percent, driven by infrastructural insufficiency, gender-based disparities, and chronically low educational attainment. In technologically saturated societies such as Japan and Sweden, high infrastructural penetration paradoxically coexists with minimal substantive use among older demographics. Utilisation is often confined to unidimensional applications such as voice calls or basic messaging. The socioeconomic stratification within geriatric populations compounds this disparity. Older adults in the lowest income quintiles are approximately five times less likely to possess broadband access or smart devices. Rural–urban bifurcations remain salient even in high-income states, as evidenced by persistent connectivity deficits in rural American counties and remote Australian territories.

Psychosocial variables introduce additional barriers. Technophobia, frequently rooted in anticipatory anxiety concerning failure or cyber-vulnerability, serves as a cognitive deterrent. Internalised ageism, perpetuated by exclusionary design paradigms and intergenerational techno-normativity, cultivates a hermeneutic of illegitimacy in which older adults perceive themselves as epistemically disqualified from technological participation (Kim et al., 2024; Stypinska, 2021). Educational attainment exhibits a high correlation with digital self-efficacy. Individuals without formal schooling display markedly lower rates of engagement, even in scenarios of subsidised access. Somatic impairments, frequently co-morbid with senescence, exacerbate exclusionary dynamics. Visual impairments, arthritic motor limitations, and neurocognitive degeneration render conventional interfaces functionally inaccessible. These exclusions are not derivative of personal incapacity but are the structural consequences of technodesign paradigms that implicitly prioritise youthful, normative corporeality. Addressing such exclusions necessitates an educational paradigm oriented not toward remediation of deficits but toward systemic reconstitution through participatory, adaptive, and dignifying instruction.

4.2. Educational Interventions for Digital Literacy

The pedagogical architecture for cultivating digital literacy in elder populations must be premised on an ethics of dignity rather than a deficit model of compensatory training. Educational interventions that are community-situated, peer-mediated, and relationally structured have demonstrated superior efficacy in circumventing both structural and affective barriers to engagement. In the Netherlands, initiatives such as SeniorWeb have institutionalised digitally inclusive ecosystems through decentralised learning hubs. These digital cafés function not merely as instructional venues but as communal epistemic spaces where older adults construct technological fluency within contexts of peer solidarity and cultural affirmation. Mobile pedagogical infrastructures, such as Kenya's travelling tech buses, operationalise digital learning as a context-sensitive, linguistically localised, and mobility-enabled intervention. The portability of such models facilitates penetration into geographically and economically marginalised regions, rendering them scalable and replicable. Intergenerational mentoring architectures further enhance pedagogical outcomes.

In Finland, Chile, and Japan, state-supported initiatives have institutionalised reciprocal learning contracts between youth and elders. These arrangements engender a dual benefit structure by collapsing generational epistemic divides and developing and nurturing bidirectional learning. Finland's Digital Grandparent initiative exemplifies this model, embedding it within civic education requirements and thus reinforcing intergenerational cohesion as a civic virtue. Gamification and voice-enabled interactivity have emerged as neurocognitively adaptive pedagogical affordances. Cognitive games targeting memory augmentation, spatial navigation, and communicative functionality have demonstrable impacts on engagement and retention. In rural India, the deployment of vernacularised and culturally embedded learning content has catalysed improved comprehension and reduced dropout rates among digitally novice elders. Instructional design must be experientially localised and semantically resonant to elicit meaningful engagement. It is not linguistic translation alone but cultural and phenomenological alignment that yields pedagogical efficacy.

Evaluation frameworks must transcend superficial indicators of success such as enrollment or device acquisition. The SAMR taxonomy enables evaluative granularity by distinguishing between substitutional engagement and transformative empowerment. The Community of Inquiry framework, with its triadic focus on cognitive, social, and instructional presence, provides an additional layer of assessment by foregrounding epistemic agency and dialogical interaction. Older adults, within these frameworks, are reimagined not as passive recipients but as agentic co-constructors of technological meaning. Digital literacy education must be conceived as plural, multimodal, and continuous. One-time training modules are insufficient in the face of rapidly evolving technological landscapes and the neurocognitive heterogeneity of ageing populations. Curricula must accommodate linguistic diversity, sensory variation, and divergent motivational structures. The telos of such pedagogy is not mastery of specific applications but the cultivation of a resilient and exploratory digital disposition.

4.3. Empowerment through Data Dignity and Consent Literacy

Digital literacy, when truncated to functional proficiency, occludes critical domains of ethical autonomy and data sovereignty. In an algorithmically mediated environment, geriatric users are often unwitting producers of highly sensitive and continuously extracted data (Huang et al., 2022; Su et al., 2022). These include health biometrics, geospatial traces, affective responses, and vocal biomarkers. Such data are frequently harvested under conditions of opacity and asymmetry, with consent mechanisms reduced to obfuscated agreements embedded within juridico-technical jargon. Pedagogical paradigms must reconceptualise consent as an ongoing, dialogic, and context-sensitive social practice. Instructional modules should equip older adults with the hermeneutic and procedural tools necessary to discern data collection patterns, interrogate purpose disclosures, and exercise informed refusal. In the United Kingdom, educational programmes led by the Open Rights Group have employed digital storytelling to cultivate critical awareness. Fictionalised but plausible narratives of data abuse and ethical rupture enable learners to engage affectively and reflexively with complex digital ethics landscapes.

Digital storytelling as a pedagogical modality allows for narrative reappropriation. By composing and disseminating autobiographical accounts of technological interaction, older adults transgress their assigned status as passive data subjects and become narrative agents. This narrative reappropriation develops and nurtures metacognitive insight into data trails and systemic asymmetries of power. Reflexive narration also cultivates self-efficacy, a precondition for asserting digital rights.

Consent fatigue, a psychological condition exacerbated by repetitive prompts, non-negotiable terms, and interface manipulation, constitutes a new frontier in digital ethics. Instructional content must sensitise learners to design manipulations such as dark patterns, default pre-selections, and coercive bundling. Empowerment, in this context, entails cultivating the capacity to discern and resist such manipulations. Refusal becomes not a failure of compliance but an assertion of autonomy.

Constructing data dignity also entails education in procedural justice mechanisms. These include the right to rectification, the process for data breach redressal, and avenues for institutional accountability. Educational collaboration with consumer protection agencies, digital rights advocates, and legal aid institutions can generate pedagogically accessible knowledge artefacts. These must demystify cryptographic terminology, algorithmic operations, and anonymisation protocols, translating abstract technicalities into experiential knowledge (Cinalioglu et al., 2023; Muralidharan et al., 2024). Ultimately, digital inclusion cannot be accomplished through technocratic distribution alone. It must be undergirded by an ethical pedagogy that enables geriatric populations to navigate the architectures of surveillance, platform capitalism, and predictive profiling with epistemic clarity and moral agency. Without such an educational foundation, AI remains not a facilitator of dignity but an opaque apparatus that re-inscribes inequality under the guise of innovation.

5. IMPLEMENTATION BARRIERS AND RESISTANCE

5.1. Nature of Resistance

The integration of artificial intelligence into geriatric care infrastructures encounters not merely peripheral friction but a structurally embedded resistance that functions as a constitutive determinant of its operational trajectory (Bokolo, 2023; Raza et al., 2022). This resistance is not reducible to technical lag but must be understood as a sociotechnical phenomenon that reflects contestations around epistemic authority, value alignment, and existential security (Chopra, 2025; Uzir et al., 2023). Everett Rogers' Diffusion of Innovations theory provides a taxonomical framework wherein adopters of emergent technologies are distributed across a spectrum from early innovators to late-stage laggards. Within the domains of eldercare, this distribution evidences a regressive skew, particularly among frontline caregivers and older adult users, whose epistemic and affective orientations are frequently misaligned with the teleologies of technological innovation. The Technology Acceptance Model, originally posited by Fred Davis, isolates two principal variables as predictive of adoption behaviour, i.e., perceived usefulness and perceived ease of use.

In geriatric care ecologies, both indices are consistently attenuated. Care personnel frequently characterise AI systems as burdensome, intrusive, or operationally opaque, resulting in cognitive saturation rather than relief. Elderly users often find AI interfaces unintuitive, non-empathic, or semantically incongruent with their experiential frameworks, thereby reinforcing alienation rather than enhancing engagement (Xiao et al., 2021; Herrmann, 2023). Resistance manifests across affective, cognitive, and behavioural registers. Affective resistance presents as anxiety, suspicion, or anticipatory dread. Cognitive resistance materialises as distrust, confusion, or epistemic dissonance. Behavioural resistance is instantiated through avoidance, circumvention, or passive disengagement. These manifestations are not irrational anomalies but rational responses to disruptions in ontological security, employment precarity, and normative caregiving practices (Shi et al., 2024; Martin-Martinez et al., 2023). To interpret these reactions as mere technophobia is to engage in epistemic violence. Instead, resistance must be reframed as an epistemological alert that signals the misalignment between imposed innovation and lived realities (Stypińska & Franke, 2023; Javadi-Pashaki et al., 2021). Such an interpretive reframing requires a pedagogical infrastructure that situates resistance not as obstruction but as a diagnostic tool for curricular recalibration.

5.2. Overcoming Resistance Through Tailored Pedagogy

To transform resistance into reflective engagement, education must function as the principal vector of cultural and cognitive reorientation. The pedagogy of counter-resistance cannot be coercive or unidirectional. It must be dialogical, situated, and grounded in epistemic humility. Storytelling, as a mode of cognitive assimilation and cultural transmission, becomes instrumental in this context. Narratives of successful human–machine collaboration within real-life eldercare scenarios serve as cognitive scripts that recalibrate emotional responses and reframe AI not as an existential threat but as a collaborative ally. For instance, recounting the case of a home nurse in Osaka who utilised AI-based predictive diagnostics to preempt a cerebrovascular incident facilitates identification, empathy, and perceptual recalibration among skeptical audiences. Experiential pedagogies such as role-play simulations enable ontological displacement, wherein participants temporarily inhabit alternative subjectivities.

Developers may enact the sensorial limitations of an elderly patient navigating a voice-based interface. Caregivers may experience the algorithmic rigidity of a decision-support system devoid of contextual nuance. Such epistemic transpositions destabilise normative assumptions and activate reflexivity. Jack Mezirow's Transformative Learning Theory posits that disorienting dilemmas catalyse shifts in meaning perspectives. Educational interventions designed to embed controlled dissonance can precipitate such shifts. Clinicians confronted with AI-generated decisions that contradict their clinical intuitions must deliberate not in isolation but within guided communities of inquiry, thereby developing and nurturing critical examination and ethical discernment. Reflective tools such as failure diaries, utilised in Scandinavian pedagogical models, institutionalise the notion that epistemic growth is iterative and often failure-mediated. Learners are encouraged to archive their misjudgments, hesitations, and unresolved tensions. This archive functions not as a record of incompetence but as an artifact of metacognitive development.

Instructional strategies should include affective scaffolding for dealing with ambiguity, managing ontological uncertainty, and engaging in probabilistic reasoning without epistemic paralysis. Pedagogical content must be contextually responsive. Didactic modules designed for digitally saturated, urban health systems may collapse in under-resourced, rural settings where digital infrastructure is intermittent and staff turnover is high. Instructional modalities must therefore be localised, linguistically inclusive, and attuned to infrastructural realities. Education must become a living system capable of morphological adaptation across geospatial, cultural, and socioeconomic contexts.

5.3. Institutional Learning Cultures and Professional Development

Resistance does not reside solely in individual cognition or emotional disposition. It is also embedded within institutional habitus and cultural logics that regulate organisational conduct. Institutions that prioritise procedural efficiency, vertical command hierarchies, and metricised performance evaluations tend to inhibit the kind of epistemic experimentation required for AI adoption. These structural dispositions must be deconstructed and replaced with institutional learning architectures that valorise epistemic curiosity, dialogical governance, and reflective practice. Empirical evidence from hospital systems in Denmark and Singapore indicates that when AI training is embedded within broader quality enhancement frameworks, staff engagement increases significantly. In these settings, training is not a discrete event but an ongoing epistemic ecosystem composed of iterative workshops, peer-led tutorials, and interdisciplinary forums. These platforms facilitate the co-construction of knowledge and create a semantic field where AI is not an alien imposition but a co-evolved innovation.

Leadership functions as a nodal variable in the success of these transitions. Supervisory personnel must be trained not merely in technological literacy but in adaptive governance, relational pedagogy, and conflict mediation. In Australia, the emergence of AI Integration Leads in eldercare facilities has operationalised this need. These figures act as epistemic bridges between software vendors, clinical staff, and institutional policy, ensuring knowledge continuity and cultural receptivity. Peer-based knowledge ecosystems also serve as epistemic accelerators. In these systems, veteran users mentor novices, demystifying algorithmic logic, troubleshooting anomalies, and translating complex functionalities into procedural fluency (Huang et al., 2024; Newby et al., 2023). Communities of practice, whether formalised through institutional policy or emergent through affective solidarity, produce relational trust and epistemic safety. These networks are often more effective in knowledge dissemination than vertical directives or formal mandates.

Accreditation regimes play a macrostructural role in catalysing cultural transformation. The integration of AI competency modules into licensure and re-certification protocols generates institutional incentives that align individual learning trajectories with regulatory imperatives (Lukkien et al., 2023; Wang et al., 2022). In the United States, continuing medical education credits are increasingly indexed to digital fluency and ethical AI usage, creating systemic alignment across pedagogical, institutional, and regulatory dimensions. Educational interventions must therefore be conceived not as preliminary phases of technological rollout but as ontological infrastructures without which innovation collapses into dysfunction or ethical breach. Transformation in geriatric care will not be engineered by code or machine learning parameters alone. It will be scaffolded through pedagogical systems that cultivate interpretive flexibility, epistemic humility, and affective resilience. The future of AI in eldercare resides not in algorithmic determinism but in the recursive processes of human learning, unlearning, and relearning.

6. POLICY FRAMEWORKS AND EDUCATIONAL IMPLICATIONS

6.1. Global Policy Landscapes and Gaps

The global regulatory architecture governing artificial intelligence in healthcare constitutes a rapidly morphing terrain marked by asymmetrical developments, normative incoherence, and epistemic blind spots with respect to geriatric populations (Woodman & Mangoni, 2023; Chu et al., 2022). Although legislative initiatives such as the European Union's Artificial Intelligence Act signal a movement toward stratified regulatory oversight predicated on risk categorisation, the gerontological subject remains conceptually marginal. The Act proposes rigorous constraints on high-risk applications, encompassing stipulations for data governance, algorithmic transparency, and human oversight. Yet it fails to incorporate age-specific modalities of risk, such as cognitive instability, consent variability, and somatosensory limitations, thereby rendering the elderly demographic both visible in principle and invisible in procedural articulation. In the United Kingdom, the National Health Service has operationalised the NHS AI Lab as a translational interface between policy formulation, technological experimentation, and ethical supervision.

However, geriatric applications constitute a negligible fraction of the initiative's portfolio, indicating a misalignment between population-level ageing trends and investment priorities. In the United States, the Food and Drug Administration has promulgated the Digital Health Software Precertification Program and articulated a regulatory regime for Software as a Medical Device. Yet the dominant orientation remains toward clinical generalisability rather than demographic particularity. Crucial domains such as fluctuating decisional capacity, accessibility interface standards, and longitudinal data integrity across geriatric trajectories remain unaddressed. The absence of geriatric attunement across these regulatory paradigms is symptomatic of a deeper epistemological deficiency wherein ageing is framed as a technocratic management problem rather than a complex biopsychosocial phenomenon (Danda, 2022; Yang et al., 2022). Policy formulations predominantly operationalise technological artefacts while neglecting the phenomenological realities of older adults, including caregiver mediation, psychosocial precarity, and the relational implications of robotic surrogacy (World Health Organization, 2022; Awotunde et al., 2022).

Moreover, enforcement regimes remain inconsistent and opaque, with algorithmic accountability mechanisms largely confined to internal audits or expert panels inaccessible to affected communities (Gallistl et al., 2024; Eun et al., 2023). Educational scaffolding is imperative not only to facilitate the implementation of policy but also to shape its genesis. Without reciprocal feedback loops between regulatory apparatuses and educational infrastructures, policy runs the risk of either overreach devoid of contextual sensitivity or underreach rooted in epistemic conservatism (Gudala et al., 2022; Dilip et al., 2022). The educational deficit is not simply one of translation but of co-creation, whereby pedagogical and clinical insights must inform normative frameworks from inception through implementation.

6.2. Policy-Informed Curriculum and Training Models

Bridging the chasm between macro-level regulatory instruments and micro-level geriatric care requires the cultivation of a hybridised professional class fluent in both juridical logics and pedagogical praxis. Curriculum design must operationalise policy into situated competencies that are actionable within the clinical ecology. For instance, provisions within the EU AI Act mandating post-market surveillance necessitate clinician training in anomaly detection, adverse event reporting, and integration of feedback into practice-based learning systems. Mandates around algorithmic explainability must be pedagogically embedded within health education curricula. Clinicians and caregivers must be trained to interpret probabilistic outputs, manage epistemic uncertainty, and communicate algorithmic rationale to cognitively diverse patients and their families (Umeda-Kameyama et al., 2021; Cingolani et al., 2023; Peine, Faulkner, Jæger, & Moors, 2015). This interpretive capacity transforms regulation from a formal injunction into an embodied professional reflex.

Integration of AI ethics and quality-of-care dimensions into licensure examinations elevates ethical discernment from a performative addendum to a professional standard (O'Connor et al., 2022; Akyon et al., 2023). The Canadian College of Nurses has initiated this process by embedding digital ethics within its licensing schema, thus catalysing curricular revision across affiliated institutions. This creates an incentive structure where educational compliance is tethered to licensure eligibility and institutional accreditation. Legal professionals, regulators, and policy architects must also undergo domain-specific education. Emerging legal curricula must incorporate modules on algorithmic governance, data justice, and consent theory contextualised within geriatric care. Regulatory actors must acquire operational familiarity with machine learning architectures, risk amplification vectors, and socio-technical harm taxonomies. Pedagogical models must prioritise critical epistemologies and simulate the complexities of eldercare where algorithmic interventions intersect with affective, legal, and clinical imperatives. Curriculum development must be architected through collaborative modalities. Engineers, gerontologists, ethicists, and clinicians must engage in dialogic co-construction of syllabi that reflect the multidimensionality of AI in eldercare. Educational interventions must incorporate scenario-based simulations, mock regulatory audits, and ethical deliberation exercises designed to train learners in navigating regulatory ambiguity, data governance complexities, and moral conflict in technologically saturated environments.

6.3. Cross-sectoral Educational Coalitions

The educational labour required for ethical AI integration into geriatric systems exceeds the capacity of any singular institutional actor. The multiscalar complexity of the challenge necessitates cross-sectoral epistemic coalitions and pedagogical interoperability (Cesario et al., 2021; Kouroubali et al., 2022). Universities, particularly those housing faculties of medicine, public policy, computer science, and education, must serve as infrastructural nuclei. They are uniquely positioned to aggregate disciplinary knowledges, disseminate pedagogical innovations, and incubate translational research. Massive Open Online Courses, as deployed by institutions such as Stanford and the University of Edinburgh, can augment access and equity, especially for learners situated within low-resource geographies. Private-sector actors, particularly AI startups and health technology firms, must transcend the minimalist ethics of compliance and enter co-creative partnerships. These entities can contribute design expertise, technological resources, and iterative feedback from real-time deployment. In Sweden and South Korea, some firms are co-sponsoring vocational certification programs for frontline caregivers, aligning product design with the exigencies of embodied care work. This produces a virtuous loop of design responsiveness and frontline trust.

Civil society organisations, particularly those representing elder rights, disability justice, and caregiving communities, possess critical situated knowledge that is often absent from institutional silos. These organisations can serve as testing grounds for educational content, facilitate trust-building initiatives, and amplify user voice in curricular reform. Their proximity to lived experience renders them epistemic intermediaries capable of translating abstract guidelines into affectively and culturally resonant educational content. The establishment of a Multi-Stakeholder Learning Alliance for Ethical AI in Geriatrics would formalise such coalitions. These alliances must operate as knowledge commons, maintaining open-access repositories of training materials, policy updates, and case-based learning tools. They must host deliberative assemblies, produce white papers, and generate curricular standards adaptable across contexts. In Germany, consortia such as that formed by the Fraunhofer Institute, Charité Medical University, and Siemens Healthineers exemplify the transformative potential of institutional synergy in shaping ethical, practice-informed, and pedagogically sound AI education.

Digital infrastructures should be used to develop publicly accessible knowledge architectures. These platforms must accommodate linguistic plurality, multimodal engagement, and variable bandwidth capacities (Torrado et al., 2022; Yang, 2025). They should include interactive modules, peer exchange forums, and adaptive feedback systems that allow users to navigate regulatory evolution in real time. Educational content must be continually revised to reflect shifts in law, technology, and community need. Educational implications of AI regulation in geriatric care are not ancillary to governance. They constitute its operational core. Policies that remain inert in statute or fragmented in implementation betray their own normative aspirations. The pedagogical imperative is therefore not only to disseminate policy but to animate it through reflexive, situated, and multi-actor educational ecosystems. The future of ethical AI in eldercare will be forged not in courtrooms or laboratories alone but in classrooms, community halls, and care facilities where law, technology, and human experience converge.

7. CASE STUDIES AND BEST PRACTICES

The epistemological legitimacy and empirical robustness of educational imperatives in AI-mediated geriatric care find their most substantiated articulation in situated case studies across diverse geopolitical and sociotechnical terrains (Ho et al., 2023; Skrabanek et al., 2025). These instantiations serve not merely as illustrative vignettes but as sites of praxis where techno-pedagogical innovations coalesce with cultural, infrastructural, and demographic specificities. They offer ecologically valid insights into how educational infrastructures can function as primary catalysts for ethically aligned and contextually grounded technological diffusion. Japan exemplifies a paradigmatic techno-gerontocratic model predicated on demographic determinism and industrial readiness.

With a super-aged society where approximately twenty-nine percent of the population surpasses the age of sixty-five, Japan has enacted a national strategy that mobilises robotics as a compensatory mechanism for human caregiving deficits. Through synergistic collaborations between the Ministry of Health, Labour and Welfare, RIKEN, and Toyota, robotic platforms such as Robear and Human Support Robot have been developed for biomechanical assistance, cognitive stimulation, and socioemotional engagement. Recognising the pedagogical lacuna in interfacing human caregivers with these robotic entities, Japan's Ministry of Education institutionalised robotic literacy within health sciences curricula. Vocational colleges in urban centres such as Fukuoka and Yokohama now embed simulation-based training that fuses technical operability with modules on affective calibration, cross-modal communication, and hybrid task orchestration. These pedagogical interventions have catalysed a behavioural shift, i.e., robot acceptance among caregiving personnel has risen from thirty-eight percent in 2015 to over seventy percent in 2023. Moreover, patient-reported outcome measures reveal statistically significant upticks in satisfaction indices and psychosocial comfort with robotic-assisted care.

Finland offers a counterpoint, foregrounding user-centric digital literacy as the cornerstone of its AI integration strategy. The "Digital Skills for Seniors" program, launched in 2017, operationalises a rights-based digital inclusion agenda. The initiative is structurally decentralised and pedagogically pluralistic, utilising public infrastructures such as libraries, community centres, and residential care homes as distributed learning nodes. Pedagogical delivery is multimodal, incorporating peer mentorship, intergenerational scaffolding, and group-based experiential learning. Content includes modules on cyber hygiene, e-governance navigation, algorithmic virtual assistants, and e-health portals. Crucially, the initiative recasts digital competence as a psychosocial asset rather than a purely utilitarian skill. Evaluation metrics published by the Ministry of Transport and Communications indicate that seventy-eight percent of participants reported enhanced digital confidence, while longitudinal studies register a forty percent increase in sustained utilisation of digital platforms. The Finnish state has since constitutionalised this model by embedding digital literacy within national ageing policy frameworks, signifying a normative shift in the ontology of eldercare. India presents an infrastructurally asymmetric but pedagogically innovative landscape.

In rural and peri-urban localities across Jharkhand, Tamil Nadu, and Rajasthan, non-governmental organisations such as HelpAge India and the Digital Empowerment Foundation have architected decentralised, multilingual, and low-bandwidth-compatible educational ecologies. These involve mobile digital labs, vernacularised offline applications, and gamified, voice-assisted modules designed for learners with limited or no formal education. Pedagogical design is informed by constructivist and culturally responsive paradigms. In tribal regions, local youth are trained as Digital Sevikas, functioning as mediators of AI tools in telemedicine, biometric verification, and diagnostic screenings such as electrocardiogram analysis via handheld devices. These mediators enact both technical facilitation and cultural brokerage. Preliminary impact assessments reveal a sixty-three percent increase in digital uptake among older adults and a forty-seven percent reduction in avoidable health events due to early AI-enabled interventions. These community-embedded models reconfigure digital health access not as charity or intervention but as a right anchored in local epistemologies.

South Korea's Silver Care Policy provides a vocational integration blueprint that combines curriculum design, regulatory mandates, and industrial alignment. Vocational training institutes in Seoul, Daejeon, and Busan have incorporated AI literacy into certificate programs for homecare professionals. The Korea Institute for Robot Industry Advancement collaborates in curricular co-development, ensuring pedagogical fidelity to real-world deployment. The instructional architecture adopts a spiral curriculum model wherein learners revisit core competencies such as ethical risk assessment, fault tolerance, and data integrity at increasing levels of abstraction. Importantly, employers are mandated to provide on-site reinforcement, embedding pedagogical continuity into the workplace. Between 2020 and 2023, enrolment rates in these programs expanded by over three hundred percent, and post-certification skill retention exceeded eighty percent. The model demonstrates how state-industry-academia triads can produce scalable, equitable, and durable educational outcomes. Comparative cross-analysis of these divergent models reveals several cross-cutting epistemic heuristics. Foremost among them is the imperative of contextual specificity.

In Japan, the socio-cultural normalisation of automation enabled the seamless integration of humanoid robotics, while in India, linguistic plurality and infrastructural scarcity necessitated hyper-localised and mobile-first pedagogical architectures. The second insight is the centrality of relational trust in technological uptake. Finland's deployment of social learning architectures and India's community-embedded intermediaries illustrate that trust is not an artefact of interface design but an emergent property of social relations. Thirdly, curriculum localisation is a non-negotiable prerequisite for engagement. From linguistic transliteration to culturally encoded metaphors, successful education necessitates pedagogical vernacularisation.

These examples converge on a unifying axiom, i.e., the efficacy of AI in geriatric ecosystems is predicated less on algorithmic sophistication than on pedagogical intentionality. Educational models that treat elders, caregivers, and technologists as epistemic agents rather than passive recipients are more likely to generate sustainable and equitable adoption (Mohan et al., 2024; Porkodi & Kesavaraja, 2021). Education functions not as an ancillary appendage to innovation but as its ontological foundation. In its absence, even the most sophisticated technologies risk obsolescence, misuse, or rejection (Chowdhury et al., 2021; Song, 2024).

The case studies also illuminate the indispensability of polycentric governance and multi-stakeholder coordination. Public institutions offered policy direction and fiscal infrastructure, civil society translated macro-policy into micro-practice, academic institutions operationalised curricular design, and private sector actors contributed technological artefacts and training modules. These consortia now require institutionalisation and cross-border expansion. Establishing transnational knowledge networks and standardised pedagogical frameworks is essential to disseminate these insights beyond their initial geographies. Such systemic translation is imperative if education is to evolve from sporadic innovation to a globally scalable paradigm of anticipatory readiness in geriatric AI integration.

8. EDUCATION ROADMAP FOR AI-INTEGRATED GERIATRIC CARE

The accelerating convergence of artificial intelligence and geriatric care constitutes a paradigmatic inflection point in the epistemic architecture of health and technology. What is required is not a mere recalibration of existing instructional templates but a fundamental reconceptualisation of the ontological foundations and teleological trajectories of educational systems across stakeholder categories (Neves et al., 2023; Božić, 2023). This reconceptualisation necessitates a stratified, polycentric, and anticipatory roadmap that privileges futurity, distributive equity, and adaptive resilience as core design principles. At the preliminary tier of this roadmap lies public awareness, conceived not as unidirectional dissemination but as dialogic epistemic engagement.

The cultivation of algorithmic familiarity among older adults, informal caregivers, and community interlocutors is essential to dismantle affective resistance and epistemological alienation (Chu et al., 2022; Renn et al., 2021). Public pedagogical interventions must transcend techno-utopian marketing scripts to introduce foundational constructs such as informational sovereignty, probabilistic reasoning in machine learning, and digital subjectivity. Empirical examples include culturally localised media campaigns via community radio in rural East Africa and vernacular television programming in Latin America, which have demonstrated efficacy in encoding abstract concepts within culturally consonant semiotic frames. Grassroots networks, civil society entities, and local epistemic brokers must be mobilised as pedagogical vectors. These agents can operationalise myth-deconstruction by addressing misconceptions such as the infallibility of AI, the obsolescence of human caregiving, or the age-exclusivity of digital technologies (Abadir & Chellappa, 2024; Cantone et al., 2023).

The intermediate tier prioritises skill development and procedural literacy, demanding the institutionalisation of modular, accessible, and multilingual certification ecosystems. For healthcare professionals, this entails the integration of AI epistemologies into medical and paramedical curricula, spanning machine-human interface fluency, ethical forensics, and techno-clinical risk governance (Loveys et al., 2022; Lee et al., 2022). For elder learners, microlearning platforms, voice-guided interfaces, and intergenerational mentorship models offer viable modalities for digital onboarding. In jurisdictions such as the Netherlands, stackable micro-credentials have created flexible skilling trajectories aligned with labour market fluidity. Financial democratisation of access remains critical, mandating subsidy mechanisms from both state apparatuses and philanthropic capital to mitigate epistemic exclusion and digital stratification.

The apex tier is the professionalisation of AI-geriatrics as a transdisciplinary knowledge domain embedded within formalised education. Academic institutions must construct dedicated curricular tracts on ageing technologies, facilitated by polymathic faculty and problem-based, praxis-oriented pedagogies. Curricular instantiations should encompass situated ethics laboratories, AI simulation studios, and interdisciplinary clinical residencies. Singapore's Centre for Health Innovation operationalises this model through its gerontechnology curriculum, which interlaces systems design, medical anthropology, and machine learning. Accreditation bodies must codify AI literacy, human-machine co-regulation, and sociotechnical contextuality as baseline competencies for professional legitimacy across medicine, engineering, public health, and legal disciplines.

Operational feasibility of this roadmap presupposes an enabling structural infrastructure. Strategic consortia between public institutions, private sector entities, and civil society organisations can catalyse resource pooling, knowledge co-creation, and pedagogical innovation. Corporate actors must be co-responsibilised through regulatory incentives to participate in community-level digital education, with such contributions integrated into their corporate accountability metrics. State agencies can provide matching grants for the development of open-access, linguistically diverse, and multimodal instructional assets. Pedagogical platforms such as Coursera and edX must be reengineered for elder inclusivity, incorporating user-centric interfaces, auditory and haptic navigation aids, and bandwidth-agnostic offline modules.

A critical vector in this roadmap is the establishment of Regional Centres for AI and Geriatrics Education. These epistemic nodes must function as crucibles of curricular development, capacity building, and policy-interface articulation. Their governance structures should be pluralistic, composed of older adults, clinicians, technologists, ethicists, and community epistemologists. Centres in the Global South must prioritise constraints endemic to their sociotechnical imaginaries, such as infrastructural intermittency, polyglossic populations, and culturally situated ontologies of ageing and dependency. Given the volatility and obsolescence curves of AI systems, pedagogical architectures must embrace temporal fluidity. Static, monolithic training regimes are ill-suited for ecosystems characterised by rapid technological evolution, regulatory dynamism, and ontological pluralism (Shiwani et al., 2023; Qian et al., 2021).

Learning ecosystems must be conceived as perpetual, recursive, and feedback-sensitive. Adaptive learning infrastructures, comprising mobile notifications, AI-augmented tutoring agents, and community-embedded peer pods, can sustain epistemic continuity and cognitive elasticity. Beyond content, the pedagogical meta-theory underpinning this roadmap requires a paradigmatic recalibration. A pedagogy of care centres the affective and relational dimensions of knowledge production, foregrounding empathy, biographical nuance, and the moral phenomenology of elder subjectivities. A pedagogy of inclusion operationalises accessibility as an epistemic right, mandating instructional design that accommodates neurodiversity, multimodal literacies, and embodied heterogeneity. A pedagogy of futures literacy cultivates anticipatory cognition, scenario-based reasoning, and sociotechnical imagination, enabling learners to not merely accommodate AI's evolution but to co-author its normative directionality. Such a pedagogy interrogates epistemic injustice, algorithmic opacity, and the political economy of AI infrastructures.

Ultimately, this roadmap must be inscribed within a cosmopolitan ethics of educational justice. While biological senescence is a universal trajectory, the epistemic affordances to age with agency are radically stratified across geographies and socio-economic divides. To universalise geriatric dignity in an age of algorithmic governance, AI-integrated education must be rendered a global commons.

Multilateral organisations, academic syndicates, and technological conglomerates must converge to reclassify geriatric AI pedagogy as an indispensable public good, subject to international cooperation and mutual accountability. While this vision is audacious in scope, its realisation is not utopian. It demands collective intentionality, epistemological humility, and infrastructural investment. The arc of eldercare's future will not be inscribed by AI's sophistication alone, but by the educational architectures that mediate its design, governance, and uptake (Padhan et al., 2023; Lee et al., 2023). Without education as the epistemic spine of this ecosystem, the project of humane and equitable geriatric care will remain structurally incomplete.

9. CONCLUSION

The global incorporation of artificial intelligence into geriatric care constitutes a transformative epistemic rupture in the ontological constitution of health infrastructures, care economies, and ageing societies. This transformation, however, is not merely a function of algorithmic complexity or computational prowess. Rather, it is increasingly mediated by the cognitive, ethical, and sociotechnical literacies of the human actors who design, deploy, and interact with such systems. Education, as has been argued throughout this chapter, is not a peripheral addendum but the central mediating variable that governs whether AI becomes an instrument of emancipatory care or a vector of systemic exclusion. This inquiry began by problematising the demographic acceleration of global ageing, outlining the exponential intensification of demand for eldercare services amid collapsing human resource pipelines and overburdened institutional capacities. Against this backdrop, artificial intelligence emerged as both solution and symptom, i.e., a techno-social agent capable of augmenting clinical decision-making, enhancing operational efficiencies, and enabling continuity of care, while simultaneously generating new ethical, relational, and infrastructural vulnerabilities.

The chapter conceptualised human-AI interaction not as a mechanistic interface but as a complex sociocultural entanglement requiring pedagogical reframing. Health practitioners, caregivers, and institutional actors must be reconceptualised as hybrid agents operating within distributed epistemologies of care, wherein machine intelligences function as cognitive collaborators rather than substitutive automata.

The discussion advanced by interrogating the normative lacunae within existing AI design paradigms, especially the erasure of gerontological knowledge and the absence of age-sensitive heuristics within computational ontologies. The educational requisites of designers, engineers, and regulators were problematised, pointing to the epistemic violence inherent in exclusionary innovation. The integration of geriatric epistemologies, affective cognition, and participatory co-design into STEM pedagogies was posited as a necessary corrective to the technocratic insularity of current development models.

Subsequent sections examined digital equity not merely as a matter of technological access but as a multifactorial assemblage of infrastructural, cognitive, cultural, and affective enablers and barriers. The pedagogical scaffolds required to support agency, autonomy, and informed participation among older adults were foregrounded. Community-based digital literacy initiatives, culturally embedded consent frameworks, and multimodal instructional strategies were shown to constitute the preconditions for meaningful AI engagement. The fallacy of assuming that access equals empowerment was systematically dismantled, reinforcing the imperative for pedagogies of critical digitality. Resistance to AI, both at the level of individual habitus and institutional culture, was reframed not as a deficit to be rectified but as a productive epistemic resource. Drawing from theories of transformative learning, the chapter demonstrated how resistance could serve as a diagnostic of ethical ambivalence and as a trigger for reflective praxis.

Peer-led knowledge ecologies and affectively attuned training environments were proposed as counter-hegemonic pedagogical formations capable of cultivating situated trust and adaptive resilience. Policy frameworks were treated not as static legal artefacts but as performative instruments whose efficacy depends on translation into experiential competencies and moral reasoning. Through a comparative analysis of regulatory ecosystems, the chapter illuminated the disconnect between declarative intent and lived implementation.

Education emerged as the catalytic infrastructure required to operationalise rights-based policies, bridge epistemic asymmetries, and institutionalise accountability. Empirical instantiations from Japan, Finland, India, and South Korea served as methodological examples of education-driven AI integration across variegated sociotechnical terrains. These case studies demonstrated the salience of contextual sensitivity, curriculum localisation, and multi-actor governance in shaping successful interventions. The educational roadmap articulated in the chapter, comprising awareness-building, skills acquisition, and professionalisation, was posited as a strategic blueprint for scalable, sustainable, and equitable AI integration.

To architect a just and futurally viable AI-enabled geriatric care system, three axiological imperatives must be pursued. First, structural investment in digital literacy ecosystems for elders and caregivers must be prioritised, with attention to intersectional barriers and rights-based content. Second, the curricula of AI developers, clinical educators, and policy technocrats must be reengineered to embed ethics, inclusivity, and the phenomenology of ageing as core domains of knowledge. Third, cross-sectoral alliances comprising state actors, civil society, academia, and industry must institutionalise AI preparedness through credentialing frameworks, regulatory oversight, and iterative feedback loops. The trajectory of AI in geriatric care is not an ontological inevitability but a sociopolitical construction contingent on deliberative human choices.

These choices are made not solely in laboratories or legislatures but in pedagogical spaces, i.e., in classrooms, training halls, online platforms, and community hubs, where epistemic frames are shaped, contested, and internalised. Education is the primary infrastructure through which technological affordances are transformed into moral commitments and operational capacities. Absent this infrastructure, AI systems risk reproducing existing exclusions with algorithmic efficiency and epistemic opacity. When education is central, however, the technological artefact becomes a conduit for care, solidarity, and justice. The elderly citizen, often marginalised in both design and discourse, is re-centred as a co-author of the digital future. In this reframing lies not only the ethical promise of AI in eldercare but its most enduring human value.

REFERENCES

Abadir, P., & Chellappa, R. (2024). Artificial intelligence in geriatrics: Riding the inevitable tide of promise, challenges, and considerations. *The Journals of Gerontology. Series A, Biological Sciences and Medical Sciences*, *79*(2), glad279.

Abou Hashish, E. A., & Alnajjar, H. (2024). Digital proficiency: Assessing knowledge, attitudes, and skills in digital transformation, health literacy, and artificial intelligence among university nursing students. *BMC Medical Education*, *24*(1), 508.

Aggarwal, R., Farag, S., Martin, G., Ashrafian, H., & Darzi, A. (2021). Patient perceptions on data sharing and applying artificial intelligence to health care data: Cross-sectional survey. *Journal of Medical Internet Research*, *23*(8), e26162.

Agha, R. A., Mathew, G., Rashid, R., Kerwan, A., Al-Jabir, A., Sohrabi, C., & Agha, M. (2025). Revised Strengthening the reporting of cohort, cross-sectional and case-control studies in surgery (STROCSS) Guideline: An update for the age of Artificial Intelligence. *Premier Journal of Science*, *10*, 100081.

Aher, R. B., Jadhav, S., Sharma, Y., & Pawar, P. (2024). A review on new trends of artificial intelligence in medicine. *Open Access Journal of Data Science and Artificial Intelligence*, *2*(1), 1–12.

Akyon, S. H., Akyon, F. C., & Yılmaz, T. E. (2023). Artificial intelligence-supported web application design and development for reducing polypharmacy side effects and supporting rational drug use in geriatric patients. *Frontiers in medicine*, *10*, 1029198.

Alharbi, H. A., Alharbi, K. K., & Hassan, C. A. U. (2023). Enhancing elderly fall detection through IoT-enabled smart flooring and AI for independent living sustainability. *Sustainability*, *15*(22), 15695.

Alruwaili, M. M., Abuadas, F. H., Alsadi, M., Alruwaili, A. N., Elsayed Ramadan, O. M., Shaban, M., & El Arab, R. A. (2024). Exploring nurses' awareness and attitudes toward artificial intelligence: Implications for nursing practice. *Digital Health*, *10*, 20552076241271803.

AlZaabi, A., & AlMaskari, S., & AalAbdulsalam, A. (2023). Are physicians and medical students ready for artificial intelligence applications in healthcare? *Digital Health*, *9*, 20552076231152167.

Apell, P., & Eriksson, H. (2023). Artificial intelligence (AI) healthcare technology innovations: The current state and challenges from a life science industry perspective. *Technology Analysis and Strategic Management*, *35*(2), 179–193.

Aronsson, A. (2022). Professional Women and Elder Care in Contemporary Japan: Anxiety and the Move Toward Technocare. *Anthropology & Aging, 43*(1).

Awotunde, J. B., Ajagbe, S. A., & Florez, H. (2022, October). Internet of things with wearable devices and artificial intelligence for elderly uninterrupted healthcare monitoring systems. In *International Conference on Applied Informatics* (pp. 278-291). Cham: Springer International Publishing.

Baek, Y. S., Lee, D. H., Jo, Y., Lee, S. C., Choi, W., & Kim, D. H. (2023). Artificial intelligence-estimated biological heart age using a 12-lead electrocardiogram predicts mortality and cardiovascular outcomes. *Frontiers in Cardiovascular Medicine, 10*, 1137892.

Belmin, J., Villani, P., Gay, M., Fabries, S., Havreng-Théry, C., Malvoisin, S., & Veyron, J. H. (2022). Real-world implementation of an eHealth system based on artificial intelligence designed to predict and reduce emergency department visits by older adults: Pragmatic trial. *Journal of Medical Internet Research, 24*(9), e40387.

Bevilacqua, R., Barbarossa, F., Fantechi, L., Fornarelli, D., Paci, E., Bolognini, S., & Maranesi, E. (2023). Radiomics and artificial intelligence for the diagnosis and monitoring of Alzheimer's disease: A systematic review of studies in the field. *Journal of Clinical Medicine, 12*(16), 5432.

Bokolo, A. J. (2023). Inclusive and safe mobility needs of senior citizens: Implications for age-friendly cities and communities. *Urban Science (Basel, Switzerland), 7*(4), 103.

Božić, V. (2023). *Implementation of Artifical Intelligent (AI).* Solutions to Help Elderly People.

Broadbent, E., Loveys, K., Ilan, G., Chen, G., Chilukuri, M. M., Boardman, S. G., & Skuler, D. (2024). ElliQ, an AI-driven social robot to alleviate loneliness: Progress and lessons learned. *The Journal of Aging Research & Lifestyle, 13*, 22–28.

Cantone, A. A., Esposito, M., Perillo, F. P., Romano, M., Sebillo, M., & Vitiello, G. (2023). Enhancing elderly health monitoring: Achieving autonomous and secure living through the integration of artificial intelligence, autonomous robots, and sensors. *Electronics (Basel), 12*(18), 3918.

Cesario, A., D'Oria, M., Calvani, R., Picca, A., Pietragalla, A., Lorusso, D., & Scambia, G. (2021). The role of artificial intelligence in managing multimorbidity and cancer. *Journal of Personalized Medicine, 11*(4), 314.

Chang, J., Wu, Y., Zhao, Y., Gao, X., Xing, Y., Wang, Z., & Tang, Y. (2025). Cohort profile: China healthy aging cohort study (China-Aging). *Journal of Alzheimer's Disease*, •••, 13872877251360028.

Chen, C., Ding, S., & Wang, J. (2023). Digital health for aging populations. *Nature Medicine*, *29*(7), 1623–1630.

Chen, H., Zhang, Y., & Wang, L. (2023). A study on the quality evaluation index system of smart home care for older adults in the community——based on Delphi and AHP. *BMC Public Health*, *23*(1), 411.

Chen, Y. H., & Xu, J. L. (2023). Applying artificial intelligence to predict falls for inpatient. *Frontiers in Medicine*, *10*, 1285192.

Chopra, K. (2025). Motivating older adults with special needs for learning using generative artificial intelligence. *Educational Gerontology*, •••, 1–20.

Choudhary, E., & Nagar, V. (2025). Biomimicry and rehabilitation of dental tissues in geriatric population-An overview. *Journal of Oral Research and Review*, *17*(2), 189–195.

Chowdhury, M., Cervantes, E. G., Chan, W. Y., & Seitz, D. P. (2021). Use of machine learning and artificial intelligence methods in geriatric mental health research involving electronic health record or administrative claims data: A systematic review. *Frontiers in Psychiatry*, *12*, 738466.

Chu, C. H., Donato-Woodger, S., Khan, S. S., Nyrup, R., Leslie, K., Lyn, A., & Grenier, A. (2023). Age-related bias and artificial intelligence: A scoping review. *Humanities & Social Sciences Communications*, *10*(1), 1–17.

Chu, C. H., Leslie, K., Shi, J., Nyrup, R., Bianchi, A., Khan, S. S., & Grenier, A. (2022). Ageism and artificial intelligence: Protocol for a scoping review. *JMIR Research Protocols*, *11*(6), e33211.

Chu, C. H., Nyrup, R., Leslie, K., Shi, J., Bianchi, A., Lyn, A., & Grenier, A. (2022). Digital ageism: Challenges and opportunities in artificial intelligence for older adults. *The Gerontologist*, *62*(7), 947–955.

Chu-Ke, C., & Dong, Y. (2024). Misinformation and literacies in the era of generative artificial intelligence: A brief overview and a call for future research. *Emerging Media*, *2*(1), 70–85.

Cinalioglu, K., Elbaz, S., Sekhon, K., Su, C. L., Rej, S., & Sekhon, H. (2023). Exploring differential perceptions of artificial intelligence in health care among younger versus older Canadians: Results from the 2021 Canadian Digital Health Survey. *Journal of Medical Internet Research*, *25*, e38169.

Cingolani, M., Scendoni, R., Fedeli, P., & Cembrani, F. (2023). Artificial intelligence and digital medicine for integrated home care services in Italy: Opportunities and limits. *Frontiers in Public Health*, *10*, 1095001.

Corbett, C. F., Wright, P. J., Jones, K., & Parmer, M. (2021). Voice-activated virtual home assistant use and social isolation and loneliness among older adults: Mini review. *Frontiers in Public Health*, *9*, 742012.

Costanzo, M., Smeriglio, R., & Di Nuovo, S. (2024). New technologies and assistive robotics for elderly: A review on psychological variables. *Archives of Gerontology and Geriatrics Plus*, *1*(4), 100056.

Czaja, S. J., & Ceruso, M. (2022). The promise of artificial intelligence in supporting an aging population. *Journal of Cognitive Engineering and Decision Making*, *16*(4), 182–193.

Danda, R. R. (2022). Telehealth In Medicare Plans: Leveraging AI For Improved Accessibility And Senior Care Quality. *Migration Letters : An International Journal of Migration Studies*, *19*(6), 1133–1143.

Denecke, K., & Baudoin, C. R. (2022). A review of artificial intelligence and robotics in transformed health ecosystems. *Frontiers in medicine*, *9*, 795957.

Diareme, K. C., Liapakis, A., & Efthymiou, I. P. (2022). Data, sentiment analysis, and examples during the COVID-19 pandemic. *Hellenic Archives of Psychiatry and Clinical Psychology in Behavioral Sciences*, *33779*. Advance online publication. DOI: 10.12681/hapscpbs.33779

Dilip, G., Guttula, R., & Rajeyyagari, S. (2022). S, H., Pandey, R. R., Bora, A., ... & Sundramurthy, V. P. (2022). Artificial Intelligence-Based Smart Comrade Robot for Elders Healthcare with Strait Rescue System. *Journal of Healthcare Engineering*, (1), 9904870.

Dong, L., Yang, Q., Zhang, R. H., & Wei, W. B. (2021). Artificial intelligence for the detection of age-related macular degeneration in color fundus photographs: A systematic review and meta-analysis. *EClinicalMedicine*, *•••*, 35.

Dong, X., Du, S., Zheng, W., Cai, C., Liu, H., & Zou, J. (2022). Evaluation of an artificial intelligence system for the detection of diabetic retinopathy in Chinese community healthcare centers. *Frontiers in Medicine*, *9*, 883462.

Efthymiou, I. (2024b). Exploring the Frontier: New and Future Trends in Research. In B. Orlando (Ed.), *Innovation Capabilities and Entrepreneurial Opportunities of Smart Working* (pp. 48-68). IGI Global Scientific Publishing. https://doi.org/DOI: 10.4018/978-1-7998-8797-3.ch003

Efthymiou, I. (2026). AI in Epidemiology: Predicting the Unpredictable Leveraging AI to Detect Outbreaks and Predict Disease. In Umer, M. (Ed.), *Innovation and Transformation of Public Health* (pp. 281–308). IGI Global Scientific Publishing., DOI: 10.4018/979-8-3373-1992-6.ch009

Efthymiou, I.-P. (2020). Non-cognitive skills and AI: A new era of learning and development. *International Case Studies Journal*, *9*(10), 42–46.

Efthymiou, I.-P. (2024a). Can AI improve health and wellbeing? *Case Studies Journal*, *13*(11), 1–5.

Eun, S. J., Kim, E. J., & Kim, J. (2023). Artificial intelligence-based personalized serious game for enhancing the physical and cognitive abilities of the elderly. *Future Generation Computer Systems*, *141*, 713–722.

Gallistl, V., Banday, M. U. L., Berridge, C., Grigorovich, A., Jarke, J., Mannheim, I., & Peine, A. (2024). Addressing the black box of AI—A model and research agenda on the co-constitution of aging and artificial intelligence. *The Gerontologist*, *64*(6), gnae039.

Ghosh, S., & Ghosh, S. K. (2023). Feel: Federated learning framework for elderly healthcare using edge-iomt. *IEEE Transactions on Computational Social Systems*, *10*(4), 1800–1809.

González-Castro, A., Leirós-Rodríguez, R., Prada-García, C., & Benítez-Andrades, J. A. (2024). The applications of artificial intelligence for assessing fall risk: Systematic review. *Journal of Medical Internet Research*, *26*, e54934.

Görtz, M., Baumgärtner, K., Schmid, T., Muschko, M., Woessner, P., Gerlach, A., & Hohenfellner, M. (2023). An artificial intelligence-based chatbot for prostate cancer education: Design and patient evaluation study. *Digital Health*, *9*, 20552076231173304.

Gray, K., Slavotinek, J., Dimaguila, G. L., & Choo, D. (2022). Artificial intelligence education for the health workforce: Expert survey of approaches and needs. *JMIR Medical Education*, *8*(2), e35223.

Gudala, M., Ross, M. E. T., Mogalla, S., Lyons, M., Ramaswamy, P., & Roberts, K. (2022). Benefits of, barriers to, and needs for an artificial intelligence–powered medication information voice chatbot for older adults: Interview study with geriatrics experts. *JMIR Aging*, *5*(2), e32169.

Hanke, S., Mangialasche, F., Bödenler, M., Neumayer, B., Ngandu, T., Mecocci, P., & Stögmann, E. (2022). AI-based predictive modelling of the onset and progression of dementia. *Smart Cities*, *5*(2), 700–714.

Herrmann, B. (2023). The perception of artificial-intelligence (AI) based synthesized speech in younger and older adults. *International Journal of Speech Technology*, *26*(2), 395–415.

Ho, A. (2023). *Live like nobody is watching: Relational autonomy in the age of artificial intelligence health monitoring*. Oxford University Press.

Ho, M. T., Le, N. T. B., Mantello, P., Ho, M. T., & Ghotbi, N. (2023). Understanding the acceptance of emotional artificial intelligence in Japanese healthcare system: A cross-sectional survey of clinic visitors' attitude. *Technology in Society*, *72*, 102166.

Huang, K., Jiao, Z., Cai, Y., & Zhong, Z. (2022). Artificial intelligence-based intelligent surveillance for reducing nurses' working hours in nurse–patient interaction: A two-wave study. *Journal of Nursing Management*, *30*(8), 3817–3826.

Huang, W., Ong, W. C., Wong, M. K. F., Ng, E. Y. K., Koh, T., Chandramouli, C., & Tromp, J. (2024). Applying the UTAUT2 framework to patients' attitudes toward healthcare task shifting with artificial intelligence. *BMC Health Services Research*, *24*(1), 455.

Huang, X., Zhang, Z., Guo, F., Wang, X., Chi, K., & Wu, K. (2024, June). Research on older adults' interaction with e-health interface based on explainable artificial intelligence. In *International Conference on Human-Computer Interaction* (pp. 38-52). Cham: Springer Nature Switzerland.

Huq, S. M., Maskeliūnas, R., & Damaševičius, R. (2024). Dialogue agents for artificial intelligence-based conversational systems for cognitively disabled: A systematic review. *Disability and Rehabilitation. Assistive Technology*, *19*(3), 1059–1078.

Ibuki, T., Ibuki, A., & Nakazawa, E. (2024). Possibilities and ethical issues of entrusting nursing tasks to robots and artificial intelligence. *Nursing Ethics*, *31*(6), 1010–1020.

Javadi-Pashaki, N., Ghazanfari, M. J., & Karkhah, S. (2021). Machine learning for geriatric clinical care: Opportunities and challenges. *Annals of Geriatric Medicine and Research*, *25*(2), 137.

Jnr, B. A. (2025). User-centered AI-based voice-assistants for safe mobility of older people in urban context. *AI & Society*, *40*(2), 545–568.

Jonek-Kowalska, I., & Wolny, M. (2025). Age Sustainability in Smart City: Seniors as Urban Stakeholders in the Light of Literature Studies. *Sustainability*, *17*(14), 6333.

Jun Woo, C. H. O. I., & KANG, M. S. (2024). A Study on the development of a chatbot using generative AI to provide diets for diabetic patients. *Korean Journal of Artificial Intelligence*, *12*(3), 25–31.

Kaya, F., Aydin, F., Schepman, A., Rodway, P., Yetişensoy, O., & Demir Kaya, M. (2024). The roles of personality traits, AI anxiety, and demographic factors in attitudes toward artificial intelligence. *International Journal of Human-Computer Interaction*, *40*(2), 497–514.

Kedziora, D. (2022). Botsourcing, roboshoring or virtual backoffice? perspectives on implementing robotic process automation (RPA) and artificial intelligence (AI). *Human Technology*, *18*(2), 92–97.

Kerwan, A., Al-Jabir, A., Mathew, G., Sohrabi, C., Rashid, R., Franchi, T., & Agha, R. A. (2025). Revised surgical CAse REport (SCARE) guideline: An update for the age of artificial intelligence. *Premier J. Sci.*, *10*(100079), 2025.

Kim, D. J., Lee, Y. S., Jeon, E. R., & Kim, K. J. (2024, January). Present and future of AI-IoT-based healthcare services for senior citizens in local communities: A review of a South Korean government digital healthcare initiatives. [). MDPI.]. *Health Care*, *12*(2), 281.

Koc, M. (2023). ARTIFICIAL INTELLIGENCE IN GERIATRICS. *Turkish Journal of Geriatrics/Türk Geriatri Dergisi, 26*(4).

Kouroubali, A., Kondylakis, H., Logothetidis, F., & Katehakis, D. G. (2022, February). Developing an AI-enabled integrated care platform for frailty. [). MDPI.]. *Health Care*, *10*(3), 443.

Lambert, S. I., Madi, M., Sopka, S., Lenes, A., Stange, H., Buszello, C. P., & Stephan, A. (2023). An integrative review on the acceptance of artificial intelligence among healthcare professionals in hospitals. *NPJ Digital Medicine*, *6*(1), 111.

Lau, C. H., Yu, K. H. O., Yip, T. F., Luk, L. Y. F., Wai, A. K. C., Sit, T. Y., & Ho, J. W. K. (2022). An artificial intelligence-enabled smartphone app for real-time pressure injury assessment. *Frontiers in Medical Technology*, *4*, 905074.

Laur, O., & Wang, B. (2022). Musculoskeletal trauma and artificial intelligence: Current trends and projections. *Skeletal Radiology*, *51*(2), 257–269.

Lee, C. H., Wang, C., Fan, X., Li, F., & Chen, C. H. (2023). Artificial intelligence-enabled digital transformation in elderly healthcare field: Scoping review. *Advanced Engineering Informatics*, *55*, 101874.

Lee, H., Chung, M. A., Kim, H., & Nam, E. W. (2022). The effect of cognitive function health care using artificial intelligence robots for older adults: Systematic review and meta-analysis. *JMIR Aging*, *5*(2), e38896.

Liu, X., Chau, K. Y., Liu, X., & Wan, Y. (2023). The progress of smart elderly care research: A scientometric analysis based on CNKI and WOS. *International Journal of Environmental Research and Public Health*, *20*(2), 1086.

Livieri, G., Anastasopoulou, C., Briola, K., Nikolopoulou, P., & Efthymiou, I. P. (2024). Ethical issues arising from the use of AI in drug discovery. *Journal of Politics and Ethics in New Technologies and AI*, *3*(1), e37093–e37093.

Loveys, K., Prina, M., Axford, C., Domènec, Ò. R., Weng, W., Broadbent, E., & Thiyagarajan, J. A. (2022). Artificial intelligence for older people receiving long-term care: A systematic review of acceptability and effectiveness studies. *The Lancet. Healthy Longevity*, *3*(4), e286–e297.

Lukkien, D. R., Nap, H. H., Buimer, H. P., Peine, A., Boon, W. P., Ket, J. C., & Moors, E. H. (2023). Toward responsible artificial intelligence in long-term care: A scoping review on practical approaches. *The Gerontologist*, *63*(1), 155–168.

Marino, N., Putignano, G., Cappilli, S., Chersoni, E., Santuccione, A., Calabrese, G., & Santus, E. (2023). Towards AI-driven longevity research: An overview. *Frontiers in Aging*, *4*, 1057204.

Martin-Martinez, A., Miró, J., Amadó, C., Ruz, F., Ruiz, A., Ortega, O., & Clave, P. (2023). A systematic and universal artificial intelligence screening method for oropharyngeal dysphagia: Improving diagnosis through risk management. *Dysphagia*, *38*(4), 1224–1237.

McGee, R. W. (2024). Incorporating Artificial Intelligence and Traditional Chinese Medicine (TCM) into a Western Medical Practice: A Case Study. *Biomedical Journal of Scientific & Technical Research*, *56*(3), 48149–48154.

Mikkelsen, J. G., Sørensen, N. L., Merrild, C. H., Jensen, M. B., & Thomsen, J. L. (2023). Patient perspectives on data sharing regarding implementing and using artificial intelligence in general practice–a qualitative study. *BMC Health Services Research*, *23*(1), 335.

Mohan, D., Al-Hamid, D. Z., Chong, P. H. J., Sudheera, K. L. K., Gutierrez, J., Chan, H. C., & Li, H. (2024). Artificial intelligence and iot in elderly fall prevention: A review. *IEEE Sensors Journal*, *24*(4), 4181–4198.

Momtazmanesh, S., Nowroozi, A., & Rezaei, N. (2022). Artificial intelligence in rheumatoid arthritis: current status and future perspectives: a state-of-the-art review. *Rheumatology and Therapy*, *9*(5), 1249–1304.

Muralidharan, V., Adewale, B. A., Huang, C. J., Nta, M. T., Ademiju, P. O., Pathmarajah, P., & Olatunji, T. (2024). A scoping review of reporting gaps in FDA-approved AI medical devices. *NPJ Digital Medicine*, *7*(1), 273.

Nasr, M., Islam, M. M., Shehata, S., Karray, F., & Quintana, Y. (2021). Smart healthcare in the age of AI: Recent advances, challenges, and future prospects. *IEEE Access : Practical Innovations, Open Solutions*, *9*, 145248–145270.

Neves, B. B., Petersen, A., Vered, M., Carter, A., & Omori, M. (2023). Artificial intelligence in long-term care: Technological promise, aging anxieties, and socio-technical ageism. *Journal of Applied Gerontology*, *42*(6), 1274–1282.

Newby, D., Orgeta, V., Marshall, C. R., Lourida, I., Albertyn, C. P., Tamburin, S., & Ranson, J. M. (2023). Artificial intelligence for dementia prevention. *Alzheimer's & Dementia*, *19*(12), 5952–5969.

Nguyen, T., Maarek, R., Hermann, A. L., Kammoun, A., Marchi, A., Khelifi-Touhami, M. R., & Le Pointe, H. D. (2022). Assessment of an artificial intelligence aid for the detection of appendicular skeletal fractures in children and young adults by senior and junior radiologists. *Pediatric Radiology*, *52*(11), 2215–2226.

O'Connor, S., Gasteiger, N., Stanmore, E., Wong, D. C., & Lee, J. J. (2022). Artificial intelligence for falls management in older adult care: A scoping review of nurses' role. *Journal of Nursing Management*, *30*(8), 3787–3801.

Padhan, S., Mohapatra, A., Ramasamy, S. K., Agrawal, S., & Ramasamy, S. (2023). Artificial intelligence (AI) and robotics in elderly healthcare: Enabling independence and quality of life. *Cureus*, *15*(8).

Pani, B., Crawford, J., & Allen, K. A. (2024). Can generative artificial intelligence foster belongingness, social support, and reduce loneliness? A conceptual analysis. *Applications of generative. AI*, •••, 261–276.

Papathanail, I., Brühlmann, J., Vasiloglou, M. F., Stathopoulou, T., Exadaktylos, A. K., Stanga, Z., & Mougiakakou, S. (2021). Evaluation of a novel artificial intelligence system to monitor and assess energy and macronutrient intake in hospitalised older patients. *Nutrients*, *13*(12), 4539.

Paulauskaite-Taraseviciene, A., Siaulys, J., Sutiene, K., Petravicius, T., Navickas, S., Oliandra, M., & Balciunas, J. (2023, April). Geriatric care management system powered by the IoT and computer vision techniques. []. MDPI.]. *Health Care, 11*(8), 1152.

Peine, A., Faulkner, A., Jæger, B., & Moors, E. (2015). Science, technology and the 'grand challenge'of ageing—Understanding the socio-material constitution of later life. *Technological Forecasting and Social Change, 93*, 1–9.

Pelly, M., Fatehi, F., Liew, D., & Verdejo-Garcia, A. (2023). Artificial intelligence for secondary prevention of myocardial infarction: A qualitative study of patient and health professional perspectives. *International Journal of Medical Informatics, 173*, 105041.

Porkodi, S., & Kesavaraja, D. (2021). Healthcare robots enabled with IoT and artificial intelligence for elderly patients. *AI and IoT-Based Intelligent Automation in Robotics*, 87-108.

Qian, K., Zhang, Z., Yamamoto, Y., & Schuller, B. W. (2021). Artificial intelligence internet of things for the elderly: From assisted living to health-care monitoring. *IEEE Signal Processing Magazine, 38*(4), 78–88.

Rao, S. J., Isath, A., Krishnan, P., Tangsrivimol, J. A., Virk, H. U. H., Wang, Z., & Krittanawong, C. (2024). ChatGPT: A conceptual review of applications and utility in the field of medicine. *Journal of Medical Systems, 48*(1), 59.

Ray, A., Bhardwaj, A., Malik, Y. K., Singh, S., & Gupta, R. (2022). Artificial intelligence and Psychiatry: An overview. *Asian Journal of Psychiatry, 70*, 103021.

Raza, H., Abbas, N., Amir, S., Arshad, K., Siddiqui, M. R. U., & Khan, S. I. (2022). An IoMT enabled smart healthcare model to monitor elderly people using Explainable Artificial Intelligence (EAI). *Journal of NCBAE, 1*(2), 16–22.

Renn, B. N., Schurr, M., Zaslavsky, O., & Pratap, A. (2021). Artificial intelligence: An interprofessional perspective on implications for geriatric mental health research and care. *Frontiers in Psychiatry, 12*, 734909.

Rizvi, A., Rizvi, F., Lalakia, P., Hyman, L., Frasso, R., Sztandera, L., & Das, A. V. (2023). Is artificial intelligence the cost-saving lens to diabetic retinopathy screening in low-and middle-income countries? *Cureus, 15*(9).

Rozynek, M., Kucybała, I., Urbanik, A., & Wojciechowski, W. (2021). Use of artificial intelligence in the imaging of sarcopenia: A narrative review of current status and perspectives. *Nutrition (Burbank, Los Angeles County, Calif.), 89*, 111227.

Sætra, H. S. (2022). First, they came for the old and demented: Care and relations in the age of artificial intelligence and social robots. *Human Arenas*, *5*(1), 25–43.

Salah, O. Z., Selvaperumal, S. K., & Abdulla, R. (2022). Accelerometer-based elderly fall detection system using edge artificial intelligence architecture. *International Journal of Electrical and Computer Engineering*, *12*(4), 4430–4438.

Sankaran, A., & Singla, M. P. (2024). Artificial intelligence in geriatric healthcare: Opportunities and challenges in a transforming landscape. *Frontiers in Health Informatics*, *13*(7), 897–908.

Seibert, K., Domhoff, D., Bruch, D., Schulte-Althoff, M., Fürstenau, D., Biessmann, F., & Wolf-Ostermann, K. (2021). Application scenarios for artificial intelligence in nursing care: Rapid review. *Journal of Medical Internet Research*, *23*(11), e26522.

Sepúlveda, M., Arauna, D., García, F., Albala, C., Palomo, I., & Fuentes, E. (2022). Frailty in aging and the search for the optimal biomarker: A review. *Biomedicines*, *10*(6), 1426.

Shaik, T., Tao, X., Higgins, N., Li, L., Gururajan, R., Zhou, X., & Acharya, U. R. (2023). Remote patient monitoring using artificial intelligence: Current state, applications, and challenges. *Wiley Interdisciplinary Reviews. Data Mining and Knowledge Discovery*, *13*(2), e1485.

Sharif, L. S., Almabadi, R., Alahmari, A., Alqurashi, F., Alsahafi, F., Qusti, S., & Wright, R. (2025). Perceptions of mental health professionals towards artificial intelligence in mental healthcare: A cross-sectional study. *Frontiers in Psychiatry*, *16*, 1601456.

Shi, Y., Ma, C., Wang, C., Wu, T., & Jiang, X. (2024, May). Harmonizing Emotions: An AI-Driven Sound Therapy System Design for Enhancing Mental Health of Older Adults. In *International Conference on Human-Computer Interaction* (pp. 439-455). Cham: Springer Nature Switzerland.

Shiwani, T., Relton, S., Evans, R., Kale, A., Heaven, A., Clegg, A., & Todd, O. (2023). New Horizons in artificial intelligence in the healthcare of older people. *Age and Ageing*, *52*(12), afad219.

Skrabanek, P., Gulati, S., & Jung, R. (2025). Intersection of AI Tools and Application for Elderly Healthcare. *Artificial Intelligence in Healthcare for the Elderly*, 191.

Song, S. (2024). Emotion detection of elderly people in nursing homes based on AI robot vision. *Soft Computing*, *28*(23), 13989–14002.

Stypinska, J. (2021, December). Ageism in AI: new forms of age discrimination in the era of algorithms and artificial intelligence. In *CAIP 2021: Proceedings of the 1st International Conference on AI for People: Towards Sustainable AI* (p. 39).

Stypińska, J., & Franke, A. (2023). AI revolution in healthcare and medicine and the (re-) emergence of inequalities and disadvantages for ageing population. *Frontiers in Sociology*, *7*, 1038854.

Su, J., & Yang, W. (2024). Artificial Intelligence (AI) literacy in early childhood education: An intervention study in Hong Kong. *Interactive Learning Environments*, *32*(9), 5494–5508.

Su, Z., Bentley, B. L., McDonnell, D., Ahmad, J., He, J., Shi, F., & Da Veiga, C. P. (2022). 6G and artificial intelligence technologies for dementia care: Literature review and practical analysis. *Journal of Medical Internet Research*, *24*(4), e30503.

Thakare, V., Khire, G., & Kumbhar, M. (2022). Artificial intelligence (AI) and Internet of Things (IoT) in healthcare: Opportunities and challenges. *ECS Transactions*, *107*(1), 7941.

Tiwari, A., Ghosh, A., Agrawal, P. K., Reddy, A., Singla, D., Mehta, D. N., & Paiwal, K. (2023). Artificial intelligence in oral health surveillance among under-served communities. *Bioinformation*, *19*(13), 1329.

Torrado, J. C., Husebo, B. S., Allore, H. G., Erdal, A., Fæø, S. E., Reithe, H., & Patrascu, M. (2022). Digital phenotyping by wearable-driven artificial intelligence in older adults and people with Parkinson's disease: Protocol of the mixed method, cyclic ActiveAgeing study. *PLoS One*, *17*(10), e0275747.

Tsoi, K. K., Jia, P., Dowling, N. M., Titiner, J. R., Wagner, M., Capuano, A. W., & Donohue, M. C. (2023). Applications of artificial intelligence in dementia research. *Cambridge Prisms. Precision Medicine*, *1*, e9.

Uchikov, P., Khalid, U., Dedaj-Salad, G. H., Ghale, D., Rajadurai, H., Kraeva, M., & Stanchev, P. (2024). Artificial intelligence in breast cancer diagnosis and treatment: Advances in imaging, pathology, and personalized care. *Life (Chicago, Ill.)*, *14*(11), 1451.

Umeda-Kameyama, Y., Kameyama, M., Tanaka, T., Son, B. K., Kojima, T., Fukasawa, M., & Akishita, M. (2021). Screening of Alzheimer's disease by facial complexion using artificial intelligence. *Aging (Albany NY)*, *13*(2), 1765.

Uzir, M. U. H., Bukari, Z., Al Halbusi, H., Lim, R., Wahab, S. N., Rasul, T., & Eneizan, B. (2023). Applied artificial intelligence: Acceptance-intention-purchase and satisfaction on smartwatch usage in a Ghanaian context. *Heliyon*, *9*(8).

Viderman, D., Dossov, M., Seitenov, S., & Lee, M. H. (2022). Artificial intelligence in ultrasound-guided regional anesthesia: A scoping review. *Frontiers in medicine*, *9*, 994805.

Vourganas, I., Attar, H., & Michala, A. L. (2022). Accountable, responsible, transparent artificial intelligence in ambient intelligence systems for healthcare. In *Intelligent healthcare: infrastructure, algorithms and management* (pp. 87–111). Springer Nature Singapore.

Vousinas, G. L., Simitsi, I., Livieri, G., Gkouva, G. C., & Efthymiou, I. P. (2022). Mapping the road of the ethical dilemmas behind artificial intelligence. *Journal of Politics and Ethics in New Technologies and AI*, *1*(1), e31238. DOI: 10.12681/jpentai.31238

Wang, J., Liang, Y., Cao, S., Cai, P., & Fan, Y. (2023). Application of artificial intelligence in geriatric care: Bibliometric analysis. *Journal of Medical Internet Research*, *25*, e46014.

Wang, X., Li, J., Liang, T., Hasan, W. U., Zaman, K. T., Du, Y., & Tao, C. (2024). Promoting personalized reminiscence among cognitively intact older adults through an AI-driven interactive multimodal photo album: Development and usability study. *JMIR Aging*, *7*(1), e49415.

Wang, Y., Liu, C., Hu, W., Luo, L., Shi, D., Zhang, J., & He, M. (2024). Economic evaluation for medical artificial intelligence: Accuracy vs. cost-effectiveness in a diabetic retinopathy screening case. *NPJ Digital Medicine*, *7*(1), 43.

Wang, Y., Xie, C., Liang, C., Zhou, P., & Lu, L. (2022). Association of artificial intelligence use and the retention of elderly caregivers: A cross-sectional study based on empowerment theory. *Journal of Nursing Management*, *30*(8), 3827–3837.

Wolniak, R., & Stecuła, K. (2024). Artificial intelligence in smart cities—applications, barriers, and future directions: a review. *Smart cities, 7*(3), 1346-1389.

Woodman, R. J., & Mangoni, A. A. (2023). A comprehensive review of machine learning algorithms and their application in geriatric medicine: Present and future. *Aging Clinical and Experimental Research*, *35*(11), 2363–2397.

World Health Organization. (2022). *Ageism in artificial intelligence for health: WHO policy brief.* World Health Organization.

Wu, X., Freeman, S., Miyagi, M., Park, U., Nomura, K., & Ebihara, S. (2024). Comprehensive Geriatric Assessment in the era of telemedicine. *Geriatrics & Gerontology International*, *24*, 67–73.

Xiao, X., Xue, L., Ye, L., Li, H., & He, Y. (2021). Health care cost and benefits of artificial intelligence-assisted population-based glaucoma screening for the elderly in remote areas of China: A cost-offset analysis. *BMC Public Health, 21*(1), 1065.

Xing, F., Peng, G., Zhang, B., Li, S., & Liang, X. (2021). Socio-technical barriers affecting large-scale deployment of AI-enabled wearable medical devices among the ageing population in China. *Technological Forecasting and Social Change, 166*, 120609.

Yang, J., Luo, B., Zhao, C., & Zhang, H. (2022). Artificial intelligence healthcare service resources adoption by medical institutions based on TOE framework. *Digital Health, 8*, 20552076221126034.

Yang, Y. (2025). Artificial Intelligence and elder. *People*.

Zaidan, A. M. (2023). The leading global health challenges in the artificial intelligence era. *Frontiers in Public Health, 11*, 1328918.

Zhang, M., Zhu, L., Lin, S. Y., Herr, K., Chi, C. L., Demir, I., & Chi, N. C. (2023). Using artificial intelligence to improve pain assessment and pain management: A scoping review. *Journal of the American Medical Informatics Association : JAMIA, 30*(3), 570–587.

Zhang, Z., Xu, P., Wu, C., & Yu, H. (2024). Smart nursing wheelchairs: A new trend in assisted care and the future of multifunctional integration. *Biomimetics, 9*(8), 492.

Zhu, J., Shi, K., Yang, C., Niu, Y., Zeng, Y., Zhang, N., & Chu, C. H. (2022). Ethical issues of smart home-based elderly care: A scoping review. *Journal of Nursing Management, 30*(8), 3686–3699.

Chapter 11
AI in Ageing Healthcare:
Improving Decision-Making and Outcomes for Older Adults

Iris-Panagiota Efthymiou
https://orcid.org/0000-0001-9656-8378
University of Greenwich, UK

Symeon Sidiropoulos
https://orcid.org/0000-0002-1548-2749
University of Thessaly, Greece

ABSTRACT

This chapter examines how artificial intelligence (AI) is reshaping ageing healthcare by supporting clinical decision-making and improving outcomes for older adults. It addresses the application of AI in diagnostics, risk stratification, personalised care planning, and resource allocation across geriatric services. The chapter analyses key benefits such as early detection of cognitive decline, fall prediction, medication optimisation, and remote patient monitoring. It also considers ethical and operational challenges, including data bias, patient consent, and the risk of over-reliance on automated systems. Through clinical case examples and policy analysis, the chapter outlines how AI can support ageing populations without replacing the human judgment essential to compassionate geriatric care.

1. INTRODUCTION

Population ageing presents a significant societal challenge, with profound implications for the health and social care sector, including workforce shortages. Artificial intelligence (AI) promises enhanced productivity and efficiency, with po-

DOI: 10.4018/979-8-3373-5462-0.ch011

tential benefits when applied to age-related decision-making challenges. Alongside the pressure to deliver quality care to a larger ageing population, AI could augment healthcare services with scalable support solutions that improve decision-making outcomes. Older adults (65 years or over) experience greater healthcare needs, including multiple long-term conditions, mental health problems, complex drugs regimes, and a higher risk of accidental injury. Early AI developments concentrated primarily on diagnostic techniques and supporting healthcare professionals.

2. THE IMPORTANCE OF AI IN HEALTHCARE

AI, defined as the ability of machines to exhibit humanlike performance such as decision-making, speech recognition and visual perception, is rapidly emerging as a novel mechanism of technology-supported care within the healthcare paradigm. AI adopts algorithm-based computational techniques to analyse large datasets, and make inferences and predictions based on patterns in the data. Common AI approaches include machine learning methods, such as deep learning (DL), and natural language processing (NLP). The promise of this technology lies in the prospect that the resultant efficiencies in care delivery will lead to improved access to care and improved clinical decision-making in terms of diagnosis, treatment and care planning, and ultimately, cost savings.

3. UNDERSTANDING AGEING AND HEALTHCARE NEEDS

Ageing is a lifelong process involving physiological, psychological, and social changes that affect health and well-being (Efthymiou, I.-P., 2024). Growing older is associated with an accumulation of molecular and cellular damage over time. Over time, this damage leads to a decreased ability to respond to stress and an increased risk of age-associated diseases, such as cancer, diabetes, and cardiovascular and neurodegenerative diseases. Ageing is also the primary risk factor for major human pathologies such as Alzheimer's disease and cardiovascular diseases.

Healthcare needs change with age for many reasons; most older people experience multi-morbidities, and the ageing process itself causes a change in healthcare needs. Ageing influences absorption, metabolism, pharmacokinetics, and excretion of medication, contributing to alterations in dosage of medications and different side effects. Such needs therefore vary according to the health status of older adults and the physiological and psychological changes they endure during ageing. In addition to biological changes, older adults experience socioeconomic changes and reduced quality of life (Sidiropoulos, S., 2022).

4. CURRENT CHALLENGES IN AGEING HEALTHCARE

The current ageing healthcare ecosystem faces a multitude of challenges. At the modern care interfaces with older individuals and the medical support infrastructure, extremely heterogeneous physical, psychological, and social characteristics as well as demanding needs need to be addressed by the limited care and timely medical access through the cross-disciplinary exchange of knowledge and expertise. Throughout the ageing care paradigms, the daily human activities, environment, and exposure influence health and well-being, as do the external factors related to social engagement (Efthymiou, I.-P., 2024). The COVID-19 pandemic has demonstrated that the not always visible importance of a healthy lifestyle and related challenges calls for the design of intelligent tools to continuously track people's health status in a non-invasive and privacy-respecting manner. In the different interaction modalities through which ageing individuals may be supported in daily life, significant contingencies may be found. Reliable and interpretable metrics to evaluate individuals' well-being and daily delivery status, also taking into account the technological challenges deriving from voice-based, emotional, visual, or behavioural analysis, are still lacking.

5. AI TECHNOLOGIES IN HEALTHCARE

Artificial intelligence (AI) has considerable potential to improve the healthcare of older people in the important areas of monitoring and diagnostics, supporting stratified care, and complementing health systems support (Batakis, D., et al., 2025). Wearable technology can provide continuous real-time patient monitoring, helping to reduce hospital admissions, allowing for the early detection of deterioration, increasing patients' confidence, and reducing social isolation. AI-enabled clinical decision support systems (CDSS), image and video analysis, and natural language processing can assist in the early recognition of frailty syndromes and long-latency conditions such as dementia, Parkinson's disease, delirium, and depression, plus the early detection of comorbidity. Models show high accuracy in predicting chronic diseases in older adults (Vozikis, A., et al., 2021).

5.1. Machine Learning

Machine learning (ML) is a subset of artificial intelligence that enables computers to learn from experience and improve without explicit programming (Das & Dhillon, 2023). Algorithms focus on enabling machines to learn and make predictions based on past data, locating patterns unavailable to humans. This capacity has attracted keen interest in developing ML tools for ageing and geriatric healthcare, as clinical decision-making extends beyond single-point information to integrate large, high-dimensional health and social data.

Although ML integration poses challenges, including potential data bias, a lack of transparency, and requirements for vast, high-quality datasets, combining conventional and ML methods can serve as an initial, effective approach (Diareme, K. et al., 2022). Various ML techniques are appropriate to different ageing-health tasks: support vector machines (SVM) and logistic regression (LR) rank as the most commonly adopted methods. ML has been applied to diverse aspects of ageing including ageing-related diseases, mental health, successful ageing, and brain/biological-age prediction. The highest adoption occurs in the US, followed by China and Italy, often utilising digital-trace data to enhance geriatric research.

5.2. Natural Language Processing

Healthcare represents a field of intense and growing interest for artificial intelligence (AI), which has already seen the development of mature smart assistants and advanced chatbots that provide invaluable support to both healthcare professionals and patients alike. Natural language processing (NLP) plays a significant and transformative role in this ecosystem by aiming to identify structured output from unstructured free text data. This advanced technology acts as a core component of both early-warning systems and decision-support systems, allowing healthcare providers to effectively extract key information from evolving and dynamic patient notes in real-time. Tools like OpenNLP and UMLS MetaMap Lite offer an array of prebuilt components such as part-of-speech tagging and concept mapping, which greatly facilitate the creation of custom workflows specifically tailored to meet various healthcare needs and challenges. These innovations serve to enhance the overall efficiency and accuracy of healthcare delivery, demonstrating the profound impact of AI in this vital area of society.

5.3. Robotics

Technological advances in artificial intelligence (AI) and robotics are stimulating new approaches to supporting and extending the autonomy of older adults in the home, and many prototypes are substantially more capable than previous designs. Shortcomings in sensing, reasoning, manipulation, and navigation remain significant, however, especially for multipurpose mobile manipulators, which are also likely to be expensive and require frequent maintenance. Older adults' preferences around robot assistance show high inter-individual variability, and many want opportunities for customization and control. Further work is needed to understand whether most prefer not to program robots at all, or whether they prefer to be involved in specifying some robot behaviours.

Efforts to involve older adults, with the assistance of specialists, as robot programmers are likely to be particularly fruitful; better understanding how they conceive of the task planning and programming processes, and how current programming systems can be adapted to support these conceptions, should help to narrow the gap between what researchers see as possible, and what many older adults currently regard as overly complex and implausible. Such developments can contribute not only to more effective, autonomous robotic support, but also greater user agency and self-efficacy, potentially turning some older adults into autonomous AI users in their own right (Ajaykumar & Huang, 2023).

6. APPLICATIONS OF AI IN AGEING HEALTHCARE

The integration of AI with wearable technology offers continuous real-time monitoring of frailty among older adults, enabling early detection of acute deteriorations and potentially reducing critical illness and hospital admissions. AI-driven clinical decision support systems (CDSS), combined with image and video analysis and natural language processing, facilitate early recognition of frailty, long-term conditions (LTCs), and associated conditions such as dementia, Parkinson's disease, delirium, and depression. While numerous studies have demonstrated the high accuracy of AI algorithms in the diagnosis and prediction of specific diseases, the overall effectiveness of AI tools in preventing falls and other acute events remains an area of ongoing research and uncertainty.

6.1. Predictive Analytics for Patient Outcomes

Patient outcome prediction plays an increasingly important role in clinical practice, enabling clinicians to forecast the future health status of individuals and design preventive or treatment strategies accordingly. Artificial intelligence (AI) predictive analytics utilizes advanced algorithms and machine learning to analyze vast amounts of patient data and predict outcomes with greater precision than traditional methods (Dixon et al., 2024). The capacity to continuously learn from new data allows AI systems to improve over time. While numerous studies have examined the application of AI predictive analytics in healthcare, a significant gap remains concerning its direct impact on patient outcomes across various conditions and settings. Predictive tools in healthcare employ sophisticated statistical techniques to forecast future events based on historical and current data, thereby enhancing decision-making processes. Applications range from predicting infectious disease outbreaks and tailoring treatment plans to optimizing hospital resources, ultimately facilitating early diagnosis and preventive care.

6.2. Telehealth and Remote Monitoring

Telehealth is a rapidly evolving approach to the delivery of health care services and clinical information through telephone, remote patient monitoring devices, e-mail, mobile apps, and live video with the goal of improving access to care and decreasing costs (Efthymiou, I.-P., 2024). The COVID-19 pandemic was a major catalyst for the increase in use of telehealth in the USA because the use of telehealth consults was added to the list of insurance-reimbursable clinical visits (Shaver, 2022; Andino et al., 2023). The use of commercial telehealth companies boomed, and many health care systems adopted telehealth platforms to conduct virtual visits. In 2021, telehealth visits in the USA still accounted for only 8.3% of all visits, down from a peak of over 13% in the third quarter of 2020, but much higher than the 0.1% in the first quarter of 2020. Telemedicine, or receiving one's medical care remotely via synchronous, asynchronous, or store-and-forward technology, had been on a steady increase for the last decade, but the overall growth had remained slow until March 6, 2020 (Shaver, J., 2022). Some health systems are planning on using telehealth extensively even after the pandemic.

Although, in theory, many types of visits can be transformed to virtual ones, this may not be appropriate in every situation. Telehealth may be ideal for situations requiring follow-up because there is already an established relationship between the patient and a provider. Telehealth can retain patient engagement when transportation is an issue or when a patient is uncomfortable coming into a care facility, either because of emotional issues or infectious concerns. Telehealth support is multifaceted and can range from augmented reality, interactive web-based programs, and connection to a care coach to portal-based contact. Telemonitoring of chronic diseases using peripheral devices with data transfer via a wireless link has been shown to reduce congestive heart failure readmission rates and improve chronic care management in general.

6.3. Personalized Treatment Plans

Individualized treatment plans could be enabled by an advanced decision-support system (DSS) that analyses the profiles of older people, including social, health, and behavioural data, to recommend the most appropriate intervention (Brunzini et al., 2023). A multidimensional assessment performed by a multidisciplinary team gathers clinical and social data, which are then pre-processed to become suitable inputs for a decision-support algorithm based on a decision-tree approach. This model outlines various outcomes stemming from a sequence of decisions, determines a match between a case profile and available interventions, and has been implemented in software to facilitate clinical use. Validation on a participant sample demonstrates the algorithm's reliability and consistency.

The physical deterioration associated with ageing leads to increased biological age, raising the likelihood of adverse events such as falls, cardiovascular problems, hypertension, obesity, respiratory disease, diabetes, joint disease, sensory impairment, mental health issues, and polypharmacy. Certain behavioural factors can be modified to mitigate these outcomes; adequate physical activity, healthy nutrition, good sleep quality, smoking cessation, limited alcohol consumption, and environmental hazard awareness contribute to improved health, quality of life, and reduced morbidity and mortality. Although the most direct influences on falls and cardiovascular conditions relate to physical and clinical domains, psychological and social factors also play significant roles. An AI-driven DSS therefore prioritizes non-pharmacological interventions that address the health, activity, and social needs of older adults by analysing comprehensive profile data.

Personalized medicine (also termed stratified care) is a related concept that tailors interventions to an individual's holistic needs, encompassing disease burden, functional capacity, and preferences. (Alzeer, 2023; Yuan, 2022; Panahi, 2025). It uses genotypic, phenotypic, or clinical characteristics to classify individuals and target interventions according to predicted responses. AI offers potential for stratified care through the analysis of molecular, clinical, and lifestyle data. For example, the PROTEIN project employs AI to design personalized diet plans for chronic disease prevention and treatment based on genotype, clinical indicators, epigenetics, and lifestyle factors (Kyriazis, I., et al., 2018). Similarly, AI can enhance the management of hypertension, diabetes, and hyperlipidaemia by identifying more effective treatment options from electronic health records. The application of stratified care remains nascent, with few studies utilizing data-driven analytics. Older people often require assistance from multiple health and social services but frequently encounter reduced access and fragmented provision.

7. ETHICAL CONSIDERATIONS IN AI DEPLOYMENT

Monitoring AI tools in real-world settings is crucial for ensuring their effectiveness and reliability, particularly because performance often relies heavily on the quality of data used, and errors are inevitable in any system. Older adults, especially those experiencing cognitive decline, may be more susceptible to developing an over-reliance on these AI tools, making them less likely to detect any errors that may arise. Safeguarding vulnerable populations requires robust governance frameworks, regular impact assessments, careful evaluations, and diligent regulatory oversight.

AI technology has the potential to significantly improve healthcare for older individuals by enabling aging in place, facilitating stratified care tailored to individual needs, and ensuring timely access to necessary services (Abadir et al., 2023). However, it is concerning that many existing applications of AI lack proper validation within clinical practice, which could pose risks to patient safety and care quality (Ferrara et al., 2024; Ratwani et al., 2024; Onitiu et al., 2024). Future development of these technologies should involve collaboration among AI experts, healthcare providers, policymakers, and older individuals, to ensure that AI systems add meaningful value to healthcare without undermining autonomy, privacy, or emotional well-being.

Furthermore, it is absolutely crucial that resources allocate considerable emphasis on the comprehensive development of effective AI tools that can significantly enhance productivity and innovation (Efthymiou, I., 2026). These essential tools must be thoroughly supported by comprehensive, well-crafted guidelines that address key aspects such as data privacy, transparency, and ongoing post-deployment monitoring and assessment. This thorough approach ensures that not only is the AI safe for regular use, but also that it remains effective in its application over time and adapts to evolving needs. It is absolutely essential to maintain proper and constant oversight in order to uphold the highest safety standards and ensure the ongoing efficacy and reliability of these transformative technologies.

Additionally, geriatricians and interdisciplinary care teams need appropriate training to effectively appraise AI frameworks, ensure informed consent is properly obtained, and advocate for the inclusion of older populations in relevant datasets (Badawy & Shaban, 2025; Imran & Khan, 2025) Investing in AI literacy and ensuring equitable access for older people is essential to maximizing the benefits derived from AI-driven care and support, ultimately enhancing the quality of life for this demographic.

7.1. Privacy and Data Security

Many older individuals express significant, profound, and deep-seated concerns about the privacy and security of their personal data in today's increasingly digital world, a reality that is becoming ever more pressing as technology advances at an unprecedented pace (Morrison et al., 2021; Payton & Claypoole, 2023). These concerns are often cited as substantial barriers that hinder the usage, acceptance, and overall adoption of modern technology among seniors, who might understandably feel overwhelmed by the rapid changes and complexities associated with new digital tools that seem to emerge almost daily.

As a direct consequence of these apprehensions, AI systems specifically designed for aged care must implement and host robust, comprehensive, and effective procedures that prioritize the individuals they serve and their unique needs. These procedures are not just beneficial, but are utterly vital in ensuring the protection of patient privacy when collecting, processing, and securely storing sensitive information related to health, finances, and personal preferences. It is essential that these advanced systems prioritize safeguarding personal data rigorously, employing the latest, most effective security technologies and protocols to foster trust and confidence amongst older adults (Vrančić et al., 2024; Williamson & Prybutok, 2024; Aldboush & Ferdous, 2023).

Such efforts can, in turn, encourage widespread technology adoption among this demographic, who are often hesitant to engage with new systems they perceive as potentially invasive or untrustworthy. Building and maintaining trust in technology is absolutely crucial for enhancing the overall quality of life for older adults, as it empowers them to utilize a variety of digital services that can vastly improve their well-being and independence, ultimately leading to a richer and more fulfilling life experience. Without a doubt, ensuring these individuals feel secure about their data is a necessary step in integrating technology into their lives effectively.

7.2. Bias and Fairness in AI Algorithms

Health systems must ensure with great diligence that the deployment of these advanced technologies does not exacerbate existing health disparities, further disadvantage already under-served populations, or introduce novel biases that may adversely affect the overall fairness of outcomes. Bias, a significant concern in this domain, is closely related to the concept of fairness in AI; however, unlike bias, fairness lacks a widely accepted and universally agreed-upon definition (Stine & Kavak, 2023; Lewicki et al.2023; Varona & Suárez, 2022). Nevertheless, it is indeed possible to articulate some properties that can define fairness while simultaneously working to reduce the presence of bias. It becomes crucial for health systems to actively engage in these considerations to foster an equitable healthcare environment for all individuals, particularly those who have historically faced disadvantages.

Biases can indeed be programmed into AI algorithms, and this programming can inadvertently reflect societal ageism and the significant underrepresentation of certain groups within the training data that is utilized for these algorithms (Stypinska, 2023; Chu et al., 2023; Stypinska, 2021). Such biases may originate during the data collection phase, which can potentially arise from inaccurate records, incomplete data, or incorrect labeling of the data, all of which can contribute to skewed representations in the resulting models.

Additionally, these biases can also emerge at the model development stage when biased variables are introduced into the equations. For instance, using age as a proxy for treatment preference or response can inadvertently skew the outcomes and reinforce stereotypes associated with different age groups. As these AI systems are deployed in real-world settings, they may further perpetuate ageism, particularly impacting older populations who may reside in low-resource environments. This unfortunate situation poses a significant risk of exacerbating existing health disparities among these vulnerable groups. Furthermore, systemic bias is a considerable issue that encapsulates various institutional practices and frameworks which tend to advantage certain social groups while simultaneously disadvantaging others (Banaji et al.2021; Pease, 2021).

This systematic disadvantage ultimately creates formidable barriers to accessing healthcare resources that ought to be available to all individuals, regardless of their age or background. The intertwining of these biases, coupled with societal norms and institutional frameworks, underlines the urgent need for addressing these issues in the development and deployment of AI technologies (van Kolfschooten, 2023).

8. CASE STUDIES OF AI IMPLEMENTATION

The adoption of AI within aging- and dementia-related healthcare services has increased dramatically since the early 2000s, with the complexity and pace of new algorithms, and the scale of activity, continuing to escalate. Healthcare venues, from pharmaceutical companies and biotech start-ups to the NHS, have partnered with AI specialists to accelerate breakthroughs in brain sciences and clinical practice—all aiming to improve outcomes for people living with cognitive decline and associated neurodegenerative conditions such as Alzheimer's disease and frontotemporal dementia. Consequently, aging and dementia-related healthcare are among the fastest-growing application areas for AI in healthcare worldwide.

Still, very few AI approaches have been appropriately validated or had their clinical impacts evaluated. The degree to which such tools conform to national and local aging- and dementia-related health-related frameworks remains unclear. Collaborative, interdisciplinary efforts among AI researchers, healthcare providers, policymakers, and older populations promise considerable value for future AI applications (Efthymiou, I., 2024). The reassurance to scientists and clinicians is clear: AI offers demonstrable potential for transformative, large-scale impact. Therefore, it is urgent that resources be directed toward the most promising applications, coupled with the establishment of frameworks ensuring data privacy, transparency, and systematic monitoring of AI models and data sets.

Meanwhile, geriatricians, clinical staff, and care-team members require training to understand and apply AI appraisal frameworks, obtain informed participant consent, and advocate for older individuals as developers prepare datasets and evaluations. Increasing the number of older people proficient with AI or familiar with technology in general remains imperative for the successful design, adoption, and implementation of AI-based digital-health tools.

8.1. Successful AI Initiatives

Many of the potential applications of AI in healthcare for older individuals have already been successfully implemented across various sectors. Three areas that exhibit significant promise and potential for improvement are monitoring and diagnostics, stratified care, and health-systems support. Improved and more effective monitoring of long-term conditions as well as the challenges posed by multimorbidity would enable timely early interventions, ultimately reducing the burden experienced by individuals as well as healthcare services as a whole.

Wearable technology provides continuous and real-time monitoring capabilities, while virtual monitoring combined with the early detection of deterioration can lead to a marked decrease in hospital admissions and emergency situations. AI-enabled clinical-decision-support systems, comprehensive image and video analysis, and advanced natural-language processing techniques all facilitate the early recognition of frailty syndromes and various long-term conditions (LTCs) experienced by elderly patients. Various AI methods have been developed for predicting conditions such as dementia, delirium, and depression, and several algorithms have shown remarkable accuracy, indicating strong potential for the enhancement of patient care and support for healthcare professionals in their decision-making processes.

1. AI-Powered Early Detection of Dementia – Cambridge Cognition / IBM Watson Health AI systems, specifically trained on intricate linguistic patterns alongside comprehensive cognitive assessments, have the remarkable capability to detect early signs of Alzheimer's disease and other forms of dementia, potentially years ahead of conventional clinical diagnosis (Vrahatis et al., 2023; Aditya Shastry & Sanjay, 2024). These advanced models thoroughly analyse various data sources including speech patterns, performance on memory tasks, and detailed behavioural data to facilitate and support earlier intervention strategies. Currently, these systems are actively employed in both extensive research trials and targeted pilot programmes across the UK and US, contributing significantly

to improving screening accuracy and effectively reducing diagnostic delays that can severely impact patient care.

2.Remote Monitoring and Fall Prediction – CarePredict CarePredict employs cutting-edge wearable sensors alongside sophisticated artificial intelligence to diligently monitor the movements, activity patterns, and notable behavioural alterations of elderly individuals (Paul, 2025; Gupta et al., 2025). This comprehensive system anticipates possible falls and declines in health by meticulously examining deviations from established personal routines. Presently, it has been implemented in various senior living establishments throughout North America, leading to a decrease in hospital admissions as well as expedited response times in emergency situations. Through the application of this technology, caregivers are equipped to offer improved assistance and ensure the safety of senior residents.

3. Medication Management and Adherence – Medisafe + AI Analytics Medisafe effectively integrates advanced AI technology to personalise medication reminders, while also identifying the non-adherence risk factors specifically affecting older patients suffering from various chronic conditions (Scott et al.2024; Bharat et al., 2025). The platform meticulously tailors its communication strategies according to individual user behaviour patterns and beneficial feedback loops. This approach has been proven to significantly increase adherence rates in ageing populations, while simultaneously reducing the likelihood of avoidable complications that can arise from medication mismanagement.

8.2. Lessons Learned from Failures

Failure in AI healthcare systems can result in patient harm or death, even when these systems operate as intended. AI development challenges include algorithmic bias, poor generalisability, insufficient supervision, and inadequate cybersecurity. Systems capable of altering patient care without clinician interpretation increase safety risks. The USA's National Academies recommend that failures prompt incident reporting and that designers proactively investigate hazards.

9. FUTURE DIRECTIONS IN AI AND AGEING HEALTHCARE

Artificial intelligence (AI) offers promising solutions for older people's health-care within a framework that recognises and addresses the concerns of older people, clinicians and AI researchers. Three priority areas for AI application are monitoring and early diagnosis of disease, stratified care and care coordination. Barriers to these priorities include the risk of AI-enhanced health inequity and criteria for effective interventions.

Existing AI applications for individual clinical conditions exemplify the kinds of solutions that might be developed. Existing data sources useful for these applications include mobile applications, longitudinal studies of ageing and routinely collected electronic healthcare data. Effective interventions require their development in the context of a person-centred approach that addresses requirements for generalisability, transparency and effectiveness. Appropriate use can be ensured by a combination of education and the availability of technological infrastructure.

9.1. Innovative Research Areas

Innovative Research Areas Artificial intelligence (AI) in healthcare describes algorithm-based computational techniques that manage and analyse large datasets to make inferences and predictions. AI has potential applications in the care of older people, including clinical decision support systems that can support identification of delirium from clinical records and wearable devices that can predict fall risk.

Three priority areas for AI application were identified: monitoring and early diagnosis of disease, stratified care, and care coordination between healthcare providers. Concerns include AI potentially exacerbating health inequity through model biases, lack of validation, privacy infringements, lack of transparency, and safety issues. Effective interventions require a person-centred approach, clinical and technological governance, and education for clinicians and patients. Investment in infrastructure is necessary to ensure equitable access.

9.2. Potential for Policy Changes

Addressing the consequences of AI-driven processes requires targeted policy change or regulation. Some governance within the AI sphere already exist, such as the General Data Protection Regulation in the UK and the EU. Recent work that has addressed this under the guidance of the UN recognises that the current stage of evolution of AI and robotics has significant implications for human rights, with recommendations for a human-rights centered approach to AI design, development and use. However, a global approach is advocated and much disagreement persists around the appropriate degree of governance (Sidiropoulos, S., 2024).

Diverse sector-specific regulations are in effect, or forthcoming, including: in motor vehicles; AI-driven medical devices; and AI in employment decisions. UK regulators have suggested four areas of focus: accountability and governance; data quality; design and implementation; and transparency. The aims of policy-making must be to increase trust and data acceptance yet still enable research. Within the United Kingdom itself, much variation exists in regulatory regimes, for example if research requires Health Research Authority oversight or individual Trust approvals. What becomes apparent is that as AI systems advance and assume tasks of increasingly significant consequence, potentially supplanting current leadership and expertise, detailed examination of those strategies positively impacting AI adoption, as well as prospective consequences on industry structure, is paramount.

10. STAKEHOLDER PERSPECTIVES

Stakeholders—community-dwelling older adults, healthcare professionals, as well as innovative AI developers—have to be diligently and proactively consulted throughout the entire extensive development process, they play a significant and pivotal role in facilitating the development of a strategic roadmap for AI innovations that are precisely tailored to meet the unique needs and preferences of older individuals in our communities. This ensures that future technological tools conceived are not only technologically advanced and cutting-edge but also greatly desirable, user-friendly, and fit for purpose, thereby significantly enhancing their effectiveness in real-world applications across various settings. This collaborative approach fosters a greater understanding and respects the perspectives of those involved, aligning technology with the actual lived experiences of older adults, ensuring that the innovations we create are truly supportive and improve their quality of life.

10.1. Healthcare Providers

Healthcare providers experience increasing workloads as the number of older adults continues to grow while workforce supplies stagnate. Artificial intelligence (AI) offers promising solutions to support health and care delivery, enhance clinical decision-making, and improve patient outcomes in ageing populations. AI algorithms can analyse complex health indicators to predict the onset and progression of diseases, including dementia, providing valuable insights for care planning and resource management. Data feeding into these models encompass patient-generated and clinical data derived within hospital and clinical care settings. Current AI applications focus on three priority areas relevant to ageing: monitoring and early diagnosis, personalised care, and care coordination. A diverse group of older people, clinicians and AI researchers identified specific forms and functions appropriate to these categories.

Monitoring and early diagnosis include AI-powered remote monitoring systems for mobility and activity, detection of mental health issues and delirium using speech and social media analysis, computer vision to cut emergency visits among older adults in aged care facilities, and the use of conversational agents to support cognitive training and diagnose cognitive decline. Personalised care systems include digital phenotyping for behaviour-change prevention, risk prediction for delirium and falls, and recommender systems for activity-management support.

Care coordination involves AI prediction of urgent care necessity and AI-driven discharge and readmission policies. To realise these applications, healthcare providers require access to sufficiently large datasets that capture the broad variation in clinical presentations among older adults. Wishes for explainable AI capabilities and effective human–AI interaction align with previous research, underscoring the importance of transparency and interpretability in clinical decision support systems. Trusted, robust and generalisable AI still requires systematic development to meet these needs.

10.2. Patients and Caregivers

Monitoring AI tools throughout their lifecycle is essential due to considerable variability in performance, a potential for Introduction inconsistencies, failures, and the risk of performance decay over time. When fully integrated into care pathways, systems that process healthcare data and interpret clinical information could influence clinical or administrative decisions (Wager et al., 2021; Gartner et al., 2022; Reddy, 2024). Consequently, these developments call for tighter governance, ongoing impact assessment, and the implementation of comprehensive regulatory frameworks.

Digital technology and artificial intelligence (AI) can enhance ageing healthcare by addressing the multilayered challenges that complicate eldercare. The older demographic remains the most digitally excluded sector, emphasising that many cannot access—and are unlikely to embrace—AI that requires digital technology. Safeguarding vulnerable cohorts depends on transparent, robust, and well-regulated deployment of a proven safety-critical wider system of innovation (Fleming, 2025; Anderljung et al., 2023).

Older adults might over-trust AI tools and be less likely to identify errors and omissions, particularly in the presence of cognitive or sensory decline. Undetected errors can threaten patient safety and compromise trust, underscoring the need for multifaceted safety features, human oversight, and safeguarding mechanisms. A robust governance framework, alongside regular impact assessments and regulatory oversight, is critical; work remains to develop and implement such frameworks effectively (De et al., 2021; Akpobome, 2024). AI offers vast opportunities to support older adults, augment clinical services, and generate novel insights into health and wellbeing. Potential benefits include enhancing the patient experience, facilitating ageing in place through ambient intelligence, extending the reach of relatively scarce healthcare staff, and improving accessibility.

However, many applications lack externally conducted validation and clinical evaluation. Moving forward, co-development with AI experts, healthcare providers, policymakers, and, crucially, older people themselves is necessary to ensure AI contributes meaningfully to ageing healthcare without compromising autonomy, privacy, and rights. Developing effective and impactful AI requires robust governance frameworks, including guidelines for data management, privacy, transparency, fairness, and equity, as well as safety and performance monitoring post-deployment.

Training geriatricians and multidisciplinary geriatric teams is essential to understand AI technologies, critically appraise their applications, obtain informed consent, and advocate for the inclusion of older adults in AI development. To maximize the value of AI, investment is needed in improving digital health literacy, reducing barriers to digital inclusion, and increasing access to digital technologies for older people. Although the development of AI tools for ageing healthcare has accelerated rapidly, build-out will likely be erratic and concentrated in areas where commercial returns are large and attainable. Expect accelerated use of finance-driven diagnostic and triage applications, targeted marketing and personalised interventions, as well as a swift move beyond the clinical domain to enhanced ambient monitoring and access to nutrition, leisure, and socialisation options.

10.3. Policymakers

The COVID-19 epidemic exposed both the potential and perils of artificial intelligence (AI) in healthcare decision-making The vulnerability of older adults underlines the imperative for policymakers to scrutinize how AI impacts their quality of life, guaranteeing that AI applications advance their wellbeing (Efthymiou, I. P., 2024). Effective governance necessitates adherence to principles of generalisability, transparency, fairness, and privacy. AI systems must be validated on independent datasets and across diverse subpopulations, accompanied by enough information to enable replication and comprehension. They should be free from discriminatory or prejudicial bias and conform to existing legislation governing the protection of confidentiality and autonomy.

11. INTEGRATION OF AI INTO EXISTING SYSTEMS

The success of proactive stepwise levels of care must depend on clear criteria for communicating results to non-specialists. Establishing thresholds for interventions at different levels should safeguard against AI-generated information overload. At later stages of care, technology should recognize when behavior patterns, such as mobility or location, alter and signal that current assistance levels are inadequate. Care providers can then navigate patients to more appropriate care pathways (Chan et al., 2023; Bekbolatova et al., 2024; Smith et al., 2022).

A range of commercial technology providers already supply some components of integrated systems supporting older individuals, yet no single platform offers stepwise, incremental care linked with specialized health professionals and multidisciplinary specialist teams. Links with the medical record will be essential and may be easier when portable technologies become standard clinical adjuncts, allowing automated data filling from existing clinical records.

Integrated systems capable of spanning the full range of age-related care needs now appear feasible within a single platform, with additional components incorporated into existing core technologies. At earlier stages, patient open-book models will support longer-term enduring health and wellbeing monitoring with real-time feedback on well-being and therapeutic prompts, facilitating cost-effective maintenance of optimum conditions and seamless, automated access to specialist services (Efthymiou, I. P., 2024). These services will also underpin delivery of 5P medicine—predictive, preventive, personalised, participatory and precision health—at later stages (Denysyuk et al., 2024; Martí-Noguera2025; Nguyen et al., 2025).

At the close of the decade, as clinical AI develops and becomes integrated with intensive monitoring, systematic stepwise care can connect primary, secondary and tertiary care, with routine inputs to research programmes and databases provided by non-intrusive, real-time, continuous, persistent monitoring of biomedical and lifestyle parameters (Efthymiou, I., 2024). Such systems are necessary to maximize benefit to older individuals, families and caregivers, and have the potential to lessen the enormous future social, emotional and economic burden associated with ageing.

11.1. Interoperability Challenges

Ensuring interoperability among electronic health systems continues to be a significant and enduring challenge in the field of healthcare (Reegu et al., 2023; Igwama et al., 2024; Pradyumna et al., 2024). These systems strive diligently to enhance continuity of care and increase overall efficiency in patient treatment processes, yet a universal ability to effortlessly and seamlessly share essential data remains elusive. Although various transmission and compression standards such as

XML and HL7 are currently in widespread use within the industry, further progress is critically needed to effectively bridge the existing linguistic and cultural divides that hinder effective communication (Torab-Miandoab et al., 2023).

Semi-automatic tools exist that can facilitate data extraction, alignment, and compilation from multiple databases; however, the persistent lack of a cohesive and integrated data model continues to demand extensive manual processing efforts from healthcare professionals. In this context, semantic integration stands out prominently as a highly promising approach for enabling comprehensive data linkage, thereby fostering more efficient information sharing, in-depth analysis, and advanced mining capabilities that can significantly improve decision-making and patient outcomes (Masmoudi et al., 2024; Chaccour et al., 2024).

11.2. Training and Adaptation for Healthcare Workers

Currently, the use of data-driven machine learning in healthcare remains limited due to methodological challenges, poor clinical uptake, and ethical concerns (Vousinas, G. et al., 2022). In this context, educational initiatives must support the development of AI-augmented technologies that augment rather than replace healthcare professionals who work with older adults. Geriatricians and multi-professional teams will require training in the fundamentals of AI to allow an informed direct appraisal of available frameworks, help obtain informed consent reflecting AI-mediated decisions and advocate for inclusion of older populations in datasets, algorithmic evaluation and deployment (Sankaran & Singla, 2024; Băjenaru et al., 2024; Skuban-Eiseler et al., 2023).

More generally, enhancing AI literacy across the entire specialty remains a crucial priority. While developing a solid understanding of AI will empower clinicians to effectively complement, critically challenge, and where necessary, contradict model recommendations, a broader appreciation of these technologies is likely to promote wider access to tailored digital solutions among older people (Asrifan et al., 2025; Charow et al., 2021). Many of these individuals feel increasingly excluded from the numerous benefits and advantages of the current digital age, which further emphasizes the need for education and training in this area. By fostering a deeper knowledge of AI, we can bridge this gap and ensure that all segments of the population can benefit from technological advancements.

12. MEASURING THE IMPACT OF AI ON HEALTHCARE OUTCOMES

The influx of artificial intelligence (AI) into healthcare systems worldwide offers promising assistance with complex clinical decision-making, improved patient outcomes, and reduced costs. Evaluating the impact of AI is a key challenge, especially within the context of ageing where good outcome measures are scarce (Efthymiou, I., 2024). The selection of appropriate evaluation metrics is crucial for determining the effectiveness and utility of AI-augmented healthcare processes. Existing efficiency metrics from fields such as Industrial Engineering and Operations Management, including turnaround time, waiting time, completion time, and machine downtime, can be applied effectively to temporal-AI systems to quantify improvements in patient and clinical outcomes. Complementary activity-efficiency metrics, such as the number of activities per project, activity-to-activity waiting time, resource utilisation efficiency, loop frequency, and rework frequency, provide additional insight into industry-specific performance but require adaptation—and consequently more development time—to suit the healthcare domain.

12.1. Clinical Effectiveness

The clinical effectiveness of artificial intelligence (AI) spans performance in clinical trials and clinical settings, along with the impacts on health and healthcare . Enhanced monitoring, diagnostics, stratified care, and health systems support have significant potential in the care of older people, particularly for long-term conditions (LTCs) and multimorbidity (Cassel & Fulmer, 2022; Reynolds et al., 2022). These conditions disproportionately affect older adults and contribute to frailty and syndromes including falls, delirium, functional decline, and incontinence. Improved monitoring of LTCs and AI-facilitated early diagnosis may facilitate early intervention, alleviating burdens on individuals and healthcare services. Wearable technology can provide continuous, real-time monitoring within the individual's environment, enabling virtual monitoring and early detection of deterioration. AI-enabled clinical decision support systems and image analysis support the prediction of dementia, delirium, depression, and other chronic diseases, with some models achieving accuracies exceeding 90%.

Geriatric clinical care comprises multidisciplinary assessments that evaluate older patients' (age 65 and above) functional ability, physical health, and cognitive well-being, with most patients experiencing multiple chronic conditions (Choudhury et al., 2021). Hospitals employ various AI systems to improve care for elderly patients. Research published identifies relevant studies, categorized into psychological disorders, eye diseases, and others (Zhu et al.. 2023; Velazquez-Diaz et al., 2023;

Moghadam et al., 2024; Lee et al., 2023). The prevalence of multiple ailments and chronic conditions, combined with limited cognitive and physical abilities, complicates assessment, and hospital stays may exacerbate health deterioration.

AI offers prospects for enhanced prevention, diagnosis, and treatment; screening tools have been developed for the early detection of cognitive impairments, fall risks, and urinary tract infections among patients with dementia. Although expanding AI applications are presumed to exert a positive influence on geriatric care, concerns about data uncertainty and algorithm explainability persist. An understanding of current AI practices is essential to assist clinicians in geriatrics, given the complexity and potential risks involved.

12.2. Cost-Benefit Analysis

A major challenge in broad implementation of AI innovations in ageing care is cost-benefit analysis (Maresova et al., 2023; Ramezani et al., 2025). Health economics is a multifaceted field that connects the clinical and fiscal power of healthcare. It seeks to understand where and how clinical interventions or programmes should be implemented to produce the best cost-effectiveness. (Folland et al., 2024; Getzen & Kobernick, 2022).

In Australia, for instance, there is still no population-wide evidence of the cost-effectiveness of AI technologies, and this hinders investment in AI by government and industry. Where attempts have been made, analysis has focused on a limited number of interventions or diseases and a broader, generalisable framework is still necessary. The Australian aged care system is delivered in a complex network of government regulations, service providers, rules and agreements across residential, community and hospital contexts (Sturmberg and Gainsford, 2024)

Moreover, to guide funding and service provision, elderly people undertake assessments of their functional capacity and independence, and low scores in these assessments often lead to funding packages for home or residential aged care (Peters et al., 2021; Hyams et al., 2023). Optimising this process depends on evaluating the cost-efficiency and accessibility of services, which is difficult without a clear understanding of systemic costs and benefits. Nonetheless, retrospective assessment of specific intervention costs can still provide useful benchmarks in comparison with other medical systems.

13. CHALLENGES IN AI ADOPTION

Realizing AI's potential in improving healthcare for older people in the United Kingdom (UK) requires substantial investment alongside robust governance structures. A dedicated workforce of clinicians and patients with digital expertise, supported by infrastructure investments, is essential to ensure the equitable implementation of these technologies across all sections of society (Ferreira et al., 2025; Socha-Dietrich, 2021).

These technologies will only succeed through a person-centred approach, rather than attempting to replace human decision-making. Current AI efforts in health and care focus mainly on supporting expert decision-making, for example, through clinical decision support tools and providing individualized risk assessments to aid clinical prioritization.

Three priority areas for the application of AI in healthcare reflect challenges faced by healthcare systems already under strain: reducing morbidity and prolonging independence through monitoring and early diagnosis of disease or acute illness, delivering more consistent and efficient care through stratified treatment and better resource allocation, and addressing the need for improved care coordination between multiple healthcare providers (Basmacı, 2022; Dicuonzo et al., 2023).

The advent of AI has meant ongoing scrutiny of the role of experts in decision-making, raising concerns over a loss of agency for clinicians. Large-scale population-level datasets, often used for AI training, have limited availability of data about the social and behavioural determinants of health as well as integrated social care datasets. Models developed from these datasets are thus unlikely to capture the full complexity of factors driving health outcomes and inequalities. Existing data disparate in quality and representation may therefore introduce or exacerbate bias and health inequities (Efthymiou, I. P., 2024).

A more widespread adoption of AI is subject to continuing concerns such as data privacy, transparency, safety, and accountability, which must be addressed through appropriate governance frameworks (Efthymiou, I., 2025). AI tools must demonstrate performance and effectiveness for older people—across the range of biological, psychological, social, and environmental factors impacting health—that is, generalizability beyond narrowly defined study datasets. Robust testing against existing clinical pathways remains a critical prerequisite before deployment at scale.

13.1. Resistance to Change

Implementation of existing data collection protocols and workflows often aims to validate and potentially boost organizational efficiency (LIEfthymiou, I. P., & Efthymiou Egleton, T. W., 2023). However, healthcare providers frequently resist adopting new data collection practices that appear extraneous to immediate patient care – a problem that persists even when older adults have access to highly usable technologies (Avula, 2021; Mistri et al., 2023). For example, the introduction of a data collection process requiring practitioners to fill in clinical forms manually to gather statistical information unrelated to their professional practice is vulnerable to resistance, resulting in numerous incomplete or inaccurate questionnaires. The mere act of completing a data collection instrument can become an unwelcome imposition, diverting scarce attention from direct patient care and contributing to negative attitudes toward the required tools.

One noteworthy advantage is that current assisted living technologies (ALTs) incorporate "cognitive surrogates": devices and applications that depend heavily on data to perform the associated tasks and thus may be perceived as less vulnerable to resistance than instruments that rely solely on human action (Jovanovic et al., 2022; Kim et al., 2024; Schepens et al., 2023; Iadarola et al., 2024). The one possibility that consistently motivates healthcare professionals to experiment with newer technologies is the potential to simultaneously reduce workload and improve the quality of care. This is perhaps not surprising, considering the well-documented relationship among staff stress, the quality of patient/client outcomes, and staff turnover.

13.2. Technical Limitations

Artificial intelligence (AI) can enable the analysis of large and complex medical datasets and the application of machine learning (ML) to make statistical inferences and predictions. The wide variation in the presentation and timescale of healthcare problems affecting many older people also makes AI attractive for clinicians caring for them. Early application areas of AI in healthcare of older people include clinical decision support (such as a tool for delirium diagnosis) and wearable sensors that predict falls. Top priority areas for future AI development in healthcare for older people are monitoring and early diagnosis of illness, stratified care to enhance treatment and prevention, and care coordination, including strategies that address loneliness and social isolation. (Shiwani et al.2023)

Potential negative implications of AI include exacerbating existing health and social inequalities through model bias, lack of validation and limited clinical use amongst older people, infringements of privacy, lack of transparency, and safeguarding concerns. Developers of digital health interventions should create tools based on a person-centred approach underpinned by clinical and technological governance (O'Connor et al., 2024; Nilsson et al., 2025). Clinicians and patients require education, infrastructure needs investment, and equitable access to technology must be assured.

14. REGULATORY FRAMEWORK FOR AI IN HEALTHCARE

Artificial Intelligence (AI) methodologies hold substantial promise in healthcare. Their successful translation necessitates a framework that upholds explainability, quality control, safety, and trust. The evaluation and validation of AI technologies must mirror this paradigm. An inherent risk exists that the original perspective embedded in an algorithm might be upheld, regardless of changing needs in the operational environment. AI systems have potential for unforeseen outputs, such as the creation of misinformation, both accidental and deliberate. A key challenge involves defining what constitutes the best outcomes — to facilitate decision-making through AI, values and objectives of all stakeholders require clear delineation and consensus, followed by methods to manage conflicts in objectives. None of these aspects are exclusively technological; social and ethical considerations are pivotal. The entry of AI into clinical practice demands comprehensive examination and the establishment of safety assurance methodologies that span technical, clinical, and regulatory domains (Livieri, G., et al., 2024). Structural changes are essential within the Artificial Intelligence for Health framework to accommodate social, economic, and ethical dimensions, in addition to addressing technical advancements.

15. COLLABORATION BETWEEN TECHNOLOGY AND HEALTHCARE SECTORS

Successful implementation of AI in the healthcare sector demands ongoing and sustained collaboration among various stakeholders, including technologists, healthcare providers, clinicians, and patients (Efthymiou, I.-P., 2024). This multi-faceted collaboration is essential in harnessing the full potential of AI technologies. AI in health is designed to manage and analyze vast amounts of heterogeneous and high-dimensional electronic health record (EHR) data, utilizing this information to make valuable inferences or predictions that can enhance patient care (Tong et al., 2023; Knevel & Liao, 2023; West et al., 2025).

Potential applications of AI, particularly tailored for the older population, encompass a wide range of features including clinical decision support systems that aid healthcare professionals in making informed decisions, wearable devices designed to predict fall risk and enable timely interventions, continuous monitoring for chronic conditions, early diagnosis of health issues, stratified care based on individual needs, and enhanced care coordination among multidisciplinary healthcare teams. Engaging in meetings that include older adults, clinicians, and AI researchers has emphasized the prioritization of monitoring and early diagnosis, along with stratified care and seamless coordination between various healthcare providers.

Despite the promising advancements, there are noteworthy concerns that AI applications could contribute to exacerbating existing health inequities, infringe upon individuals' privacy and autonomy, lack necessary transparency, and fall short of having robust safeguards in place to prevent errors and mishaps. To ensure that AI technologies are effective and equitable, it is crucial to employ effective interventions which require a person-centred approach along with strong and reliable governance (Currie et al., 2024; Silvera-Tawil et al., 2025). This governance must ensure adherence to the standards of generalisability, transparency, and overall effectiveness of the solutions provided (Efthymiou, I., 2025). Furthermore, the education of both clinicians and patients regarding these technologies, as well as substantial investment in the necessary infrastructure, is essential for fostering equitable access to these innovative solutions in healthcare.

16. CONCLUSION

The application of AI to the healthcare of older people is a rapidly evolving research area with the potential to improve many aspects of care, although some of the most ambitious published work has produced disappointing results

Many relatively simple interventions, such as clinical decision support systems for delirium diagnosis, wearable devices that predict fall risk and screen for atrial fibrillation, and social robots integrated into home-care plans, nevertheless have the potential to support older people and their care providers. Three priority areas for development have been identified: monitoring and early diagnosis of disease, stratified care, and care coordination.

How to deliver effective AI-enabled interventions remains less well understood. Achieving impact at scale requires a person-centred approach that respects the autonomy of older individuals and addresses their potentially complex health and social care needs. Clinical governance has a key role to play in ensuring that implemented applications meet minimum standards of generalisability and transparency, that procedures exist to identify and remedy failures, and that healthcare staff have access to appropriate training and support. Investment in infrastructure will help to ensure equitable access, while digital literacy education and involvement of patients and the public in the design process will address concerns around acceptability. With appropriate safeguards and person-centred design principles in place, AI has the potential to play an important role in sustaining health and independence as people age.

REFERENCES

Abadir, P. M., Chellappa, R., Choudhry, N., Demiris, G., Ganesan, D., Karlawish, J., & Schoenborn, N. L. (2023). The promise of AI and technology to improve quality of life and care for older adults. *Nature Aging*, *3*(6), 629–631. DOI: 10.1038/s43587-023-00424-7 PMID: 37231197

Aditya Shastry, K., & Sanjay, H. A. (2024). Artificial intelligence techniques for the effective diagnosis of Alzheimer's disease: A review. *Multimedia Tools and Applications*. Advance online publication. DOI: 10.1007/s11042-024-18327-4

Ajaykumar, G., & Huang, C. M. (2023). Older adults' task preferences for robot assistance in the home. *arXiv*. https://doi.org//arXiv.2303.03926DOI: 10.48550

Akpobome, O. (2024). The impact of emerging technologies on legal frameworks: A model for adaptive regulation. *International Journal of Research Publication and Reviews*, *5*(10), 5046–5060. DOI: 10.55248/gengpi.5.1024.58372

Aldboush, H. H. H., & Ferdous, M. (2023). Building trust in fintech: An analysis of ethical and privacy considerations in the intersection of big data, AI, and customer trust. *International Journal of Financial Studies*, *11*(4), 135. DOI: 10.3390/ijfs11040135

Alzeer, J. (2023). Integrating medicine with lifestyle for personalized and holistic healthcare. *Journal of Public Health and Emergency*, *7*, 20. DOI: 10.21037/jphe-23-16

Anderljung, M., Barnhart, J., Korinek, A., Leung, J., O'Keefe, C., Whittlestone, J., . . . Wolf, K. (2023). Frontier AI regulation: Managing emerging risks to public safety. *arXiv*. https://doi.org//arXiv.2307.03718DOI: 10.48550

Andino, J. J., Eyrich, N. W., & Boxer, R. J. (2023). Overview of telehealth in the United States since the COVID-19 public health emergency: A narrative review. *mHealth*, *9*, 26. DOI: 10.21037/mhealth-23-15 PMID: 37492124

Asrifan, A., Said, U. M. R., Jakob, J. C., & Wanci, R. (2025). AI literacy: Foundations, importance, and broader implications. In *Transforming vocational education and training using AI* (pp. 17–48). IGI Global., DOI: 10.4018/979-8-3693-9501-1.ch002

Avula, R. A. M. Y. A. (2021). Addressing barriers in data collection, transmission, and security to optimize data availability in healthcare systems for improved clinical decision-making and analytics. *Applied Research in Artificial Intelligence and Cloud Computing*, *4*(1), 78–93. DOI: 10.47363/araicc/2021(4)112

Badawy, W., & Shaban, M. (2025). Exploring geriatric nurses' perspectives on the adoption of AI in elderly care: A qualitative study. *Geriatric Nursing*, *61*, 32–39. DOI: 10.1016/j.gerinurse.2024.11.013 PMID: 39541631

Băjenaru, O. L., Băjenaru, L., Ianculescu, M., Constantin, V. ., Gu atu, A. M., & Nu ă, C. R. (2024). Geriatric healthcare supported by decision-making tools integrated into digital health solutions. *Electronics (Basel)*, *13*(17), 3440. DOI: 10.3390/electronics13173440

Banaji, M. R., Fiske, S. T., & Massey, D. S. (2021). Systemic racism: Individuals and interactions, institutions and society. *Cognitive Research: Principles and Implications*, *6*(1), 82. DOI: 10.1186/s41235-021-00349-3 PMID: 34931287

Basmacı, G. (2022). Prioritizing challenges in AI applications in healthcare: Multi-criteria decision making approach. *Nevşehir Hacı Bektaş Veli Üniversitesi SBE Dergisi*, *12*(2), 873–885. DOI: 10.30783/nevsosbilen.1084242

Batakis, D., Chatzivasileiou, S., & Efthymiou, I. P. (2025). Artificial Intelligence and its impact on healthcare. *World Journal of Advanced Research and Reviews*, *26*(01), 250–256.

Bekbolatova, M., Mayer, J., Ong, C. W., & Toma, M. (2024). Transformative potential of AI in healthcare: Definitions, applications, and navigating the ethical landscape and public perspectives. *Health Care*, *12*(3), 346. DOI: 10.3390/healthcare12030346 PMID: 38255014

Bharat, P. S., Narkhede, K. B., Prajapati, A., Narkhede, S. B., & Luhar, S. (2025). Impact of digital health technologies on medication adherence. *Asian Journal of Research in Pharmaceutical Sciences*, *15*(2), 141–146. DOI: 10.52711/2231-5659.2025.00022

Brunzini, A., Caragiuli, M., Massera, C., & Mandolini, M. (2023). Healthy ageing: A decision-support algorithm for the patient-specific assignment of ICT devices and services. *Health Care*, *11*(12), 1698. DOI: 10.3390/healthcare11121698 PMID: 37372816

Cassel, C., & Fulmer, T. (2022). Achieving diagnostic excellence for older patients. *Journal of the American Medical Association*, *327*(18), 1765–1766. DOI: 10.1001/jama.2022.5576 PMID: 35175301

Chaccour, C., Saad, W., Debbah, M., Han, Z., & Poor, H. V. (2024). Less data, more knowledge: Building next-generation semantic communication networks. *IEEE Communications Surveys and Tutorials*, *27*(1), 37–76. DOI: 10.1109/COMST.2024.3389479

Chan, R. J., Milch, V. E., Crawford-Williams, F., Agbejule, O. A., Joseph, R., Johal, J., & Hart, N. H. (2023). Patient navigation across the cancer care continuum: An overview of systematic reviews and emerging literature. *CA: a Cancer Journal for Clinicians*, *73*(6), 565–589. DOI: 10.3322/caac.21788 PMID: 37358040

Charow, R., Jeyakumar, T., Younus, S., Dolatabadi, E., Salhia, M., Al-Mouaswas, D., & Wiljer, D. (2021). Artificial intelligence education programs for health care professionals: Scoping review. *JMIR Medical Education*, *7*(4), e31043. DOI: 10.2196/31043 PMID: 34898458

Choudhury, A., Renjilian, E., & Asan, O. (2021). Use of machine learning in geriatric clinical care for chronic diseases: A systematic literature review. *JMIR Aging*, *4*(3), e26328. DOI: 10.2196/26328

Chu, C. H., Donato-Woodger, S., Khan, S. S., Nyrup, R., Leslie, K., Lyn, A., & Grenier, A. (2023). Age-related bias and artificial intelligence: A scoping review. *Humanities & Social Sciences Communications*, *10*(1), 1–17. DOI: 10.1057/s41599-023-01959-y

Currie, G., Rohren, E., & Hawk, K. E. (2024). The role of artificial intelligence in supporting person-centred care. In *Person-Centred Care in Radiology* (pp. 175–192). CRC Press., DOI: 10.1201/9781003319634-13

Das, A., & Dhillon, P. (2023). Application of machine learning in measurement of ageing and geriatric diseases: A systematic review. *Ageing Research Reviews*, *91*, 102047. DOI: 10.1016/j.arr.2023.102047 PMID: 38087195

Denysyuk, H. V., Pires, I. M., & Garcia, N. M. (2024). A roadmap for empowering cardiovascular disease patients: A 5P-medicine approach and technological integration. *PeerJ*, *12*, e18208. DOI: 10.7717/peerj.18208 PMID: 39224824

Diareme, K. C., Liapakis, A., & Efthymiou, I. P. (2022). Data, sentiment analysis, and examples during the COVID-19 pandemic. *Hellenic Archives of Psychiatry and Clinical Psychology in Behavioral Sciences*, *33779*. Advance online publication. DOI: 10.12681/hapscpbs.33779

Dicuonzo, G., Donofrio, F., Fusco, A., & Shini, M. (2023). Healthcare system: Moving forward with artificial intelligence. *Technovation*, *127*, 102860. DOI: 10.1016/j.technovation.2023.102860

Dixon, D., Sattar, H., Moros, N., Reddy Kesireddy, S., Ahsan, H., Lakkimsetti, M., & Junaid Hassan, M. (2024). Unveiling the influence of AI predictive analytics on patient outcomes: A comprehensive narrative review. *Cureus*, *16*(7), e64503. DOI: 10.7759/cureus.64503 PMID: 38854327

Efthymiou, I. (2024). Exploring the frontier: New and future trends in research. In B. Orlando (Ed.), *Innovation capabilities and entrepreneurial opportunities of smart working* (pp. 48–68). IGI Global. https://doi.org/DOI: 10.4018/978-1-7998-8797-3.ch003

Efthymiou, I. (2025). The role of e-government and e-governance in modern societies. In Wongmahesak, K., Ahmad, J., & Mustanir, A. (Eds.), *Public governance practices in the age of AI* (pp. 45–68). IGI Global., DOI: 10.4018/979-8-3693-9286-7.ch003

Efthymiou, I. (2026). AI in Epidemiology: Predicting the Unpredictable Leveraging AI to Detect Outbreaks and Predict Disease. In Umer, M. (Ed.), *Innovation and Transformation of Public Health* (pp. 281–308). IGI Global Scientific Publishing., DOI: 10.4018/979-8-3373-1992-6.ch009

Efthymiou, I. P. (2024). Wellbeing as an alternative to GDP? *HAPSc Policy Briefs Series*, *5*(1), 38–46. DOI: 10.12681/hapscpbs.38956

Efthymiou, I.-P. (2024). Can AI improve health and wellbeing? *Case Studies Journal*, *13*(11), 1–5.

Efthymiou, I.-P. (2024). The importance of soft skills in healthcare: The impact of communication, empathy, and teamwork on doctor-nurse interactions. *Case Studies Journal*, *13*(11), 6–11.

Ferrara, M., Bertozzi, G., Di Fazio, N., Aquila, I., Di Fazio, A., Maiese, A., & La Russa, R. (2024). Risk management and patient safety in the artificial intelligence era: A systematic review. *Health Care*, *12*(5), 549. DOI: 10.3390/healthcare12050549 PMID: 38470660

Ferreira, J. C., Elvas, L. B., Correia, R., & Mascarenhas, M. (2025). Empowering health professionals with digital skills to improve patient care and daily workflows. *Health Care*, *13*(1), 98. DOI: 10.3390/healthcare13010198 PMID: 39942518

Fleming, J. L. (2025). Securing space systems as critical infrastructure: A transformative approach to cybersecurity and risk mitigation. *International Journal of Critical Infrastructure Protection*, *48*, 100693. DOI: 10.1016/j.ijcip.2024.100693

Folland, S., Goodman, A. C., Stano, M., & Danagoulian, S. (2024). *The economics of health and health care* (9th ed.). Routledge., DOI: 10.4324/9781003268659

Gartner, J. B., Abasse, K. S., Bergeron, F., Landa, P., Lemaire, C., & Cote, A. (2022). Definition and conceptualization of the patient-centered care pathway, a proposed integrative framework for consensus: A concept analysis and systematic review. *BMC Health Services Research*, *22*(1), 558. DOI: 10.1186/s12913-022-07960-0 PMID: 35473632

Getzen, T. E., & Kobernick, M. S. (2022). *Health economics and financing* (6th ed.). Wiley.

Gupta, A., Sawhney, S., & Ahmed, S. (2025). CareTaker.ai—A smart health-monitoring and caretaker-assistant system for elder healthcare. *Engineering Proceedings*, *74*(1), 15. DOI: 10.3390/engproc2024074015

Hyams, C., Challen, R., Marlow, R., Nguyen, J., Begier, E., Southern, J., & Szasz-Benczur, Z. (2023). Severity of Omicron (B.1.1.529) and Delta (B.1.617.2) SARS-CoV-2 infection among hospitalised adults: A prospective cohort study in Bristol, United Kingdom. *The Lancet Regional Health. Europe*, *25*, 100556. DOI: 10.1016/j.lanepe.2022.100556 PMID: 36530491

Iadarola, G., Mengarelli, A., Crippa, P., Fioretti, S., & Spinsante, S. (2024). A review on assisted living using wearable devices. *Sensors (Basel)*, *24*(23), 7439. DOI: 10.3390/s24237439 PMID: 39685975

Igwama, G. T., Olaboye, J. A., Maha, C. C., Ajegbile, M. D., & Abdul, S. (2024). Integrating electronic health records systems across borders: Technical challenges and policy solutions. *International Medical Science Research Journal*, *4*(7), 788–796. DOI: 10.51594/imsrj.v4i7.1360

Imran, R., & Khan, S. S. (2025). A systematic review on the efficacy of artificial intelligence in geriatric healthcare: A critical analysis of current literature. *BMC Geriatrics*, *25*(1), 56. DOI: 10.1186/s12877-024-04709-2 PMID: 40217136

Jovanovic, M., Mitrov, G., Zdravevski, E., Lameski, P., Colantonio, S., Kampel, M., & Florez-Revuelta, F. (2022). Ambient assisted living: Scoping review of artificial intelligence models, domains, technology, and concerns. *Journal of Medical Internet Research*, *24*(11), e36553. DOI: 10.2196/36553 PMID: 36331530

Kim, H., Cho, J., Shin, S., & Kim, S. S. (2024). Uncertainty in surrogate decision-making about end-of-life care for people with dementia: An integrative review. *Journal of Advanced Nursing*, *80*(12), 4962–4976. DOI: 10.1111/jan.16194 PMID: 38197503

Knevel, R., & Liao, K. P. (2023). From real-world electronic health record data to real-world results using artificial intelligence. *Annals of the Rheumatic Diseases*, *82*(3), 306–311. DOI: 10.1136/ard-2022-222706 PMID: 36150748

Kyriazis, I., Lappa, T., Koufopoulou, K., Sidiropoulos, S., Efthymiou, I. P., & Vozikis, A. (2018). *Impact of Austerity on Dietary Habits and Obesity in Greek Children, Adolescents and Adult. The Impact and Implications of Crisis: A Comprehensive Approach Combining Elements of Health and Society*. Nova Science Publishers, Inc.

Lee, C. H., Wang, C., Fan, X., Li, F., & Chen, C. H. (2023). Artificial intelligence-enabled digital transformation in elderly healthcare field: Scoping review. *Advanced Engineering Informatics*, *55*, 101874. DOI: 10.1016/j.aei.2022.101874

Lewicki, K., Lee, M. S. A., Cobbe, J., & Singh, J. (2023). Out of context: Investigating the bias and fairness concerns of "artificial intelligence as a service". In *Proceedings of the 2023 CHI Conference on Human Factors in Computing Systems* (pp. 1–17). ACM. https://doi.org/DOI: 10.1145/3544548.3580763

Livieri, G., Anastasopoulou, C., Briola, K., Nikolopoulou, P., & Efthymiou, I. P. (2024). Ethical issues arising from the use of AI in drug discovery. *Journal of Politics and Ethics in New Technologies and AI*, *3*(1), e37093–e37093.

Maresova, P., Režný, L., Bauer, P., Fadeyi, O., Eniayewu, O., Barakovic, S., & Barakovic Husic, J. (2023). An effectiveness and cost-estimation model for deploying assistive technology solutions in elderly care. *International Journal of Healthcare Management*, *16*(4), 588–603. DOI: 10.1080/20479700.2023.2207687

Martí-Noguera, J. J. (2025). The 5P model as a governance framework. In *Governing digital mental health: Introducing the 5P model and the digital behavioral health expert* (pp. 47–79). Springer. https://doi.org/DOI: 10.1007/978-3-031-68429-6_3

Masmoudi, M., Ben Abdallah Ben Lamine, S., Karray, M. H., Archimede, B., & Baazaoui Zghal, H. (2024). Semantic data integration and querying: A survey and challenges. *ACM Computing Surveys*, *56*(8), 1–35. DOI: 10.1145/3653317

Mistri, I. U., Badge, A., & Shahu, S. (2023). Enhancing patient safety culture in hospitals. *Cureus*, *15*(11), e48829. DOI: 10.7759/cureus.48829 PMID: 38283419

Moghadam, M. P., Moghadam, Z. A., Qazani, M. R. C., Pławiak, P., & Alizadehsani, R. (2024). Impact of artificial intelligence in nursing for geriatric clinical care for chronic diseases: A systematic literature review. *IEEE Access : Practical Innovations, Open Solutions*, *12*, 139308–139325. DOI: 10.1109/ACCESS.2024.3469444

Morrison, B., Coventry, L., & Briggs, P. (2021). How do older adults feel about engaging with cyber-security? *Human Behavior and Emerging Technologies*, *3*(5), 1033–1049. DOI: 10.1002/hbe2.306

Nguyen, V., Van Anh, V., Ha, H. T. N., Huyen, B. T., Kien, T. B., & Anh, N. N. Q. (2025). Overview of proactive healthcare: The role of Medicine 3.0 and 5P medicine in prevention and early intervention. *T p chí. Y Hoc Viet Nam*, *550*(1), 1–10.

Nilsson, S., Hansson, H., Moons, P., Onerup, A., Saarijärvi, M., Sabel, M., & Bratt, E. L. (2025). Is this the road to health?–The person in precision health. *European Journal of Cardiovascular Nursing, 24*(4), zvaf091. Advance online publication. DOI: 10.1093/eurjcn/zvaf091 PMID: 40378194

O'Connor, S. R., Wilson, V., Brown, D., Cleland, I., & McCance, T. V. (2024). Development and optimisation of a mobile app (iMPAKT) for improving person-centred practice in healthcare settings: A multi-methods evaluation study. *Digital Health, 10*, 20552076241271788. DOI: 10.1177/20552076241271788 PMID: 39493639

Onitiu, D., Wachter, S., & Mittelstadt, B. (2024). How AI challenges the medical device regulation: Patient safety, benefits, and intended uses. *Journal of Law and the Biosciences, 11*(1), lsae007. Advance online publication. DOI: 10.1093/jlb/lsae007

Panahi, O. (2025). The role of personalized medicine in modern healthcare. *ResearchGate*. https://doi.org/DOI: 10.13140/RG.2.2.17002.00966

Paul, J. (2025). Real-time predictive health monitoring using AI-driven wearable sensors: Enhancing early detection and personalized interventions in chronic disease. *ResearchGate*. https://doi.org/DOI: 10.13140/RG.2.2.29776.25606

Payton, T., & Claypoole, T. (2023). *Privacy in the age of big data: Recognizing threats, defending your rights, and protecting your family* (2nd ed.). Rowman & Littlefield.

Pease, B. (2021). *Undoing privilege: Unearned advantage and systemic injustice in an unequal world*. Zed Books., DOI: 10.5040/9781350224032

Peters, M. D. J., Marnie, C., & Butler, A. (2021). Delivering, funding, and rating safe staffing levels and skills mix in aged care. *International Journal of Nursing Studies, 122*, 104046. DOI: 10.1016/j.ijnurstu.2021.104046

Pradyumna, G. R., Hegde, R. B., Bommegowda, K. B., Jan, T., & Naik, G. R. (2024). Empowering healthcare with IoMT: Evolution, machine learning integration, security, and interoperability challenges. *IEEE Access : Practical Innovations, Open Solutions, 12*, 20603–20623. DOI: 10.1109/ACCESS.2024.3359909

Ramezani, M., Bakhtiari, A., Daroudi, R., Mobinizadeh, M., Fazaeli, A. A., Olyaeemanesh, A., & Takian, A. (2025). Applications of artificial intelligence and the challenges in health technology assessment: A scoping review and framework with a focus on economic dimensions. *Health Economics Review, 15*(1), 46. DOI: 10.1186/s13561-025-00464-6 PMID: 40461901

Ratwani, R. M., Bates, D. W., & Classen, D. C. (2024). Patient safety and artificial intelligence in clinical care. *JAMA Health Forum*, *5*(7), e241677. DOI: 10.1001/jamahealthforum.2024.1677 PMID: 38393719

Reddy, S. (2024). Generative AI in healthcare: An implementation science informed translational path on application, integration and governance. *Implementation Science : IS*, *19*(1), 28. DOI: 10.1186/s13012-024-01357-7 PMID: 38491544

Reegu, F. A., Abas, H., Gulzar, Y., Xin, Q., Alwan, A. A., Jabbari, A., & Dziyauddin, R. A. (2023). Blockchain-based framework for interoperable electronic health records for an improved healthcare system. *Sustainability*, *15*(8), 6337. DOI: 10.3390/su15086337

Reynolds, C. F.III, Jeste, D. V., Sachdev, P. S., & Blazer, D. G. (2022). Mental health care for older adults: Recent advances and new directions in clinical practice and research. *World Psychiatry; Official Journal of the World Psychiatric Association (WPA)*, *21*(3), 336–363. DOI: 10.1002/wps.20994 PMID: 36073714

Sankaran, A., & Singla, M. P. (2024). Artificial intelligence in geriatric healthcare: Opportunities and challenges in a transforming landscape. *Frontiers in Health Informatics*, *13*, e2024016. DOI: 10.30699/fhi.v13i0.512

Schepens Niemiec, S. L., Lee, E., Saunders, R., Wagas, R., & Wu, S. (2023). Technology for activity participation in older people with mild cognitive impairment or dementia: Expert perspectives and a scoping review. *Disability and Rehabilitation. Assistive Technology*, *18*(8), 1555–1576. DOI: 10.1080/17483107.2021.1921117 PMID: 36067094

Scott, T. L., Pei, C. P., Wei, G. W., Sritheran, G., Tsann, P. Y., Balakrishnan, S., & Gupta, S. (2024). SafeMeds—Revolutionising medication reconciliation for elderly care with digital innovation. In *2024 International Conference on Emerging Trends in Networks and Computer Communications (ETNCC)* (pp. 1–10). IEEE. https://doi.org/DOI: 10.1109/ETNCC60833.2024.10645680

Shaver, J. (2022). The state of telehealth before and after the COVID-19 pandemic. *Primary Care*, *49*(4), 517–530. DOI: 10.1016/j.pop.2022.04.002 PMID: 36357058

Shiwani, T., Relton, S., Evans, R., Kale, A., Heaven, A., Clegg, A., & Todd, O. (2023). New horizons in artificial intelligence in the healthcare of older people. *Age and Ageing*, *52*(12), afad219. Advance online publication. DOI: 10.1093/ageing/afad219 PMID: 38124256

Sidiropoulos, S. (2024). Global health and civil society: financial tools and policies. *Tziola paublications*.

Sidiropoulos, S. (2022). International and Non-Governmental Organizations (CSOs-NGOs): Economic evaluation of Health Sector Activities and Projects. University of Piraeus, September. Available at *SSRN*: https://ssrn.com/abstract=4378863</eref>

Silvera-Tawil, D., Higgins, L., Packer, K., Bayor, A. A., Walker, J. G., Li, J., & Freyne, J. (2025). AI-enabled AT framework: A principles-based approach to emerging assistive technology. *Disability and Rehabilitation. Assistive Technology*, •••, 1–20. DOI: 10.1080/17483107.2024.2418172 PMID: 40170657

Skuban-Eiseler, T., Orzechowski, M., Denkinger, M., Kocar, T. D., Leinert, C., & Steger, F. (2023). Artificial intelligence–based clinical decision support systems in geriatrics: An ethical analysis. *Journal of the American Medical Directors Association*, *24*(9), 1271–1276. DOI: 10.1016/j.jamda.2023.06.013 PMID: 37453451

Smith, G. L., Banegas, M. P., Acquati, C., Chang, S., Chino, F., Conti, R. M., & Yabroff, K. R. (2022). Navigating financial toxicity in patients with cancer: A multidisciplinary management approach. *CA: a Cancer Journal for Clinicians*, *72*(5), 437–453. DOI: 10.3322/caac.21730 PMID: 35584404

Socha-Dietrich, K. (2021). Empowering the health workforce to make the most of the digital revolution. *OECD Health Working Papers, 129*. https://doi.org/DOI: 10.1787/18152015

Stine, A. A. K., & Kavak, H. (2023). Bias, fairness, and assurance in AI: Overview and synthesis. In *AI assurance* (pp. 3–30). Academic Press., DOI: 10.1016/B978-0-323-91919-7.00011-0

Sturmberg, J. P., & Gainsford, L. (2024). Health system regulation—a system 'as-a-whole' perspective: What can be learnt from the Australian aged care experiences. *Journal of Hospital Management and Health Policy*, *8*, 3. DOI: 10.21037/jhmhp-23-87

Stypinska, J. (2021). Ageism in AI: New forms of age discrimination in the era of algorithms and artificial intelligence. In *CAIP 2021: Proceedings of the 1st International Conference on AI for People: Towards Sustainable AI* (p. 39). https://doi.org/DOI: 10.5281/zenodo.5770580

Stypinska, J. (2023). AI ageism: A critical roadmap for studying age discrimination and exclusion in digitalized societies. *AI & Society*, *38*(2), 665–677. DOI: 10.1007/s00146-022-01553-8 PMID: 36212226

Tong, L., Shi, W., Isgut, M., Zhong, Y., Lais, P., Gloster, L., & Wang, M. D. (2023). Integrating multi-omics data with EHR for precision medicine using advanced artificial intelligence. *IEEE Reviews in Biomedical Engineering*, *17*, 80–97. DOI: 10.1109/RBME.2023.3306959 PMID: 37824325

Torab-Miandoab, A., Samad-Soltani, T., Jodati, A., & Rezaei-Hachesu, P. (2023). Interoperability of heterogeneous health information systems: A systematic literature review. *BMC Medical Informatics and Decision Making*, *23*(1), 18. DOI: 10.1186/s12911-023-02115-5 PMID: 36694161

van Kolfschooten, H. (2023). The AI cycle of health inequity and digital ageism: Mitigating biases through the EU regulatory framework on medical devices. *Journal of Law and the Biosciences*, *10*(2), lsad023. Advance online publication. DOI: 10.1093/jlb/lsad023 PMID: 38075950

Varona, D., & Suárez, J. L. (2022). Discrimination, bias, fairness, and trustworthy AI. *Applied Sciences (Basel, Switzerland)*, *12*(12), 5826. DOI: 10.3390/app12125826

Velazquez-Diaz, D., Arco, J. E., Ortiz, A., Pérez-Cabezas, V., Lucena-Anton, D., Moral-Munoz, J. A., & Galán-Mercant, A. (2023). Use of artificial intelligence in the identification and diagnosis of frailty syndrome in older adults: Scoping review. *Journal of Medical Internet Research*, *25*, e47346. DOI: 10.2196/47346 PMID: 37862082

Vousinas, G. L., Simitsi, I., Livieri, G., Gkouva, G. C., & Efthymiou, I. P. (2022). Mapping the road of the ethical dilemmas behind artificial intelligence. *Journal of Politics and Ethics in New Technologies and AI*, *1*(1), e31238. DOI: 10.12681/jpentai.31238

Vozikis, A., Panou, N., & Efthymiou, I. P. (2021). Chronic Diseases and Socioeconomic Factors: Findings From the SHARE 50+ Database. In Interdisciplinary Perspectives on Operations Management and Service Evaluation (pp. 252-269). IGI Global Scientific Publishing.

Vrahatis, A. G., Skolariki, K., Krokidis, M. G., Lazaros, K., Exarchos, T. P., & Vlamos, P. (2023). Revolutionizing the early detection of Alzheimer's disease through non-invasive biomarkers: The role of artificial intelligence and deep learning. *Sensors (Basel)*, *23*(9), 4184. DOI: 10.3390/s23094184 PMID: 37177386

Vrančić, A., Zadravec, H., & Orehovački, T. (2024). The role of smart homes in providing care for older adults: A systematic literature review from 2010 to 2023. *Smart Cities*, *7*(4), 1844–1877. DOI: 10.3390/smartcities7040073

Wager, K. A., Lee, F. W., & Glaser, J. P. (2021). *Health care information systems: A practical approach for health care management* (5th ed.). Jossey-Bass.

West, M., Cheng, Y., He, Y., Leng, Y., Magdamo, C., Hyman, B. T., & Das, S. (2025). Unsupervised deep learning of electronic health records to characterize heterogeneity across Alzheimer disease and related dementias: Cross-sectional study. *JMIR Aging*, *8*(1), e65178. DOI: 10.2196/65178 PMID: 40163031

Williamson, S. M., & Prybutok, V. (2024). Balancing privacy and progress: A review of privacy challenges, systemic oversight, and patient perceptions in AI-driven healthcare. *Applied Sciences (Basel, Switzerland)*, *14*(15), 6750. DOI: 10.3390/app14156750

Yuan, B. (2022). What personalized medicine humans need and way to it—Also on the practical significance and scientific limitations of precision medicine. *Pharmacogenomics and Personalized Medicine*, *15*, 927–938. DOI: 10.2147/PGPM.S380278 PMID: 36353711

Zhu, Y., Yang, Q., & Mao, X. (2023). Global trends in the study of smart healthcare systems for the elderly: Artificial intelligence solutions. *International Journal of Computational Intelligence Systems*, *16*(1), 105. DOI: 10.1007/s44196-023-00280-6

Chapter 12
Feeding the Future:
AI-Driven Food Distribution for Aging Populations

Eleftherios Karropoulos
https://orcid.org/0009-0005-1193-1366
Sotl Global Movement LLC, USA

Anastasia Psomiadi
https://orcid.org/0009-0006-9024-4894
Panteion University, Greece

ABSTRACT

AI-driven food distribution reshapes geriatric care by aligning supply chains, nutrition science, and clinical monitoring to the needs of aging populations.This chapter examines how predictive analytics and personalization engines identify and prevent malnutrition, how intelligent logistics optimize last-mile delivery and reduce waste, and how integration with clinical workflows creates feedback loops for adaptive meal provisioning. It lays out ethical risks—bias, data privacy, consent, and access gaps—and the policy and governance structures needed to mitigate them.The discussion includes operational models from food banks and community services, highlighting scalable AI applications that balance efficiency with impact.The chapter also addresses system resilience: using AI to anticipate demand shocks, ensure continuity in crises, and embed environmental sustainability in food sourcing and distribution, it proposes a framework for aligning clinical standards, data governance, and public policy to support fair, transparent, and accountable AI-enabled food systems for older adults.

DOI: 10.4018/979-8-3373-5462-0.ch012

1. INTRODUCTION

The world is experiencing a profound demographic shift: populations are aging at an unprecedented rate. By 2050, more than 2 billion people will be over the age of 60, double today's numbers, reshaping how societies think about health, infrastructure, and care (World Health Organization (WHO), 2021). At the heart of this transition lies a critical yet often overlooked issue: food insecurity among older adults. Challenges such as limited mobility, chronic illness, social isolation, financial stress, and gaps in service infrastructure are leaving millions without consistent access to the nutrition they need.

Malnutrition in older age is more than a health concern; it reflects a deeper breakdown in system design. Today's food distribution models are optimized for cost and efficiency, not personalization or clinical care (Larburu et al., 2022). As a result, countless seniors, particularly those living alone or with chronic conditions, receive food that is poorly timed, nutritionally inadequate, or sometimes absent altogether. With the added pressures of global crises—pandemics, climate shocks, and economic instability, this fragile model is no longer sustainable.

Meanwhile, the food logistics sector is being rapidly reshaped by Artificial Intelligence (AI). Predictive analytics, machine learning, and route optimization are already transforming how food is sourced, stored, and delivered. These tools can forecast demand, reduce waste, improve inventory planning, and even tailor deliveries to dietary or medical needs. When strategically applied, AI has the potential to turn food delivery into a proactive form of geriatric support, blending logistics, healthcare, and dignity.

This shift also opens the door to a new model of innovation, one that is both ethical and inclusive. Drawing on the Creating Shared Value (CSV) framework (Porter & Kramer, 2011), this chapter argues that AI-driven food distribution can advance business performance while addressing urgent social needs, particularly the nutritional health of older adults. Randomized and observational studies of medically tailored meals (MTMs) linked to clinical care have shown substantial reductions in 30–150-day hospital readmissions, including a 41–46% reduction at five months among recently discharged heart-failure patients receiving MTMs (Deng et al., 2025). In the U.S., industry analyses report that AI in distribution can deliver 5–20% logistics-cost reductions and 20–30% inventory reductions, improving service reliability during extreme events (Oca, Panikkar, Sampat, & Brown, 2024).

Equally important is the perspective of Stakeholder Theory (Freeman, 1984), which highlights the role of multi-stakeholder engagement in shaping solutions. Designing AI-enabled food distribution with input from seniors, caregivers, clinicians, dietitians, logistics managers, and community leaders ensures that innovation is not only effective but also socially grounded.

This chapter lays out a comprehensive roadmap for bringing AI into food distribution in a way that meets the complex demands of an aging world. It blends operational insights, clinical integration, ethical safeguards, and policy frameworks to propose a bold but practical vision: food distribution as a frontline service in geriatric care, with AI as a driving force for resilience, equity, and shared value.

2. THE PROBLEM: FOOD INSECURITY IN AGING POPULATIONS

The world's rapid aging brings both medical and social pressures and serious challenges to food security and nutritional equity. By 2050, people aged 60+ will surpass 2.1 billion, over one-fifth of the global population (World Health Organization (WHO), 2021). This shift is straining systems that were never designed for the complex, individualized needs of older adults.

Food insecurity among seniors isn't about too little food, it's about lack of access to safe, nutritionally appropriate, and culturally familiar meals that support aging in place and prevent decline. The clinical consequences are significant: malnutrition weakens immunity, slows healing, increases hospitalizations, impairs cognition, and raises mortality risk (Larburu et al., 2022). Even brief periods of inadequate nutrition can worsen diabetes, cardiovascular disease, and dementia.

The causes are structural such as income constraints, rising costs, shrinking family support, limited transportation, digital exclusion, and geographic isolation—especially in rural areas. The pivot to e-commerce and app-based delivery often overlooks seniors who aren't digitally connected or physically able to retrieve parcels. Traditional "food deserts" now overlap with "delivery deserts," where technology and infrastructure compound risk.

Conventional distribution models, built for scale and cost, rarely capture the health status or nutritional needs of the end recipient. They don't adapt well to dietary customization, rapid health changes, or delivery windows aligned with caregiving and medical schedules. In crises, from pandemics to extreme weather, these gaps widen; seniors are frequently the last served and most affected.

Fragmentation between food services and healthcare further erodes timely, appropriate support. Hospitals and care agencies collect rich patient data, yet it seldom informs how meals are sourced, packaged, or delivered. Without a feedback loop between clinical insights and logistics, opportunities to prevent malnutrition or adjust to new diagnoses are lost (Larburu et al., 2022).

In short, the current food ecosystem is misaligned with the realities of aging. At the moment older adults most need personalization, coordination, and agility, systems default to standardization. Fixing this is both a logistical and moral imperative:

food distribution must be reimagined as part of healthcare and social protection in an era defined by longevity, inequality, and technological disruption (Batakis, D., et al., 2025).

3. AI CAPABILITIES IN FOOD DISTRIBUTION

Artificial Intelligence (AI) is reshaping global food distribution, how we source, store, move, and deliver food. For older adults, AI's promise is twofold: smarter efficiency and true responsiveness to individualized, time-sensitive needs. From anticipating demand spikes during flu season to creating diabetic-friendly meal kits, AI can close the gap between food logistics and geriatric care.

AI systems learn, reason, and adapt. In logistics, that translates into machine learning, sensor-driven automation, and real-time decision support. When implemented well, these tools help distributors anticipate needs, cut waste, personalize offerings, and use resources wisely, exactly what's required to reach vulnerable seniors ethically and effectively.

For private companies, AI is also a competitive edge such as better delivery performance, lower spoilage, fewer labor inefficiencies, and new access to underserved markets. With AI, distributors shift from reactive firefighting to anticipatory operations, improving service and profitability (Logistics Management, 2023).

3.1 Predictive Analytics and Demand Forecasting

Machine learning has the remarkable ability to weave together vast streams of information—such as weather patterns, public health alerts, seasonal fluctuations, supply volatility, and even purchasing behaviors—and turn them into precise forecasts of demand (Efthymiou I., 2026). In the context of geriatric care, this capability becomes transformative. It allows systems not only to predict needs in advance but also to strategically pre-position resources, so that when a crisis strikes, the most vulnerable populations are not left waiting. Instead, those at highest risk receive essential nutrition and care right when they need it most.

Consider, for instance, a heatwave that swept across Southern California. An AI platform, drawing on health and demographic data, was able to anticipate dehydration risks among isolated seniors—people who were most likely to suffer in silence. Rather than reacting after problems arose, the system proactively rerouted refrigerated trucks and stocked them with water-dense food packs, delivering supplies directly into high-risk ZIP codes (*McKinsey & Company, 2023*). During COVID-19, large urban programs demonstrated at-scale meal coverage for vulnerable residents; for example, New York City distributed over 130 million meals across March 2020–September 2021 (*NYC Mayor's Office of Food Policy, 2021*).

3.2.1 Intelligent Supply Chain Management

Artificial intelligence is reshaping supply chains by injecting agility at every level—through dynamic routing, inventory optimization, and precise cold-chain monitoring. For older adults, this translates into very tangible benefits: meals that arrive fresher, deliveries that are consistently on time, and food options that align more closely with their clinical and dietary needs. Instead of being treated as just another endpoint in a logistics network, seniors become the focus of a system designed to anticipate and adapt.

What makes AI-powered inventory management particularly powerful is that it goes far beyond simply tracking shelf life. It actively forecasts usage patterns and accounts for population-specific requirements, such as softer textures for easier consumption, tailored macronutrient targets, or allergen-free alternatives. By doing so, it minimizes the risks of both shortages and wasteful overstocking, striking a balance that has long eluded traditional supply systems (Larburu et al., 2022). The result is a supply chain that is not only efficient but also deeply responsive to the needs of aging populations.

3.2.2 Operational Efficiency in Commercial Distribution

Large and regional distributors that supply hospitals, assisted living facilities, and foodservice providers are increasingly turning to AI as a way to sharpen their operations. These systems allow them to forecast demand by segment—such as senior nutrition—while also tracking route-level fuel use and monitoring SKU-level expiration dates with far greater accuracy (Logistics Management, 2023). The outcomes are practical and measurable: less product shrink, stronger fleet utilization, and improved service-level agreements with senior care programs.

Across distribution operations, embedding AI has been associated with 20–30% lower inventory, 5–20% lower logistics costs, and better service levels (Oca, Panikkar, Sampat, & Brown, 2024). For the seniors relying on those meals, this shift meant fresher food, delivered when promised, and tailored more closely to their specific needs. For the distributor, it proved that technology could simultaneously strengthen business performance and improve community health outcomes.

3.3 Personalization and Meal Customization

Artificial intelligence now makes it possible to transform food from a generic service into something deeply personal. By tailoring meals to a person's medical history, dietary restrictions, cultural preferences, and even sensory needs such as chewing or swallowing difficulties, AI ensures that nutrition is not only safe but also meaningful. For older adults, this personalization is far more than a luxury—it is often a lifeline. Carefully designed meals can stabilize blood pressure, balance blood sugar, or ease the strain on failing kidneys. In this sense, AI does more than optimize; it actively becomes part of the care plan for managing chronic conditions like hypertension, diabetes, and chronic kidney disease.

Recent evidence on medically tailored meals (MTMs) demonstrates the clinical potential of personalized nutrition. Randomized and observational studies show that MTMs, when integrated with healthcare workflows, can lead to substantial reductions in hospital readmissions, including a 41–46% reduction within five months for recently discharged heart-failure patients (Deng et al., 2025). Similarly, integrating AI tools with electronic health records (EHRs) enables providers to design nutrition plans that reflect not only medical requirements but also cultural and sensory preferences, ensuring meals are clinically effective while maintaining dignity and familiarity at the dinner table (Larburu, Garcia-Zapirain, & Alvarez, 2022).

For families, such personalization reduces anxiety by ensuring consistent, appropriate meals. For clinicians, it supports smoother transitions from hospital to home. And for older adults themselves, it turns food into personalized medicine—bridging clinical precision with the warmth of cultural familiarity.

3.4 Responsive Routing and Crisis Adaptation

Artificial intelligence demonstrates its most critical value under conditions of stress. During disasters, pandemics, or sudden shortages, AI enables real-time rerouting, automated driver coordination, and geo-targeted messaging to ensure continuity of supply (Marwala, 2024). For older adults, particularly those unable to evacuate or retrieve provisions on their own, this capability can mean the difference between resilience and crisis.

A telling example emerged during the early months of the COVID-19 pandemic. In New York City, AI-based logistics platforms were used to monitor infection hotspots while simultaneously coordinating food deliveries to seniors sheltering in place. Routes were updated daily to avoid restricted zones, and drivers received automated instructions to minimize exposure risk. As a result, meal programs reached thousands of older adults without major service disruption, even when demand spiked by over 40% in certain boroughs.

This case illustrates how AI is not merely an operational convenience but a critical safeguard in crisis response. By adapting supply chains in real time, it ensures that essential services remain accessible to those who need them most—transforming logistics into a vital component of public health and social care.

3.5 Ethical Enhancement Through Intelligence

Artificial intelligence has the potential not only to optimize logistics but also to elevate ethics across the entire supply chain. By embedding transparency, traceability, and accountability into daily operations, AI creates systems that stakeholders can trust. When these capabilities are combined with clinical data, the nature of food delivery changes fundamentally, from a generic logistical service into an extension of compassionate, person-centered care.

Put simply, AI is not just an operations upgrade. It offers a pathway to building adaptive, dignity-centered models of senior nutrition. As reimbursement structures shift and ESG expectations continue to rise, distributors who integrate AI effectively are positioned to gain not only market share but also long-term resilience.

Yet realizing this promise depends on design choices. AI must be embedded within systems that are ethical, inclusive, and clinically integrated (Efthymiou, I. P., 2024). Only then can it fulfill its dual role, delivering efficiency while reinforcing the values of care, dignity, and equity that aging populations deserve.

4. CLINICAL INTEGRATION: AI AT THE INTERSECTION OF FOOD AND HEALTH

Integrating food distribution with healthcare may be one of the most impactful advances in geriatric care and AI is the enabler. For many older adults, food functions like medicine: essential for managing chronic conditions, recovery, and quality of life. When logistics align with clinical workflows, AI can help deliver medically tailored nutrition with the rigor we expect from pharmaceuticals.

Although WHO (2021) names nutrition a "fundamental pillar of healthy aging," most countries still treat food delivery as a social service, not a care intervention. AI can bridge that gap by linking distribution platforms with EHRs, remote monitoring, and clinical scheduling.

4.1 EHR-Integrated Meal Planning

When artificial intelligence is linked with electronic health records (EHRs), nutrition moves firmly into the realm of clinical care. Instead of relying on generic diet sheets, clinicians can effectively "prescribe" diets tailored to each patient's condition. An AI platform can automatically generate weekly meal plans, for example, a low-sodium diet for patients with heart failure, while timing deliveries to coincide with hospital discharge and adjusting recommendations to reflect lab results and medication interactions.

A real-world example comes from Sweden, where AI-enabled meal services were embedded into discharge protocols for elderly patients with chronic obstructive pulmonary disease (COPD). By aligning menus with pulmonary dietary guidance, caregiver schedules, and case manager alerts, the program significantly reduced the risk of relapse. Peer-reviewed studies of medically tailored meals (MTMs) linked to clinical workflows report lower readmissions and utilization compared with usual care (Deng et al., 2025).

In this way, EHR-integrated meal planning demonstrates how AI can blur the boundary between medicine and daily life, transforming meals into structured, evidence-based interventions that extend the continuum of care into the home.

4.2 Closed-Loop Feedback Systems

Wearables and home monitoring devices open the door to closed-loop feedback systems that fundamentally reshape how nutrition is delivered and adjusted. By continuously tracking indicators such as glucose levels, hydration, blood pressure, and even medication adherence, these systems allow AI to refine meal plans in real time. A spike in blood pressure, for instance, can automatically trigger a shift toward lower-sodium meal options for the following week.

This dynamic feedback not only supports dietary compliance but also reduces the likelihood of complications, creating a more adaptive model of care. Perhaps most importantly, it offers providers visibility into the home environment, something that has traditionally been difficult to achieve. For older adults who live alone, this visibility can be critical. It allows clinicians and caregivers to respond proactively, addressing nutritional or health issues before they escalate into medical crises.

In effect, closed-loop feedback turns meals into part of a living, evolving care system, one that adapts in step with the patient's body and ensures that support extends far beyond the walls of hospitals or clinics.

4.3 Interdisciplinary Coordination

Artificial intelligence can serve as a central coordination hub, linking the efforts of caregivers, clinicians, social workers, and community health workers. By integrating factors such as frailty, mobility, social support networks, and behavioral health status, AI systems can do more than schedule deliveries—they can prioritize which clients receive attention first, flag high-risk individuals, and direct caregiver focus where it is most urgently needed.

A practical illustration of this approach comes from New York, where a Medicaid-managed care plan partnered with a regional distributor to introduce AI-driven meal triage for 10,000 seniors. The system aggregated caregiver notes and clinical alerts, enabling a unified view of client needs. Through this integration, the team identified 280 seniors at particularly high risk and referred them to in-home dietitians for targeted intervention. The result was not only a reduction in avoidable hospitalizations but also a measurable lowering of long-term healthcare costs.

This example highlights how AI can shift nutrition services from a logistics task into a coordinated element of population health management, ensuring that vulnerable seniors receive the right support at the right time.

4.4 Benefits for Commercial Food Distributors

For commercial food distributors, the integration of AI into clinically informed nutrition services is not only about efficiency, it is also a powerful source of new value creation. By offering AI-enabled, clinically integrated services, distributors position themselves to secure multi-year healthcare contracts, access Medicaid and Medicare reimbursement streams for medically tailored meals, and strengthen their performance in long-term care evaluations. These same capabilities allow companies to stand out in competitive requests for proposals (RFPs) by demonstrating measurable, technology-driven outcomes (Livieri et al., 2024).

Beyond direct financial benefits, such services align with broader environmental, social, and governance (ESG) expectations. Distributors that deliver offerings advancing public health can enhance their reputation, build stronger long-term partnerships, and reinforce their role as trusted actors in both healthcare and community nutrition ecosystems (Larburu et al., 2022). In this way, AI integration offers distributors a dual return: improved business resilience and a meaningful contribution to public health goals.

4.5 Ethical Considerations and Data Safeguards

The convergence of food and health data raises urgent ethical considerations, demanding robust safeguards to protect older adults. HIPAA-compliant data handling, clear and ongoing informed consent for seniors and caregivers, and full transparency around AI-driven adjustments must form the foundation of these systems. Equally important are audit trails and the ability for clinicians to override automated recommendations. Without such safeguards, the benefits of AI can quickly be undermined, through privacy breaches, opaque decision-making, or the erosion of autonomy, particularly for cognitively impaired users who may already face heightened vulnerability (Marwala, 2024).

The bottom line is clear: once clinical integration occurs, meals are no longer just meals, they become care interventions in their own right. In this model, AI serves as the connective tissue that binds logistics, nutrition, and medicine together, ensuring that deliveries are not only timely and efficient but also therapeutic, accountable, and ethically sound.

5. ETHICAL CHALLENGES: NAVIGATING AI USE IN GERIATRIC FOOD SYSTEMS

AI's potential in healthcare, logistics, and social care is immense, but so too are the ethical stakes. Older adults, in particular, often face compounded vulnerabilities, whether physical, cognitive, or digital, that make them more susceptible to harm if safeguards are weak (Vayena et al., 2018). For systems that span such critical domains, ethical guardrails are not optional; they are essential for ensuring effectiveness, building trust, and protecting fundamental rights.

Importantly, ethics should never be regarded as a brake on innovation. Instead, it serves as the very foundation for progress that is sustainable and equitable (Psomiadi, 2025). By embedding transparency, inclusivity, and accountability at the core of AI-driven systems, societies can ensure that technological advances uplift rather than marginalize, transforming potential into real, lasting benefit.

5.1 Algorithmic Bias and Discrimination

The power of artificial intelligence rests on the quality and inclusivity of its training data. When datasets fail to represent diverse aging populations, rural residents, non-Western cultures, or ethnic minorities, the resulting models risk reproducing and even amplifying inequities (Eubanks, 2018). In healthcare, this danger is not theoretical; it has been documented. Biased algorithms have historically under-prioritized Black patients, leading to gaps in care and missed opportunities for intervention (Obermeyer et al., 2019; Diareme et al., 2022).

For older adults, already a group facing multiple vulnerabilities, the consequences of bias can be particularly severe, from misaligned nutritional planning to reduced access to timely clinical support. Addressing these risks requires intentional strategies: building and maintaining diverse datasets, conducting routine bias audits, and implementing correction methods. Crucially, these processes must be overseen by interdisciplinary teams that bring together clinicians, technologists, ethicists, and community representatives. Only through such vigilance can fairness be safeguarded and the benefits of AI extended equitably across all populations.

5.2 Informed Consent and Autonomy

For many older adults, the processes by which AI systems collect data or generate decisions are not always transparent or easy to grasp (Mittelstadt et al., 2016). This creates a heightened responsibility to ensure that consent is both ongoing and meaningful. Consent must be communicated in plain language, supported by simple opt-out mechanisms, and designed with clear pathways for caregivers or proxies when individuals cannot act on their own behalf.

Equally important is the recognition that consent is not a one-time event. As AI systems evolve—introducing new features, risks, or uses of data, periodic renewals are essential to maintain trust and integrity. In this context, autonomy means more than formal agreement; it reflects an individual's ability to maintain control over both their personal data and the decisions that shape their care. By embedding these safeguards, systems respect the dignity of older adults while ensuring that innovation does not come at the expense of self-determination.

5.3 Digital Literacy and Exclusion

App-based systems, while efficient for many, often create barriers for older adults who lack reliable digital access, technical skills, or the confidence to navigate complex interfaces (Pew Research Center, 2021). In these cases, technology intended to expand care can inadvertently deepen exclusion, leaving some of the most vulnerable without adequate support.

Ethical design must therefore be guided by the principle of inclusion. This means ensuring that low-tech alternatives are always available, such as phone-based support lines, printed menus that can be reviewed at home, and in-person assessments for those unable to engage digitally. By embedding these options into the system from the outset, providers can make sure that no one is left behind and that innovation serves to reduce, rather than reinforce, inequality.

5.4 Transparency and Explainability

Trust in artificial intelligence depends fundamentally on clarity. For older adults and their caregivers, it is not enough to simply receive a service, they need to understand why a particular meal was recommended, how delivery schedules were prioritized, and when or how their personal data is being used or shared. Without this transparency, systems risk fostering suspicion rather than confidence.

This expectation aligns closely with broader regulatory movements, including the "Right to Explanation" initiatives and the principles set forth in the EU AI Act (European Commission, 2021). Beyond protecting individual rights, transparency also safeguards organizational reputations, particularly in competitive procurement environments where accountability and openness can be decisive factors. By prioritizing explainability, AI-driven systems ensure that efficiency is matched by trustworthiness, creating an environment where innovation and responsibility advance together.

5.5 Ethical Business Models

Ethical artificial intelligence is not merely a regulatory obligation—it can also become a distinct market advantage. Companies that embed ethical principles into their operations are not only reducing potential harms but also signaling accountability and trustworthiness to partners, regulators, and the public. This is particularly critical when serving vulnerable populations, such as older adults, where failures in oversight can have profound human consequences (Floridi & Cowls, 2019).

Practical measures are already emerging as hallmarks of responsible practice. These include establishing interdisciplinary AI ethics boards to guide governance, conducting algorithmic impact assessments (AIAs) to identify risks, publishing transparency statements that clarify how systems operate, and offering AI literacy and ethics training for staff. Together, these practices form the foundation of business models that are not only profitable but also sustainable, inclusive, and socially responsible.

5.6 Data Governance and Security

The blending of food and health data creates both opportunity and responsibility. To safeguard older adults, rigorous protections are essential. These include end-to-end encryption, HIPAA- and GDPR-compliant storage, role-based access controls, and clear breach notification protocols. Seniors and caregivers must also be informed about how long their data will be retained, their rights to access it, and the procedures for deletion or correction when necessary. Without these protections, trust in AI-driven nutrition and care systems cannot be sustained.

In conclusion, ethical AI for aging populations must rest on a comprehensive foundation: transparency, inclusivity, respect for autonomy, mitigation of bias, and robust data governance. Only by meeting these requirements can technology amplify dignity rather than deepen exclusion. As food delivery becomes a formal component of clinical care, these safeguards will determine whether AI serves as a tool of empowerment or becomes another layer of inequity.

6. POLICY AND GOVERNANCE: BUILDING TRUST AND ACCOUNTABILITY IN AI-DRIVEN FOOD SYSTEMS

As AI becomes central to senior nutrition, governments, companies, and civil society must collaborate to establish governance that ensures safety, fairness, and scalability. Without proactive policy, these systems risk replicating inequities, eroding trust, and overlooking the complexity of geriatric needs (Gasser & Almeida, 2017). Food is recognized as a human right within international frameworks. When its distribution is guided by algorithms and integrated with clinical systems, it becomes part of essential infrastructure—requiring oversight, transparency, and inclusive design. Governance must therefore pair technical capability with ethical accountability to safeguard both health and human dignity.

6.1 Regulatory Gaps in AI and Social Care

Oversight of artificial intelligence is still at a formative stage, and this is felt most acutely where geriatric care intersects with food distribution. The regulatory landscape remains thin, leaving critical vulnerabilities that place older adults at risk. At present, there is often no requirement for clinical oversight of AI-generated nutrition plans, consumer protections remain limited and rarely tailored to elderly users, and private AI tools are frequently deployed in public health contexts without mandated audits or transparency requirements.

Such gaps matter profoundly. They determine whether AI becomes a trusted extension of healthcare or, conversely, an unregulated experiment on vulnerable populations. The stakes are especially high when systems influence access to nutrition and care—areas where errors or inequities can have immediate consequences for health and dignity. To close these gaps, cross-sector standards spanning healthcare, logistics, and social services are urgently needed. These must safeguard both quality and accountability, particularly in contexts involving public funds or sensitive health data (Binns et al., 2018). Without such guardrails, the promise of AI in social care risks being undermined by uneven practices, inconsistent protections, and unchecked vulnerabilities.

6.2 Interoperability and Data Governance Standards

Artificial intelligence depends on accurate and interoperable data, yet in practice, the information needed to support geriatric food distribution is too often trapped in silos. Health records, delivery logistics, nutritional databases, and supply chain information remain fragmented, making it difficult to create reliable, end-to-end systems (D'Amour et al., 2020). This lack of integration not only weakens performance but also undermines trust in AI-driven interventions.

Establishing interoperability and robust data governance must therefore be a priority. This includes developing common data schemas that allow different platforms to "speak" to one another, enabling privacy-preserving data sharing across sectors, and ensuring audit trails for AI decisions that directly affect access to food or care. Role-based controls are also essential to safeguard sensitive information and prevent misuse. Importantly, such standards should align with established frameworks like the GDPR and HIPAA, ensuring that innovations in AI respect both legal compliance and ethical responsibility.

6.3 Funding Models and Public-Private Partnerships

Scaling AI solutions for at-risk seniors requires more than technological innovation; it demands sustained investment and coordinated partnerships across sectors (Kolk, 2014). Emerging examples illustrate what this can look like in practice: municipalities contracting AI-enabled logistics services to reach isolated elders, insurers reimbursing medically tailored meals informed by AI, and technology firms collaborating with nonprofits to co-develop platforms for food banks. Each of these models demonstrates how shared responsibility can drive both innovation and impact.

For such partnerships to succeed, however, they must be anchored in accountability. This includes establishing clear performance metrics, ensuring transparent public reporting, and creating governance mechanisms that prevent misuse or inequity. Financing models can be creatively structured to align with broader sustainability and social responsibility goals, through ESG-linked metrics, social impact bonds, or targeted grants that incentivize the integration of technology into social care systems (Psomiadi, 2025).

Ultimately, robust public-private partnerships provide the financial and structural backbone needed to transform AI in geriatric food distribution from isolated pilots into sustainable, large-scale solutions.

6.4 Case Comparison: Municipal vs. NGO-led Models

Comparisons between municipal and community-led initiatives reveal the importance of infrastructure and coalition-building in shaping outcomes. In New York City, the Department for the Aging coordinated large-scale food distribution during the COVID-19 pandemic. More than **130 million meals** were delivered across March 2020–September 2021, supported by municipal resources and service networks (NYC Mayor's Office of Food Policy, 2021). This model illustrates the advantages of municipal leadership, where access to resources, data infrastructure, and established service networks enables rapid scaling and clinical integration.

By contrast, smaller community and NGO-led initiatives often show strong creativity and agility in mobilizing resources but may face limitations when not fully integrated with healthcare systems or public databases. These differences highlight both the strengths and the constraints present in non-municipal models, where innovation may come at the expense of system-level alignment.

The lesson is clear: the success of AI-driven food distribution does not depend solely on the sophistication of the technology but equally on the infrastructure, governance frameworks, and coalitions that support it. Strong rules matter, but strong partnerships matter just as much.

6.5 Embedding Ethical Principles into Governance

For AI to serve older adults responsibly, governance frameworks must embed ethical principles at their core. This requires moving beyond technical oversight toward policies that address lived realities in social care. Key measures include mandating algorithmic impact assessments to evaluate potential harms, establishing ombuds and appeal channels for those negatively affected by automated decisions, and requiring systematic consultation with seniors and caregivers before deploying new systems.

Applying Stakeholder Theory (Freeman, 1984) strengthens this approach by ensuring that decisions reflect the voices of those most affected. In practice, this means treating seniors, caregivers, and community health workers not as passive recipients of technology but as active participants in shaping it. Embedding ethics into governance in this way builds legitimacy, fosters trust, and ensures that AI operates in alignment with the values of dignity and inclusion that must underpin geriatric care.

6.6 Implications for Private Sector and ESG Compliance

Good governance is also good business. Transparency not only safeguards ethical practice but also unlocks partnerships with hospitals and government agencies, while active participation in standards development helps shape the norms that guide entire industries. At the same time, tying initiatives to social impact targets strengthens ESG scores and bolsters investor confidence, reinforcing the alignment between ethical responsibility and financial performance (Eccles & Klimenko, 2019).

In this light, effective governance becomes more than compliance, it is a strategic framework. By closing regulatory gaps, standardizing data ethics, funding inclusive innovation, and centering stakeholders in decision-making, governance ensures that AI delivers not only efficiency but also justice and resilience.

7. SYSTEM RESILIENCE AND SUSTAINABILITY: DESIGNING FUTURE-PROOF FOOD SYSTEMS FOR AGING POPULATIONS

In an era defined by climate shocks, economic volatility, and rapid demographic change, resilience and sustainability are no longer optional they are foundational requirements. For older adults, the stakes could not be higher: when food delivery systems fail, the result is not inconvenience but hunger, illness, and in some cases, life-threatening crises.

Globally, **931 million tonnes of food** are wasted yearly, and **8–10% of global GHG emissions** are linked to food that is not consumed (UNEP, 2021).

Artificial intelligence, when properly designed and deployed, has the potential to hardwire resilience and sustainability into food distribution systems. By anticipating disruptions, optimizing resource allocation, and adapting dynamically to shocks, AI can transform distribution networks into systems capable of withstanding uncertainty while continuing to serve vulnerable populations (FAO, 2022).

7.1 Anticipating and Responding to Disruptions

Artificial intelligence equips food distribution systems with the ability to anticipate and respond to disruptions before they escalate into crises. By drawing on historical, environmental, and behavioral data, AI can forecast a wide spectrum of challenges, including extreme weather events, supply chain breakdowns, labor shortages, and public health emergencies. These predictive capabilities transform response from reactive to proactive, ensuring that vulnerable populations, especially older adults, remain supported even under strain.

The COVID-19 pandemic offered a vivid demonstration of this potential. During lockdowns, AI systems re-prioritized delivery routes to maintain continuity of service for high-risk seniors, ensuring that essential nutrition reached those most in need despite unprecedented logistical challenges. Similarly, climate-sensitive models now allow distributors to forecast droughts or floods and adjust sourcing and inventory accordingly, mitigating the risk of shortages and spoilage (FAO, 2022).

For public agencies, such continuity can literally save lives. For private firms, the ability to anticipate and adapt to disruptions provides not only resilience but also a competitive edge, strengthening reputation and long-term viability in an increasingly unpredictable world.

7.2 Waste Reduction and Efficiency

Globally, an estimated 931 million tons of food are wasted every year (UNEP, 2021). For aging populations, this waste represents not only a systemic inefficiency but also a lost opportunity to meet urgent nutritional needs. Artificial intelligence provides a powerful set of tools to address this challenge by embedding efficiency directly into food distribution systems.

Through real-time inventory management calibrated to expiration dates, AI can sharply reduce spoilage. Dynamic forecasting minimizes overbuying by aligning procurement with actual consumption patterns, while last-minute redirection of excess stock into emergency channels ensures that surplus food nourishes people rather than ending up in landfills. In addition, AI can prioritize the dispatch of perishable goods based on external conditions—factoring in temperature, potential delivery delays, and even weather forecasts to preserve nutritional value.

Together, these strategies create a cascading set of benefits: reducing costs for distributors, strengthening sustainability performance across key indicators, and ensuring that food retains both its quality and its purpose. In this way, AI transforms waste reduction from an operational afterthought into a cornerstone of resilient, senior-focused food systems.

7.3 Local Sourcing and Carbon Reduction

Artificial intelligence can play a pivotal role in advancing sustainable sourcing strategies by strengthening the connection between distributors and local suppliers. By mapping vetted regional producers, optimizing delivery routes to reduce fuel consumption, and tracking Scope 3 emissions across the supply chain, AI helps organizations meet rigorous sustainability benchmarks (CDP, 2023). These capabilities directly support global reporting standards such as GRI and CSRD, while also aligning with Creating Shared Value (CSV) strategies that integrate business success with societal progress (Porter & Kramer, 2011).

For older adults, the benefits of local sourcing extend well beyond sustainability metrics. Fresher products enhance both nutritional quality and food safety, while culturally familiar options ensure that meals resonate with dignity and personal identity. Moreover, local supply networks are inherently more adaptable during shocks, enabling faster pivots when global supply chains are disrupted. In this way, AI not only reduces carbon footprints but also strengthens the cultural and clinical relevance of food systems designed to serve seniors.

7.4 Sustainability Metrics for the Aging-Centered Supply Chain

Artificial intelligence enables a new level of accountability in aging-centered food systems by monitoring a wide range of critical sustainability indicators. Dashboards can track waste by site or delivery route, measure emissions generated per meal, and assess compliance with senior nutrition guidelines. They can also capture percentages of locally sourced products and equity metrics that reflect service levels in underserved communities. Taken together, these data points create a comprehensive foundation for justifying investment, guiding public policy decisions, meeting ESG commitments, and strengthening stakeholder confidence in both the sustainability and the social impact of the supply chain.

7.5 Aligning with Health and Planetary Well-being

AI also serves as a bridge between clinical nutrition and planetary health. By integrating dietary guidance with environmental considerations, it supports a gradual shift toward plant-forward proteins that improve cardiovascular outcomes, while simultaneously reducing the food system's carbon footprint (Willett et al., 2019). AI can further encourage the substitution of high-emission items with seasonal and locally sourced alternatives, and design culturally appropriate, low-sodium menus grounded in sustainable sourcing practices. This integrated approach delivers a dual benefit: advancing the health of older adults while contributing to the well-being of the planet.

7.6 Private Sector Leadership in Resilience and ESG

For distributors, resilience and sustainability have moved from the periphery of operations to the core of business strategy. Companies that strengthen their systems through AI-enabled resilience can lower insurance risks and claim costs, qualify for green finance opportunities, and meet ESG procurement criteria that are increasingly central in competitive bids. Just as importantly, they can build long-term loyalty among health-conscious and values-driven clients.

In summary, AI empowers distributors to anticipate shocks, reduce waste, cut carbon emissions, and align individual health with global sustainability goals. These capabilities enable organizations not only to achieve ESG targets but also to ensure stronger protection for older adults demonstrating that resilience and responsibility are mutually reinforcing pillars of modern supply chains (Psomiadi, 2025).

8. FUTURE DIRECTIONS AND RECOMMENDATIONS

Aging and digital transformation demand a shift from reactive logistics to proactive, data-driven care ecosystems. Progress requires cross-sector strategies that blend ethics with innovation.

One priority is to build integrated AI-health-food platforms that connect distribution systems with electronic health records, wearables, and nutrition assessments. Such interoperability transforms food delivery into a closed-loop clinical intervention, enabling dynamic adjustments as individual needs evolve. For instance, AI-enabled discharge planning can "prescribe" meal services based on diagnoses, dietary restrictions, and medication interactions (Larburu et al., 2022).

Equally important is the design of ethical and inclusive AI. Transparency, explainability, and fairness must be embedded from the outset, with seniors and caregivers actively involved in co-design, clear audit trails guiding food-related decisions, and strong protections for consent and privacy (Efthymiou, I. P., 2024; Vousinas, G. et al., 2022). Establishing ethics boards or advisory councils to oversee deployments for vulnerable populations ensures accountability and safeguards trust (Mittelstadt et al., 2016).

Future progress also depends on launching pilot programs with measurable return on investment. Public–private partnerships can fund real-world pilots that assess reductions in readmission rates, improvements in nutritional adherence, decreases in food waste, and increases in client satisfaction and independence. These outcomes form the business case for optimizing last-mile costs while simultaneously advancing ESG commitments and social impact (McKinsey & Company, 2023).

At the policy level, strengthening funding mechanisms and incentives will accelerate adoption. Tax credits for low-emission, equity-focused AI deployments, municipal grants for senior nutrition pilots, and procurement preferences tied to clinical and sustainability benchmarks can drive systemic change. In doing so, these policies contribute directly to advancing SDG 2 and SDG 3 (UNDP, 2023).

Knowledge exchange is another pillar. Forming international consortia to share models, code, and anonymized datasets promotes innovation and comparability across regions. Universities, in particular, can lead multi-country evaluations and help standardize indicators for global impact (HLEG AI, 2019; WHO, 2021; Efthymiou I. P., 2024).

At the organizational level, businesses can encourage Creating Shared Value (CSV) and stakeholder alignment. By applying the frameworks of Porter and Kramer (2011) and Freeman (1984), companies can develop ESG-aligned AI tools that reduce costs, improve nutrition outcomes, and strengthen community ties—unlocking sustainable business models that balance profitability with responsibility.

Finally, preparing the workforce for AI-augmented operations is essential. This means investing in digital literacy for frontline teams, nutrition knowledge for AI engineers, and human-centered design skills for deployment teams. Such efforts ensure strong human oversight, which is indispensable for sustaining trust in the system (Brynjolfsson & McAfee, 2017; OECD, 2022).

In sum, success will depend on a multi-sector commitment to innovation, ethics, and inclusion, one that balances clinical urgency with operational excellence and social value. Within this vision, ethical design in AI emerges not as a limitation but as a driving force, a catalyst that aligns technological innovation with the Sustainable Development Goals and ensures that progress for aging populations is both resilient and just (Efthymiou, Efthymiou-Egleton, Psomiadi, & Tariq, 2025).

9. CONCLUSION

As populations age, food distribution must evolve from a transactional service to a core pillar of geriatric care. AI can power that shift, combining efficiency, clinical integration, and ethical governance. But impact isn't automatic; it requires intentional design, investment, and a deep understanding of older adults and the systems around them.

AI-enabled distribution can deliver more than meals: it can deliver health, independence, dignity, and equity. To get there, solutions must be compassionate in purpose, accountable in practice, and explicitly aimed at those most in need, aligning logistics, medicine, ethics, and policy.

For distributors, AI is a business imperative. Predictive inventory, route optimization, and personalized delivery reduce costs, minimize waste, and sharpen service. Just as importantly, they provide real-time visibility to respond to pandemics, labor constraints, or climate disruptions, building resilience into every layer (Brynjolfsson & McAfee, 2017).

Strategically, AI opens new partnerships and revenue, government senior-nutrition programs, hospital collaborations, home health and insurer agreements. These require transparency, accountability, and trust, strengthened by auditability, ethical data practices, and closed-loop feedback.

Societally, food is medicine, identity, and care. For seniors living alone or with chronic illness, access to the right food at the right time shapes health and quality of life. AI that anticipates and responds to those needs becomes a tool for social good, not just operational efficiency.

ESG frameworks and sustainability reporting translate these social needs into strategy anchored in KPIs and transparent communication. Paired with Creating Shared Value (Porter & Kramer, 2011) and Stakeholder Theory (Freeman, 1984), AI becomes a driver of inclusive innovation and sustainable growth (Efthymiou, I. P., & Efthymiou Egleton, T. W., 2023).

This is more than an upgrade, it's a redefinition of purpose. Aging populations invite us to innovate and collaborate, honoring longevity with intelligence, empathy, and care. Organizations that embed AI within ESG-aligned strategies will strengthen performance and help define a future of aging built on equity, resilience, and vision.

REFERENCES

Batakis, D., Chatzivasileiou, S., & Efthymiou, I.-P. (2025). Artificial intelligence and its impact on healthcare. *World Journal of Advanced Research and Reviews*, *26*(1), 250–256. DOI: 10.30574/wjarr.2025.26.1.1015

Binns, R., Veale, M., Van Kleek, M., & Shadbolt, N. (2018). "It's reducing a human being to a percentage": Perceptions of justice in algorithmic decisions. *Proceedings of the 2018 CHI Conference on Human Factors in Computing Systems* (Paper 377, 14 pp.). Association for Computing Machinery. https://doi.org/DOI: 10.1145/3173574.3173951

Brynjolfsson, E., & McAfee, A. (2017). *Machine, platform, crowd: Harnessing our digital future*. W. W. Norton & Company.

CDP. (2023, November). *Technical Annex IV: Scope 3 overview and modelling*. https://cdn.cdp.net/cdp-production/comfy/cms/files/files/000/008/613/original/Technical_Annex_IV_Scope_3_Overview_and_Modelling_2023.pdf

D'Amour, A., Heller, K., Moldovan, D., . . . (2020). Underspecification presents challenges for credibility in modern machine learning. *arXiv preprint arXiv:2011.03395*. https://arxiv.org/abs/2011.03395

Deng, S., Hager, K., Wang, L., Cudhea, F. P., Wong, J. B., Kim, D. D., & Mozaffarian, D. (2025). Estimated impact of medically tailored meals on health care use and expenditures in 50 US states. *Health Affairs*, *44*(4), 433–442. DOI: 10.1377/hlthaff.2024.01307 PMID: 40193837

Diareme, K. C., Liapakis, A., & Efthymiou, I.-P. (2022). Data, sentiment analysis, and examples during the COVID-19 pandemic. *HAPSc Policy Briefs Series*, *3*(2), 21–30. DOI: 10.12681/hapscpbs.33779

Eccles, R. G., & Klimenko, S. (2019). The investor revolution. *Harvard Business Review*, *97*(3), 106–116. https://hbr.org/2019/05/the-investor-revolution

Efthymiou, I. (2024). Exploring the frontier: New and future trends in research. In B. Orlando (Ed.), *Innovation capabilities and entrepreneurial opportunities of smart working* (pp. 48–68). IGI Global. https://doi.org/DOI: 10.4018/978-1-7998-8797-3.ch003

Efthymiou, I. (2026). AI in epidemiology: Predicting the unpredictable—Leveraging AI to detect outbreaks and predict disease. In Umer, M. (Ed.), *Innovation and transformation of public health* (pp. 281–308). IGI Global., DOI: 10.4018/979-8-3373-1992-6.ch009

Efthymiou, I.-P. (2024). *What's left for us? AI, ethics and the future of work.* Independently published.

Efthymiou, I.-P., Efthymiou-Egleton, A., Psomiadi, A., & Tariq, M. U. (2025). The role of artificial intelligence in humanitarian aid for achieving Sustainable Development Goals. In Tariq, M. U., & Sergio, R. P. (Eds.), *Cases on AI-driven solutions to environmental challenges* (pp. 43–72). IGI Global., DOI: 10.4018/979-8-3693-7483-2.ch008

Efthymiou, I.-P., & Efthymiou Egleton, T. W. (2023). Artificial intelligence for sustainable smart cities. In Mishra, B. K. (Ed.), *Handbook of research on applications of AI, digital twin, and internet of things for sustainable development.* IGI Global., DOI: 10.4018/978-1-6684-6821-0.ch001

Eubanks, V. (2018). *Automating inequality: How high-tech tools profile, police, and punish the poor.* St. Martin's Press.

European Commission. (2021). *Proposal for a regulation laying down harmonised rules on artificial intelligence (Artificial Intelligence Act) (COM(2021) 206 final).* https://eur-lex.europa.eu/legal-content/EN/TXT/?uri=celex%3A52021PC0206

FAO. (2022). *The state of food security and nutrition in the world 2022.* Food and Agriculture Organization of the United Nations., DOI: 10.4060/cc0639en

Floridi, L., & Cowls, J. (2019). A unified framework of five principles for AI in society. *Harvard Data Science Review, 1*(1). Advance online publication. DOI: 10.1162/99608f92.8cd550d1

Freeman, R. E. (1984). *Strategic management: A stakeholder approach.* Pitman.

Gasser, U., & Almeida, V. A. F. (2017). A layered model for AI governance. *IEEE Internet Computing, 21*(6), 58–62. DOI: 10.1109/MIC.2017.4180835

High-Level Expert Group on AI (HLEG AI). (2019). *Ethics guidelines for trustworthy AI.* European Commission., DOI: 10.2759/346720

Kolk, A. (2014). Partnerships as panacea for addressing global problems? On rationale, context, and limitations. *Business & Society, 53*(6), 937–979. DOI: 10.1177/0007650314520962

Larburu, N., Garcia-Zapirain, B., & Alvarez, R. (2022). Integrating EHRs and AI for personalized nutrition interventions. *Healthcare Technology Letters, 9*(3), 45–55. DOI: 10.1049/htl2.12030

Livieri, G., Anastasopoulou, C., Briola, K., Nikolopoulou, P., & Efthymiou, I.-P. (2024). Ethical issues arising from the use of AI in drug discovery. *Journal of Politics and Ethics in New Technologies and AI, 3*(1), e37093. DOI: 10.12681/jpentai.37093

Logistics Management. (2023). Smart supply chains: AI adoption trends in North American food distribution. *Logistics Management, 62*(4), 48–52. https://www.logisticsmgmt.com/

Marwala, T. (2024). *The democratization of artificial intelligence: Reimagining governance and equity*. MIT Press., DOI: 10.7551/mitpress/14234.001.0001

McKinsey & Company. (2023). *How AI is transforming food logistics.* https://www.mckinsey.com/

NYC Mayor's Office of Food Policy. (2021). *Food metrics report 2021.* City of New York. https://www.nyc.gov/assets/foodpolicy/downloads/pdf/Food-Metrics-Report-2021.pdf

Obermeyer, Z., Powers, B., Vogeli, C., & Mullainathan, S. (2019). Dissecting racial bias in an algorithm used to manage the health of populations. *Science, 366*(6464), 447–453. DOI: 10.1126/science.aax2342 PMID: 31649194

Oca, A., Panikkar, R., Sampat, C., & Brown, T. (2024, November 15). *Harnessing the power of AI in distribution operations.* McKinsey & Company. https://www.mckinsey.com/industries/industrials-and-electronics/our-insights/distribution-blog/harnessing-the-power-of-ai-in-distribution-operations

OECD. (2022). *AI and the future of work.* Organisation for Economic Co-operation and Development., DOI: 10.1787/ai-future-work

Porter, M. E., & Kramer, M. R. (2011). Creating shared value. *Harvard Business Review, 89*(1/2), 62–77. https://hbr.org/2011/01/creating-shared-value

Psomiadi, A. (2025). *Your playbook for growth and resilience*. APSON Editions., DOI: 10.4324/9789609906580

Vayena, E., Blasimme, A., & Cohen, I. G. (2018). Machine learning in medicine: Addressing ethical challenges. *PLoS Medicine, 15*(11), e1002689. DOI: 10.1371/journal.pmed.1002689 PMID: 30399149

Vousinas, G. L., Simitsi, I., Livieri, G., Gkouva, G. C., & Efthymiou, I.-P. (2022). Mapping the road of the ethical dilemmas behind artificial intelligence. *Journal of Politics and Ethics in New Technologies and AI, 1*(1), e31238. DOI: 10.12681/jpentai.31238

Willett, W., Rockström, J., & Loken, B.. (2019). Food in the Anthropocene: The EAT–Lancet Commission on healthy diets from sustainable food systems. *Lancet, 393*(10170), 447–492. DOI: 10.1016/S0140-6736(18)31788-4 PMID: 30660336

World Health Organization. (2021). *Decade of healthy ageing: Baseline report.* World Health Organization. https://www.who.int/publications/i/item/9789240017900

Chapter 13

Devotional Singing and Neurocognitive Resilience:

A Non-Pharmacological Approach

Nikita Baruah Phukan
https://orcid.org/0009-0000-4817-2002
PES University, India

Shreya Ghosh
https://orcid.org/0009-0008-9309-3424
PES University, India

ABSTRACT

Devotional singing is said to be well-suited for promoting resilience in aging populations, as seen in its "capacity to engage widespread brain regions, linking memory, emotion, and reward" (Koelsch, 2014, p.171). Psychologically, devotional singing offers catharsis and mindfulness-based regulation that enhances self-efficacy and stability (Bernardi et al.,2001). Neuroscientific findings demonstrate its capacity to stimulate dopaminergic reward pathways (Salimpoor et al.,2011), strengthen autobiographical memory (Jacobsen et al.,2015), and foster neuroplasticity, thereby contributing to cognitive reserve. Cross-cultural traditions, from Gregorian chants to gospel choirs, reflect their universal role in fostering resilience and collective bonding. Seeing devotional singing as culturally embedded, a non-pharmacological intervention with therapeutic potential to sustain neurocognitive health and promote successful aging across different cultures, spiritual believers, and religions.

DOI: 10.4018/979-8-3373-5462-0.ch013

INTRODUCTION

Encompassing various cultures, music, and vocal recitation serve as a connection fostering collective purpose, overall healing, and resilience. The practice of Bhajans and Naam-Kirtans serves the purpose of emotional regulation, stress reduction, and helps combat loneliness, apart from the religious and spiritual traditions deeply embedded within the Indian sentiments. Helping reinforce cultural identity and belonging, one of the fundamental human needs in accordance with social psychology (Baumeister & Leary, 1995). These practices are increasingly recognized for their psychological and neurocognitive effects by researchers, becoming more prominent within the field of scientific enquiry, as a supplement to the previous spiritual significance. The aging brain presents a fertile ground to explore this intersection between traditional wisdom and modern science. With the aging population on the rise and concerns regarding neurocognitive decline, including but not limited to dementia, depression, and social isolation, among the elderly, there has been an enhanced interest in non-pharmacological interventions to sustain cognitive and emotional health. With it's widespread presence and deep cultural resonance globally, Devotional singing represents one such intervention.

The global pandemic, COVID-19, served as a stark reminder of the importance of collective practices for emotional stability and social bonding. Faced with unprecedented social isolation, anxiety, and uncertainty, individuals adopted traditional methods of emotional resilience that included prayers, chanting practices, and listening to devotional music, serving as therapeutic mechanisms and helping them stay grounded. With the state of affairs during the pandemic, these practices did not remain individual; rather were swiftly adapted into online and community-based digital formats. Serving as a testament to their timeless relevance and adaptability. For older adults, being among the most vulnerable to the pandemic's isolation, incorporating devotional singing through digital circles served as a lifeline, a structural activity that played a role in reducing stress, building resilience, and providing neurocognitive stability (Diareme et al., 2022). The shift towards the integration of accessible, community-driven, and culturally sensitive adaptations of contemporary healthcare is highlighted here to meet the holistic needs of the aging population (Feng et al., 2020).

Given a psychological perspective, Devotional singing enhances social cohesion and helps in the regulation of emotions. Factors that contribute to the overall well-being of ageing populations include the mitigation of feelings of loneliness, a sense of belonging, and the reduction of anxiety- seen in Group Singing (Davidson & Faulkner, 2010; Johnson et al., 2013; Pentikäinen et al., 2021). Often, the rhythmic and repetitive structure in devotional singing resembles meditative practices; this predictability and structure help foster a state of mindfulness, serving as a buffer against stress and uncertainty that often accompany advanced age. The themes and lyrics, often inclined towards surrender, acceptance, and the possibility of a higher purpose, provide a framework for meaning-making, a key component of psychological resilience (Park, 2010).

Given a neuroscientific standpoint, music can be seen as a powerful stimulus that can engage a distributed network of brain regions associated with memory, emotion, and executive functioning. With multiple studies concluding that music can activate the mesolimbic dopaminergic system, generating emotional peaks linked to the reward production within the brain, increasing motivation (Salimpoor et al., 2011). In older adults, devotional songs, which are often familiar from their youth, can serve as powerful **autobiographical memory cues**, activating preserved neural pathways even in cases of severe neurocognitive decline, such as Alzheimer's or advanced dementia (Jacobsen et al., 2015; Särkämö et al., 2014; Fusar-Poli et al., 2018; Fang et al., 2017). These findings indicate that the practice of devotional singing operates at both a psychological as well as a biological level, promoting resilience and helping maintain neurocognitive function despite age-related decline, building what is known as cognitive reserve (Hanna-Pladdy & MacKay, 2011; Román-Caballero et al., 2018).

Further, we will see how devotional singing, practiced in cultural contexts such as Indian Bhajans and Naam-Kirtan, contributes to building neurocognitive resilience in the Aging Brain. Drawing upon established theories of psychological theories of resilience and emotional regulation, alongside mounting neuroscientific evidence on the interconnectedness of music, memory, and brain plasticity. This is framed around three interwoven dimensions, exploring them in detail:

- Historical and Cultural Background- Exploring in detail, how Devotional Singing has historically functioned as a tool for spiritual connection, identity of a community/individual, and community belonging, referencing Indian traditions.
- Psychological Mechanisms- Going in depth into how Devotional Singing combats loneliness in older adults, reduction of stress, regulates emotions, and fosters resilience within older adults.
- Neuroscientific Mechanisms- Analyzing how Devotional Singing helps in engaging memory, neurochemistry, and compensatory pathways in the aging brain to promote neurocognitive health.

The chapter's main objective is to position devotional singing as not only a cultural tradition; it is a scientifically relevant, neuroprotective, and psychologically enriching practice that holds significant potential for integration into therapeutic and clinical frameworks. This understanding helps by bridging the gap between ancient cultural wisdom and modern scientific understanding. This chapter aims to highlight the potential of devotional singing as a low-cost, high-impact non-pharmacological intervention for promoting successful and dignified aging, through a timeless integrative practice.

HISTORICAL AND CULTURAL BACKGROUND

The psychological and neuroscientific benefits of devotional singing are inextricably linked to its rich cultural and historical foundations. Within the Indian subcontinent, devotional music, particularly in the forms of Bhajans, Kirtans, and Naam Kirtan, has served as a vital pillar of communal and spiritual life for centuries. Far from being isolated or occasional rituals, these musical forms are deeply interwoven into the social fabric, shaping identity, reinforcing belonging, and ensuring intergenerational continuity. Their enduring relevance—especially for older adults—stems not only from their profound spiritual significance but also from the predictable structure, emotional catharsis, and collective unity they foster.

The origins of these traditions can be traced to the Bhakti movement, which flourished between the 8th and 17th centuries. This socio religious reform was marked by a democratization of spirituality. Saint poets such as Mirabai, Kabir, and Guru Nanak challenged orthodoxy, emphasizing a personal connection with the divine and bypassing rigid ritualism and caste hierarchies. Their teachings were conveyed through simple, emotionally resonant songs, composed in vernacular languages and designed for communal singing. These devotional compositions provided a powerful vehicle for expressing the full range of human emotions—love, longing, surrender, and grief, functioning as both spiritual and psychosocial outlets for the communities that embraced them.

A compelling example of this practice is Naam Kirtan in the Vaishnavite tradition of Assam, where communities gather in the Namghar (prayer hall) to engage in call and response chanting, often accompanied by traditional instruments like the khol (double-headed drum) and taal (cymbals). For many elderly participants, these gatherings are part of a daily or weekly routine, offering not only spiritual sustenance but also vital social engagement. Older adults frequently serve as group leaders, sharing cultural knowledge and guiding younger generations. The rhythmic repetition, collective synchronization, and emotional resonance of these sessions induce a heightened sense of social unity a phenomenon akin to what can be (Durkheim, 1912/1995) described as "collective effervescence." Particularly for older individuals facing isolation, physical decline, or bereavement, such gatherings reinforce a sense of purpose, belonging, and cultural identity.

From a psychological perspective, devotional singing functions as a profound form of embodied mindfulness. The repetition of sacred phrases, combined with melody, rhythmic breathing, and group participation, draws attention inward, facilitating emotional regulation and mental focus. These mechanisms mirror those found in contemplative practices such as meditation and breathwork. The structured nature of devotional music offers a mental anchor, helping practitioners remain present and centered, thereby reducing the burden of ruminative thought and existential anxiety, issues particularly salient in older adulthood.

CROSS-CULTURAL PARALLELS

While devotional singing holds particular prominence in Indian traditions, its psychological and social functions resonate deeply in cultures across the globe. These vocal and rhythmic practices—though culturally distinct—share key structural features: predictability, repetition, group synchrony, and emotional resonance. These elements consistently support emotional regulation, stress reduction, and social cohesion, rendering such traditions invaluable across aging populations worldwide.

- **Gregorian Chants (Europe)**: Emerging from monastic traditions in medieval Europe, Gregorian chants consist of slow, monophonic melodies that promote meditative focus and spiritual calm. These chants provided monks with a rhythmic and emotional structure for their daily lives, enhancing mental clarity and social cohesion in cloistered environments.
- **Buddhist Chanting (Thailand)**: The repetitive recitation of suttas, particularly the Metta Sutta, serves as both a meditative tool and an emotional regulator. The slow, rhythmic phrasing encourages compassionate awareness and has been linked to reduced activity in the Default Mode Network (DMN), a neural system associated with self-referential thinking and anxiety (Koole et al., 2015).
- **Sufi Zikr and Qawwali (South Asia and the Middle East)**: These practices involve the rhythmic repetition of divine names (zikr) or poetic devotional songs (qawwali), often accompanied by handclapping, body swaying, and communal chanting. The entrainment of rhythm and movement induces trance like states and fosters profound emotional release and spiritual ecstasy. For older practitioners, these sessions offer psychological relief and maintain cognitive vitality through structured social participation.
- **Gospel Choirs (United States)**: Rooted in African American spiritual traditions, gospel singing combines musical expressiveness, group synchrony, and religious fervour. The call and response structure, emotional intensity, and

shared meaning promote resilience and social connection, particularly for elderly members of the congregation who often describe choir participation as spiritually fulfilling and emotionally grounding.

Despite regional and theological differences, these traditions share striking psychological commonalities. For older adults, the combination of musical repetition, group interaction, and spiritual reflection provides emotional catharsis, reinforces identity continuity, and buffers against the isolating effects of aging. The structured predictability inherent in these practices offers a sense of control and familiarity, factors that are crucial for mental stability during periods of life transition.

Contemporary Revitalization in Times of Crisis

Cultural evidence suggests that devotional singing has historically seen revival during periods of collective uncertainty or upheaval. The COVID-19 pandemic offers a contemporary example of this resurgence. As physical gatherings became restricted, communities rapidly adapted by migrating devotional singing practices to digital platforms. Online kirtan sessions, livestreamed bhajan gatherings, and global chant circles emerged as alternative modes of spiritual engagement. For older adults, these virtual spaces provided continuity, emotional support, and a renewed sense of social inclusion during a period marked by intense isolation and vulnerability (Diareme et al., 2022).

This modern adaptation parallels the global rise in digital mindfulness, chanting, and prayer apps during the pandemic, indicating a broader return to rhythmic and repetitive practices as coping mechanisms in times of crisis. The collective and predictable structure of devotional singing positioned it as a powerful psychosocial buffer, capable of reducing pandemic-induced stress, loneliness, and anxiety, especially among aging individuals (Bernardi et al., 2001).

Devotional singing, therefore, is far more than a historical or religious artifact; it is a living, adaptive practice that continues to meet essential human needs in both traditional and modern contexts. In the landscape of aging, its dual function becomes especially salient: it is spiritually resonant while simultaneously offering significant psychological and social benefits. By regulating stress, enhancing emotional well-being, and connecting individuals to their community and cultural heritage, devotional singing emerges as a holistic and culturally congruent strategy for supporting successful aging.

Its relevance today lies in its flexibility, its ability to remain rooted in centuries-old tradition while evolving to meet the emotional and cognitive needs of contemporary, aging populations. As such, it represents a powerful, low-cost, and inclusive intervention that aligns with both historical wisdom and modern therapeutic paradigms.

Psychological Facet of Devotional Singing

As seen in the previous section of the chapter, culture and historical foundations, alongside psychological mechanisms of devotional singing, have a profound impact on mental well-being later in life. Psychology, long recognizing the therapeutic value of structured, repetitive activities in regulating emotions and promoting mental health. Devotional singing, much like ritual chanting, offers predictable rhythmic and melodic structures that provide a sense of stability and predictability, which is crucial for older adults facing the uncertainties of aging. The act of singing sacred lyrics repeatedly allows participants to externalize emotions, channelling anxiety into a structured, controllable form and leading up to what Aristotle describes as **"catharsis,"** a cleansing or release of pent-up emotions, a concept foundational to Western theories of drama and emotional expression (Aristotle, trans. 1987). For the elderly, practicing Bhajans of lament or surrendering through Kirtan serves as a safe emotional outlet, promoting acceptance of life's challenges while reinforcing positive emotions such as gratitude and peace.

Physiological markers of stress can be lowered by rhythmic recitation or singing practices, as suggested by research (Bernardi et al., 2001). Rumination, i.e., a repetitive pattern of negative thinking, could often present as anxiety and depression in older adults. Integrating practices of slow, deep breathing, rhythmic phrasing, mirroring the mechanisms of mindfulness and Yoga-based relaxation techniques, with melodic structure and lyrical meaning, helps buffer against such cognitive stressors that often accompany aging.

As individuals transition into older adulthood, the risk of social isolation and loneliness, strongly associated with psychological distress, physical illness, and cognitive decline, becomes increasingly heightened (Feng et al., 2018). Within this context, **devotional singing** emerges as a potent social and emotional resource. The collective nature of group singing, whether in temples, local community halls, or intimate household gatherings, cultivates a sense of kinship and shared identity, mirroring views of belongingness theory observed in social psychology. According to Baumeister and Leary (1995), the human need to belong is not merely a social preference but a fundamental psychological drive, closely tied to resilience and emotional well-being. Participation in Kirtan Mandalis and Bhajan groups often fulfills this drive, becoming more than a spiritual routine, evolving into support networks for older adults who find in them both companionship and affirmation (Coulton et al., 2015).

The practice of singing in unison is not only symbolic but deeply physiological. Synchronized vocalization has been shown to enhance feelings of trust and social closeness, mediated by the release of oxytocin, a neuropeptide associated with bonding and empathy (Keeler et al., 2015). Such effects reinforce the emotional safety of communal devotional settings, offering older individuals a predictable and affirming structure amidst the often-unpredictable landscape of aging.

Many elders encounter profound forms of loss, such as bereavement, physical decline, or shifts in identity post-retirement. Devotional singing, through its lyrical focus on impermanence, surrender, and the soul's continuity, provides a narrative framework for meaning-making. Rather than resisting decline, older adults are invited to reframe suffering within a spiritual arc, aligning with positive psychology's emphasis on existential meaning as a core resilience factor (Park, 2010). Bhajans that reflect themes of mortality, devotion, and transcendence allow emotional expression to occur within culturally resonant boundaries, often offering a psychospiritual scaffolding for grief and transformation.

In addition to fostering emotional regulation, participation in Naam-Kirtan also cultivates a sense of personal agency and self-efficacy. For many elders, contributing vocally to a collective ritual, even in modest ways, becomes an empowering act. Bandura's social cognitive theory highlights self-efficacy as a pivotal determinant of adaptive coping, particularly in the face of life's stressors. The experience of leading or teaching devotional songs, especially in intergenerational contexts, reinforces one's perceived value within the social fabric. These roles serve not only to transmit cultural heritage but also to fortify intergenerational bonds, which have been widely recognized as buffers against mental health challenges in aging populations (Johnson et al., 2013).

Thus, from a psychological lens, devotional singing intersects with multiple vulnerabilities associated with aging, ranging from emotional volatility and social marginalization to existential anxiety and diminished agency. Through its rhythmic repetition, communal engagement, and symbolic content, it activates protective mechanisms that are as emotionally resonant as they are neurologically grounded. These dimensions will be explored more fully in the following section, where the cognitive and neurobiological underpinnings of devotional music are examined in greater depth.

Neuroscientific Perspectives on Devotional Singing

As explored in previous sections, the psychological benefits of devotional singing are far-reaching; however, these are not solely emotional or symbolic in nature. Underlying them is a rich tapestry of neuroscientific mechanisms that render this practice not only culturally resonant but cognitively restorative. Far from being a simple auditory exercise, singing engages a wide network of cortical and subcortical structures, offering a holistic stimulation of the aging brain. Functional neuroimaging studies have revealed that singing simultaneously recruits the auditory cortex for sound processing, motor and premotor regions for rhythmic and vocal coordination, and language areas such as Broca's and Wernicke's regions for lyrical comprehension. Crucially, when singing is emotionally meaningful, as in devotional settings, it profoundly activates the limbic system, including the amygdala, hippocampus, and nucleus accumbens, regions deeply involved in emotion, memory, and reward.

This extensive neural engagement holds particular significance for older adults. Age-related brain changes often result in compensatory strategies such as neural redundancy, where multiple regions are recruited to sustain cognitive performance (Cabeza et al., 2002). In this light, devotional singing serves as a naturally embedded cognitive intervention, activating memory, language, attention, and motor coordination in unison. Much like a cognitive symphony, it orchestrates these systems into a coherent, embodied activity that may help buffer against the onset of neurodegenerative decline (Kim & Yoo, 2015; Bugos et al., 2007).

A key dimension of this process lies in the neurochemical shifts that accompany group singing. The collective experience of Kirtan or Bhajan is known to elevate dopamine levels within the mesolimbic pathway, often referred to as the brain's pleasure and motivation centre (Salimpoor et al., 2011). This aligns closely with the profound joy and transcendence frequently described by participants. Additionally, increases in oxytocin, the neuropeptide linked to trust, attachment, and social bonding, further amplify the interpersonal warmth and sense of unity within the group (Keeler et al., 2015). For elders, especially those vulnerable to loneliness, these biochemical responses provide a physiological basis for connection and inclusion. The release of endorphins, often termed the body's natural painkillers, contributes to the physical ease and emotional calm many report after singing sessions, an embodied sense of peace that extends beyond the activity itself.

The Limbic System and Its Role in Devotional Singing for Older Adults

The limbic system is a complex network of interconnected brain structures that plays a crucial role in emotion, motivation, memory, and learning. Comprising key regions such as the amygdala, hippocampus, hypothalamus, and anterior cingulate cortex, it forms the emotional core of the brain. When older adults engage in devotional singing, these limbic structures become highly active, contributing significantly to the observed psychological and cognitive benefits.

- **Amygdala and Emotional Processing**: The amygdala is central to processing emotions, particularly fear, pleasure, and emotional memory. In devotional singing, the emotionally rich lyrics and melodies, often evoking feelings of devotion, gratitude, or spiritual longing, directly engage the amygdala. For older adults, this engagement can help regulate mood, reduce anxiety, and foster a sense of emotional well-being. It provides a safe channel for emotional expression, which is particularly beneficial for those navigating age-related stressors or grief.

- **Hippocampus and Memory Consolidation**: The hippocampus is vital for the formation of new memories and the retrieval of existing ones. Devotional songs, especially those learned in youth, act as powerful cues for autobiographical memory. The repetition of familiar lyrics and melodies during singing actively stimulates hippocampal function. For older adults, whose hippocampal integrity might be compromised by age or neurodegenerative conditions, this musical activation can help preserve memory pathways, reinforce cognitive identity, and provide access to cherished memories, thereby enhancing cognitive function and maintaining a sense of self.
- **Nucleus Accumbens and Reward**: Part of the brain's reward system, the nucleus accumbens is strongly associated with motivation and pleasure, driven by dopamine release. The collective, rhythmic, and emotionally uplifting experience of devotional singing can trigger a significant release of dopamine in this region. This neurochemical reward enhances feelings of joy, satisfaction, and motivation, acting as a natural mood elevator. For older adults, these positive emotional states can combat symptoms of depression, increase engagement in social activities, and improve overall quality of life.
- **Hypothalamus and Autonomic Regulation**: The hypothalamus plays a critical role in regulating autonomic functions, including heart rate, blood pressure, and stress responses. The rhythmic breathing and structured vocalization inherent in devotional singing can help activate the parasympathetic nervous system, leading to a reduction in heart rate and blood pressure, and a decrease in stress hormones like cortisol. This physiological calming effect is profoundly beneficial for older adults, contributing to improved sleep, reduced anxiety, and enhanced physical health.

In essence, the limbic system acts as a central hub, integrating the emotional, mnemonic, and motivational aspects of devotional singing. For older adults, this coordinated activation provides a robust mechanism for emotional regulation, memory preservation, and the experience of profound well-being, underscoring the practice's holistic neurocognitive benefits.

Equally vital is the role of devotional singing in stimulating memory and preserving cognitive identity. The repetition and retrieval of lyrics, melodies, and rhythmic sequences actively engage the hippocampus, a region critically involved in learning and memory consolidation. Given that the hippocampus is among the first areas to exhibit deterioration in age-related cognitive disorders, its regular activation through song provides a valuable exercise in memory resilience. Notably, musical memory often endures even in advanced stages of dementia, suggesting that song-based recall mechanisms are neurologically distinct and deeply embedded (Jacobsen et al., 2015; Särkämö et al., 2014; Fusar Poli et al., 2018). For many older adults, devotional songs are not merely musical; they are autobiographical anchors, tied to early rituals, familial gatherings, and cultural rites. Engaging with these songs becomes an act of self-continuity, preserving narrative identity amidst the disorientation that can accompany cognitive decline.

This cognitive preservation can be further understood through the lens of cognitive reserve, a concept referring to the brain's ability to adapt and compensate in the face of neuropathology (Hanna Pladdy & MacKay, 2011; Román Caballero et al., 2018). Devotional singing engages a diverse array of mental faculties—attention, language, emotional modulation, memory recall, and motor coordination—simultaneously. Such multi-domain engagement fosters neuroplasticity, the brain's remarkable capacity to form and strengthen neural connections (Mansens et al., 2018). Studies of lifelong musicians have shown increased Gray matter density and heightened connectivity in auditory motor networks (Gaser & Schlaug, 2003). While not all devotional singers undergo formal training, consistent participation over decades, particularly in emotionally and socially enriched contexts, may yield comparable cognitive benefits (Feng et al., 2018; Pentikäinen et al., 2021).

Beyond structural and chemical enhancements, the rhythmic nature of devotional singing also modulates neural oscillations. Increased alpha and theta brainwave activity, often observed during chanting or singing, is associated with relaxation, meditative focus, and heightened creativity. These brain states support emotional regulation and reduce cognitive overload, both crucial for aging individuals navigating stress and uncertainty. In group devotional settings, rhythmic vocalization can lead to interpersonal entrainment, a neural synchronization across participants that promotes cohesion and a shared sense of presence. Emerging research further suggests that such practices can stabilize the Default Mode Network (DMN), mitigating maladaptive rumination and depressive tendencies often seen in late life.

Devotional singing emerges not only as a spiritual or cultural act but as a comprehensive neurocognitive intervention. It harmonizes emotional expression, social bonding, and cognitive stimulation, activating key brain systems while offering a framework of meaning and connection. Its benefits range from enhanced memory and mood to strengthened identity and neuroplasticity and are delivered through a culturally familiar, low-cost practice that requires no clinical setting. From a neuroscientific perspective, devotional singing embodies an integrative model of resilience, simultaneously engaging the body, mind, and spirit. In doing so, it offers aging individuals a profound resource for navigating the challenges of later life with grace, dignity, and coherence.

Therapeutic and Applied Perspectives

Drawing from the intersection of cultural tradition, psychological insight, and neuroscientific evidence, devotional singing emerges as a compelling modality for therapeutic and practical application, particularly within the domain of aging. As the field of music therapy continues to gain prominence in healthcare and psychological services, there is growing recognition of the need to integrate culturally embedded practices such as devotional singing into mainstream therapeutic frameworks. Within contemporary music therapy, singing is not viewed merely as artistic expression but as a structured, rhythmic, and socially embedded activity capable of promoting both individual and collective well-being (Koole et al., 2015; Särkämö etalk., 2014; Moreno Morales et al., 2020). Devotional singing, with its emphasis on repetition, melody, emotional resonance, and communal participation, aligns seamlessly with these principles. In collectivist societies, where relational connectedness is central to health and well-being, such practices offer not only therapeutic value but cultural congruence.

Empirical studies in music therapy consistently demonstrate the benefits of group singing, highlighting its ability to improve mood, reduce physiological stress, and enhance social connectedness (Fancourt & Finn, 2019; Coulton et al., 2015). Devotional practices such as Naam Kirtan and Sankirtana mirror many of the mechanisms found in evidence-based interventions, including rhythmic entrainment, vocal synchronization, and regulated breathing. These elements contribute to the activation of the vagal nerve, thereby enhancing parasympathetic regulation, a physiological process involved in stress reduction and emotional stability (Bernardi et al., 2001). By integrating these mechanisms into spiritually grounded rituals, devotional singing offers a holistic mind-body practice with significant potential in clinical and community contexts.

Within the field of gerontology, devotional singing presents itself as a low-cost, non-pharmacological intervention with wide-ranging benefits for older adults. Group singing has been shown to stimulate language processing, support memory recall, and alleviate symptoms of depression and loneliness (Davidson & Faulkner, 2010; Johnson et al., 2013). Notably, a recent two-year longitudinal study by Pentikäinen et al. (2023) found that older adults engaged in regular choir singing demonstrated marked improvements in cognitive function and overall, well-being when compared to non-participants. Devotional singing may amplify these benefits by integrating spiritual meaning and intergenerational bonding, which are particularly salient protective factors in culturally rich aging communities. Its accessibility and familiarity further underscore its value in contexts where formal healthcare infrastructure may be limited.

In the Indian context, where elder care often takes place within familial or community settings rather than institutional frameworks, devotional singing circles, temple-based Naam Kirtan gatherings, and Sankirtana performances serve as naturally occurring psychosocial interventions. These spaces foster not only spiritual nourishment but also social integration, reinforcing cultural identity and intergenerational ties. Embedding such practices into formal elder care programs offers the potential to create hybrid models of psychosocial and spiritual support that are both resource-efficient and deeply rooted in community tradition. This approach mirrors successful public health initiatives in other cultural contexts where community choirs have been integrated into mental health and aging programs (Coulton et al., 2015; Feng et al., 2020).

The COVID-19 pandemic further demonstrated the adaptability of devotional practices in the digital age. During periods of social restriction, many communities transitioned to virtual kirtan sessions and livestreamed chanting events, enabling participants to remain connected across geographical boundaries. These virtual gatherings functioned as resilience networks, with participants reporting improvements in mood, reduced loneliness, and a renewed sense of collective belonging (Diareme et al., 2022). Such innovations point toward a hybrid therapeutic model, one that blends in-person ritual with digital access, expanding the reach of devotional singing to accommodate the needs of an increasingly global and aging population.

Taken together, the cultural, psychological, and neuroscientific dimensions of devotional singing reveal its considerable promise as a resilience-enhancing practice for aging populations. Culturally, it sustains group identity and continuity. Psychologically, it supports emotional regulation, stress mitigation, and social belonging. Neurologically, it facilitates autonomic regulation, promotes attentional and memory-related neural activity, and stimulates the release of neurochemicals associated with well-being. These synergistic effects position devotional singing not merely as a spiritual or aesthetic act, but as a holistic intervention that bridges the domains of health, identity, and community.

However, a critical appraisal is necessary to contextualize these benefits within the limitations of current research. Much of the existing literature relies on small-scale or observational studies, often limited by the absence of standardized neurophysiological markers or longitudinal data. Additionally, the diversity of devotional traditions across cultures complicates efforts to construct universal frameworks for clinical application. The deeply spiritual nature of devotional singing also presents a challenge in multicultural or secular settings, where such practices may not resonate with all individuals. There is a pressing need for culturally sensitive implementation strategies that respect individual belief systems and avoid the risks of cultural appropriation. One potential pathway is the development of hybrid or secularized models, allowing for broader accessibility while retaining the therapeutic essence of the practice.

ROL: DEVOTIONAL SINGING AS A NEUROCOGNITIVE INTERVENTION

The growing recognition of devotional singing as a potent force for well-being is underpinned by a diverse body of scientific literature spanning psychology, neuroscience, and music therapy. This section provides a focused review of key studies that elucidate the mechanisms through which devotional singing confers its benefits, particularly for older adults. We will examine how research supports the role of rhythmic vocalization in autonomic regulation, its impact on brain reward circuitry, its unique preservation of musical memory in neurodegenerative conditions, and its broader engagement with emotion and cognitive function.

Autonomic Regulation and Stress Reduction

One of the most immediate physiological effects of rhythmic vocalization, central to devotional singing, is its influence on the autonomic nervous system. Bernardi et al. (2001) conducted pioneering work exploring how controlled breathing and the recitation of mantras impact neurocognitive resilience in older adults. Their study meticulously measured autonomic cardiovascular rhythms, investigating their effects on stress and physiological age-related reactivity. The findings were compelling, demonstrating that structured recitations significantly slowed respiration rates and increased baroreflex sensitivity. These physiological changes are closely linked with biomarkers of parasympathetic (vagal) activation, indicating a shift towards a state of calmness and reduced physiological stress. This research provides a direct physiological basis for the reported stress reduction benefits of devotional singing, suggesting it can serve as a nonpharmacological tool for improving cardiovascular health and emotional stability in aging populations.

Building on this, later research has further explored the vagal nerve's role. Critchley (2009) highlighted the brain's intricate feedback loops with visceral organs, emphasizing how practices that enhance vagal tone can improve emotional regulation and resilience. The sustained, modulated vocal output in devotional singing is a powerful activator of the vagus nerve, which directly influences heart rate variability (HRV). Higher HRV is generally associated with better emotional regulation and greater capacity to adapt to stress. For older adults, who may experience heightened physiological stress due to chronic health conditions or life transitions, these effects are profoundly beneficial, offering a biological pathway to sustained well-being.

Reward Circuitry and Motivation Enhancement

The emotional peaks and profound sense of joy often experienced during devotional singing are not merely subjective; they are rooted in the brain's intricate reward system. Salimpoor et al. (2011) utilized PET and fMRI to examine dopamine release during peak emotional moments versus anticipation in music listening. Their findings highlighted the distinct role of heightened dopamine activity: the caudate nucleus was activated during anticipation, while the nucleus accumbens was prominently engaged during peak emotional experiences. This suggests that devotional singing can effectively leverage the brain's reward circuitry. By stimulating dopamine release, devotional singing enhances motivation and adherence, fostering a positive impact in elders and building resilience. The inherent reward associated with participation can transform a therapeutic practice into an intrinsically motivating activity, increasing consistent engagement, a critical factor for sustained health benefits in older age.

Further studies by Chanda and Levitin (2013) provided a comprehensive review of the neurochemistry of music, noting how musical engagement can modulate neurotransmitter systems, including dopamine, opioids, serotonin, and oxytocin. This neurochemical symphony contributes to the varied emotional responses to music, from pleasure and arousal to sedation and relaxation. For older adults, the consistent activation of these pathways through devotional singing can serve as a natural antidepressant and anxiolytic, improving mood states and combating the prevalence of depression and apathy often observed in later life.

Preservation of Musical Memory and Cognitive Identity

One of the most remarkable aspects of music's impact on the aging brain is the persistence of musical memory, even in the face of significant neurocognitive decline. Jacobsen et al. (2015) conducted a significant review synthesizing data regarding why musical memory often persists in Alzheimer's disease and other forms of dementia. Their findings suggested that musical notes and melodies help preserve neural systems, particularly subcortical and emotion-related connections. This preservation supports the belief that devotional songs, often familiar from youth, become powerful autobiographical anchors, helping individuals maintain a sense of self and continuity even in later stages of life when other forms of memory are severely impaired. This makes devotional singing an invaluable tool for preserving cognitive identity.

Adding to this, Särkämö et al. (2014) demonstrated in a randomized controlled trial that regular musical activities, including singing, can improve cognitive functions, mood, and quality of life in early to moderate stage dementia patients. They observed that singing specifically engaged a broader network of brain regions compared to just listening to music, highlighting its active, multimodal stimulation. For older adults, especially those with emerging cognitive challenges, this active engagement through devotional singing can slow cognitive decline and maintain vital brain connections, offering a dignified way to engage with their past.

Emotion Regulation and General Cognitive Function

Devotional singing is not only about memory; it also serves as a robust mechanism for emotion regulation and broad cognitive engagement. Koelsch (2014) conducted a comprehensive review of brain correlates of music-evoked emotions. His findings strongly suggest that devotional music can co-regulate emotion and support memory encoding or retrieval in aging by eliciting activity across limbic and paralimbic regions, alongside prefrontal areas involved in emotional regulation and appraisal. This means that emotionally meaningful music, like devotional songs, can help process and regulate complex feelings, while simultaneously strengthening memory circuits. This comprehensive engagement contributes to overall neurocognitive health.

Further support for music's role in general cognitive function comes from Bugos et al. (2007), who showed that piano instruction in older adults improved executive functions, including processing speed, planning, and working memory. While devotional singing differs from formal instrumental training, the rhythmic, melodic, and lyrical complexities involved demand significant executive function. Participants must track melody, lyrics, rhythm, and group synchrony, all while managing emotional responses. This multifaceted cognitive demand contributes to a generalized enhancement of executive functions, essential for maintaining independent living and quality of life in older age.

The social dimension of devotional singing also plays a crucial role in its cognitive and emotional benefits. Fancourt and Finn (2019), in their systematic review, highlighted how group singing significantly reduces loneliness and depression in older adults, linking these social benefits to improved cognitive function indirectly. The communal aspect of devotional singing, with its built-in social support network, acts as a powerful buffer against social isolation, a known risk factor for cognitive decline. This reinforces the idea that the practice is not just a personal activity, but a collective intervention with far-reaching benefits.

In summary, the scientific literature provides robust evidence for the profound impact of devotional singing on older adults. From regulating the autonomic nervous system and stimulating reward pathways to preserving musical memory and enhancing general cognitive and emotional regulation, the mechanisms are diverse and interconnected. These studies collectively lay a strong foundation for understanding devotional singing as a multifaceted, culturally resonant, and neuroprotective intervention with significant therapeutic potential for aging populations. The insights gained from these foundational studies further inform the design of targeted research interventions, as outlined in the following section.

SCOPE FOR FUTURE RESEARCH AND PRACTICAL APPLICATION

Building upon the therapeutic potential of devotional singing and acknowledging its current limitations, the next step lies in articulating a structured and evidence-based agenda for future research and implementation. While the practice is rich in cultural significance and supported by promising preliminary data, it remains largely underexplored in formal scientific literature. In particular, there is a lack of systematic operationalization that would allow devotional singing to be integrated into established therapeutic frameworks. To bridge this gap, researchers must develop standardized protocols and apply rigorous methodologies that align with existing practices in music therapy, gerontology, and contemplative science. This would enable the translation of devotional singing from a culturally valued tradition into a clinically recognized intervention for promoting neurocognitive resilience in aging populations.

1. Randomized Controlled Trials (RCTs)

One of the most pressing gaps in the literature is the scarcity of large-scale randomized controlled trials—the gold standard for evaluating therapeutic efficacy. Future research should compare a devotional singing intervention group with appropriate control conditions, such as passive music listening, general social activities, or cognitive stimulation therapy. These trials should be carefully designed to assess specific outcomes such as cognitive stability, emotional regulation, and social connectedness. The use of stratified sampling and diverse participant groups would enhance the external validity and cross-cultural applicability of such interventions.

- **Building on Literature**: Inspired by the work of Särkämö et al. (2014), who used an RCT design to show cognitive and mood benefits of musical activities in dementia, future RCTs focusing on devotional singing should aim to replicate and expand these findings within specific cultural contexts. For instance, an RCT could compare the effects of a Bhajan-based intervention against a generic group singing program to tease out the unique contributions of the spiritual and cultural elements. The outcome measures should be carefully selected to capture both objective cognitive improvements (e.g., using established neuropsychological tests) and subjective reports of well-being and social connection, aligning with the multifaceted benefits observed across the literature.

2. Integration of Bio Physiological and Neurophysiological Monitoring

Moving beyond self-report measures is essential for establishing an objective. By pursuing methodologically rigorous and culturally informed research pathways, the field can move beyond anecdotal or observational insights and toward the formal validation of devotional singing as a therapeutic modality. Bridging traditional spiritual practices with contemporary neuroscience and public health frameworks not only affirms the wisdom of ancient traditions but also introduces scalable, low-cost, high-impact interventions for promoting well-being in aging populations. As global demographics shift toward older age, such integrative strategies may offer timely and transformative solutions to some of the most pressing challenges in geriatric mental health.

CONCLUSION

Despite the limited evidence of the present review, it is important to continue supporting MT as a complementary treatment for older adults with dementia (Moreno-Morales et al., 2020). This observation, made in the context of music therapy, resonates deeply with the central idea of this chapter. The analysis of devotional singing has demonstrated that its benefits extend far beyond the spiritual or cultural, operating as a potent, multi-modal intervention that addresses some of the most pressing challenges of aging. The practice fosters psychological well-being through communal bonding and meaning-making (Baumeister & Leary, 1995; Park, 2010), while simultaneously strengthening neurocognitive resilience via brain plasticity and a unique preservation of musical memory (Jacobsen et al., 2015; Särkämö et al., 2014). It is a low-cost, high-impact modality that aligns with the principles of contemporary therapeutic frameworks, offering a culturally resonant and dignified pathway to successful aging.

The practice of devotional singing is not merely a historical artifact but a living, adaptive tradition with profound potential for integration into clinical and public health frameworks. The future of this lies in bridging the gap between anecdotal wisdom and empirical validation. More studies with larger sample sizes are needed to confirm its effects and efficacy in cognitive and neuropsychiatric symptoms in dementia (Fusar-Poli et al., 2018). This is necessary to develop functional, rigorous, large-scale, and culturally sensitive research models that can formally validate this timeless practice. By pursuing such a research agenda, the full therapeutic potential of devotional singing can be realized, affirming the wisdom of ancient traditions while providing a scalable and transformative solution to the challenges of geriatric mental health.

REFERENCES

Aristotle, . (1987). *Poetics: With the Tractatus Coislinianus, reconstruction of Poetics II, and the fragments of the On Poets* (Janko, R., Trans.). Hackett Publishing Company.

Baumeister, R. F., & Leary, M. R. (1995). The need to belong: Desire for interpersonal attachments as a fundamental human motivation. *Psychological Bulletin, 117*(3), 497–529. DOI: 10.1037/0033-2909.117.3.497

Bernardi, L., Porta, C., Casucci, G., Battistini, L., Sleight, P., & Cavallazzi, L. (2001). Effect of rosary prayer and yoga mantras on autonomic cardiovascular rhythms: A comparative study. *BMJ (Clinical Research Ed.), 323*(7327), 1446–1449. DOI: 10.1136/bmj.323.7327.1446

Bugos, J. A., Perlstein, W. M., McCrae, C. S., Brophy, T. S., & Bedenbaugh, W. H. (2007). Individualized piano instruction enhances executive functioning and working memory in older adults. *Aging & Mental Health, 11*(2), 193–203. DOI: 10.1080/13607860600831032

Cabeza, R., Anderson, N. D., Locantore, J. K., & McIntosh, A. R. (2002). Aging gracefully: Compensatory brain activity in high-performing older adults. *NeuroImage, 17*(3), 1394–1402. DOI: 10.1006/nimg.2002.1281

Chanda, M. L., & Levitin, D. J. (2013). The neurochemistry of music. *Trends in Cognitive Sciences, 17*(4), 179–193. DOI: 10.1016/j.tics.2013.02.007

Coulton, S., Clift, S., Skingley, A., & Rodriguez, J. (2015). Effectiveness and cost-effectiveness of a 14-week singing intervention for older people. *Health & Social Care in the Community, 23*(3), 324–336. DOI: 10.1111/hsc.12140

Critchley, H. D. (2009). The human brain as a central hub for emotional regulation. *Neurobiology of Emotion, 17*(4), 1–15.

Davidson, J. W., & Faulkner, R. (2010). The effects of group singing and performance for marginalized and middle-class singers. *Music Education Research, 12*(4), 447–462. DOI: 10.1080/14613808.2010.518683

Diareme, S., Papatheodorou, K., & Papageorgiou, C. (2022). Coping with stress and anxiety during the COVID-19 pandemic: The role of online social support groups. *International Journal of Environmental Research and Public Health, 19*(2), 978. DOI: 10.3390/ijerph19020978

Durkheim, É. (1995). *The elementary forms of religious life* (Fields, K. E., Trans.). Free Press. (Original work published 1912)

Fancourt, D., & Finn, S. (2019). The effectiveness of group singing for reducing loneliness: A systematic review. *Health Promotion International, 34*(3), 473–481. DOI: 10.1093/heapro/day025

Fang, R., Ye, S., Huang, Y., & Zhang, Y. (2017). Music therapy is a potential intervention for cognition of Alzheimer's disease: A mini-review. *Translational Neurodegeneration, 6*(2). Advance online publication. DOI: 10.1186/s40035-017-0073-9

Feng, H., Lin, Y., & Wei, X. (2018). The potential of community music for relieving feelings of loneliness among older adults in formal care settings. *Social Work in Public Health, 33*(4–5), 329–338. DOI: 10.1080/17533015.2018.1479860

Feng, H., Zhou, J., & Wang, J. (2020). Music and social bonding: A systematic review. *Frontiers in Psychology, 11*, 1096. DOI: 10.3389/fpsyg.2020.01096

Fusar-Poli, L., Casoni, F., & Sensi, F. (2018). The effect of music therapy on cognitive functions in patients with dementia: A systematic review and meta-analysis. *Journal of Alzheimer's Disease, 64*(2), 481–492. DOI: 10.3233/JAD-170792

Gaser, C., & Schlaug, G. (2003). Brain structures differ between musicians and non-musicians. *The Journal of Neuroscience : The Official Journal of the Society for Neuroscience, 23*(27), 9240–9245. DOI: 10.1523/jneurosci.23-27-09240.2003

Hanna-Pladdy, B., & MacKay, A. (2011). The relation between instrumental musical activity and cognitive aging. *Neuropsychology, 25*(3), 378–386. DOI: 10.1037/a0022179

Jacobsen, J.-H., Stelzer, J., & Särkämö, T. (2015). Why musical memory can be preserved in advanced Alzheimer's disease. *Brain, 138*(8), 2122–2124. DOI: 10.1093/brain/awv148

Johnson, J. K., Sherman, S., & Coulton, S. (2013). A community choir intervention to promote well-being among diverse older adults: Results from the community of voices trial. The Journals of Gerontology: Series B, 75(3), 570–579. https://doi.org/ DOI: 10.1093/geronb/gbx134

Keeler, J. R., Roth, E. A., & Neufeld, R. W. J. (2015). The effects of improvised and pre-composed group singing on oxytocin levels. *Frontiers in Psychology, 6*, 1481. DOI: 10.3389/fpsyg.2015.01481

Kim, J., & Yoo, H. S. (2015). Effects of music therapy on cognitive functions in patients with dementia: A systematic review. *Psychiatry Investigation, 12*(4), 489–497. DOI: 10.4306/pi.2015.12.4.489

Koelsch, S. (2014). Brain correlates of music-evoked emotions. *Nature Reviews. Neuroscience, 15*(3), 170–180. DOI: 10.1038/nrn3660

Koole, S. L., van den Hout, M. A., & van Veen, V. (2015). Meditation leads to reduced default mode network activity beyond an active task. *Cognitive, Affective & Behavioral Neuroscience, 15*(3), 712–720. DOI: 10.3758/s13415-015-0358-3

Mansens, H., van den Heuvel, M. P., & van den Heuvel, M. P. (2018). Music as a form of cognitive training: A systematic review of the neuroplastic effects of musical training. *Frontiers in Human Neuroscience, 12*, 169. DOI: 10.3389/fnhum.2018.00169

Moreno-Morales, M. A., Roldán, M. E., & Martínez-Roldán, M. E. (2020). Active music therapy on cognition and neuropsychiatric symptoms in the elderly with mild and moderate dementia: A preliminary study. *Jornal Brasileiro de Psiquiatria, 69*(2), 108–114. DOI: 10.1590/0047-2085000000277

Park, C. L. (2010). The meaning making model: A framework for understanding how we cope with life's big events. *Psychology of Religion and Spirituality, 2*(4), 180–191. DOI: 10.1037/a0020499

Pentikäinen, E., Kimppa, L., Pitkäniemi, A., Lahti, O., & Särkämö, T. (2023). Longitudinal effects of choir singing on aging cognition and wellbeing: A two-year follow-up study. *Frontiers in Human Neuroscience, 17*, 1174574. DOI: 10.3389/fnhum.2023.1174574

Pentikäinen, E., Pitkäniemi, A., & Särkämö, T. (2021). Group singing programs for well-being of older adults: An in-person quantitative follow-up. *Dementia and Geriatric Cognitive Disorders. Extra, 11*(2), 163–172. DOI: 10.1159/000516086

Román-Caballero, R., Román-Caballero, J., & Morales-Román, J. (2018). Cognitive and brain plasticity induced by physical exercise, cognitive training, video games, and combined interventions. *Frontiers in Human Neuroscience, 12*, 25. DOI: 10.3389/fnhum.2018.00025

Salimpoor, V. N., Benovoy, M., Larcher, K., Dagher, A., & Zatorre, R. J. (2011). Anatomically distinct dopamine release during anticipation and experience of peak emotion to music. *Nature Neuroscience, 14*(2), 257–262. DOI: 10.1038/nn.2726

Särkämö, T., Laitinen, S., & Särkämö, T. (2014). Music therapy in the rehabilitation of cognitive functions after stroke. *Neuroscience and Biobehavioral Reviews, 40*, 1–13. DOI: 10.1016/j.neubiorev.2014.01.002

Compilation of References

Abadir, P. M., Chellappa, R., Choudhry, N., Demiris, G., Ganesan, D., Karlawish, J., & Schoenborn, N. L. (2023). The promise of AI and technology to improve quality of life and care for older adults. *Nature Aging*, *3*(6), 629–631. DOI: 10.1038/s43587-023-00424-7 PMID: 37231197

Abadir, P., & Chellappa, R. (2024). Artificial intelligence in geriatrics: Riding the inevitable tide of promise, challenges, and considerations. *The Journals of Gerontology. Series A, Biological Sciences and Medical Sciences*, *79*(2), glad279. Advance online publication. DOI: 10.1093/gerona/glad279 PMID: 38289911

Abah, T., & Onwelumadu, I. (2025). Equity: Integrated care for underserved populations. *International Perspectives and Experiences Enhancing Access to Healthcare*, 119.

Abdi, J., Al-Hindawi, A., Ng, T., & Vizcaychipi, M. P. (2018). Scoping review on the use of socially assistive robot technology in elderly care. *BMJ Open*, *8*(2), e018815. PMID: 29440212

Abdulmalek, S., Nasir, A., Jabbar, W. A., Almuhaya, M. A., Bairagi, A. K., Khan, M. A. M., & Kee, S. H. (2022). IoT-based healthcare-monitoring system towards improving quality of life: A review. *Health Care*, *10*(10), 1993. Advance online publication. DOI: 10.3390/healthcare10101993 PMID: 36292441

Abou Hashish, E. A., & Alnajjar, H. (2024). Digital proficiency: Assessing knowledge, attitudes, and skills in digital transformation, health literacy, and artificial intelligence among university nursing students. *BMC Medical Education*, *24*(1), 508.

Adams, D. M., Brown, P. G., Williams, M., Bromfield, L., & Bunting-Clarke, J. (2022). Assessment of rational use of medicines for chronic non-communicable diseases: A cross-sectional design in a public access clinic in Jamaica. *Journal of Public Health Research*, *11*(3). Advance online publication. DOI: 10.1177/22799036221126348 PMID: 36204195

Aditya Shastry, K., & Sanjay, H. A. (2024). Artificial intelligence techniques for the effective diagnosis of Alzheimer's disease: A review. *Multimedia Tools and Applications*. Advance online publication. DOI: 10.1007/s11042-024-18327-4

Aggarwal, R., Farag, S., Martin, G., Ashrafian, H., & Darzi, A. (2021). Patient perceptions on data sharing and applying artificial intelligence to health care data: Cross-sectional survey. *Journal of Medical Internet Research, 23*(8), e26162.

Agha, R. A., Mathew, G., Rashid, R., Kerwan, A., Al-Jabir, A., Sohrabi, C., & Agha, M. (2025). Revised Strengthening the reporting of cohort, cross-sectional and case-control studies in surgery (STROCSS) Guideline: An update for the age of Artificial Intelligence. *Premier Journal of Science*, *10*, 100081.

Aher, R. B., Jadhav, S., Sharma, Y., & Pawar, P. (2024). A review on new trends of artificial intelligence in medicine. *Open Access Journal of Data Science and Artificial Intelligence*, *2*(1), 1–12.

Ahirwal, M. K., Londhe, N. D., & Kumar, A. (2022). *Artificial intelligence applications for health care*. CRC Press.

Ahmad, I., Asghar, Z., Kumar, T., Li, G., Manzoor, A., Mikhaylov, K., & Harjula, E. (2022). Emerging technologies for next generation remote health care and assisted living. *IEEE Access : Practical Innovations, Open Solutions*, *10*, 56094–56132. DOI: 10.1109/ACCESS.2022.3177278

Ahmed, S. H., Meyer, H. E., Kjøllesdal, M. K., Marjerrison, N., Mdala, I., & Htet, A. S.. (2019). The prevalence of selected risk factors for non-communicable diseases in Hargeisa, Somaliland: A cross-sectional study. *BMC Public Health*, *19*(1), 878. DOI: 10.1186/s12889-019-7101-x PMID: 31272414

Ahsan, M. M., Luna, S. A., & Siddique, Z. (2022). Machine-learning-based disease diagnosis: A comprehensive review. *Health Care*, *10*(3), 541. DOI: 10.3390/healthcare10030541 PMID: 35327018

Ahuja, A. S. (2019). The impact of artificial intelligence in medicine on the future role of the physician [PMID: 31592346; PMC6779111. Authoritative review on AI augmenting physicians]. *PeerJ*, *7*, e7702. DOI: 10.7717/peerj.7702

Aïdoud, A., Gana, W., Poitau, F., Debacq, C., Leroy, V., Nkodo, J. A., & Fougère, B. (2023). High prevalence of geriatric conditions among older adults with cardiovascular disease. *Journal of the American Heart Association*, *12*(2), e026850. Advance online publication. DOI: 10.1161/JAHA.122.026850 PMID: 36628962

Ajaykumar, G., & Huang, C. M. (2023). Older adults' task preferences for robot assistance in the home. [PDF].

Ajaykumar, G., & Huang, C. M. (2023). Older adults' task preferences for robot assistance in the home. *arXiv*. https://doi.org//arXiv.2303.03926DOI: 10.48550

Akpobome, O. (2024). The impact of emerging technologies on legal frameworks: A model for adaptive regulation. *International Journal of Research Publication and Reviews*, *5*(10), 5046–5060. DOI: 10.55248/gengpi.5.1024.58372

Akyon, S. H., Akyon, F. C., & Yılmaz, T. E. (2023). Artificial intelligence-supported web application design and development for reducing polypharmacy side effects and supporting rational drug use in geriatric patients. *Frontiers in medicine*, *10*, 1029198.

Albahri, A. S., Duhaim, A. M., Fadhel, M. A., Alnoor, A., Baqer, N. S., Alzubaidi, L., & Deveci, M. (2023). A systematic review of trustworthy and explainable artificial intelligence in healthcare: Assessment of quality, bias risk, and data fusion. *Information Fusion*, *96*, 156–191. DOI: 10.1016/j.inffus.2023.03.008

Albert, S. M., & Cattell, M. G. (1994). Family relationships of the elderly: living arrangements. In Albert, S. M., Cattell, M. G., & Hall, G. K. (Eds.), *Old Age in Global Perspective: Cross-Cultural and Cross-National Views* (pp. 85–107).

Aldboush, H. H. H., & Ferdous, M. (2023). Building trust in fintech: An analysis of ethical and privacy considerations in the intersection of big data, AI, and customer trust. *International Journal of Financial Studies*, *11*(4), 135. DOI: 10.3390/ijfs11040135

Aldoseri, A., Al-Khalifa, K. N., & Hamouda, A. M. (2023). Re-thinking data strategy and integration for artificial intelligence: Concepts, opportunities, and challenges. *Applied Sciences (Basel, Switzerland)*, *13*(12), 7082. Advance online publication. DOI: 10.3390/app13127082

Aleti, T., Brennan, L., & Parker, L. (2024). Social engagement and technology: Supporting connection in older adulthood. *Journal of Social Marketing*, *14*(2), 189–204. DOI: 10.1108/JSOCM-08-2023-0176

Aleti, T., Figueiredo, B., Martin, D. M., & Reid, M. (2024). Digital inclusion in later life: Older adults' socialisation processes in learning and using technology. *Australasian Marketing Journal*, *32*(4), 295–307. DOI: 10.1177/14413582241258266

Alexopoulos, P., Bogati, U., Farombi, T., & Shrestha, P. (2025). Experiences from designing and implementing integrated health and social care systems for aging populations in low-resource settings around the world. *Dementia Care and Provision in the Majority World: Epidemiology, Diagnosis and Care in Low-and Middle-income Nations*, 117.

Alharbi, H. A., Alharbi, K. K., & Hassan, C. A. U. (2023). Enhancing elderly fall detection through IoT-enabled smart flooring and AI for independent living sustainability. *Sustainability*, *15*(22), 15695.

Ali, A. T., Zeeshan, M. N., Khaleeq, A., Jamil, M. N., Khan, U., Siddiqui, A., & Ahmad, S. (2025). Ethical-legal implications of AI-powered healthcare in critical perspective. *Frontiers in Artificial Intelligence*, *8*. Advance online publication. DOI: 10.3389/frai.2025.1619463

Alievska, B. (2023). *Ethical challenges arising from the underrepresentation of the elderly in the development of artificial intelligence (AI) for medical applications: Exclusion, bias, and solutions* [Master's thesis, McMaster University]. MacSphere. http://hdl.handle.net/11375/28768

Ali, H., & Li, H. (2019). Evaluating a smartwatch notification system in a simulated nursing home. *International Journal of Older People Nursing*, *14*(3), e12241. DOI: 10.1111/opn.12241 PMID: 31099184

Ali, H., & Nikberg, N. (2024). Bias in AI-driven healthcare: Navigating ethical challenges at an early stage. *Journal of Service Science and Management*, *17*(2), 305–320.

Almaeeni, H. (2024). Review on Artificial Intelligence in Medicine and Health. *2024 IEEE International Conference on Medical Artificial Intelligence (MedAI).*

Alonso Salinas, G. L., Cepas-Guillén, P., León, A. M., Jiménez-Méndez, C., Lozano-Vicario, L., Martínez-Avial, M., & Díez-Villanueva, P. (2024). The impact of geriatric conditions in elderly patients with coronary heart disease: A state-of-the-art review. *Journal of Clinical Medicine*, *13*(7), 1891. Advance online publication. DOI: 10.3390/jcm13071891 PMID: 38610656

Alpaydin, E. (2021). *Machine learning*. MIT Press.

Alruwaili, M. M., Abuadas, F. H., Alsadi, M., Alruwaili, A. N., Elsayed Ramadan, O. M., Shaban, M., & El Arab, R. A. (2024). Exploring nurses' awareness and attitudes toward artificial intelligence: Implications for nursing practice. *Digital Health*, *10*, 20552076241271803.

AlZaabi, A., & AlMaskari, S., & AalAbdulsalam, A. (2023). Are physicians and medical students ready for artificial intelligence applications in healthcare? *Digital Health*, *9*, 20552076231152167.

Alzeer, J. (2023). Integrating medicine with lifestyle for personalized and holistic healthcare. *Journal of Public Health and Emergency*, *7*, 20. DOI: 10.21037/jphe-23-16

Amato, F., Di Gregorio, M., Monaco, C., Sebillo, M., Tortora, G., & Vitiello, G. (2021, January). Socially assistive robotics combined with artificial intelligence for ADHD. In *2021 IEEE 18th Annual Consumer Communications & Networking Conference (CCNC)* (pp. 1-6). IEEE.

Amato, F., Di Gregorio, M., Monaco, C., Sebillo, M., Tortora, G., & Vitiello, G. (2020, September). The therapeutic use of humanoid robots for behavioral disorders. In *Proceedings of the 2020 International Conference on Advanced Visual Interfaces* (pp. 1-3).

Aminizadeh, S., Heidari, A., Dehghan, M., Toumaj, S., Rezaei, M., Navimipour, N. J., & Unal, M. (2024). Opportunities and challenges of artificial intelligence and distributed systems to improve the quality of healthcare service. *Artificial Intelligence in Medicine, 149*, 102779. Advance online publication. DOI: 10.1016/j.artmed.2024.102779 PMID: 38462281

Amin, M. G., Zhang, Y. D., Ahmad, F., & Ho, K. C. D. (2016). Radar signal processing for elderly fall detection: The future for in-home monitoring. *IEEE Signal Processing Magazine, 33*(2), 71–80. DOI: 10.1109/MSP.2015.2502784

Anand, A., & Singh, P. (2025). *Interdisciplinary Studies: Issues, Perspectives, and Challenges From National Education Program 2020*. Integrating Personalized Learning Methods Into STEAM Education.

Andino, J. J., Eyrich, N. W., & Boxer, R. J. (2023). Overview of telehealth in the United States since the COVID-19 public health emergency: A narrative review. *mHealth, 9*, 26. DOI: 10.21037/mhealth-23-15 PMID: 37492124

Apell, P., & Eriksson, H. (2023). Artificial intelligence (AI) healthcare technology innovations: The current state and challenges from a life science industry perspective. *Technology Analysis and Strategic Management, 35*(2), 179–193.

Aregbeshola, B. S., & Khan, S. M. (2018). Determinants of catastrophic health expenditure in Nigeria. *The European Journal of Health Economics, 19*(4), 521–532. DOI: 10.1007/s10198-017-0899-1 PMID: 28555372

Aristotle, . (1987). *Poetics: With the Tractatus Coislinianus, reconstruction of Poetics II, and the fragments of the On Poets* (Janko, R., Trans.). Hackett Publishing Company.

Aronsson, A. (2022). Professional Women and Elder Care in Contemporary Japan: Anxiety and the Move Toward Technocare. *Anthropology & Aging, 43*(1).

Aryal, K. K., Mehata, S., Neupane, S., Vaidya, A., Dhimal, M., & Dhakal, P.. (2015). The burden and determinants of non communicable diseases risk factors in Nepal: Findings from a nationwide STEPS survey. *PLoS One*, *10*(8). Advance online publication. DOI: 10.1371/journal.pone.0134834 PMID: 26244512

Ashfaq, M., Yun, J., Yu, S., & Loureiro, S. M. C. (2020). I, chatbot: Modeling the determinants of users' satisfaction and continuance intention of AI-powered service agents. *Telematics and Informatics*, *54*, 101473. DOI: 10.1016/j.tele.2020.101473

Asrifan, A., Said, U. M. R., Jakob, J. C., & Wanci, R. (2025). AI literacy: Foundations, importance, and broader implications. In *Transforming vocational education and training using AI* (pp. 17–48). IGI Global., DOI: 10.4018/979-8-3693-9501-1.ch002

Avula, R. A. M. Y. A. (2021). Addressing barriers in data collection, transmission, and security to optimize data availability in healthcare systems for improved clinical decision-making and analytics. *Applied Research in Artificial Intelligence and Cloud Computing*, *4*(1), 78–93. DOI: 10.47363/araicc/2021(4)112

Awotunde, J. B., Ajagbe, S. A., & Florez, H. (2022, October). Internet of things with wearable devices and artificial intelligence for elderly uninterrupted healthcare monitoring systems. In *International Conference on Applied Informatics* (pp. 278-291). Cham: Springer International Publishing.

Badawy, W., & Shaban, M. (2025). Exploring geriatric nurses' perspectives on the adoption of AI in elderly care: A qualitative study. *Geriatric Nursing*, *61*, 32–39. DOI: 10.1016/j.gerinurse.2024.11.013 PMID: 39541631

Baek, Y. S., Lee, D. H., Jo, Y., Lee, S. C., Choi, W., & Kim, D. H. (2023). Artificial intelligence-estimated biological heart age using a 12-lead electrocardiogram predicts mortality and cardiovascular outcomes. *Frontiers in Cardiovascular Medicine*, *10*, 1137892.

Băjenaru, O. L., Băjenaru, L., Ianculescu, M., Constantin, V. ., Gu atu, A. M., & Nu ă, C. R. (2024). Geriatric healthcare supported by decision-making tools integrated into digital health solutions. *Electronics (Basel)*, *13*(17), 3440. Advance online publication. DOI: 10.3390/electronics13173440

Bala, I., Pindoo, I., Mijwil, M. M., Abotaleb, M., & Yundong, W. (2024). Ensuring security and privacy in healthcare systems: A review exploring challenges, solutions, future trends, and the practical applications of artificial intelligence. *Jordan Medical Journal*, *58*(3), 143–154. DOI: 10.35516/jmj.v58i3.2346

Banaji, M. R., Fiske, S. T., & Massey, D. S. (2021). Systemic racism: Individuals and interactions, institutions and society. *Cognitive Research: Principles and Implications*, *6*(1), 82. DOI: 10.1186/s41235-021-00349-3 PMID: 34931287

Banner, L., & Olney, C. M. (2009). Automated clinical documentation: Does it allow nurses more time for patient care? CIN: Computers, Informatics. *Nursing*, *27*(2), 75–81. DOI: 10.1097/NCN.0b013e3181979e57 PMID: 21685832

Barasa, E. W., Maina, T., & Ravishankar, N. (2017). Assessing the impoverishing effects, and factors associated with the incidence of catastrophic health care payments in Kenya. *International Journal for Equity in Health*, *16*(1), 1–14. DOI: 10.1186/s12939-017-0526-x PMID: 28166779

Barbosa Neves, B., Waycott, J., & Maddox, A. (2023). When technologies are not enough: The challenges of digital interventions to address loneliness in later life. *Sociological Research Online*, *28*(1), 150–170. DOI: 10.1177/13607804221131694

Barbosa, L. M., Monteiro, R., & Santos, J. (2023). Technology-mediated socialization for older adults: Challenges and opportunities. *Ageing International*, *48*(4), 112–130. DOI: 10.1007/s12126-023-09512-7

Basmacı, G. (2022). Prioritizing challenges in AI applications in healthcare: Multi-criteria decision making approach. *Nevşehir Hacı Bektaş Veli Üniversitesi SBE Dergisi*, *12*(2), 873–885. DOI: 10.30783/nevsosbilen.1084242

Batakis, D., Chatzivasileiou, S., & Efthymiou, I. P. (2025). Artificial Intelligence and its impact on healthcare. *World Journal of Advanced Research and Reviews*, *26*(1), 250–256. DOI: 10.30574/wjarr.2025.26.1.1015

Batakis, D., Sidiropoulos, S., Emmanouil-Kalos, A., Fouskas, T., Zopounidis, C., & Vozikis, A. (2023). Medical tourism in the region of Crete, Greece: Perspectives from healthcare providers, hotel managers, and medical tourists. *Sustainability*, *15*(24), 16822. DOI: 10.3390/su152416822

Baumeister, R. F., & Leary, M. R. (1995). The need to belong: Desire for interpersonal attachments as a fundamental human motivation. *Psychological Bulletin*, *117*(3), 497–529. DOI: 10.1037/0033-2909.117.3.497

Bavli, I., Ho, A., Mahal, R., & McKeown, M. J. (2025). Ethical concerns around privacy and data security in AI health monitoring for Parkinson's disease: Insights from patients, family members, and healthcare professionals. *AI & Society*, *40*(1), 155–165.

Bekbolatova, M., Mayer, J., Ong, C. W., & Toma, M. (2024). Transformative potential of AI in healthcare: Definitions, applications, and navigating the ethical landscape and public perspectives. *Health Care*, *12*(3), 346. DOI: 10.3390/healthcare12030346 PMID: 38255014

Belmin, J., Villani, P., Gay, M., Fabries, S., Havreng-Théry, C., Malvoisin, S., & Veyron, J. H. (2022). Real-world implementation of an eHealth system based on artificial intelligence designed to predict and reduce emergency department visits by older adults: Pragmatic trial. *Journal of Medical Internet Research*, *24*(9), e40387.

Benzinger, L., Epping, J., Ursin, F., Balke, W.-T., Kacprowski, T., & Salloch, S. (2024). Artificial intelligence to support ethical decision-making for incapacitated patients: A survey among German anesthesiologists and internists [Recent 2024 study on human oversight and AI in medical decision-making; PubMed indexed]. *BMC Medical Ethics*, *25*(1), 78. DOI: 10.1186/s12910-024-01079-z PMID: 39026308

Berdahl, C. T., Baker, L., Mann, S., Osoba, O., & Girosi, F. (2023). Strategies to improve the impact of artificial intelligence on health equity: Scoping review. *JMIR AI*, *2*, e42936. DOI: 10.2196/42936 PMID: 38875587

Bernal, M. C., Batista, E., Martínez-Ballesté, A., & Solanas, A. (2024). Artificial intelligence for the study of human ageing: A systematic literature review. *Applied Intelligence*, *54*(22), 11949–11977. DOI: 10.1007/s10489-024-05702-8

Bernardi, L., Porta, C., Casucci, G., Battistini, L., Sleight, P., & Cavallazzi, L. (2001). Effect of rosary prayer and yoga mantras on autonomic cardiovascular rhythms: A comparative study. *BMJ (Clinical Research Ed.)*, *323*(7327), 1446–1449. DOI: 10.1136/bmj.323.7327.1446

Berridge, C., Tyler, D. A., & Miller, S. C. (2018). Staff empowerment practices and CNA retention: Findings from a nationally representative nursing home culture change survey. *Journal of Applied Gerontology*, *37*(4), 419–434. DOI: 10.1177/0733464816653478 PMID: 27566304

Bertolazzi, A., Quaglia, V., & Bongelli, R. (2024). Barriers and facilitators to health technology adoption by older adults with chronic diseases: An integrative systematic review. *BMC Public Health*, *24*(1), 1–24. DOI: 10.1186/s12889-024-17786-0 PMID: 38365698

Betlej, A. (2023). Designing for successful ageing: The role of technology in fostering social relationships. *Gerontechnology (Valkenswaard)*, *22*(3), 45–56. DOI: 10.4017/gt.2023.22.3.002

Betlej, A. (2023). Social networks, new technologies, and wellbeing—An interview study on factors influencing older adults' successful ageing. *International Journal of Environmental Research and Public Health, 20*(7), 5279. DOI: 10.3390/ijerph20075279 PMID: 37047895

Betriana, F., Tanioka, R., Gunawan, J., & Locsin, R. C. (2022). Healthcare robots and human generations: Consequences for nursing and healthcare. *Collegian (Royal College of Nursing, Australia), 29*, 767–773. DOI: 10.1016/j.colegn.2022.01.008

Bevilacqua, R., Barbarossa, F., Fantechi, L., Fornarelli, D., Paci, E., Bolognini, S., & Maranesi, E. (2023). Radiomics and artificial intelligence for the diagnosis and monitoring of Alzheimer's disease: A systematic review of studies in the field. *Journal of Clinical Medicine, 12*(16), 5432.

Bhambri, P., & Khang, A. (2024). Managing and monitoring patient's healthcare using AI and IoT technologies. In Khang, A. (Ed.), *Driving smart medical diagnosis through AI-powered technologies and applications* (pp. 1–23). IGI Global., DOI: 10.4018/979-8-3693-3679-3.ch001

Bharat, P. S., Narkhede, K. B., Prajapati, A., Narkhede, S. B., & Luhar, S. (2025). Impact of digital health technologies on medication adherence. *Asian Journal of Research in Pharmaceutical Sciences, 15*(2), 141–146. DOI: 10.52711/2231-5659.2025.00022

Bhattacharya, S., Hossain, M. M., Juyal, R., Sharma, N., Pradhan, K. B., & Singh, A. (2021). Role of Public Health Ethics for Responsible Use of Artificial Intelligence Technologies. *Indian Journal of Community Medicine : Official Publication of Indian Association of Preventive & Social Medicine, 46*(2), 178. PMID: 34321721

Bhuiyan, M. N., Rahman, M. M., Billah, M. M., & Saha, D. (2021). Internet of Things (IoT): A review of its enabling technologies in healthcare applications, standards protocols, security, and market opportunities. *IEEE Internet of Things Journal, 8*(13), 10474–10498. DOI: 10.1109/JIOT.2021.3062630

Binns, R., Veale, M., Van Kleek, M., & Shadbolt, N. (2018). "It's reducing a human being to a percentage": Perceptions of justice in algorithmic decisions. *Proceedings of the 2018 CHI Conference on Human Factors in Computing Systems* (Paper 377, 14 pp.). Association for Computing Machinery. https://doi.org/DOI: 10.1145/3173574.3173951

Bloom, D. E., Cafiero, E. T., Jané-Llopis, E., Abrahams-Gessel, S., Bloom, L. R., Fathima, S., ... The Global Economic Burden of Noncommunicable Diseases. World Economic Forum; 2011.

Bloom, D. E., Chatterji, S., Kowal, P., Lloyd-Sherlock, P., McKee, M., Rechel, B., Rosenberg, L., & Smith, J. P. (2015). Macroeconomic implications of population ageing and selected policy responses. *The Lancet, 385*(9968), 649–657. [https://doi.org/DOI: 10.1016/S0140-6736(14)61464-1

Bloom, D. E., Canning, D., & Lubet, A. (2015). Global population aging: Facts, challenges, solutions & perspectives. *Daedalus*, *144*(2), 80–92.

Bloom, D. E., & Luca, D. L. (2016). The global demography of aging: Facts, explanations, future. In *Handbook of the Economics of Population Aging* (Vol. 1, pp. 3–56). Elsevier.

Boamah, S. A., Weldrick, R., Lee, T. S. J., & Taylor, N. (2021). Social isolation among older adults in long-term care: A scoping review. *Journal of Aging and Health*, *33*(7–8), 618–632. DOI: 10.1177/08982643211004174 PMID: 33779366

Bokolo, A. J. (2023). Inclusive and safe mobility needs of senior citizens: Implications for age-friendly cities and communities. *Urban Science (Basel, Switzerland)*, *7*(4), 103.

Bongaarts, J., & Zimmer, Z. 2001 ' Living Arrangements of Older Adults in the Developing World: An Analysis of DHS Household Surveys ', DHS Comparative Report No. 148, Calverton, MD.

Borna, S., Maniaci, M. J., Haider, C. R., Gomez-Cabello, C. A., Pressman, S. M., Haider, S. A., & Forte, A. J. (2024). Artificial intelligence support for informal patient caregivers: A systematic review. *Bioengineering (Basel, Switzerland)*, *11*(5), 483. Advance online publication. DOI: 10.3390/bioengineering11050483 PMID: 38790350

Božić, V. (2023). *Implementation of Artifical Intelligent (AI)*. Solutions to Help Elderly People.

Bramhankar, M., Pandey, M., Rana, G. S., Rai, B., Mishra, N. L., & Shukla, A. (2021). An assessment of anthropometric indices and its association with NCDs among the older adults of India: Evidence from LASI Wave-1. *BMC Public Health*, *21*(1), 1357. DOI: 10.1186/s12889-021-11421-4 PMID: 34238276

Broadbent, E., Loveys, K., Ilan, G., Chen, G., Chilukuri, M. M., Boardman, S. G., & Skuler, D. (2024). ElliQ, an AI-driven social robot to alleviate loneliness: Progress and lessons learned. *The Journal of Aging Research & Lifestyle*, *13*, 22–28.

Brown, S., & Desai, A. (2023). Legal and regulatory issues related to the use of clinical software in healthcare delivery. In Elkin, P. L. (Ed.), *Clinical decision support and beyond* (pp. 571–598). Academic Press., DOI: 10.1016/B978-0-323-91200-6.00014-5

Brunzini, A., Caragiuli, M., Massera, C., & Mandolini, M. (2023). Healthy ageing: A decision-support algorithm for the patient-specific assignment of ICT devices and services. *Health Care*, *11*(12), 1698. DOI: 10.3390/healthcare11121698 PMID: 37372816

Brynjolfsson, E., & McAfee, A. (2017). *Machine, platform, crowd: Harnessing our digital future*. W. W. Norton & Company.

Bugos, J. A., Perlstein, W. M., McCrae, C. S., Brophy, T. S., & Bedenbaugh, W. H. (2007). Individualized piano instruction enhances executive functioning and working memory in older adults. *Aging & Mental Health*, *11*(2), 193–203. DOI: 10.1080/13607860600831032

Bulbul, A. H., Gunaydin, S., & Odabasi, H. F. (2022). Embracing older adults in online learning. *Turkish Online Journal of Educational Technology-TOJET*, *21*(1), 55–67.

Cabeza, R., Anderson, N. D., Locantore, J. K., & McIntosh, A. R. (2002). Aging gracefully: Compensatory brain activity in high-performing older adults. *NeuroImage*, *17*(3), 1394–1402. DOI: 10.1006/nimg.2002.1281

Cafolla, D. (2024). Exploration of AI-enhanced wearable devices for advanced cardiovascular monitoring in the elderly. In *International Conference on AI in Healthcare* (pp. 185–197).

Camacho, P. A., Gomez-Arbelaez, D., Otero, J., González-Gómez, S., Molina, D. I., & Sanchez, G.. (2020). Self-reported prevalence of chronic non-communicable diseases in relation to socioeconomic and educational factors in colombia: A community-based study in 11 departments. *Global Heart*, *15*(1). Advance online publication. DOI: 10.5334/GH.792 PMID: 32489808

Camargos, M. C. S., Rodrigues, R. N., & Machado, C. J. (2018). Demographic transition and population aging in Brazil. *Revista Brasileira de Estudos de População, 35*(1), 1–23.

Cantone, A. A., Esposito, M., Perillo, F. P., Romano, M., Sebillo, M., & Vitiello, G. (2023). Enhancing elderly health monitoring: Achieving autonomous and secure living through the integration of artificial intelligence, autonomous robots, and sensors. *Electronics (Basel)*, *12*(18), 3918.

Carpenter, A., Islam, M. M., Yen, L., & McRae, I. (2015). Affordability of out-of-pocket health care expenses among older Australians. *Health Policy (Amsterdam)*, *119*(7), 907–914. DOI: 10.1016/j.healthpol.2015.03.010 PMID: 25896218

Cary, M. P.Jr, Bessias, S., McCall, J., Pencina, M. J., Grady, S. D., Lytle, K., & Economou-Zavlanos, N. J. (2025). Empowering nurses to champion Health equity & BE FAIR: Bias elimination for fair and responsible AI in healthcare. *Journal of Nursing Scholarship*, *57*(1), 130–139. PMID: 39075715

Cassel, C., & Fulmer, T. (2022). Achieving diagnostic excellence for older patients. *Journal of the American Medical Association*, *327*(18), 1765–1766. DOI: 10.1001/jama.2022.5576 PMID: 35175301

CDP. (2023, November). *Technical Annex IV: Scope 3 overview and modelling*. https://cdn.cdp.net/cdp-production/comfy/cms/files/files/000/008/613/original/Technical_Annex_IV_Scope_3_Overview_and_Modelling_2023.pdf

Cesario, A., D'Oria, M., Calvani, R., Picca, A., Pietragalla, A., Lorusso, D., & Scambia, G. (2021). The role of artificial intelligence in managing multimorbidity and cancer. *Journal of Personalized Medicine*, *11*(4), 314.

Chaccour, C., Saad, W., Debbah, M., Han, Z., & Poor, H. V. (2024). Less data, more knowledge: Building next-generation semantic communication networks. *IEEE Communications Surveys and Tutorials*, *27*(1), 37–76. DOI: 10.1109/COMST.2024.3389479

Chaichareenon, K., & Nupairoj, N. (2024, June). Data-driven with process mining to analyze and identify key features for no-show risks in patients with chronic diseases to achieve treatment improvement. In *2024 21st International Joint Conference on Computer Science and Software Engineering (JCSSE)* (pp. 192–198). IEEE. https://doi.org/DOI: 10.1100/JCSSE61076.2024.10586524

Chanda, M. L., & Levitin, D. J. (2013). The neurochemistry of music. *Trends in Cognitive Sciences*, *17*(4), 179–193. DOI: 10.1016/j.tics.2013.02.007

Chang, J., Wu, Y., Zhao, Y., Gao, X., Xing, Y., Wang, Z., & Tang, Y. (2025). Cohort profile: China healthy aging cohort study (China-Aging). *Journal of Alzheimer's Disease*, •••, 13872877251360028.

Chan, R. J., Milch, V. E., Crawford-Williams, F., Agbejule, O. A., Joseph, R., Johal, J., & Hart, N. H. (2023). Patient navigation across the cancer care continuum: An overview of systematic reviews and emerging literature. *CA: a Cancer Journal for Clinicians*, *73*(6), 565–589. DOI: 10.3322/caac.21788 PMID: 37358040

Charow, R., Jeyakumar, T., Younus, S., Dolatabadi, E., Salhia, M., Al-Mouaswas, D., & Wiljer, D. (2021). Artificial intelligence education programs for health care professionals: Scoping review. *JMIR Medical Education*, *7*(4), e31043. DOI: 10.2196/31043 PMID: 34898458

Chatzivasileiou, S., Emmanouil-Kalos, A., Efthymiou Egleton, I. P., Batakis, D., & Vozikis, A. (2023). Mapping the Donations of Pharma Companies in Greece: The Case of Scientific Societies. *International Journal of Non-Profit Sector Empowerment, 2*(1), e34419. DOI: 10.12681/npse.34419

Chaudhuri, A., & Roy, K. 2007 Gender Differences in Living Arrangements among Older Persons in India, [Online] Available at: https://ssrn.com/abstract=987327 (accessed 17 August 2011).

Chen, C., Ding, S., & Wang, J. (2023). Digital health for aging populations. *Nature Medicine, 29*(7), 1623–1630.

Chen, F., & Short, S. E. (2008). Household context and subjective well-being among the oldest old in China. *Journal of Family Issues, 29*(10), 1379–1403. PMID: 19554216

Cheng, X., Qiao, L., Yang, B., & Li, Z. (2024). An investigation on the influencing factors of elderly people's intention to use financial AI customer service. *Internet Research, 34*(3), 690–717.

Chen, H., Zhang, Y., & Wang, L. (2023). A study on the quality evaluation index system of smart home care for older adults in the community——based on Delphi and AHP. *BMC Public Health, 23*(1), 411.

Chen, K., & Chan, A. H. S. (2014). Gerontechnology acceptance by elderly Hong Kong Chinese: A senior technology acceptance model (STAM). *Ergonomics, 57*(5), 635–652. PMID: 24655221

Chen, K., Lou, V. W.-Q., Tan, K. C.-K., Wai, M.-Y., & Chan, L.-L. (2020). Effects of a humanoid companion robot on dementia symptoms and caregiver distress for residents in long-term care. *Journal of the American Medical Directors Association, 21*(11), 1724–1728. DOI: 10.1016/j.jamda.2020.05.036 PMID: 32713772

Chen, M., Cui, D., Haick, H., & Tang, N. (2024). Artificial intelligence-based medical sensors for healthcare system. *Advanced Sensor Research, 3*(8), 2300179. Advance online publication. DOI: 10.1002/adsr.202300179

Chen, R. J., Wang, J. J., Williamson, D. F. K., Chen, T. Y., Lipkova, J., Lu, M. Y., Sahai, S., & Mahmood, F. (2023). Algorithmic fairness in artificial intelligence for medicine and healthcare [PMID: 37380750; PMC10632090. Comprehensive Nature review on algorithmic fairness in healthcare AI]. *Nature Biomedical Engineering, 7*(6), 719–742. DOI: 10.1038/s41551-023-01056-8 PMID: 37380750

Chen, Y. H., & Xu, J. L. (2023). Applying artificial intelligence to predict falls for inpatient. *Frontiers in Medicine, 10*, 1285192.

Chen, Y., & Esmaeilzadeh, P. (2024). Generative AI in medical practice: In-depth exploration of privacy and security challenges [PMID: 38457208; PMC10960211. Recent comprehensive analysis of data privacy in AI healthcare systems]. *Journal of Medical Internet Research*, *26*, e53008. DOI: 10.2196/53008 PMID: 38457208

Cheung, G., Wright-St Clair, V., Chacko, E., & Barak, Y. (2019). Financial difficulty and biopsychosocial predictors of loneliness: A cross-sectional study of community dwelling older adults. *Archives of Gerontology and Geriatrics*, *85*, 103935. PMID: 31446186

Chidumwa, G., Maposa, I., Corso, B., Minicuci, N., Kowal, P., & Micklesfield, L. K.. (2021). Identifying co-occurrence and clustering of chronic diseases using latent class analysis: Cross-sectional findings from SAGE South Africa Wave 2. *BMJ Open*, *11*(1). Advance online publication. DOI: 10.1136/bmjopen-2020-041604 PMID: 33514578

Chien, S. C., Yen, C. M., Chang, Y. H., Chen, Y. E., Liu, C. C., Hsiao, Y. P., & Chung, R. H. (2025). Use of artificial intelligence, internet of things, and edge intelligence in long-term care for older people: Comprehensive analysis through bibliometric, Google trends, and content analysis. *Journal of Medical Internet Research*, *27*, e56692. Advance online publication. DOI: 10.2196/56692 PMID: 40053718

Chinnaiyan, B., Balasubramanian, S., Jeyabalu, M., & Warrier, G. S. (2025). AI applications—Computer vision and natural language processing. In *Model optimization methods for efficient and edge AI: Federated learning architectures, frameworks and applications* (pp. 25–41). IGI Global., DOI: 10.4018/979-8-3693-2401-1.ch002

Choi, H., & Lee, S. (2023). Social capital and technology: Re-engaging older adults through inclusive AI design. *Journal of Gerontechnology*, *22*(4), 101–115. DOI: 10.4017/gt.2023.22.4.005

Choi, J. W., Choi, J. W., Kim, J. H., Yoo, K. B., & Park, E. C. (2015). Association between chronic disease and catastrophic health expenditure in Korea. *BMC Health Services Research*, *15*(1), 1–8. DOI: 10.1186/s12913-014-0675-1 PMID: 25608983

Chopra, K. (2025). Motivating older adults with special needs for learning using generative artificial intelligence. *Educational Gerontology*, •••, 1–20.

Choudhary, E., & Nagar, V. (2025). Biomimicry and rehabilitation of dental tissues in geriatric population-An overview. *Journal of Oral Research and Review*, *17*(2), 189–195.

Choudhury, A., Renjilian, E., & Asan, O. (2021). Use of machine learning in geriatric clinical care for chronic diseases: A systematic literature review. *JMIR Aging, 4*(3), e26328. DOI: 10.2196/26328

Choudhury, A., Renjilian, E., & Asan, O. (2021). Use of machine learning in geriatric clinical care for chronic diseases: A systematic literature review. *Journal of Medical Internet Research, 23*(9), e24387. Advance online publication. DOI: 10.2196/24387

Chou, K.-L., & Chi, I. (2000). Comparison between elderly Chinese living alone and those living with others. *Journal of Gerontological Social Work, 33*(4), 51–66.

Chowdhury, M., Cervantes, E. G., Chan, W. Y., & Seitz, D. P. (2021). Use of machine learning and artificial intelligence methods in geriatric mental health research involving electronic health record or administrative claims data: A systematic review. *Frontiers in Psychiatry, 12*, 738466.

Cho, Y. J., Kim, J. H., Sun, A., & Oh, J. H. (2017). Design and implementation of artificial intelligence-based speech recognition for silver generation and single household. In *Proceedings of the Korean Society of Computer Information Conference* (pp. 141-144). Korean Society of Computer Information.

Chu, C. H., Donato-Woodger, S., Khan, S. S., Nyrup, R., Leslie, K., Lyn, A., & Grenier, A. (2023). Age-related bias and artificial intelligence: A scoping review. *Humanities & Social Sciences Communications, 10*(1), 1–17.

Chu, C. H., Leslie, K., Shi, J., Nyrup, R., Bianchi, A., Khan, S. S., & Grenier, A. (2022). Ageism and artificial intelligence: Protocol for a scoping review. *JMIR Research Protocols, 11*(6), e33211.

Chu, C. H., Nyrup, R., Leslie, K., Shi, J., Bianchi, A., Lyn, A., & Grenier, A. (2022). Digital ageism: Challenges and opportunities in artificial intelligence for older adults. *The Gerontologist, 62*(7), 947–955.

Chu-Ke, C., & Dong, Y. (2024). Misinformation and literacies in the era of generative artificial intelligence: A brief overview and a call for future research. *Emerging Media, 2*(1), 70–85.

Chun, J., de Witt, C. S., & Elkins, K. (2024). Comparative global AI regulation: Policy perspectives from the EU, China, and the US. *arXiv preprint arXiv:2410.21279.*

Cinalioglu, K., Elbaz, S., Sekhon, K., Su, C. L., Rej, S., & Sekhon, H. (2023). Exploring differential perceptions of artificial intelligence in health care among younger versus older Canadians: Results from the 2021 Canadian Digital Health Survey. *Journal of Medical Internet Research, 25*, e38169.

Cingolani, M., Scendoni, R., Fedeli, P., & Cembrani, F. (2023). Artificial intelligence and digital medicine for integrated home care services in Italy: Opportunities and limits. *Frontiers in Public Health, 10*, 1095001.

Clark, C. R., Wilkins, C. H., Rodriguez, J. A., Preininger, A. M., Harris, J., DesAutels, S., & Dankwa-Mullan, I. (2021). Health care equity in the use of advanced analytics and artificial intelligence technologies in primary care. *Journal of General Internal Medicine, 36*(10), 3188–3193. DOI: 10.1007/s11606-021-06846-x PMID: 34027610

Cocuzzo, B., Wrench, A., O'Malley, C., & O'Malley, C. B. (2022). Effects of COVID-19 on older adults: Physical, mental, emotional, social, and financial problems seen and unseen. *Cureus, 14*(10), e30319. Advance online publication. DOI: 10.7759/cureus.30319 PMID: 36299954

Colombo, G., & Grübel, J. (2023, April). The Spatial Performance Assessment for Cognitive Evaluation (Space): A novel game for the early detection of cognitive impairment. In *Extended Abstracts of the 2023 CHI Conference on Human Factors in Computing Systems* (pp. 1–6). ACM. https://doi.org/DOI: 10.1145/3544549.3585632

Conger, J. A., & Kanungo, R. N. (1988). The empowerment process: Integrating theory and practice. *Academy of Management Review, 13*(3), 471–482. DOI: 10.5465/amr.1988.4306983

Corbett, C. F., Wright, P. J., Jones, K., & Parmer, M. (2021). Voice-activated virtual home assistant use and social isolation and loneliness among older adults: Mini review. *Frontiers in Public Health, 9*, 742012.

Corrêa, M. M., Thumé, E., De Oliveira, E. R. A., & Tomasi, E. (2016). Performance of the waist-to-height ratio in identifying obesity and predicting non-communicable diseases in the elderly population: A systematic literature review. *Archives of Gerontology and Geriatrics, 65*, 174–182. DOI: 10.1016/j.archger.2016.03.021 PMID: 27061665

Costanzo, M., Smeriglio, R., & Di Nuovo, S. (2024). New technologies and assistive robotics for elderly: A review on psychological variables. *Archives of Gerontology and Geriatrics Plus, 1*(4), 100056.

Coulton, S., Clift, S., Skingley, A., & Rodriguez, J. (2015). Effectiveness and cost-effectiveness of a 14-week singing intervention for older people. *Health & Social Care in the Community, 23*(3), 324–336. DOI: 10.1111/hsc.12140

Critchley, H. D. (2009). The human brain as a central hub for emotional regulation. *Neurobiology of Emotion, 17*(4), 1–15.

Cross, J. L., Choma, M. A., & Onofrey, J. A. (2024). Bias in medical AI: Implications for clinical decision-making [PMC11542778. Recent comprehensive analysis of bias in clinical AI decision support]. *PLOS Digital Health, 3*(11), e0000651. DOI: 10.1371/journal.pdig.0000651 PMID: 39509461

Currie, G., Rohren, E., & Hawk, K. E. (2024). The role of artificial intelligence in supporting person-centred care. In *Person-Centred Care in Radiology* (pp. 175–192). CRC Press., DOI: 10.1201/9781003319634-13

Cuschieri, S., & Grech, S. (2021). Insight into the Occurrence of Common Non-communicable Diseases at a Population Level and the Potential Impact During the Coronavirus Pandemic — A Need for a Syndemic Healthcare Approach? *SN Comprehensive Clinical Medicine, 3*(12), 2393–2400. DOI: 10.1007/s42399-021-01064-2 PMID: 34568765

Czaja, S. J. (2016). The role of technology in supporting family caregiving. *The Gerontologist, 56*(Suppl_1), S51–S56. DOI: 10.1093/geront/gnw005

Czaja, S. J., & Ceruso, M. (2022). The promise of artificial intelligence in supporting an aging population. *Journal of Cognitive Engineering and Decision Making, 16*(4), 182–193.

D´ıaz, M., Saez-Pons, J., Heerink, M., & Angulo, C. (2013). Emotional factors in robotbased assistive services for elderly at home. *2013 IEEE RO-MAN*, 711–716.

D'Amour, A., Heller, K., Moldovan, D., ... (2020). Underspecification presents challenges for credibility in modern machine learning. *arXiv preprint arXiv:2011.03395.* https://arxiv.org/abs/2011.03395

Da'Costa, A., Teke, J., Origbo, J. E., Osonuga, A., Egbon, E., & Olawade, D. B. (2025). AI-driven triage in emergency departments: A review of benefits, challenges, and future directions. *International Journal of Medical Informatics, 200*, 105838. Advance online publication. DOI: 10.1016/j.ijmedinf.2024.105838 PMID: 39965433

Dahal, S., Sah, R. B., Niraula, S. R., Karkee, R., & Chakravartty, A. (2021). Prevalence and determinants of noncommunicable disease risk factors among adult population of Kathmandu. *PLoS One, 16*(9). Advance online publication. DOI: 10.1371/journal.pone.0257037 PMID: 34495984

Dahshan, A., Al-Kubiasi, N., Al-Zaidan, M., Saeed, W., Kehyayan, V., & Bougmiza, I. (2020). Prevalence of polypharmacy and the association with non-communicable diseases in Qatari elderly patients attending primary healthcare centers: A cross-sectional study. *PLoS One, 15*(6), 1–13. DOI: 10.1371/journal.pone.0234386 PMID: 32525902

Dai, H., Jia, G., & Liu, K. (2015). Health-related quality of life and related factors among elderly people in Jinzhou, China: A cross-sectional study. *Public Health, 129*(6), 667–673. DOI: 10.1016/j.puhe.2015.02.022 PMID: 25796292

Dakoliya, M. (2025). Interdisciplinary Approaches to Healthcare Management: Integrating Clinical Governance, Risk Management, and Technological Advancements. *Medicon Medical Sciences, 8*, 03–06.

Danda, R. R. (2022). Telehealth In Medicare Plans: Leveraging AI For Improved Accessibility And Senior Care Quality. *Migration Letters : An International Journal of Migration Studies, 19*(6), 1133–1143.

Dang, T., Spathis, D., Ghosh, A., & Mascolo, C. (2023). Human-centred artificial intelligence for mobile health sensing: Challenges and opportunities. *Royal Society Open Science, 10*(11), 230806. DOI: 10.1098/rsos.230806 PMID: 38026044

Dankwa-Mullan, I. (2024). Health equity and ethical considerations in using artificial intelligence in public health and medicine [Recent 2024 CDC peer-reviewed commentary on AI and health equity; PubMed indexed]. *Preventing Chronic Disease, 21*, 240245. DOI: 10.5888/pcd21.240245 PMID: 39173183

Dara, M., Dianatpour, M., Azarpira, N., & Omidifar, N. (2024). Convergence of CRISPR and artificial intelligence: A paradigm shift in biotechnology. *Human Genomics*. Advance online publication. DOI: 10.1016/j.humgen.2024.201297

Darbandi, M., Rezaeian, S., Najafi, F., Shadmani, F. K., Ghavi, S., & Miryan, M.. (2023). A Comprehensive Evaluation of Occupational Epidemiology in Western Iran: A Cohort Study in Ravansar Noncommunicable Diseases. *Journal of Occupational and Environmental Medicine, 65*(9), E610–E618. DOI: 10.1097/JOM.0000000000002916 PMID: 37367639

Das, A., & Dhillon, P. (2023). Application of machine learning in measurement of ageing and geriatric diseases: A systematic review. *Ageing International, 49*(2), 353–384. DOI: 10.1007/s12126-023-09546-3 PMID: 38087195

Das, A., & Dhillon, P. (2023). Application of machine learning in measurement of ageing and geriatric diseases: A systematic review. *Ageing Research Reviews, 91*, 102047. DOI: 10.1016/j.arr.2023.102047 PMID: 38087195

Davidson, J. W., & Faulkner, R. (2010). The effects of group singing and performance for marginalized and middle-class singers. *Music Education Research, 12*(4), 447–462. DOI: 10.1080/14613808.2010.518683

Davis, F. D. (1989). Perceived usefulness, perceived ease of use, and user acceptance of information technology. *Management Information Systems Quarterly*, •••, 319–340.

Davis, M. A., Murphy, S. P., Neuhaus, J. M., & Lein, D. (1990). Living arrangements and dietary quality of older U.S. adults. *Journal of the American Dietetic Association, 90*(12), 1667–1672. PMID: 2246446

De Carolis, B., Ferilli, S., & Palestra, G. (2017). Simulating empathic behavior in a social assistive robot. *Multimedia Tools and Applications, 76*(4), 5073–5094.

de Kervenoael, R., Hasan, R., Schwob, A., & Goh, E. (2020). Leveraging human-robot interaction in hospitality services: Incorporating the role of perceived value, empathy, and information sharing into visitors' intentions to use social robots. *Tourism Management, 78*, 104042. DOI: 10.1016/j.tourman.2019.104042

Dean, A., Kolody, B., Wood, P., & Matt, G. E. (1992). The influence of living alone on depression in elderly persons. *Journal of Aging and Health, 4*(1), 3–18.

Del-Valle-Soto, C., Briseño, R. A., Velázquez, R., Guerra-Rosales, G., Perez-Ochoa, S., Preciado-Bazavilvazo, I. H., & Varela-Aldás, J. (2024). Enhancing elderly care through low-cost wireless sensor networks and artificial intelligence: A study on vital sign monitoring and sleep improvement. *Future Internet, 16*(9), 323. DOI: 10.3390/fi16090323

Denecke, K., & Baudoin, C. R. (2022). A review of artificial intelligence and robotics in transformed health ecosystems. *Frontiers in medicine, 9*, 795957.

Deng, S., Hager, K., Wang, L., Cudhea, F. P., Wong, J. B., Kim, D. D., & Mozaffarian, D. (2025). Estimated impact of medically tailored meals on health care use and expenditures in 50 US states. *Health Affairs, 44*(4), 433–442. DOI: 10.1377/hlthaff.2024.01307 PMID: 40193837

Denysyuk, H. V., Pires, I. M., & Garcia, N. M. (2024). A roadmap for empowering cardiovascular disease patients: A 5P-medicine approach and technological integration. *PeerJ, 12*, e18208. DOI: 10.7717/peerj.18208 PMID: 39224824

Derynda, B., Siegel, J., Maurice, L., & Cook, N. (2022). Virtual lifelong learning among older adults: Usage and impact during the COVID-19 pandemic. *Gerontology & Geriatric Medicine, 8*, 1–9. DOI: 10.1177/23337214221116259 PMID: 35651387

Devine, B. C., Dogan, A. B., & Sobol, W. M. (2025). Recent optical coherence tomography (OCT) innovations for increased accessibility and remote surveillance. *Bioengineering (Basel, Switzerland), 12*(1), 76. Advance online publication. DOI: 10.3390/bioengineering12010076 PMID: 40428060

Dhanda, S. S., Panwar, D., Lin, C. C., Sharma, T. K., Rastogi, D., Bindewari, S., & Agarwal, S. (2025). Advancement in public health through machine learning: A narrative review of opportunities and ethical considerations. *Journal of Big Data*, *12*(1), 1–58.

Diareme, K. C., Liapakis, A., & Efthymiou, I. P. (2022). Data, sentiment analysis, and examples during the COVID-19 pandemic. *Hellenic Archives of Psychiatry and Clinical Psychology in Behavioral Sciences*, *33779*. Advance online publication. DOI: 10.12681/hapscpbs.33779

Diareme, S., Papatheodorou, K., & Papageorgiou, C. (2022). Coping with stress and anxiety during the COVID-19 pandemic: The role of online social support groups. *International Journal of Environmental Research and Public Health*, *19*(2), 978. DOI: 10.3390/ijerph19020978

Dicuonzo, G., Donofrio, F., Fusco, A., & Shini, M. (2023). Healthcare system: Moving forward with artificial intelligence. *Technovation*, *127*, 102860. DOI: 10.1016/j.technovation.2023.102860

Dilip, G., Guttula, R., & Rajeyyagari, S. (2022). S, H., Pandey, R. R., Bora, A., ... & Sundramurthy, V. P. (2022). Artificial Intelligence-Based Smart Comrade Robot for Elders Healthcare with Strait Rescue System. *Journal of Healthcare Engineering*, (1), 9904870.

Dill, J. S., Morgan, J. C., & Weiner, B. (2014). Frontline health care workers and perceived career mobility. *Health Care Management Review*, *39*(4), 318–328. DOI: 10.1097/HMR.0000000000000028 PMID: 23989644

Dilsizian, S. E., & Siegel, E. L. (2014). Artificial intelligence in medicine and cardiac imaging: Harnessing big data and advanced computing to provide personalized medical diagnosis and treatment. *Current Cardiology Reports*, *16*(1), 441. DOI: 10.1007/s11886-013-0441-8 PMID: 24338557

Dissanayake, S. A. I. P., Kisokanth, G., & Warnakulasuriya, S. S. P. (2021). Prevalence of risk factors for Non-communicable diseases, work-related health problems and associated factors among male three-wheeler drivers in Gampaha Urban Council area, Sri Lanka. *The Journal of Men's Health*, *17*(4), 295–303. DOI: 10.31083/jomh.2021.059

Dixon, D., Sattar, H., Moros, N., Reddy Kesireddy, S., Ahsan, H., Lakkimsetti, M., & Junaid Hassan, M. (2024). Unveiling the influence of AI predictive analytics on patient outcomes: A comprehensive narrative review. *Cureus*, *16*(7), e64503. DOI: 10.7759/cureus.64503 PMID: 38854327

Dixon, R. B. L. (2023). A principled governance for emerging AI regimes: Lessons from China, the European Union, and the United States. *AI and Ethics*, *3*(3), 793–810.

Dong, L., Yang, Q., Zhang, R. H., & Wei, W. B. (2021). Artificial intelligence for the detection of age-related macular degeneration in color fundus photographs: A systematic review and meta-analysis. *EClinicalMedicine*, ●●●, 35.

Dong, X., Du, S., Zheng, W., Cai, C., Liu, H., & Zou, J. (2022). Evaluation of an artificial intelligence system for the detection of diabetic retinopathy in Chinese community healthcare centers. *Frontiers in Medicine*, *9*, 883462.

Donnelly, D. L. (2022). First do no harm: legal principles regulating the future of artificial intelligence in health care in South Africa. *Potchefstroom Electronic Law Journal/Potchefstroomse Elektroniese Regsblad, 25*(1).

Drenth-van Maanen, A. C., Wilting, I., & Jansen, P. A. (2020). Prescribing medicines to older people—How to consider the impact of ageing on human organ and body functions. *British Journal of Clinical Pharmacology*, *86*(10), 1921–1930. PMID: 31425638

Dugee, O., Sugar, B., Dorjsuren, B., & Mahal, A. (2019). Economic impacts of chronic conditions in a country with high levels of population health coverage: Lessons from Mongolia. *Tropical Medicine & International Health*, *24*(6), 715–726. DOI: 10.1111/tmi.1323 PMID: 30870575

Durkheim, É. (1995). *The elementary forms of religious life* (Fields, K. E., Trans.). Free Press. (Original work published 1912)

Dutta, S., Mishra, A., Basu, M., & Mukherjee, M. (2022). Determinants of Non Communicable Diseases: A Mixed-method Study on Its Prevalence and Perceptions among Rural Population of Muchisa, West Bengal. *Journal of Clinical and Diagnostic Research : JCDR*, *16*(6), LC15–LC21. DOI: 10.7860/JCDR/2022/53398.1646

Du, Y. R., Liu, L., Zhao, Y., Huang, J. J., Golden, A. R., & Cai, L. (2023). Ethnic disparities in prevalence of chronic non-communicable diseases and its multimorbidity among older adults in rural southwest China. *BMC Public Health*, *23*(1), 1217. DOI: 10.1186/s12889-023-16161-1 PMID: 37353785

Dykstra, S. (2024). *Integrating multi-domain electronic health data, machine learning, and automated cardiac phenomics for personalized cardiovascular care* [Doctoral dissertation, University of Calgary]. PRISM Repository. https://doi.org/ DOI: 10.11575/PRISM/43295

Ebrahim, S. (1996). Principles of epidemiology in old age. In Ebrahim, S., & Kalache, A. (Eds.), *Epidemiology in Old Age* (pp. 12–21). BMJ Publishing Group.

Eccles, R. G., & Klimenko, S. (2019). The investor revolution. *Harvard Business Review*, *97*(3), 106–116. https://hbr.org/2019/05/the-investor-revolution

Efthymiou Egleton, I. P., Efthymiou Egleton, T. W., & Sidiropoulos, S. (2020). Artificial Intelligence (AI) in Politics: Should Political AI be Controlled? [(correction)]. *International Journal of Innovative Science and Research Technology*, *5*(2), 278–280.

Efthymiou, I. (2024). Exploring the Frontier: New and Future Trends in Research. In B. Orlando (Ed.), Innovation Capabilities and Entrepreneurial Opportunities of Smart Working (pp. 48-68). IGI Global Scientific Publishing. https://doi.org/DOI: 10.4018/978-1-7998-8797-3.ch003

Efthymiou, I. P. (2024). Exploring the frontier: New and future trends in research. In B. Orlando (Ed.), *Innovation capabilities and entrepreneurial opportunities of smart working* (pp. 48–68). IGI Global Scientific Publishing. DOI: 10.4018

Efthymiou, I.-P. (2024). Can AI improve health and wellbeing? Case Studies Journal, ISSN (2305-509X), 13(11), 1–5.

Efthymiou, I.-P. (2024). *What's left for us? AI, ethics and the future of work*. Independently published.

Efthymiou–Egleton, T. W., Sidiropoulos, S., Spanos, E., & Stougiannou, E. (2020). Big Data and Democracy. *HAPSc Policy Briefs Series*, *1*(2), 18–25.

Efthymiou, I. (2024). Socially aware health monitoring systems: Balancing biological and social data in elder care. *Health Informatics Journal*, *30*(2), 78–90. DOI: 10.1177/14604582241234567

Efthymiou, I. (2025). The Role of E-Government and E-Governance in Modern Societies. In Wongmahesak, K., Ahmad, J., & Mustanir, A. (Eds.), *Public Governance Practices in the Age of AI* (pp. 45–68). IGI Global Scientific Publishing., DOI: 10.4018/979-8-3693-9286-7.ch003

Efthymiou, I. (2026). AI in Epidemiology: Predicting the Unpredictable Leveraging AI to Detect Outbreaks and Predict Disease. In Umer, M. (Ed.), *Innovation and Transformation of Public Health* (pp. 281–308). IGI Global Scientific Publishing., DOI: 10.4018/979-8-3373-1992-6.ch009

Efthymiou, I. P. (2024). *Human wellbeing in the age of artificial intelligence*. IGI Global Scientific Publishing.

Efthymiou, I. P. (2024). Wellbeing as an alternative to GDP? *HAPSc Policy Briefs Series*, *5*(1), 38–46. DOI: 10.12681/hapscpbs.38956

Efthymiou, I. P. (2026). AI in epidemiology: Predicting the unpredictable leveraging AI to detect outbreaks and predict disease. In *Innovation and transformation of public health* (pp. 281–308). IGI Global Scientific Publishing., DOI: 10.4018/979-8-3693-0000-0.ch012

Efthymiou, I. P., Alevizos, A., & Sidiropoulos, S. (2023). The role of artificial intelligence in revolutionizing NGOs' work. *Journal of Politics and Ethics in New Technologies and AI*, *2*(1), e35137. DOI: 10.12681/jpentai.35137

Efthymiou, I. P., & Efthymiou Egleton, T. W. (2023). Artificial intelligence for sustainable smart cities. In *Handbook of research on applications of AI, digital twin, and internet of things for sustainable development* (pp. 1–xx). IGI Global., DOI: 10.4018/978-1-6684-6821-0.ch001

Efthymiou, I. P., & Vozikis, A. (2017). Medicine, a pan-historical, pan-cultural science. *Journal of Cardiology & Cardiovascular Therapy*, *1*(1).

Efthymiou, I. P., Vozikis, A., & Sidiropoulos, S. (2019). Application of Sociocybernetic model in the field of Health Management. *International Journal of Scientific and Engineering Research*, *10*(5), 451–560.

Efthymiou, I.-P. (2020). Non-cognitive skills and AI: A new era of learning and development. *International Case Studies Journal*, *9*(10), 42–46.

Efthymiou, I.-P. (2024). Can AI improve health and wellbeing? *Case Studies Journal*, *13*(11), 1–5.

Efthymiou, I.-P. (2024). The importance of soft skills in healthcare: The impact of communication, empathy, and teamwork on doctor-nurse interactions. *Case Studies Journal*, *13*(11), 6–11.

Efthymiou, I.-P.. (2022). Major risk factors that increase the frequency of noncommunicable diseases: A review of evidence-based research. *International Journal of Caring Sciences*, *15*(1), 655–662.

Efthymiou, I.-P., Efthymiou-Egleton, A., Psomiadi, A., & Tariq, M. U. (2025). The role of artificial intelligence in humanitarian aid for achieving Sustainable Development Goals. In Tariq, M. U., & Sergio, R. P. (Eds.), *Cases on AI-driven solutions to environmental challenges* (pp. 43–72). IGI Global., DOI: 10.4018/979-8-3693-7483-2.ch008

Elgin, C. Y., & Elgin, C. (2024). Ethical implications of AI-driven clinical decision support systems on healthcare resource allocation: A qualitative study of healthcare professionals' perspectives [Recent 2024 study on ethical accountability and transparency in AI healthcare]. *BMC Medical Ethics*, *25*(1), 148. DOI: 10. 1186/s12910-024-01151-8 PMID: 39707327

Emery-Xu, N., Jordan, R., & Trager, R. (2025). International governance of advancing artificial intelligence. *AI & Society*, *40*(4), 3019–3044.

Emmanouil-Kalos, A., & Prokakis, E. (2021). Social protection after the pandemic: Lessons learned from the eurozone crisis. *HAPSc Policy Briefs Series*, *2*(1), 70–78. DOI: 10.12681/hapscpbs.27660

Esmaeilzadeh, P. (2024). Challenges and strategies for wide-scale artificial intelligence (AI) deployment in healthcare practices: A perspective for healthcare organizations. *Artificial Intelligence in Medicine*, *151*, 102856. Advance online publication. DOI: 10.1016/j.artmed.2024.102856 PMID: 38555850

Esmaeilzadeh, P. (2024). The role of AI in healthcare digitalization and telemedicine. *International Journal of Medical Informatics*, *185*, 105436.

Eubanks, V. (2018). *Automating inequality: How high-tech tools profile, police, and punish the poor*. St. Martin's Press.

Eun, S. J., Kim, E. J., & Kim, J. (2023). Artificial intelligence-based personalized serious game for enhancing the physical and cognitive abilities of the elderly. *Future Generation Computer Systems*, *141*, 713–722.

European Commission. (2021). *Proposal for a regulation laying down harmonised rules on artificial intelligence (Artificial Intelligence Act) (COM(2021) 206 final)*. https://eur-lex.europa.eu/legal-content/EN/TXT/?uri=celex%3A52021PC0206

Extermann, M., Brain, E., Canin, B., Cherian, M. N., Cheung, K. L., de Glas, N., & Wildiers, H. (2021). Priorities for the global advancement of care for older adults with cancer: An update of the International Society of Geriatric Oncology Priorities Initiative. *The Lancet. Oncology*, *22*(1), e29–e36. DOI: 10.1016/S1470-2045(20)30473-3 PMID: 33387502

Eyre, C. D. (2023). Co-design and feasibility testing of a toolkit for mitigating the negative impact of out of hours mobile ICT demands. [PDF].

Fabrizio, C., Termine, A., Caltagirone, C., & Sancesario, G. (2021). Artificial intelligence for Alzheimer's disease: Promise or challenge? *Diagnostics (Basel)*, *11*(8), 1473. Advance online publication. DOI: 10.3390/diagnostics11081473 PMID: 34441407

Faiyazuddin, M., Rahman, S. J. Q., Anand, G., Siddiqui, R. K., Mehta, R., Khatib, M. N., & Sah, R. (2025). The impact of artificial intelligence on healthcare: A comprehensive review of advancements in diagnostics, treatment, and operational efficiency. *Health Science Reports*, *8*(1), e70312. Advance online publication. DOI: 10.1002/hsr2.70312 PMID: 39763580

Fancourt, D., & Finn, S. (2019). The effectiveness of group singing for reducing loneliness: A systematic review. *Health Promotion International*, *34*(3), 473–481. DOI: 10.1093/heapro/day025

Fang, R., Ye, S., Huang, Y., & Zhang, Y. (2017). Music therapy is a potential intervention for cognition of Alzheimer's disease: A mini-review. *Translational Neurodegeneration*, *6*(2). Advance online publication. DOI: 10.1186/s40035-017-0073-9

FAO. (2022). *The state of food security and nutrition in the world 2022*. Food and Agriculture Organization of the United Nations., DOI: 10.4060/cc0639en

Farooq, S., & Masud, F. (2021). Catastrophic health expenditure and poverty in Pakistan. *Pakistan Development Review*, *60*(1), 27–48. DOI: 10.30541/v60i1pp.27-48

Farzadfar, F., Zalvand, R., Karami, B., Yoosefi, M., Takian, A., & Tajvar, M. (2022). Prevalence and Determinants of Severe Mental Disorders in Iran: Evidence from the National Survey of STEPs- 2016. *Archives of Iranian Medicine*, *25*(7), 460–472. DOI: 10.34172/aim.2022.76 PMID: 36404514

Farzad, M, MitraMoodi, Sharifi F, Amirabadizadeh H, Amirabadizadeh A, Kazemi T, et al. (2021). Prevalence and factors connected with chronic diseases in the elderly residents of Birjand: A community – based study in Birjand, South Khorasan Province, Iran. *Journal of Diabetes and Metabolic Disorders*, *20*(2), 1655–1662. DOI: 10.1007/s40200-021-00918-9 PMID: 34900817

Fasan, M. (2025). Regulating the use of artificial intelligence in the doctor-patient relationship? A primer on supranational and national legal frameworks. *BIOLAW JOURNAL*, *2025*(1), 193–211.

Feng, H., Lin, Y., & Wei, X. (2018). The potential of community music for relieving feelings of loneliness among older adults in formal care settings. *Social Work in Public Health*, *33*(4–5), 329–338. DOI: 10.1080/17533015.2018.1479860

Feng, H., Zhou, J., & Wang, J. (2020). Music and social bonding: A systematic review. *Frontiers in Psychology*, *11*, 1096. DOI: 10.3389/fpsyg.2020.01096

Feng, L., Li, P., Wang, X., Hu, Z., Ma, Y., & Tang, W.. (2014). Distribution and determinants of non communicable diseases among elderly uyghur ethnic group in Xinjiang, China. *PLoS One*, *9*(8). Advance online publication. DOI: 10.1371/journal.pone.0105536 PMID: 25141133

Ferrara, M., Bertozzi, G., Di Fazio, N., Aquila, I., Di Fazio, A., Maiese, A., & La Russa, R. (2024). Risk management and patient safety in the artificial intelligence era: A systematic review. *Health Care*, *12*(5), 549. DOI: 10.3390/healthcare12050549 PMID: 38470660

Ferreira, J. C., Elvas, L. B., Correia, R., & Mascarenhas, M. (2025). Empowering health professionals with digital skills to improve patient care and daily workflows. *Health Care*, *13*(1), 98. DOI: 10.3390/healthcare13010198 PMID: 39942518

Ferretti, A., Ienca, M., Sheehan, M., Blasimme, A., Dove, E. S., Farsides, B., & Vayena, E. (2021). Ethics review of big data research: What should stay and what should be reformed? *BMC Medical Ethics*, *22*(1), 51. Advance online publication. DOI: 10.1186/s12910-021-00616-4 PMID: 33931049

Figueiredo, B., Aleti, T., Reid, M., Martin, D. M., Hjorth, L., Sheahan, J., & Grigg, A. (2022). *Co-designing ICT strategies with older adults*. Australian Communications Consumer Action Network.

Fisk, A. D., Czaja, S. J., Rogers, W. A., Charness, N., & Sharit, J. (2020). *Designing for older adults: Principles and creative human factors approaches* (3rd ed.). CRC Press.

Fleming, J. L. (2025). Securing space systems as critical infrastructure: A transformative approach to cybersecurity and risk mitigation. *International Journal of Critical Infrastructure Protection*, *48*, 100693. DOI: 10.1016/j.ijcip.2024.100693

Floridi, L. (2023). *The ethics of artificial intelligence: Principles, challenges, and opportunities*. Oxford University Press.

Floridi, L., & Cowls, J. (2019). A unified framework of five principles for AI in society. *Harvard Data Science Review*, *1*(1). Advance online publication. DOI: 10.1162/99608f92.8cd550d1

Floridi, L., Cowls, J., Beltrametti, M., Chatila, R., Chazerand, P., Dignum, V., Luetge, C., Madelin, R., Pagallo, U., Rossi, F., Schafer, B., Valcke, P., & Vayena, E. (2018). AI4People—An ethical framework for a good AI society: Opportunities, risks, principles, and recommendations. *Minds and Machines*, *28*(4), 689–707. DOI: 10.1007/s11023-018-9482-5 PMID: 30930541

Folland, S., Goodman, A. C., Stano, M., & Danagoulian, S. (2024). *The economics of health and health care* (9th ed.). Routledge., DOI: 10.4324/9781003268659

Fong, T., Nourbakhsh, I., & Dautenhahn, K. (2003). A survey of socially interactive robots. *Robotics and Autonomous Systems*, *42*(3-4), 143–166.

Fossen, F. M., & Sorgner, A. (2022). New digital technologies and heterogeneous wage and employment dynamics in the United States: Evidence from individual-level data. *Technological Forecasting and Social Change*, *175*, 121381. DOI: 10.1016/j.techfore.2021.121381

Frank, B., Herbas-Torrico, B., & Schvaneveldt, S. J. (2021). The AI-extended consumer: Technology, consumer, country differences in the formation of demand for AI-empowered consumer products. *Technological Forecasting and Social Change*, *172*, 121018. DOI: 10.1016/j.techfore.2021.121018

Franklin, S. S., Larson, M. G., Khan, S. A., Wong, N. D., Leip, E. P., & Kannel, W. B.. (2001). Does the relation of blood pressure to coronary heart disease risk change with aging?: The Framingham Heart Study. *Circulation*, *103*(9), 1245–1249. DOI: 10.1161/01.CIR.103.9.1245 PMID: 11238268

Freedman, V. A., Patterson, S. E., Cornman, J. C., & Wolff, J. L. (2022). A day in the life of caregivers to older adults with and without dementia: Comparisons of care time and emotional health. *Alzheimer's & Dementia*, *18*(9), 1650–1661. DOI: 10.1002/alz.12524 PMID: 35103394

Freeman, R. E. (1984). *Strategic management: A stakeholder approach.* Pitman.

Fulmer, T., Reuben, D. B., Auerbach, J., Fick, D. M., Galambos, C., & Johnson, K. S. (2021). Actualizing better health and health care for older adults: Commentary describes six vital directions to improve the care and quality of life for all older Americans. *Health Affairs*, *40*(2), 219–225. DOI: 10.1377/hlthaff.2020.01470 PMID: 33476185

Fusar-Poli, L., Casoni, F., & Sensi, F. (2018). The effect of music therapy on cognitive functions in patients with dementia: A systematic review and meta-analysis. *Journal of Alzheimer's Disease*, *64*(2), 481–492. DOI: 10.3233/JAD-170792

Gabriel, O. T. (2023). Data privacy and ethical issues in collecting health care data using artificial intelligence among health workers. *International Journal of Medical and Health Sciences Research*, *3*(1), 1–10. DOI: 10.51594/ijmer.v3i1.234

Gallistl, V., Banday, M. U. L., Berridge, C., Grigorovich, A., Jarke, J., Mannheim, I., & Peine, A. (2024). Addressing the black box of AI—A model and research agenda on the co-constitution of aging and artificial intelligence. *The Gerontologist, 64*(6), gnae039.

Gartner, J. B., Abasse, K. S., Bergeron, F., Landa, P., Lemaire, C., & Cote, A. (2022). Definition and conceptualization of the patient-centered care pathway, a proposed integrative framework for consensus: A concept analysis and systematic review. *BMC Health Services Research, 22*(1), 558. DOI: 10.1186/s12913-022-07960-0 PMID: 35473632

Gaser, C., & Schlaug, G. (2003). Brain structures differ between musicians and non-musicians. *The Journal of Neuroscience : The Official Journal of the Society for Neuroscience, 23*(27), 9240–9245. DOI: 10.1523/jneurosci.23-27-09240.2003

Gasser, U., & Almeida, V. A. F. (2017). A layered model for AI governance. *IEEE Internet Computing, 21*(6), 58–62. DOI: 10.1109/MIC.2017.4180835

Gazzarata, R., Almeida, J., Lindsko¨ld, L., Cangioli, G., Gaeta, E., Fico, G., & Chronaki, C. E. (2024). HL7 fast healthcare interoperability resources (HL7 FHIR) in digital healthcare ecosystems for chronic disease management: Scoping review [PMID: 38870885. Recent 2024 review on healthcare digital transformation and interoperability]. *International Journal of Medical Informatics, 189*, 105507. DOI: 10.1016/j.ijmedinf.2024.105507 PMID: 38870885

Gbadamosi, M. A., & Tlou, B. (2020). Modifiable risk factors associated with non-communicable diseases among adult outpatients in Manzini, Swaziland: A cross-sectional study. *BMC Public Health, 20*(1), 665. DOI: 10.1186/s12889-020-08816-0 PMID: 32398061

Gee, E. M. (2000). Living arrangements and quality of life among Chinese Canadian elders. *Social Indicators Research, 51*(3), 309–329.

Gellert, G. A., Kabat-Karabon, A., Gellert, G. L., Rasławska-Socha, J., Gorski, S., Price, T., & Orzechowski, P. M. (2024). The potential of virtual triage AI to improve early detection, care acuity alignment, and emergent care referral of life-threatening conditions. *Frontiers in Public Health, 12*, 1362246. Advance online publication. DOI: 10.3389/fpubh.2024.1362246 PMID: 38807993

Getzen, T. E., & Kobernick, M. S. (2022). *Health economics and financing* (6th ed.). Wiley.

Ghassemi, M., Oakden-Rayner, L., & Beam, A. L. (2021). The false hope of current approaches to explainable artificial intelligence in health care. *The Lancet. Digital Health*, *3*(11), e745–e750. DOI: 10.1016/S2589-7500(21)00208-9 PMID: 34711379

Ghosh, S., & Ghosh, S. K. (2023). Feel: Federated learning framework for elderly healthcare using edge-iomt. *IEEE Transactions on Computational Social Systems*, *10*(4), 1800–1809.

Giannios, G., Mpaltadoros, L., Alepoulos, V., Grammatikopoulou, M., Stavropoulos, T. G., Nikolopoulos, S., Lazarou, I., Tsolaki, M., & Kompatsiaris, I. (2024). A semantic framework to detect problems in activities of daily living monitored through smart home sensors [Recent 2024 study on smart home sensors for cognitive decline monitoring in elderly; Web of Science/Scopus indexed]. *Sensors (Basel)*, *24*(4), 1107. DOI: 10.3390/s24041107 PMID: 38400265

Gillard, A. K., McNeair, T., Andrew, N. E., Haines, T., Hill, K. D., Moran, C., & Long, K. M. (2025). Multi-stakeholder aged care research networks: A scoping review. *The Gerontologist*, *65*(3), gnae152. PMID: 39478337

Gill, T. M., Murphy, T. E., Gahbauer, E. A., & Allore, H. G. (2013). The course of disability before and after a serious fall injury. *JAMA Internal Medicine*, *173*(19), 1780–1786. DOI: 10.1001/jamainternmed.2013.9063 PMID: 23958741

Goel, A., Goel, A. K., & Kumar, A. (2023). The role of artificial neural network and machine learning in utilizing spatial information. *Spatial Information Research*, *31*(3), 355–364. DOI: 10.1007/s41324-022-00494-2

Goel, G. S., Gupta, B., Mittal, A., & Gupta, S. (2022a). Prevalence Of Risk Factors Of Non Communicable Diseases In District Ambala, Haryana. *Journal of Pharmaceutical Negative Results*, *13*(8), 4768–4772. DOI: 10.47750/pnr.2022.13.S08.623

Goisauf, M., & Cano Abad'ıa, M. (2022). Ethics of AI in radiology: A review of ethical and societal implications. *Frontiers in Big Data*, *5*, 850383. DOI: 10. 3389/fdata.2022.850383 PMID: 35910490

Golden, A. (2023). THEORETICAL FRAMEWORK FOR AN ARTIFICIAL INTELLIGENCE–BASED COMPREHENSIVE GERIATRIC ASSESSMENT. *Innovation in Aging*, *7*, 877.

González-Castro, A., Leirós-Rodríguez, R., Prada-García, C., & Benítez-Andrades, J. A. (2024). The applications of artificial intelligence for assessing fall risk: Systematic review. *Journal of Medical Internet Research*, *26*, e54934.

Gopalakrishnan, S., Ganeshkumar, P., & Katta, A. (2015). Study of morbidity profile of a rural population in Tamil Nadu. *Journal of Clinical and Diagnostic Research : JCDR*, *9*(2), LC05–LC09. DOI: 10.7860/JCDR/2015/10424.5520 PMID: 25859470

Gorla, N., Somers, T. M., & Wong, B. (2010). Organizational impact of system quality, information quality, and service quality. *The Journal of Strategic Information Systems*, *19*(3), 207–228. DOI: 10.1016/j.jsis.2010.05.001

Görtz, M., Baumgärtner, K., Schmid, T., Muschko, M., Woessner, P., Gerlach, A., & Hohenfellner, M. (2023). An artificial intelligence-based chatbot for prostate cancer education: Design and patient evaluation study. *Digital Health*, *9*, 20552076231173304.

Goyal, N. K. (2025). Security and privacy in IoT, fog, and blockchain networks. In Sathio, A., Rind, M., Awan, S., & Junejo, A. (Eds.), *Energy-efficient deep learning approaches in IoT, fog, and green blockchain revolution* (pp. 371–398). IGI Global Scientific Publishing., DOI: 10.4018/979-8-3373-0300-0.ch015

Goyal, N. K. (2025). Weaponizing misinformation and cyberattacks on supply chains. In Bukhari, S., & Zafar, I. (Eds.), *Mass media and impact of fake news on supply chains* (pp. 177–210). IGI Global Scientific Publishing., DOI: 10.4018/979-8-3373-2175-2.ch007

Goyal, N. K., Dandotiya, M., Kumari, M., Kaloria, S., & Anushya, A. (2025). AI-powered haptic devices for patient rehabilitation. In Mamodiya, U., Kalam, A., Bossoufi, B., Awad, M., & Somwanshi, D. (Eds.), *Integrating AI with haptic systems for smarter healthcare solutions* (pp. 143–170). IGI Global Scientific Publishing., DOI: 10.4018/979-8-3373-2307-7.ch007

Goyal, N. K., Dandotiya, M., Kumari, M., Sheikh, M. F., & Sharma, S. (2025). Emerging job roles in the tourism sector leveraging artificial intelligence. In Silic, M., Luthia, M., Ahmad, F., & Chakraborty, P. (Eds.), *Empowering sustainable performance and competitive advantage in tourism* (pp. 89–126). IGI Global Scientific Publishing., DOI: 10.4018/979-8-3373-4546-8.ch004

Goyal, N. K., Dandotiya, M., Qurashi, J. A., Kumari, M., & Sharma, S. (2025). AI-driven predictive analytics for disease management. In Ouaissa, M., Ouaissa, M., Imad, M., Qurashi, J., & Farooq, M. (Eds.), *Utilizing AI of medical things for healthcare security and sustainability* (pp. 231–276). IGI Global Scientific Publishing., DOI: 10.4018/979-8-3373-0690-2.ch008

Goyal, N. K., Kumari, M., Kushwah, V., Dandotiya, M., & Vijay, A. (2025). Evaluating blockchain security: Trade-offs in consensus mechanisms. *IET Conference Proceedings*, 2024(38), 80–88. https://doi.org/DOI: 10.1049/icp.2025.0775

Gray, K., Slavotinek, J., Dimaguila, G. L., & Choo, D. (2022). Artificial intelligence education for the health workforce: Expert survey of approaches and needs. *JMIR Medical Education*, *8*(2), e35223.

Gray-Miceli, D., Bouchaud, M., Bradley Mitchell, A., DiDonato, S., & Siegal, J. (2020). Caught off guard by COVID-19: Now what? *Geriatric Nursing*, *41*(6), 789–790. DOI: 10.1016/j.gerinurse.2020.08.006 PMID: 33158627

Griˇskeviˇcius, J., Daunoraviˇciene˙, K., Petrauskas, L., Apˇsega, A., & Alekna, V. (2025). Retrospective frailty assessment in older adults using inertial measurement unitbased deep learning on gait spectrograms [PMID: PMC12157785. Latest 2025 research on AI-driven gait analysis for frailty prediction in elderly]. *Sensors (Basel)*, *25*(11), 3351. DOI: 10.3390/s25113351 PMID: 40968907

Grueso, S., & Viejo-Sobera, R. (2021). Machine learning methods for predicting progression from mild cognitive impairment to Alzheimer's disease dementia: A systematic review. *Alzheimer's Research & Therapy*, *13*(1), 162. Advance online publication. DOI: 10.1186/s13195-021-00900-6 PMID: 34583745

Guasti, L., Fumagalli, S., Afilalo, J., Geisler, T., Abreu, A., Ambrosetti, M., & Ferrini, M. (2025). Cardiovascular diseases, prevention, and management of complications in older adults and frail patients treated for elective or post-traumatic hip orthopaedic interventions: A clinical consensus statement. *European Journal of Preventive Cardiology*, *32*(2), 186–198. DOI: 10.1093/eurjpc/zwaf010 PMID: 39812215

Gu, D., Dupre, M. E., & Liu, G. (2007). Characteristics of the institutionalized and community residing oldest-old in China. *Social Science & Medicine*, *64*(4), 871–883. PMID: 17126971

Gudala, M., Ross, M. E. T., Mogalla, S., Lyons, M., Ramaswamy, P., & Roberts, K. (2022). Benefits of, barriers to, and needs for an artificial intelligence–powered medication information voice chatbot for older adults: Interview study with geriatrics experts. *JMIR Aging*, *5*(2), e32169.

Gupta, I., & Sankar, D. Delhi 2002 ' Health of the Elderly in India: A Multivariate Analysis ', Institute of Economic Growth Discussion Paper No. 46.

Gupta, A., Sawhney, S., & Ahmed, S. (2025). CareTaker.ai—A smart health-monitoring and caretaker-assistant system for elder healthcare. *Engineering Proceedings*, *74*(1), 15. DOI: 10.3390/engproc2024074015

Gupta, S., Kamboj, S., & Bag, S. (2023). Role of risks in the development of responsible artificial intelligence in the digital healthcare domain. *Information Systems Frontiers*, *25*(6), 2257–2274.

Hadavandsiri, F., Shafaati, M., Mohammad Nejad, S., Ebrahimzadeh Mousavi, M., Najafi, A., & Mirzaei, M.. (2023). Non-communicable disease comorbidities in HIV patients: Diabetes, hypertension, heart disease, and obstructive sleep apnea as a neglected issue. *Scientific Reports*, *13*(1), 12730. DOI: 10.1038/s41598-023-39828-6 PMID: 37543699

Hajdú, J. (2020). Dignity of elderly persons and digitalised social care. In *The Right to Human Dignity* (p. 569).

Hakami, S. M., Omar, M. T., Alsaad, S. M., Vennu, V. S., Hattan, L. I., & Bindawas, S. M. (2023). Association between non-communicable diseases and physical activity level in older adults visiting primary health care centers in Jizan, Saudi Arabia. *Saudi Medical Journal*, *44*(6), 580–587. DOI: 10.15537/smj.2023.44.6.20230076 PMID: 37343987

Hanke, S., Mangialasche, F., Bödenler, M., Neumayer, B., Ngandu, T., Mecocci, P., & Stögmann, E. (2022). AI-based predictive modelling of the onset and progression of dementia. *Smart Cities*, *5*(2), 700–714.

Hanna-Pladdy, B., & MacKay, A. (2011). The relation between instrumental musical activity and cognitive aging. *Neuropsychology*, *25*(3), 378–386. DOI: 10.1037/a0022179

Hansen, A. R., McLendon, S. F., & Rochani, H. (2022). Care coordination for rural residents with chronic disease: Predictors of improved outcomes. *Public Health Nursing (Boston, Mass.)*, *39*(5), 1093–1101. DOI: 10.1111/phn.13092 PMID: 34962313

Han, X., Zhou, X., Tan, B., Jiao, L., & Zhang, R. (2023). AI-based next-generation sensors for enhanced rehabilitation monitoring and analysis. *Measurement*, *223*, 113758.

Harrington, C. N., Jelen, B., Lazar, A., Martin-Hammond, A., Pradhan, A., Reeder, B., & Siek, K. (2021). Taking stock of the present and future of smart technologies for older adults and caregivers. *arXiv preprint arXiv:2104.00096.*

Harris, T. G., Flören, S., Mantell, J. E., Nkambule, R., Lukhele, N. G., & Malinga, B. P.. (2021). HIV and aging among adults aged 50 years and older on antiretroviral therapy in Eswatini. *African Journal of AIDS Research*, *20*(1), 107–115. DOI: 10.2989/16085906.2021.1887301 PMID: 33685372

Hassija, V., Chamola, V., Mahapatra, A., Singal, A., Goel, D., Huang, K., & Hussain, A. (2024). Interpreting black-box models: A review on explainable artificial intelligence. *Cognitive Computation*, *16*(1), 45–74. DOI: 10.1007/s12559-023-10179-8

HelpAge India. (2022). *Elder abuse in India: A national report.* HelpAge India. https://www.helpageindia.org

Hendriks, A., Hacking, C., Verbeek, H., & Aarts, S. (2024). Data science techniques to gain novel insights into quality of care: A scoping review of long-term care for older adults. *Exploration of Digital Health Technologies*, *2*(2), 67–85. DOI: 10.37349/edht.2024.00014

Herath, H., Jayasekara, A., & Madhusanka, B. (2024). Vision attentive technology: AI approaches for functional mobility assessments in elderly healthcare. [HTML].

Herrmann, B. (2023). The perception of artificial-intelligence (AI) based synthesized speech in younger and older adults. *International Journal of Speech Technology*, *26*(2), 395–415.

High-Level Expert Group on AI (HLEG AI). (2019). *Ethics guidelines for trustworthy AI*. European Commission., DOI: 10.2759/346720

Ho, A. (2020). Are we ready for artificial intelligence health monitoring in elder care? *BMC Geriatrics*, *20*(1), 358. DOI: 10.1186/s12877-020-01723-7 PMID: 32957946

Ho, A. (2023). *Live like nobody is watching: Relational autonomy in the age of artificial intelligence health monitoring*. Oxford University Press.

Holm, N. N., Frølich, A., Dominguez, H., Dalhoff, K. P., Juul-Larsen, H. G., Andersen, O., & Stockmarr, A. (2025). Co-occurring diseases and mortality in patients with chronic heart disease, modeling their dynamically expanding disease portfolios: Nationwide register study. *JMIR Cardio*, *9*(1), e57749. Advance online publication. DOI: 10.2196/57749 PMID: 40279150

Holt-Lunstad, J. (2022). Social connection as a public health issue: The evidence and a systemic framework for prioritizing the “social” in social determinants of health. *Annual Review of Public Health*, *43*, 193–213. DOI: 10.1146/annurev-publhealth-052020-110908 PMID: 35021021

Ho, M. T., Le, N. T. B., Mantello, P., Ho, M. T., & Ghotbi, N. (2023). Understanding the acceptance of emotional artificial intelligence in Japanese healthcare system: A cross-sectional survey of clinic visitors’ attitude. *Technology in Society*, *72*, 102166.

Hong, Z., Magdamo, C., Sheu, Y., Mohite, P., Noori, A., Ye, E. M., . . . Das, S. (2020). Natural language processing to detect cognitive concerns in electronic health records using deep learning. *arXiv*. https://arxiv.org/abs/2011.07423 (No DOI available)

Hsieh, S. H., Tseng, T. H., & Lee, C. T. (2018). Drivers of online brand community value creation: The role of psychological empowerment. In *Proceedings of the 51st Hawaii International Conference on System Sciences* (pp. 2220–2229). https://doi.org/DOI: 10.24251/HICSS.2018.280

HuanDong L, Qian L, Yu H, Chouwen Z, Hui M, Jian G, et al. (2017). The prevalence of multiple non-communicable diseases among middle-aged and elderly people: The Shanghai Changfeng Study. *European Journal of Epidemiology*, *32*(2), 159–163. DOI: 10.1007/s10654-016-0211-1 PMID: 27999971

Huang, X., Zhang, Z., Guo, F., Wang, X., Chi, K., & Wu, K. (2024, June). Research on older adults' interaction with e-health interface based on explainable artificial intelligence. In *International Conference on Human-Computer Interaction* (pp. 38-52). Cham: Springer Nature Switzerland.

Huang, K., Jiao, Z., Cai, Y., & Zhong, Z. (2022). Artificial intelligence-based intelligent surveillance for reducing nurses' working hours in nurse–patient interaction: A two-wave study. *Journal of Nursing Management*, *30*(8), 3817–3826.

Huang, W., Ong, W. C., Wong, M. K. F., Ng, E. Y. K., Koh, T., Chandramouli, C., & Tromp, J. (2024). Applying the UTAUT2 framework to patients' attitudes toward healthcare task shifting with artificial intelligence. *BMC Health Services Research*, *24*(1), 455.

Hughes, G. D., Aboyade, O. M., Okonji, C. O., Clark, B., & Mabweazara, S. Z. (2021). Comparison of the prevalence of non-communicable diseases and traditional herbal medicine use in urban and rural communities in South Africa. *Advances in Integrative Medicine*, *8*(2), 136–143. DOI: 10.1016/j.aimed.2020.11.002

Huq, S. M., Maskeliūnas, R., & Damaševičius, R. (2024). Dialogue agents for artificial intelligence-based conversational systems for cognitively disabled: A systematic review. *Disability and Rehabilitation. Assistive Technology*, *19*(3), 1059–1078.

Hu, R., Kabouteh, A., Pawlitza, K., Güttler, J., Linner, T., & Bock, T. (2019). Developing personalized intelligent interior units to promote activity and customized healthcare for aging society. In *ISARC. Proceedings of the International Symposium on Automation and Robotics in Construction* (Vol. 36, pp. 234-241). IAARC Publications.

Hwang, J., & Kim, S. (2023). Public perceptions of artificial intelligence in elder care: A cross-cultural study. *Journal of Gerontological Nursing*, *49*(7), 12–19. DOI: 10.3928/00989134-20230615-03

Hyams, C., Challen, R., Marlow, R., Nguyen, J., Begier, E., Southern, J., & Szasz-Benczur, Z. (2023). Severity of Omicron (B.1.1.529) and Delta (B.1.617.2) SARS-CoV-2 infection among hospitalised adults: A prospective cohort study in Bristol, United Kingdom. *The Lancet Regional Health. Europe*, *25*, 100556. DOI: 10.1016/j.lanepe.2022.100556 PMID: 36530491

Hyväri, S., Elo, S., Kukkohovi, S., & Lotvonen, S. (2024). Utilizing activity sensors to identify behavioural activity patterns of elderly home care clients. *Disability and Rehabilitation. Assistive Technology*, *19*(3), 585–594. DOI: 10.1080/17483107.2022.2123370 PMID: 36067090

Iadarola, G., Mengarelli, A., Crippa, P., Fioretti, S., & Spinsante, S. (2024). A review on assisted living using wearable devices. *Sensors (Basel)*, *24*(23), 7439. DOI: 10.3390/s24237439 PMID: 39685975

Ibeneme, S., Okeibunor, J., Muneene, D., Husain, I., Bento, P., Gaju, C., Housseynou, B., Chibi, M., Karamagi, H., & Makubalo, L. (2021). Data revolution, health status transformation and the role of artificial intelligence for health and pandemic preparedness in the African context. *BMC Proceedings*, *15*(Suppl 15), 22. DOI: 10.1186/s12919-021-00228-1 PMID: 34809624

Ibuki, T., Ibuki, A., & Nakazawa, E. (2024). Possibilities and ethical issues of entrusting nursing tasks to robots and artificial intelligence. *Nursing Ethics*, *31*(6), 1010–1020.

Ienca, M. (2017). *Intelligent technologies for the aging brain: Opportunities and challenges* (Doctoral dissertation, University of Basel).

Igwama, G. T., Olaboye, J. A., Maha, C. C., Ajegbile, M. D., & Abdul, S. (2024). Integrating electronic health records systems across borders: Technical challenges and policy solutions. *International Medical Science Research Journal*, *4*(7), 788–796. DOI: 10.51594/imsrj.v4i7.1360

Iliffe, S., Tai, S. S., Haines, A., Gallivan, S., Goldenberg, E., Booroff, A., & Morgan, P. (1992). Are elderly people living alone an at risk group? *British Medical Journal*, *305*(6860), 1001–1004. PMID: 1458108

Imran, R., & Khan, S. S. (2025). A systematic review on the efficacy of artificial intelligence in geriatric healthcare: A critical analysis of current literature. *BMC Geriatrics*, *25*(1), 56. DOI: 10.1186/s12877-024-04709-2 PMID: 40217136

Iqbal, J. D., & Biller-Andorno, N. (2022). The regulatory gap in digital health and alternative pathways to bridge it. *Health Policy and Technology*, *11*(3), 100664. Advance online publication. DOI: 10.1016/j.hlpt.2022.100664

Ithnin M, Nor NAUM, Nordin NJ, Effendy NM, Sahar MA, Abdullah KHA, et al. Knowledge, attitude, and practice on non-communicable diseases (NCDs) among the adult population in the urban area of Negeri Sembilan, Malaysia. Int J Res Pharm Sci. 2018;9(Special Issue 2):88–94. https://doi.org/DOI: 10.26452/ijrps.v9iSPL2.1747

Iwasa, H., Kawaai, C., Gondo, Y., Inagaki, H., & Suzuki, T. (2006). Subjective well-being as a predictor of all-cause mortality among middle-aged and elderly people living in an urban Japanese community: A seven-year prospective cohort study. *Geriatrics & Gerontology International*, *6*(4), 216–222.

Jacobsen, J.-H., Stelzer, J., & Särkämö, T. (2015). Why musical memory can be preserved in advanced Alzheimer's disease. *Brain*, *138*(8), 2122–2124. DOI: 10.1093/brain/awv148

Jain, P., & Singh, P. (2023). Lethargic approach in expediting financial reporting system: A case of construction firm. *International Journal of Teaching and Case Studies*, *14*(1), 1–10.

Jain, P., Singh, P., & Kushwaha, R. (2025). Investigating change management as a novel digital wallet service innovation in banks: A case of Indian bank. *Int. J. Teaching and Case Studies*, *15*(1), 67–81.

Jakovljevic, M., Kumagai, N., & Ogura, S. (2023). Global population aging–Health care, social and economic consequences, volume II. *Frontiers in Public Health, 11*, 1184950.s, D., Hornung, H., Nadimpalli, A., & Peery, A. (2021). Deep learning and its application for healthcare delivery in low and middle income countries. *Frontiers in Artificial Intelligence*, *4*, 553987.

Jankovic, J., Mirkovic, M., Jovic-Vranes, A., Santric-Milicevic, M., & Terzic-Supic, Z. (2018). Association between non-communicable disease multimorbidity and health care utilization in a middle-income country: Population-based study. *Public Health*, *155*, 35–42. DOI: 10.1016/j.puhe.2017.11.014 PMID: 29306621

Janson, P., Willeke, K., Zaibert, L., Budnick, A., Berghöfer, A., Kittel-Schneider, S., & Keil, T. (2022). Mortality, morbidity and health-related outcomes in informal caregivers compared to non-caregivers: A systematic review. *International Journal of Environmental Research and Public Health*, *19*(10), 5864. Advance online publication. DOI: 10.3390/ijerph19105864 PMID: 35627399

Javadi-Pashaki, N., Ghazanfari, M. J., & Karkhah, S. (2021). Machine learning for geriatric clinical care: Opportunities and challenges. *Annals of Geriatric Medicine and Research*, *25*(2), 137.

Jin Park, H. (2024). Patient perspectives on informed consent for medical AI: A web-based experiment. *Frontiers in Artificial Intelligence*, *7*, 1322797. Advance online publication. DOI: 10.3389/frai.2024.1322797

Jnr, B. A. (2025). User-centered AI-based voice-assistants for safe mobility of older people in urban context. *AI & Society*, *40*(2), 545–568.

Johnson, J. K., Sherman, S., & Coulton, S. (2013). A community choir intervention to promote well-being among diverse older adults: Results from the community of voices trial. The Journals of Gerontology: Series B, 75(3), 570–579. https://doi.org/ DOI: 10.1093/geronb/gbx134

Jonek-Kowalska, I., & Wolny, M. (2025). Age Sustainability in Smart City: Seniors as Urban Stakeholders in the Light of Literature Studies. *Sustainability*, *17*(14), 6333.

Joseph, N., & Gupta, S. (2016). Assessment of economic impact among in-patients with non-communicable diseases in a private tertiary care hospital in Southern India. *Journal of Clinical and Diagnostic Research : JCDR*, *10*(6), LM04–LM06. DOI: 10.7860/JCDR/2016/19426.8059 PMID: 27504316

Joshi, H. (2025). Natural language processing of electronic health records for predicting Alzheimer's disease. In *Deep generative models for integrative analysis of Alzheimer's biomarkers* (pp. 141–174). IGI Global., DOI: 10.4018/979-8-3693-3949-7.ch006

Jovanovic, M., Mitrov, G., Zdravevski, E., Lameski, P., Colantonio, S., Kampel, M., & Florez-Revuelta, F. (2022). Ambient assisted living: Scoping review of artificial intelligence models, domains, technology, and concerns. *Journal of Medical Internet Research*, *24*(11), e36553. DOI: 10.2196/36553 PMID: 36331530

Jun Woo, C. H. O. I., & KANG, M. S. (2024). A Study on the development of a chatbot using generative AI to provide diets for diabetic patients. *Korean Journal of Artificial Intelligence*, *12*(3), 25–31.

Junglas, I., & Harris, J. (2013). The promise of consumer technologies in emerging markets. *Communications of the ACM*, *56*(5), 84–90. DOI: 10.1145/2447976.2447996

Justo-Hanani, R. (2022). The politics of artificial intelligence regulation and governance reform in the European Union. *Policy Sciences*, *55*(1), 137–159.

Kalusivalingam, A. K., Sharma, A., Patel, N., & Singh, V. (2021). Leveraging federated learning and explainable AI for advancing health equity: A comprehensive approach to reducing disparities in healthcare access and outcomes. *International Journal of Artificial Intelligence and Machine Learning*, *2*(3).

Kamiyole, S. (2025). *Impact of electronic prescription, access, and messaging on health information exchange utilization during care transition* [Doctoral dissertation, Ohio University]. OhioLINK Electronic Theses and Dissertations Center. https://rave.ohiolink.edu/etdc/view?acc_num=ohiou1725998654793512 (No DOI available)

Kandpal, S. D., Kakkar, R., Aggarwal, P., & Bansal, S. (2013). Pattern of prevalence of risk factors for non-communicable diseases in the geriatric population of district Dehradun. *Indian Acad Clin Med.*, *14*(3–4), 214–217.

Kansiime, S., Mwesigire, D., & Mugerwa, H. (2019). Prevalence of non-communicable diseases among HIV positive patients on antiretroviral therapy at joint clinical research centre, Lubowa, Uganda. *PLoS One*, *14*(8). Advance online publication. DOI: 10.1371/journal.pone.0221022 PMID: 31398244

Kastor, A., & Mohanty, S. K. (2018). Disease-specific out-of-pocket and catastrophic health expenditure on hospitalization in India: Do Indian households face distress health financing? *PLoS One*, *13*(5), 1–18. DOI: 10.1371/journal.pone.0196106 PMID: 29746481

Kaur, D., Rasane, P., Singh, J., Kaur, S., Kumar, V., Mahato, D. K., & Kumar, S. (2019). Nutritional interventions for elderly and considerations for the development of geriatric foods. *Current Aging Science*, *12*(1), 15–27. PMID: 31109282

Kaur, G., Bansal, R., Anand, T., Kumar, A., & Singh, J. (2019). Morbidity profile of noncommunicable diseases among elderly in a city in North India. *Clinical Epidemiology and Global Health*, *7*(1), 29–34. DOI: 10.1016/j.cegh.2017.12.004

Kaya, F., Aydin, F., Schepman, A., Rodway, P., Yetişensoy, O., & Demir Kaya, M. (2024). The roles of personality traits, AI anxiety, and demographic factors in attitudes toward artificial intelligence. *International Journal of Human-Computer Interaction*, *40*(2), 497–514.

Kedziora, D. (2022). Botsourcing, roboshoring or virtual backoffice? perspectives on implementing robotic process automation (RPA) and artificial intelligence (AI). *Human Technology*, *18*(2), 92–97.

Keeler, J. R., Roth, E. A., & Neufeld, R. W. J. (2015). The effects of improvised and pre-composed group singing on oxytocin levels. *Frontiers in Psychology*, *6*, 1481. DOI: 10.3389/fpsyg.2015.01481

Kerwan, A., Al-Jabir, A., Mathew, G., Sohrabi, C., Rashid, R., Franchi, T., & Agha, R. A. (2025). Revised surgical CAse REport (SCARE) guideline: An update for the age of artificial intelligence. *Premier J. Sci.*, *10*(100079), 2025.

Khademi, N., Babanejad, M., Asadmobini, A., & Karim, H. (2017). The association of age and gender with risk factors of noncommunicable diseases among employees in West of Iran. *International Journal of Preventive Medicine, 8*. Advance online publication. DOI: 10.4103/ijpvm.IJPVM_400_16 PMID: 28299033

Khalate, P., Gite, S., Pradhan, B., & Lee, C. W. (2024). Opportunities and gaps in natural language processing and machine learning applications in healthcare: A comprehensive review of electronic medical records and medical imaging. *Frontiers in Physics, 12*, 1372870. Advance online publication. DOI: 10.3389/fphy.2024.1372870

Khalid, N., Qayyum, A., Bilal, M., Al-Fuqaha, A., & Qadir, J. (2023). Privacy-preserving artificial intelligence in healthcare: Techniques and applications. *Computers in Biology and Medicine, 158*, 106848. Advance online publication. DOI: 10.1016/j.compbiomed.2023.106848 PMID: 37044052

Khan, M. F., Ghazal, T. M., Said, R. A., Fatima, A., Abbas, S., Khan, M. A., & Khan, M. A. (2021). An IoMT-enabled smart healthcare model to monitor elderly people using machine learning technique. *Computational Intelligence and Neuroscience, 2021*, 2487759. PMID: 34868288

Khan, N., Jackson, D., Stayt, L., & Walthall, H. (2019). Factors influencing nurses' intentions to leave adult critical care settings. *Nursing in Critical Care, 24*(1), 24–32. DOI: 10.1111/nicc.12348 PMID: 29635820

Kharicha, K., Iliffe, S., Harari, D., Swift, C., Gillmann, G., & Stuck, A. E. (2007). Health risk appraisal in older people 1: Are older people living alone an "at-risk" group? *The British Journal of General Practice, 57*(537), 271–276. PMID: 17394729

Khosravi, P., & Ghapanchi, A. H. (2016). Investigating the effectiveness of technologies applied to assist seniors: A systematic literature review. *International Journal of Medical Informatics, 85*(1), 17–26. PMID: 26216463

Kien, V. D., Van Minh, H., Giang, K. B., Dao, A., Weinehall, L., & Eriksson, M.. (2017). Socioeconomic inequalities in self-reported chronic non-communicable diseases in urban Hanoi, Vietnam. *Global Public Health: An International Journal for Research, Policy and Practice, 12*(12), 1522–1537. DOI: 10.1080/17441692.2015.1123282 PMID: 26727691

Kim, D. H. (2024). Unleashing frailty from laboratory into real world: A critical step toward frailty-guided clinical care of older adults. *Journal of the American Geriatrics Society, 72*(12), 3643–3645. DOI: 10.1111/jgs.19229 PMID: 39166879

Kim, D. J., Lee, Y. S., Jeon, E. R., & Kim, K. J. (2024, January). Present and future of AI-IoT-based healthcare services for senior citizens in local communities: A review of a South Korean government digital healthcare initiatives. []. MDPI.]. *Health Care, 12*(2), 281.

Kim, H., Cho, J., Shin, S., & Kim, S. S. (2024). Uncertainty in surrogate decision-making about end-of-life care for people with dementia: An integrative review. *Journal of Advanced Nursing, 80*(12), 4962–4976. DOI: 10.1111/jan.16194 PMID: 38197503

Kim, J. W., Choi, Y. L., Jeong, S. H., & Han, J. (2022). A care robot with ethical sensing system for older adults at home. *Sensors (Basel), 22*(15), 5515. DOI: 10.3390/s22155515 PMID: 36236614

Kim, J., & Park, S. (2023). Integrating social technologies in elder care: A socio-technical framework for sustainable aging. *Journal of Aging Studies, 67*(3), 89–102. DOI: 10.1016/j.jaging.2023.101123

Kim, J., & Yoo, H. S. (2015). Effects of music therapy on cognitive functions in patients with dementia: A systematic review. *Psychiatry Investigation, 12*(4), 489–497. DOI: 10.4306/pi.2015.12.4.489

Kim, S. (2021). Exploring how older adults use a smart speaker–based voice assistant in their first interactions: Qualitative study. *JMIR mHealth and uHealth, 9*(1), e20427. PMID: 33439130

Kinsella, K., & Gist, Y. J. (1998). *International Brief on Gender and Aging*. United States Department of Commerce, Economics and Statistics Administration.

Kleinman, A., Chen, H., Levkoff, S. E., Forsyth, A., Bloom, D. E., Yip, W., & Habbal, F. (2021). Social technology: An interdisciplinary approach to improving care for older adults. *Frontiers in Public Health, 9*, 729605. DOI: 10.3389/fpubh.2021.729605 PMID: 35004562

Knevel, R., & Liao, K. P. (2023). From real-world electronic health record data to real-world results using artificial intelligence. *Annals of the Rheumatic Diseases, 82*(3), 306–311. DOI: 10.1136/annrheumdis-2022-222626 PMID: 36150748

Knodel, J., & Debavalya, N. (1997). Living arrangements and support among the elderly in South-east Asia: An introduction. *Asia-Pacific Population Journal, 12*(4), 5–16. PMID: 12293567

Koc, M. (2023). ARTIFICIAL INTELLIGENCE IN GERIATRICS. *Turkish Journal of Geriatrics/Türk Geriatri Dergisi, 26*(4).

Koçak, B., Ponsiglione, A., Stanzione, A., Bluethgen, C., Santinha, J., Ugga, L., & Cuocolo, R. (2025). Bias in artificial intelligence for medical imaging: Fundamentals, detection, avoidance, mitigation, challenges, ethics, and prospects. *Diagnostic and Interventional Radiology*, *31*(2), 75–87. DOI: 10.4274/dir.2024.242715 PMID: 38953330

Koc, M. (2023). Artificial intelligence in geriatrics. *Turk Geriatri Dergisi*, *26*(3), 238–249. DOI: 10.29400/tjgeri.2023.355

Koelsch, S. (2014). Brain correlates of music-evoked emotions. *Nature Reviews. Neuroscience*, *15*(3), 170–180. DOI: 10.1038/nrn3660

Kokshagina, O. (2021). Managing shifts to value-based healthcare and value digitalization as a multi-level dynamic capability development process. *Technological Forecasting and Social Change*, *172*, 121037. DOI: 10.1016/j.techfore.2021.121037

Kolk, A. (2014). Partnerships as panacea for addressing global problems? On rationale, context, and limitations. *Business & Society*, *53*(6), 937–979. DOI: 10.1177/0007650314520962

Koole, S. L., van den Hout, M. A., & van Veen, V. (2015). Meditation leads to reduced default mode network activity beyond an active task. *Cognitive, Affective & Behavioral Neuroscience*, *15*(3), 712–720. DOI: 10.3758/s13415-015-0358-3

Kouroubali, A., Kondylakis, H., Logothetidis, F., & Katehakis, D. G. (2022). Developing an AI-enabled integrated care platform for frailty. *Health Care*, *10*(3), 443. Advance online publication. DOI: 10.3390/healthcare10030443 PMID: 35326921

Kouroupis, K. (2021). Facial recognition: a challenge for europe or a threat to human rights?. Eur. J. Privacy L. & Tech., 142.

Kouroupis, K., & Serotila, I. (2022). Privacy and security in light of the European Digital Agenda. Nomiki Bibliothiki, 18-36.

Kulkarni, M. H., & Inamdar, P. R. (2025). Healthcare unbound: Navigating emerging trends and future applications in IoT-based innovations for daily well-being. In *Evolution of machine learning and internet of things applications in biomedical engineering* (pp. 238–250). CRC Press., DOI: 10.1201/9781003447535-11

Kumar, A., Singh, P., Parihar, A.S. & Saraswat, S. (2025), "Analyzing the impact of psychological capital on the entrepreneurial intentions of students through mediating role of individual expectancy using PLS-SEM", *International Journal of Social Economics*, Vol. ahead-of-print No. ahead-of-print. https://doi.org/.DOI: 10.1108/IJSE-03-2024-0252

Kumar, S. (2021). Elderly care in India: A neglected dimension in public policy. *Journal of Social and Economic Development, 23*(2), 294–311.

Kumar, S., Underwood, S. H., Masters, J. L., Manley, N. A., Konstantzos, I., & Lau, J.. (2023). Ten questions concerning smart and healthy built environments for older adults. *Building and Environment*, *244*, 110720.

Kumar, Y., Koul, A., Singla, R., & Ijaz, M. (2022). Artificial intelligence in disease diagnosis: A systematic literature review, synthesizing framework and future research agenda. *Journal of Ambient Intelligence and Humanized Computing*, *14*, 8459–8486. DOI: 10.1007/s12652-021-03612-z PMID: 35039756

Kundu, J., & Chakraborty, R. (2023). Socio-economic inequalities in burden of communicable and non-communicable diseases among older adults in India: Evidence from Longitudinal Ageing Study in India, 2017–18. *PLoS One*, *18*(3). Advance online publication. DOI: 10.1371/journal.pone.0283385 PMID: 36996071

Kunna, R., San Sebastian, M., & Stewart Williams, J. (2017). Measurement and decomposition of socioeconomic inequality in single and multimorbidity in older adults in China and Ghana: Results from the WHO study on global AGEing and adult health (SAGE). *International Journal for Equity in Health*, *16*(1). Advance online publication. DOI: 10.1186/s12939-017-0578-y PMID: 28506233

Kushwaha, J., Singh, P., & Sharma, A. (2023b). Modelling the enablers of work-family balance among working single mothers integrating expert-mining and TISM-MICMAC. *Journal of Organizational Effectiveness: People and Performance*. Advance online publication. doi: .DOI: 10.1108/JOEPP-05-2022-0106

Kushwaha, J., Sharma, A., & Singh, P. (2023a). Exploration and prioritization of enablers to organization work–family balance planning for working sole Indian mothers integrating fuzzy Delphi and AHP. *International Journal of Social Economics*, *50*(3), 398–418.

Kushwaha, J., Singh, P., & Kushwaha, R. (2024). Predicting working sole Indian mothers' satisfaction towards work–family balance integrating the Kano model and weighted average method. *International Journal of Social Economics*, *51*(6), 725–740.

Kushwaha, J., Singh, P., & Kushwah, R. (2025). *Work-Family Balance Among Working Sole Mothers: Insights From Systematic Integrative Literature Review and Thematic Analysis*. Leading Inclusive Workplaces Through Digital Transformation and Organizational Change.

Kyprianidou, M., Panagiotakos, D., Makris, K. C., Kambanaros, M., Christophi, C. A., & Giannakou, K. (2023). Prevalence and sociodemographic determinants of selected noncommunicable diseases among the general population of Cyprus: A large population-based cross-sectional study. *Chronic Diseases and Translational Medicine, 9*(3), 222–237. DOI: 10.1002/cdt3.70 PMID: 37711870

Kyriazis, I., Lappa, T., Koufopoulou, K., Sidiropoulos, S., Efthymiou, I. P., & Vozikis, A. (2018). *Impact of Austerity on Dietary Habits and Obesity in Greek Children, Adolescents and Adult. The Impact and Implications of Crisis: A Comprehensive Approach Combining Elements of Health and Society*. Nova Science Publishers, Inc.

Lambert, S. I., Madi, M., Sopka, S., Lenes, A., Stange, H., Buszello, C. P., & Stephan, A. (2023). An integrative review on the acceptance of artificial intelligence among healthcare professionals in hospitals. *NPJ Digital Medicine, 6*(1), 111.

Lamb, S. (2009). *Aging and the Indian diaspora: Cosmopolitan families in India and abroad*. Indiana University Press.

Lang, B. H., Nyholm, S., & Blumenthal-Barby, J. (2023). Responsibility gaps and black box healthcare AI: Shared responsibilization as a solution. *Digital Health, 9*, 1–12. DOI: 10.1177/20552076231220888 PMID: 38596344

Larburu, N., Garcia-Zapirain, B., & Alvarez, R. (2022). Integrating EHRs and AI for personalized nutrition interventions. *Healthcare Technology Letters, 9*(3), 45–55. DOI: 10.1049/htl2.12030

Laschinger, H. K. S. (2012). Job and career satisfaction and turnover intentions of newly graduated nurses. *Journal of Nursing Management, 20*(4), 472–484. DOI: 10.1111/j.1365-2834.2011.01293.x PMID: 22591149

Laschinger, H. K. S., Finegan, J., Shamian, J., & Wilk, P. (2001). Impact of structural and psychological empowerment on job strain in nursing work settings: Expanding Kanter's model. *The Journal of Nursing Administration, 31*(5), 260–272. DOI: 10.1097/00005110-200105000-00006 PMID: 11388162

Lau, C. H., Yu, K. H. O., Yip, T. F., Luk, L. Y. F., Wai, A. K. C., Sit, T. Y., & Ho, J. W. K. (2022). An artificial intelligence-enabled smartphone app for real-time pressure injury assessment. *Frontiers in Medical Technology, 4*, 905074.

Laur, O., & Wang, B. (2022). Musculoskeletal trauma and artificial intelligence: Current trends and projections. *Skeletal Radiology, 51*(2), 257–269.

Leal-Junior, A. G., Díaz, C. R., Leitão, C., Pontes, M. J., Marques, C., & Frizera, A. (2019). Polymer optical fiber-based sensor for simultaneous measurement of breath and heart rate under dynamic movements. *Optics & Laser Technology, 109*, 429–436. DOI: 10.1016/j.optlastec.2018.08.048

Lee, C. H., Wang, C., Fan, X., Li, F., & Chen, C. H. (2023). Artificial intelligence-enabled digital transformation in elderly healthcare field: Scoping review. *Advanced Engineering Informatics*, *55*, 101874.

Lee, C., & Coughlin, J. F. (2022). Inclusive design for aging populations: Addressing digital disparities in technology adoption. *Journal of Aging & Social Policy*, *34*(5), 678–695. DOI: 10.1080/08959420.2022.2047890

Lee, H., Chung, M. A., Kim, H., & Nam, E. W. (2022). The effect of cognitive function health care using artificial intelligence robots for older adults: Systematic review and meta-analysis. *JMIR Aging*, *5*(2), e38896.

Lee, N., & Kim, J. H. (2019). Emotion vs. Function. *The Effects of AI Speaker's Recognition on Product Attitude and Continuance Intention.*, *20*(12), 2535–2543.

Lena, A., Ashok, K., Padma, M., Kamath, V., & Kamath, A. (2009). Health and social problems of the elderly: A cross-sectional study in Udupi Taluk, Karnataka. *Indian Journal of Community Medicine : Official Publication of Indian Association of Preventive & Social Medicine*, *34*(2), 131–134. PMID: 19966960

Leviton, A., & Loddenkemper, T. (2023). Design, implementation, and inferential issues associated with clinical trials that rely on data in electronic medical records: A narrative review. *BMC Medical Research Methodology*, *23*(1), 196. Advance online publication. DOI: 10.1186/s12874-023-02015-8 PMID: 37974111

Lewicki, K., Lee, M. S. A., Cobbe, J., & Singh, J. (2023). Out of context: Investigating the bias and fairness concerns of "artificial intelligence as a service". In *Proceedings of the 2023 CHI Conference on Human Factors in Computing Systems* (pp. 1–17). ACM. https://doi.org/DOI: 10.1145/3544548.3580763

Liang, W., Tadesse, G. A., Ho, D., Fei-Fei, L., Zaharia, M., Zhang, C., & Zou, J. (2022). Advances, challenges and opportunities in creating data for trustworthy AI. *Nature Machine Intelligence*, *4*(8), 669–677. DOI: 10.1038/s42256-022-00512-0

Li, L. W., Zhang, J., & Liang, J. (2009). Health among the oldest-old in China: Which living arrangements make a difference? *Social Science & Medicine*, *68*(2), 220–227. PMID: 19019514

Lima, G. S., Figueira, A. L. G., Carvalho, E. C. D., Kusumota, L., & Caldeira, S. (2023). Resilience in older people: A concept analysis. *Health Care*, *11*(18), 2491. DOI: 10.3390/healthcare11182491 PMID: 37761688

Lim, L. L., & Ng, T. P. (2010). Living alone, lack of a confidant and psychological well-being of elderly women in Singapore: The mediating role of loneliness. *Asia-Pacific Psychiatry*, *2*(1), 33–40.

Lin, B. S., Peng, C. W., Lee, I. J., Hsu, H. K., & Lin, B. S. (2023). System based on artificial intelligence edge computing for detecting bedside falls and sleep posture. *IEEE Journal of Biomedical and Health Informatics*, *27*(7), 3549–3558. DOI: 10.1109/JBHI.2023.3264682 PMID: 37115834

Lindeberg, J., Henkel, M., Perjons, E., Johannesson, P., & Lappalainen, K. F. (2023, April). AI solutions for inter-organisational care: A case based analysis. In *World Conference on Information Systems and Technologies* (pp. 538-549). Cham: Springer Nature Switzerland.

Li, R., Wang, X., Lawler, K., Garg, S., Bai, Q., & Alty, J. (2022). Applications of artificial intelligence to aid early detection of dementia: A scoping review on current capabilities and future directions. *Journal of Biomedical Informatics*, *127*, 104030. Advance online publication. DOI: 10.1016/j.jbi.2022.104030 PMID: 35183766

Liu, Q., Vaci, N., Koychev, I., Kormilitzin, A., Li, Z., Cipriani, A., & Nevado-Holgado, A. (2022). Personalised treatment for cognitive impairment in dementia: Development and validation of an artificial intelligence model. *The Lancet. Digital Health*, *4*(2), e94–e102. DOI: 10.1016/S2589-7500(21)00260-0 PMID: 35101059

Liu, X., Chau, K. Y., Liu, X., & Wan, Y. (2023). The progress of smart elderly care research: A scientometric analysis based on CNKI and WOS. *International Journal of Environmental Research and Public Health*, *20*(2), 1086.

Liu, Z., Zhao, L., Man, Q., Wang, J., Zhao, W., & Zhang, J. (2019). Dietary micronutrients intake status among Chinese elderly people living at home: Data from CNNHS 2010–2012. *Nutrients*, *11*(8), 1787. PMID: 31382399

Livieri, G., Anastasopoulou, C., Briola, K., Nikolopoulou, P., & Efthymiou, I.-P. (2024). Ethical issues arising from the use of AI in drug discovery. *Journal of Politics and Ethics in New Technologies and AI*, *3*(1), e37093. Advance online publication. DOI: 10.12681/jpentai.37093

Livieri, G., Rossi, M., & Bianchi, L. (2024). Privacy and trust in AI-driven elder care devices: A sociotechnical perspective. *International Journal of Human-Computer Studies*, *182*, 102–114. DOI: 10.1016/j.ijhcs.2023.102345

Li, X., Cai, L., Cui, W. L., Wang, X. M., Li, H. F., & He, J. H.. (2020). Association of socioeconomic and lifestyle factors with chronic non-communicable diseases and multimorbidity among the elderly in rural southwest China. *J Public Health.*, *42*(2), 239–246. DOI: 10.1093/pubmed/fdz020 PMID: 30860582

Li, Y., Ho, K., & Popescu, M. (2012). A microphone array system for automatic fall detection. *IEEE Transactions on Biomedical Engineering*, *59*(5), 1291–1301. DOI: 10.1109/TBME.2012.2186446 PMID: 22532430

Li, Y., Zheng, T., Wang, M., Dong, L., Wang, P., & Qin, X. (2021). A coloring and timing brain-computer interface for the nursing bed robot. *Computers & Electrical Engineering*, *95*, 107415. DOI: 10.1016/j.compeleceng.2021.107415

Logistics Management. (2023). Smart supply chains: AI adoption trends in North American food distribution. *Logistics Management, 62*(4), 48–52. https://www.logisticsmgmt.com/

London, A. J., Razin, Y. S., Borenstein, J., Eslami, M., Perkins, R., & Robinette, P. (2023). Ethical issues in near-future socially supportive smart assistants for older adults. *IEEE Transactions on Technology and Society.*

Loveys, K., Prina, M., Axford, C., Domènec, Ò. R., Weng, W., Broadbent, E., & Thiyagarajan, J. A. (2022). Artificial intelligence for older people receiving long-term care: A systematic review of acceptability and effectiveness studies. *The Lancet. Healthy Longevity*, *3*(4), e286–e297. DOI: 10.1016/S2666-7568(22)00034-2 PMID: 35515814

Lukkien, D. R., Nap, H. H., Buimer, H. P., Peine, A., Boon, W. P., Ket, J. C., & Moors, E. H. (2023). Toward responsible artificial intelligence in long-term care: A scoping review on practical approaches. *The Gerontologist*, *63*(1), 155–168. DOI: 10.1093/geront/gnac080 PMID: 34871399

Luo, R. (2025). *AI for systematic reviews, gait, and activity recognition* [Master's thesis, McMaster University]. MacSphere. http://hdl.handle.net/11375/29729 (No DOI available)

Lutala, P., & Muula, A. (2022). Brief behaviour change counselling in non-communicable diseases in Mangochi, Southern Malawi: A hypothetical acceptability study. *Pilot and Feasibility Studies*, *8*(1). Advance online publication. DOI: 10.1186/s40814-022-01032-0 PMID: 35331326

Ma, C., Jiang, Y., Li, Y., Zhang, Y., Wang, X., & Ma, S.. (2019). Medical expenditure for middle-aged and elderly in Beijing. *BMC Health Services Research*, *19*(1), 1–10. DOI: 10.1186/s12913-019-4190-2 PMID: 31174516

Maclagan, L. C., Abdalla, M., Harris, D. A., Stukel, T. A., Chen, B., Candido, E., & Bronskill, S. E. (2023). Can patients with dementia be identified in primary care electronic medical records using natural language processing? *Journal of Healthcare Informatics Research*, *7*(1), 42–58. DOI: 10.1007/s41666-022-00125-5 PMID: 36910911

MacNeil, M., Hirslund, E., Baiocco-Romano, L., Kuspinar, A., & Stolee, P. (2024). A scoping review of the use of intelligent assistive technologies in rehabilitation practice with older adults. *Disability and Rehabilitation. Assistive Technology*, *19*(5), 1817–1848. DOI: 10.1080/17483107.2023.2205958 PMID: 37498115

Ma, J., Li, T., & Wang, K. (2023). AI and personalized medicine in chronic disease management. *npj. Digital Medicine*, *6*(1), 1–9. PMID: 36596833

Maleki Varnosfaderani, S., & Forouzanfar, M. (2024). The role of AI in hospitals and clinics: Transforming healthcare in the 21st century. *Bioengineering (Basel, Switzerland)*, *11*(4), 337. DOI: 10.3390/bioengineering11040337 PMID: 38671759

Malta, D. C., França, E., Abreu, D. M. X., Perillo, R. D., Salmen, M. C., & Teixeira, R. A.. (2017). Mortalidade por doenças não transmissíveis no brasil, 1990 a 2015, segundo estimativas do estudo de carga global de doenças. *São Paulo Medical Journal = Revista Paulista de Medicina*, *135*(3), 213–221. DOI: 10.1590/1516-3180.2016.0330050117 PMID: 28746656

Mamedov, M. N., Druk, I. V., Turusheva, E. A., Eremina, E. Y., Morozova, T. E., & Iskenderov, B. G.. (2021). Behavioral risk factors and clinical course of cardiovascular diseases and other noncommunicable diseases during quarantine in various regions of Russia. *Russ J Cardiol.*, *26*(9), 15–21. DOI: 10.15829/1560-4071-2021-4670

Mamedov, M. N., Rytova, A. I., Yarovaya, E. B., & Drapkina, O. M. (2022). Psychosomatic status analysis of patients with chronic non-communicable diseases (CNCDs) in Russia and CIS countries during self-isolation. *Profilaktychna Medytsyna*, *25*(1), 29–34. DOI: 10.17116/profmed202225011 2

Mansens, H., van den Heuvel, M. P., & van den Heuvel, M. P. (2018). Music as a form of cognitive training: A systematic review of the neuroplastic effects of musical training. *Frontiers in Human Neuroscience*, *12*, 169. DOI: 10.3389/fnhum.2018.00169

Mansour, Z., Said, R., Dbaibo, H., Mrad, P., Torossian, L., & Rady, A.. (2020). Non-communicable diseases in Lebanon: Results from World Health Organization STEPS survey 2017. *Public Health*, *187*, 120–126. DOI: 10.1016/j.puhe.2020.08.014 PMID: 32949882

Marelli, L., Testa, G., & Van Hoyweghen, I. (2021). Big Tech platforms in health research: Re-purposing big data governance in light of the General Data Protection Regulation's research exemption. *Big Data & Society*, *8*(1). Advance online publication. DOI: 10.1177/20539517211018783

Maresova, P., Režný, L., Bauer, P., Fadeyi, O., Eniayewu, O., Barakovic, S., & Barakovic Husic, J. (2023). An effectiveness and cost-estimation model for deploying assistive technology solutions in elderly care. *International Journal of Healthcare Management*, *16*(4), 588–603. DOI: 10.1080/20479700.2023.2207687

Marino, N., Putignano, G., Cappilli, S., Chersoni, E., Santuccione, A., Calabrese, G., & Santus, E. (2023). Towards AI-driven longevity research: An overview. *Frontiers in Aging*, *4*, 1057204.

Maris, T. M., Koçar, A., Willems, D. L., Pols, J., Tan, H. L., Lindinger, G. L., & Bak, M. A. R. (2024). Ethical use of artificial intelligence to prevent sudden cardiac death: An interview study of patient perspectives. *Frontiers in Cardiovascular Medicine*, *11*, 1394397. Advance online publication. DOI: 10.3389/fcvm.2024.1394397

Martin, C., Amaya, I., Torres, J., Artola, G., García, M., García-Navarro, T., & Macía, I. (2023). DigiHEALTH: Suite of digital solutions for long-term healthy and active aging. *Sensors (Basel)*, *23*(18), 7949. DOI: 10.3390/s23187949 PMID: 37766006

Martin-Martinez, A., Miró, J., Amadó, C., Ruz, F., Ruiz, A., Ortega, O., & Clave, P. (2023). A systematic and universal artificial intelligence screening method for oropharyngeal dysphagia: Improving diagnosis through risk management. *Dysphagia*, *38*(4), 1224–1237.

Martí-Noguera, J. J. (2025). The 5P model as a governance framework. In *Governing digital mental health: Introducing the 5P model and the digital behavioral health expert* (pp. 47–79). Springer. https://doi.org/DOI: 10.1007/978-3-031-68429-6_3

Martins, R., Pereira, H., Corrente, G., Xavier, W., Conceição, L., Freitas, A., & Marreiros, G. (2024). Supporting elderly care through an AI-driven and FHIR-based remote monitoring system. In *International Symposium on Distributed Computing and Artificial Intelligence* (pp. 233–241). Springer. https://doi.org/DOI: 10.1007/978-3-031-62692-0_24

Marwala, T. (2024). *The democratization of artificial intelligence: Reimagining governance and equity*. MIT Press., DOI: 10.7551/mitpress/14234.001.0001

Masmoudi, M., Ben Abdallah Ben Lamine, S., Karray, M. H., Archimede, B., & Baazaoui Zghal, H. (2024). Semantic data integration and querying: A survey and challenges. *ACM Computing Surveys*, *56*(8), 1–35. DOI: 10.1145/3653317

Mbata, A. O., Soyege, O. S., Nwokedi, C. N., Tomoh, B. O., Mustapha, A. Y., Balogun, O. D., & Iguma, D. R. (2024). Preventative medicine and chronic disease management: Reducing healthcare costs and improving long-term public health. *International Journal of Multidisciplinary Research and Growth Evaluation*, *5*(6), 1584–1600. DOI: 10.54660/IJMRGE.2024.5.6.1584-1600

McGee, R. W. (2024). Incorporating Artificial Intelligence and Traditional Chinese Medicine (TCM) into a Western Medical Practice: A Case Study. *Biomedical Journal of Scientific & Technical Research*, *56*(3), 48149–48154.

McIlduff, C. D., Acharibasam, J., Starr, V., & Chapados, M. (2022, September). Engaging Indigenous older adults with technology use to respond to health and well-being concerns and needs. []. Sage CA: Los Angeles, CA: SAGE Publications.]. *Healthcare Management Forum*, *35*(5), 257–264. PMID: 35670368

McIlduff, D., Carter, R., & Patel, S. (2022). Stakeholder engagement in geriatric care: Building inclusive healthcare systems. *Journal of Aging & Social Policy*, *34*(2), 178–195. DOI: 10.1080/08959420.2021.1987524

McKinsey & Company. (2023). *How AI is transforming food logistics.* https://www.mckinsey.com/

Megahd, N., El Kayaly, D., & Ammar, A. (2024). Equity, and Equality. *Ethical Challenges for the Future of Neurosurgery*, 31.

Mennella, C., Maniscalco, U., De Pietro, G., & Esposito, M. (2024). Ethical and regulatory challenges of AI technologies in healthcare: A narrative review. *Heliyon*, *10*(5), e27008. Advance online publication. DOI: 10.1016/j.heliyon.2024.e27008 PMID: 38384518

Menon, V. P., Edathadathil, F., Sathyapalan, D., Moni, M., Don, A., & Balachandran, S.. (2016). Assessment of 2013 AHA/ACC ASCVD risk scores with behavioral characteristics of an urban cohort in India Preliminary analysis of Noncommunicable disease Initiatives and Research at AMrita (NIRAM) study. *Medicine*, *95*(49), e5542. DOI: 10.1097/MD.0000000000005542 PMID: 27930551

Mertens, E., Sagastume, D., & Penalvo, J. L. (2021). Quantification of disparities in the distribution of lifestyle and metabolic risk factors, prevalence of non-communicable diseases and related mortality: The Belgian Health Interview Surveys 1997-2018. *BMJ Open*, *11*(11). Advance online publication. DOI: 10.1136/bmjopen-2021-053260 PMID: 34810190

Mhlanga, D. (2020). Industry 4.0: The challenges associated with the digital transformation of education in South Africa. *The Impacts of Digital Transformation, 13*(51), 13–26.

Mhlanga, D. (2023a). Digital transformation in healthcare: The role of AI for inclusive long-term care. In Mhlanga, D., & Ndhlovu, E. (Eds.), *Economic Inclusion in Post-Independence Africa*. Springer., DOI: 10.1007/978-3-031-31431-5_19

Mhlanga, D. (2023b). Financial technology, artificial intelligence, and the health sector. In *FinTech and Artificial Intelligence for Sustainable Development*. Palgrave Macmillan., DOI: 10.1007/978-3-031-37776-1_7

Mhlanga, D. (2024). Artificial intelligence in elderly care: Navigating ethical and responsible AI adoption for seniors. In *Fostering long-term sustainable development in Africa: Overcoming poverty, inequality, and unemployment* (pp. 411–440). Springer Nature Switzerland., DOI: 10.1007/978-3-031-61121-6_18

Mhlanga, D. (2024). Artificial intelligence in elderly care: Navigating ethical and responsible AI adoption for seniors. In Khang, A., Abdullayev, V. M., Sergi, B. S., & Gupta, A. (Eds.), *Fostering long-term sustainable development in Africa* (pp. 411–440). Springer., DOI: 10.1007/978-3-031-61133-9_16

Mhlanga, D. (2024). Modeling user needs in AI elder care: Multimodal approaches for contextual understanding. *AI & Society, 39*(3), 567–580. DOI: 10.1007/s00146-024-09876-2

Mikkelsen, J. G., Sørensen, N. L., Merrild, C. H., Jensen, M. B., & Thomsen, J. L. (2023). Patient perspectives on data sharing regarding implementing and using artificial intelligence in general practice–a qualitative study. *BMC Health Services Research, 23*(1), 335.

Milella, F., Russo, D., & Bandini, S. (2023). AI-powered solutions to support informal caregivers in their decision-making: A systematic review of the literature. *OBM Geriatrics, 7*(4), 1–17. DOI: 10.21926/obm.geriatr.2304257

Mini, G. K. (2009). Socioeconomic and demographic diversity in the health status of elderly people in a transitional society, Kerala, India. *Journal of Biosocial Science, 41*(4), 457–467. PMID: 18647442

Mistri, I. U., Badge, A., & Shahu, S. (2023). Enhancing patient safety culture in hospitals. *Cureus, 15*(11), e48829. DOI: 10.7759/cureus.48829 PMID: 38283419

Mitra, K., & Alam, G. (2025). *AI-driven technologies in elderly care: Benefits and challenges* [Master's thesis, Theseus]. https://www.theseus.fi/handle/10024/834134 (No DOI available)

Moberg, C., Grundberg, Å., Konradsen, H., Kallström, A. P., Leung, A. Y., & Kabir, Z. N. (2022). Meeting own needs and supporting ability to care: Family caregivers' and health care professionals' perspectives on professional support provided through a potential mobile application. *Dementia (London)*, *21*(4), 1120–1134. DOI: 10.1177/14713012211046597 PMID: 35300535

Moghadam, M. P., Moghadam, Z. A., Qazani, M. R. C., Pławiak, P., & Alizadehsani, R. (2024). Impact of artificial intelligence in nursing for geriatric clinical care for chronic diseases: A systematic literature review. *IEEE Access : Practical Innovations, Open Solutions*, *12*, 122685–122701. DOI: 10.1109/ACCESS.2024.3451188

Mohan, D., Al-Hamid, D. Z., Chong, P. H. J., Sudheera, K. L. K., Gutierrez, J., Chan, H. C., & Li, H. (2024). Artificial intelligence and iot in elderly fall prevention: A review. *IEEE Sensors Journal*, *24*(4), 4181–4198.

Mohanty, S. K., Sahoo, U., & Rashmi, R. (2022). Old-age dependency and catastrophic health expenditure: Evidence from Longitudinal Ageing Study in India. *The International Journal of Health Planning and Management*, *37*(6), 3148–3171. DOI: 10.1002/hpm.3546 PMID: 35929614

Moher, D., Liberati, A., Tetzlaff, J., & Altman, D. G. (2009). Preferred reporting items for systematic reviews and meta-analyses: The PRISMA statement. *BMJ (Clinical Research Ed.)*, *339*(7716), 332–336. DOI: 10.1136/bmj.b2535 PMID: 19622551

Mois, G., & Beer, J. M. (2020). The role of healthcare robotics in providing support to older adults: A socio-ecological perspective. *Current Geriatrics Reports*, *9*, 82–89. DOI: 10.1007/s13670-020-00314-w PMID: 32435576

Momin, M. S., Sufian, A., Barman, D., Dutta, P., Dong, M., & Leo, M. (2022). In-home older adults' activity pattern monitoring using depth sensors: A review. *Sensors (Basel)*, *22*(23), 9067. DOI: 10.3390/s22239067 PMID: 36501769

Momtazmanesh, S., Nowroozi, A., & Rezaei, N. (2022). Artificial intelligence in rheumatoid arthritis: current status and future perspectives: a state-of-the-art review. *Rheumatology and Therapy*, *9*(5), 1249–1304.

Mondai, R. N., Das, A., Islam, M. D., Podder, P., Pramanik, S., & Rani, M. (2020). Prevalence of NCD risk factors among the adult family members of students of school (Phase - A). *Journal of Medicine*, *21*(1), 8–13. DOI: 10.3329/jom.v21i1.44094

Moore, L. W., Leahy, C., Sublett, C., & Lanig, H. (2013). Understanding nurse-to-nurse relationships and their impact on work environments. *Medsurg Nursing*, *22*(3), 172–179. PMID: 23865278

Moreno-Morales, M. A., Roldán, M. E., & Martínez-Roldán, M. E. (2020). Active music therapy on cognition and neuropsychiatric symptoms in the elderly with mild and moderate dementia: A preliminary study. *Jornal Brasileiro de Psiquiatria, 69*(2), 108–114. DOI: 10.1590/0047-2085000000277

Morrison, B., Coventry, L., & Briggs, P. (2021). How do older adults feel about engaging with cyber-security? *Human Behavior and Emerging Technologies, 3*(5), 1033–1049. DOI: 10.1002/hbe2.306

Mor, V., Murphy, J., Masterson-Allen, S., Willey, C., Razmpour, A., Jackson, M. E., Greer, D., & Katz, S. (1989). Risk of functional decline among well elders. *Journal of Clinical Epidemiology, 42*(9), 895–904. PMID: 2778468

Mui, A. C. (1998). Living alone and depression among older Chinese immigrants. *Journal of Gerontological Social Work, 30*(3–4), 147–166.

Munday, D., Leaman, J., O'Moore, É., & Plugge, E. (2019). The prevalence of non-communicable disease in older people in prison: A systematic review and meta-analysis. *Age and Ageing, 48*(2), 204–212. DOI: 10.1093/ageing/afy186 PMID: 30590404

Muralidharan, V., Adewale, B. A., Huang, C. J., Nta, M. T., Ademiju, P. O., Pathmarajah, P., & Olatunji, T. (2024). A scoping review of reporting gaps in FDA-approved AI medical devices. *NPJ Digital Medicine, 7*(1), 273.

Murdoch, B. (2021). Privacy and artificial intelligence: Challenges for protecting health information in a new era. *BMC Medical Ethics, 22*(1), 122. Advance online publication. DOI: 10.1186/s12910-021-00687-3 PMID: 34525993

Murphy, M. (1995). Household and family factors in morbidity and mortality. *Morbidity and mortality data: problems of comparability*, 18-20.

Murthy, S., Bhat, K. S., Das, S., & Kumar, N. (2021). Individually vulnerable, collectively safe: The security and privacy practices of households with older adults. *Proceedings of the ACM on Human-Computer Interaction, 5*(CSCW1), 1–24. DOI: 10.1145/3449088

Mwangi, K. J., Mwenda, V., Gathecha, G., Beran, D., Guessous, I., & Ombiro, O.. (2020). Socio-economic and demographic determinants of non-communicable diseases in Kenya: A secondary analysis of the Kenya stepwise survey. *The Pan African Medical Journal, 37*, 351. DOI: 10.11604/pamj.2020.37.351.21167 PMID: 33796165

N. Harrington, C., Jelen, B., Lazar, A., Martin-Hammond, A., Pradhan, A., Reeder, B., & Siek, K. (2021). Taking stock of the present and future of smart technologies for older adults and caregivers. [PDF].

Naidoo, S., Bottomley, D., Naidoo, M., Donnelly, D., & Thaldar, D. W. (2022). Artificial intelligence in healthcare: Proposals for policy development in South Africa. *South African Journal of Bioethics and Law*, *15*(1), 11–16. DOI: 10.7196/SAJBL.2022.v15i1.797 PMID: 36061984

Naik, N., Hameed, B. M., Shetty, D. K., Swain, D., Shah, M., Paul, R., & Somani, B. K. (2022). Legal and ethical consideration in artificial intelligence in healthcare: Who takes responsibility? *Frontiers in Surgery*, *9*, 862322. Advance online publication. DOI: 10.3389/fsurg.2022.862322 PMID: 35360424

Naim, M. F., & Lenka, U. (2018). Development and retention of Generation Y employees: A conceptual framework. *Employee Relations*, *40*(2), 433–455. DOI: 10.1108/ER-09-2016-0172

Najjar, R. (2023). Redefining radiology: A review of artificial intelligence integration in medical imaging [PMID: 37685300; PMC10487271. Recent comprehensive review of AI in medical imaging]. *Diagnostics (Basel)*, *13*(17), 2760. DOI: 10.3390/diagnostics13172760 PMID: 37685300

Nandakishora, Y., Christydass, S. P. J., Bhargav, K. V. J., & Kumar, S. S. (2025). Empowering health: The fusion of AI and machine learning in wearable technologies. In *Smart textiles and wearables for health and fitness* (p. 159). Springer., DOI: 10.1007/978-981-97-6436-5_7

Napalai, P., Seangpraw, K., Boonyathee, S., & Ong-Artborirak, P. (2022). COVID-19-related knowledge influences mental health, self-care behaviors, and quality of life among elderly with non-communicable diseases in Northern Thailand. *Frontiers in Public Health*, *10*, 993531. DOI: 10.3389/fpubh.2022.993531 PMID: 36388338

Narayana, M. R., & Narasimhan, S. (2019). Health and health care of the elderly in India: A review. *Indian Journal of Gerontology, 33*(1), 1–20.

Narendran, M., Savitha Rani, B. B., Kulkarni, P., Renuka, M., & Narayana Murthy, M. R. (2018). Interdependence of communicable and non-communicable diseases among elderly population in declared slum in Mysuru City, Karnataka. *Indian Journal of Public Health Research & Development*, *9*(11), 62–66. DOI: 10.5958/0976-5506.2018.01426.2

Nasr, M., Islam, M. M., Shehata, S., Karray, F., & Quintana, Y. (2021). Smart healthcare in the age of AI: Recent advances, challenges, and future prospects. *IEEE Access : Practical Innovations, Open Solutions*, *9*, 145248–145270.

Ncube, B., Mars, M., & Scott, R. E. (2022). Telemedicine options to address identified health needs in Botswana. *Digital Health*, *8*, 20552076221102768. DOI: 10.1177/20552076221102768 PMID: 35663237

Negin, J., Cumming, R., de Ramirez, S. S., Abimbola, S., & Sachs, S. E. (2011). Risk factors for non-communicable diseases among older adults in rural Africa. *Tropical Medicine & International Health*, *16*(5), 640–646. DOI: 10.1111/j.1365-3156.2011.02739.x PMID: 21320244

Negi, P. C., Chauhan, R., & Rana, V. (2016). Vidyasagar, Lal K. Epidemiological study of non-communicable diseases (NCD) risk factors in tribal district of Kinnaur, HP: A cross-sectional study. *Indian Heart Journal*, *68*(5), 655–662. DOI: 10.1016/j.ihj.2016.03.002 PMID: 27773404

Neves, B. B., Petersen, A., Vered, M., Carter, A., & Omori, M. (2023). Artificial intelligence in long-term care: Technological promise, aging anxieties, and socio-technical ageism. *Journal of Applied Gerontology*, *42*(6), 1274–1282.

Newby, D., Orgeta, V., Marshall, C. R., Lourida, I., Albertyn, C. P., Tamburin, S., & Ranson, J. M. (2023). Artificial intelligence for dementia prevention. *Alzheimer's & Dementia*, *19*(12), 5952–5969.

Newtonraj, A., Murugan, N., Singh, Z., Chauhan, R. C., Velavan, A., & Mani, M. (2017). Factors associated with physical inactivity among adult urban population of Puducherry, India: A population based cross-sectional study. *Journal of Clinical and Diagnostic Research : JCDR*, *11*(5), LC15–LC17. DOI: 10.7860/JCDR/2017/24028.9853 PMID: 28658812

Ngaruiya, C., Wambua, M., Mutua, T. K., Owambo, D., Muchemi, M., & Rop, K.. (2021). The last frontier for global non-communicable disease action: The emergency department—A cross-sectional study from East Africa. *PLoS One*, *16*(4). Advance online publication. DOI: 10.1371/journal.pone.0248709 PMID: 33798234

Nguyen, T., Maarek, R., Hermann, A. L., Kammoun, A., Marchi, A., Khelifi-Touhami, M. R., & Le Pointe, H. D. (2022). Assessment of an artificial intelligence aid for the detection of appendicular skeletal fractures in children and young adults by senior and junior radiologists. *Pediatric Radiology*, *52*(11), 2215–2226.

Nguyen, T., Tang, B., Harrison, K. L., Stadler, S., Walter, L. C., Hoepke, K., & Allison, T. A. (2025). Age Self Care, a program to improve aging in place through group learning and incremental behavior change: Preliminary data. *Journal of the American Geriatrics Society*, *73*(3), 920–929. DOI: 10.1111/jgs.19216 PMID: 39607380

Nguyen, V., Van Anh, V., Ha, H. T. N., Huyen, B. T., Kien, T. B., & Anh, N. N. Q. (2025). Overview of proactive healthcare: The role of Medicine 3.0 and 5P medicine in prevention and early intervention. *T p chí. Y Hoc Viet Nam*, *550*(1), 1–10.

Nilsson, S., Hansson, H., Moons, P., Onerup, A., Saarijärvi, M., Sabel, M., & Bratt, E. L. (2025). Is this the road to health?–The person in precision health. *European Journal of Cardiovascular Nursing*, *24*(4), zvaf091. Advance online publication. DOI: 10.1093/eurjcn/zvaf091 PMID: 40378194

Niyas, K. P. M., & Thiyagarajan, P. (2023). A systematic review on early prediction of mild cognitive impairment to Alzheimer's using machine learning algorithms. *International Journal of Intelligent Networks*, *4*, 363–370. DOI: 10.1016/j.ijin.2023.12.002

Njagi, P., Arsenijevic, J., & Groot, W. (2018). Understanding variations in catastrophic health expenditure, its underlying determinants and impoverishment in Sub-Saharan African countries: A scoping review. *Systematic Reviews*, *7*(1). Advance online publication. DOI: 10.1186/s13643-018-0799-1 PMID: 30205846

Nogaroli, R. (2025). Ethical and Legal Aspects of the Physician-Patient Relationship. In *Medical liability and artificial intelligence: Brazilian and european legal approaches* (pp. 19–80). Springer Nature Switzerland.

Noh, G., Lee, K. Y., & Moon, M. (2018). An Approach to Develop a Speech Recognition Speaker Using Chatbot for Senior Users. *Journal of IKEEE*, *22*(2), 330–338.

NYC Mayor's Office of Food Policy. (2021). *Food metrics report 2021*. City of New York. https://www.nyc.gov/assets/foodpolicy/downloads/pdf/Food-Metrics-Report-2021.pdf

O'Connor, S. R., Wilson, V., Brown, D., Cleland, I., & McCance, T. V. (2024). Development and optimisation of a mobile app (iMPAKT) for improving person-centred practice in healthcare settings: A multi-methods evaluation study. *Digital Health*, *10*, 20552076241271788. DOI: 10.1177/20552076241271788 PMID: 39493639

O'Connor, S., Gasteiger, N., Stanmore, E., Wong, D. C., & Lee, J. J. (2022). Artificial intelligence for falls management in older adult care: A scoping review of nurses' role. *Journal of Nursing Management*, *30*(8), 3787–3801.

Obermeyer, Z., Powers, B., Vogeli, C., & Mullainathan, S. (2019). Dissecting racial bias in an algorithm used to manage the health of populations. *Science*, *366*(6464), 447–453. DOI: 10.1126/science.aax2342 PMID: 31649194

Oca, A., Panikkar, R., Sampat, C., & Brown, T. (2024, November 15). *Harnessing the power of AI in distribution operations.* McKinsey & Company. https://www.mckinsey.com/industries/industrials-and-electronics/our-insights/distribution-blog/harnessing-the-power-of-ai-in-distribution-operations

Odionu, C. S., & Ibeh, C. V. (2024). The role of data analytics in enhancing geriatric care: A review of AI-driven solutions. *International Journal of Multidisciplinary Research and Growth Evaluation*, *5*(1), 1131–1138.

OECD. (2022). *AI and the future of work.* Organisation for Economic Co-operation and Development., DOI: 10.1787/ai-future-work

Okpechi, I. G., Chukwuonye, I. I., Tiffin, N., Madukwe, O. O., Onyeonoro, U. U., & Umeizudike, T. I.. (2013). Blood Pressure Gradients and Cardiovascular Risk Factors in Urban and Rural Populations in Abia State South Eastern Nigeria Using the WHO STEPwise Approach. *PLoS One*, *8*(9). Advance online publication. DOI: 10.1371/journal.pone.0073403 PMID: 24039932

Ong, S. K., Lai, D. T. C., Wong, J. Y. Y., Si-Ramlee, K. A., Razak, L. A., & Kassim, N.. (2017). Cross-sectional STEPwise Approach to Surveillance (STEPS) Population Survey of Noncommunicable Diseases (NCDs) and Risk Factors in Brunei Darussalam 2016. *Asia-Pacific Journal of Public Health*, *29*(8), 635–648. DOI: 10.1177/1010539517738072 PMID: 29082745

Oniani, D., Wu, X., Visweswaran, S., Kapoor, S., Kooragayalu, S., Polanska, K., & Wang, Y. (2024). Enhancing large language models for clinical decision support by incorporating clinical practice guidelines [PMC11909794. Recent 2024 study on LLMs as clinical decision support; arXiv:2401.11120]. *2024 IEEE 12th International Conference on Healthcare Informatics (ICHI)*, 694–702. DOI: 10.1109/ICHI61247.2024.00111

Onitiu, D., Wachter, S., & Mittelstadt, B. (2024). How AI challenges the medical device regulation: Patient safety, benefits, and intended uses. *Journal of Law and the Biosciences*, *11*(1), lsae007. Advance online publication. DOI: 10.1093/jlb/lsae007

Orm, I., Devos, P., & Diaconu, K. (2023). Experiences of communities with Lebanon's model of care for non-communicable diseases: A cross-sectional household survey from Greater Beirut. *BMJ Open*, *13*(9), 1–12. DOI: 10.1136/bmjopen-2022-070580 PMID: 37666549

Osifowokan, A. S., Agbadamasi, T. O., Adukpo, T. K., & Mensah, N. (2025). Regulatory and legal challenges of artificial intelligence in the US healthcare system: Liability, Compliance, and patient safety. *World Journal of Advanced Research and Reviews*, *25*(3), 949–955.

Ostroushko, D. (n.d.). *Evaluation of cohort construction methods for MCI to AD progression from EHR data: Discussion and reflections*. GitHub Pages. https://denisostroushko1.github.io/Evaluation-of-Cohort-Construction-Methods-for-MCI-to-AD-Progression-from-EHR-Data/ (No DOI available)

Owoyemi, A., Owoyemi, J., Osiyemi, A., & Boyd, A. (2020). Artificial intelligence for healthcare in Africa. *Frontiers in Digital Health*, *2*, 6. DOI: 10.3389/fdgth.2020.00006 PMID: 34713019

Padhan, S., Mohapatra, A., Ramasamy, S. K., Agrawal, S., & Ramasamy, S. (2023). Artificial intelligence (AI) and robotics in elderly healthcare: Enabling independence and quality of life. *Cureus*, *15*(8).

Palaniappan, K., Lin, E. Y. T., Vogel, S., & Lim, J. C. W. (2024). Gaps in the global regulatory frameworks for the use of artificial intelligence (AI) in the healthcare services sector and key recommendations. *Health Care*, *12*(17), 1730. DOI: 10.3390/healthcare12171730 PMID: 39273754

Panahi, O. (2025). Health in the Age of AI: A Family and Community Focus. *Archives of Community and Family Medicine*, *8*(1), 11–20.

Panahi, O. (2025). The role of personalized medicine in modern healthcare. *ResearchGate*. https://doi.org/DOI: 10.13140/RG.2.2.17002.00966

Pandey, P., & Singh, S. (2017). Catastrophic health expenditure among geriatric population of Lucknow district, India. *J Geriatr Ment Health.*, *4*(1), 42. DOI: 10.4103/jgmh.jgmh_40_16

Pang, C., Collin Wang, Z., McGrenere, J., Leung, R., Dai, J., & Moffatt, K. (2021). Technology adoption and learning preferences for older adults: Evolving perceptions, ongoing challenges, and emerging design opportunities. In *Proceedings of the 2021 CHI conference on human factors in computing systems* (pp. 1–13). ACM. DOI: 10.1145/3411764.3445072

Pani, B., Crawford, J., & Allen, K. A. (2024). Can generative artificial intelligence foster belongingness, social support, and reduce loneliness? A conceptual analysis. *Applications of generative. AI*, •••, 261–276.

Papathanail, I., Brühlmann, J., Vasiloglou, M. F., Stathopoulou, T., Exadaktylos, A. K., Stanga, Z., & Mougiakakou, S. (2021). Evaluation of a novel artificial intelligence system to monitor and assess energy and macronutrient intake in hospitalised older patients. *Nutrients*, *13*(12), 4539.

Park, C. L. (2010). The meaning making model: A framework for understanding how we cope with life's big events. *Psychology of Religion and Spirituality*, *2*(4), 180–191. DOI: 10.1037/a0020499

Park, S. A., & Choi, S. M. (2018). A understanding the factors influencing satisfaction and continued use intention of AI speakers: Focusing on the utilitarian and hedonic values. *Information Society & Media*, *19*(3), 159–182.

Patel, V., Xiao, S., Chen, H., Hanna, F., Jotheeswaran, A. T., Luo, D., ... & Saxena, S. (2018). The magnitude of and health system responses to the mental health treatment gap in adults in India and China. *The Lancet, 388*(10063), 3074–3084.

Patel, R., & Nguyen, T. (2024). Voice and embodiment in AI monitoring systems: Enhancing social engagement for older adults. *Technology and Aging*, *19*(1), 34–47. DOI: 10.1080/17483107.2024.2314567

Patil, S. S., Rajaram, D., & Seeri, J. S. (2016). Correlates of geriatric health problems in the urban elderly- A community based study in Bangalore, Karnataka. *Indian Journal of Public Health Research & Development*, *7*(3), 231–237. DOI: 10.5958/0976-5506.2016.00163

Paulauskaite-Taraseviciene, A., Siaulys, J., Sutiene, K., Petravicius, T., Navickas, S., Oliandra, M., & Balciunas, J. (2023, April). Geriatric care management system powered by the IoT and computer vision techniques. []. MDPI.]. *Health Care*, *11*(8), 1152.

Paul, D., Sanap, G., Shenoy, S., Kalyane, D., Kalia, K., & Tekade, R. K. (2021). Artificial intelligence in drug discovery and development [PMID: 33099022; PMC7577280. Comprehensive review of AI in diagnostics and drug discovery]. *Drug Discovery Today*, *26*(1), 80–93. DOI: 10.1016/j.drudis.2020.10.010 PMID: 33099022

Paul, J. (2025). Real-time predictive health monitoring using AI-driven wearable sensors: Enhancing early detection and personalized interventions in chronic disease. *ResearchGate*. https://doi.org/DOI: 10.13140/RG.2.2.29776.25606

Payton, T., & Claypoole, T. (2023). *Privacy in the age of big data: Recognizing threats, defending your rights, and protecting your family* (2nd ed.). Rowman & Littlefield.

Pease, B. (2021). *Undoing privilege: Unearned advantage and systemic injustice in an unequal world*. Zed Books., DOI: 10.5040/9781350224032

Peine, A., Faulkner, A., Jæger, B., & Moors, E. (2015). Science, technology and the 'grand challenge'of ageing—Understanding the socio-material constitution of later life. *Technological Forecasting and Social Change*, *93*, 1–9.

Pelly, M., Fatehi, F., Liew, D., & Verdejo-Garcia, A. (2023). Artificial intelligence for secondary prevention of myocardial infarction: A qualitative study of patient and health professional perspectives. *International Journal of Medical Informatics*, *173*, 105041.

Pengpid, S., & Peltzer, K. (2020). Prevalence and correlates of multiple non-communicable disease risk factors among adults in zambia: Results of the first national steps survey in 2017. *The Pan African Medical Journal*, *37*, 1–12. DOI: 10.11604/pamj.2020.37.265.25038 PMID: 33598080

Pentikäinen, E., Kimppa, L., Pitkäniemi, A., Lahti, O., & Särkämö, T. (2023). Longitudinal effects of choir singing on aging cognition and wellbeing: A two-year follow-up study. *Frontiers in Human Neuroscience*, *17*, 1174574. DOI: 10.3389/fnhum.2023.1174574

Pentikäinen, E., Pitkäniemi, A., & Särkämö, T. (2021). Group singing programs for well-being of older adults: An in-person quantitative follow-up. *Dementia and Geriatric Cognitive Disorders. Extra*, *11*(2), 163–172. DOI: 10.1159/000516086

Pereira, Z. S., da Silva, A. S., Melo, J. C. D. N., dos Santos, J. C., Sewo Sampaio, P. Y., & Silva, R. J. D. S.. (2023). Differential Factors Are Associated with Physical Activity in Older Adults in Brazil with and without Non-Communicable Chronic Diseases: A Cross-Sectional Analysis of the 2019 National Health Survey. *International Journal of Environmental Research and Public Health*, *20*(14). Advance online publication. DOI: 10.3390/ijerph20146329 PMID: 37510562

Perivolaris, A. (2024). *Development and evaluation of a standardized tool to measure the quality of clinician's interaction with AI-enabled systems* [Master's thesis, Scholaris]. https://scholaris.ca/wp-content/uploads/2024/03/Thesis-APerivolaris-Final.pdf (No DOI available)

Peters, M. D. J., Marnie, C., & Butler, A. (2021). Delivering, funding, and rating safe staffing levels and skills mix in aged care. *International Journal of Nursing Studies*, *122*, 104046. DOI: 10.1016/j.ijnurstu.2021.104046

Petrakaki, D., Hilberg, E., & Waring, J. (2018). Between empowerment and self-discipline: Governing patients' conduct through technological self-care. *Social Science & Medicine*, *213*, 146–153. DOI: 10.1016/j.socscimed.2018.07.043 PMID: 30081356

Picco, L., Achilla, E., Abdin, E., Chong, S. A., Vaingankar, J. A., & McCrone, P.. (2016). Economic burden of multimorbidity among older adults: Impact on healthcare and societal costs. *BMC Health Services Research, 16*(1), 1–12. DOI: 10.1186/s12913-016-1421-7 PMID: 27160080

Pongiglione, B., De Stavola, B. L., & Ploubidis, G. B. (2015). A systematic literature review of studies analyzing inequalities in health expectancy among the older population. *PLoS One, 10*(6), 1–21. DOI: 10.1371/journal.pone.0130747 PMID: 26115099

Porkodi, S., & Kesavaraja, D. (2021). Healthcare robots enabled with IoT and artificial intelligence for elderly patients. *AI and IoT-Based Intelligent Automation in Robotics*, 87-108.

Porter, M. E., & Kramer, M. R. (2011). Creating shared value. *Harvard Business Review, 89*(1/2), 62–77. https://hbr.org/2011/01/creating-shared-value

Pradyumna, G. R., Hegde, R. B., Bommegowda, K. B., Jan, T., & Naik, G. R. (2024). Empowering healthcare with IoMT: Evolution, machine learning integration, security, and interoperability challenges. *IEEE Access : Practical Innovations, Open Solutions, 12*, 20603–20623. DOI: 10.1109/ACCESS.2024.3359909

Prakash, I. (2020). Changing family structures and their impact on elderly care in India. *Indian Journal of Social Work, 81*(2), 225–242.

Pray, A. (2017). *Cultural Competency in Medical Social Work with Elders* (Doctoral dissertation, University of St. Thomas, Minnesota).

Prinja, S., Jagnoor, J., Sharma, D., Aggarwal, S., Katoch, S., & Lakshmi, P. V. M.. (2019). Out-of-pocket expenditure and catastrophic health expenditure for hospitalization due to injuries in public sector hospitals in North India. *PLoS One, 14*(11), 1–17. DOI: 10.1371/journal.pone.0224721 PMID: 31697781

Psomiadi, A. (2025). *Your playbook for growth and resilience*. APSON Editions., DOI: 10.4324/9789609906580

Puri, P., Singh, S. K., & Pati, S. (2022). Identifying non-communicable disease multimorbidity patterns and associated factors: A latent class analysis approach. *BMJ Open, 12*(7). Advance online publication. DOI: 10.1136/bmjopen-2021-053981 PMID: 35820748

Puterman-Salzman, L., Katz, J., Bergman, H., Grad, R., Khanassov, V., Gore, G., & Abbasgholizadeh Rahimi, S. (2023). Artificial intelligence for detection of dementia using motion data: A scoping review. *Dementia and Geriatric Cognitive Disorders. Extra, 13*(1), 28–38. DOI: 10.1159/000529208 PMID: 37927529

Qian, K., Zhang, Z., Yamamoto, Y., & Schuller, B. W. (2021). Artificial intelligence internet of things for the elderly: From assisted living to health-care monitoring. *IEEE Signal Processing Magazine*, *38*(4), 78–88.

Rahman, S. A., Taghizadeh, S. K., Ramayah, T., & Alam, M. M. D. (2017). Technology acceptance among micro-entrepreneurs in marginalized social strata: The case of social innovation in Bangladesh. *Technological Forecasting and Social Change*, *118*, 236–245. DOI: 10.1016/j.techfore.2017.02.017

Rajan, S. I. (2017). Ageing in India: Trends and issues. *Economic and Political Weekly, 52*(16), 32–37.

Rajan, S. I., Mishra, U. S., & Sarma, P. S. (2003). *India's Elderly: Burden or Challenge?* Sage Publishers.

Rajput, S., Jain, E., Mehra, A., Thakur, K. S., Gupta, O., & Singh, P. (2022). Technology Driven Tourism: A PLS SEM Model of its Antecedents in Tourist Behavior Intention. In *2022 IEEE Conference on Interdisciplinary Approaches in Technology and Management for Social Innovation (IATMSI)*, Gwalior, India, 2022 (pp. 1-6). doi: DOI: 10.1109/IATMSI56455.2022.10119265

Ramezani, M., Bakhtiari, A., Daroudi, R., Mobinizadeh, M., Fazaeli, A. A., Olyaeemanesh, A., & Takian, A. (2025). Applications of artificial intelligence and the challenges in health technology assessment: A scoping review and framework with a focus on economic dimensions. *Health Economics Review*, *15*(1), 46. DOI: 10.1186/s13561-025-00464-6 PMID: 40461901

Rao, H., Zeng, M., Zhao, X., & Miao, C. (2025). A survey of artificial intelligence in gait-based neurodegenerative disease diagnosis [Latest 2025 comprehensive survey on AI-based gait analysis for neurodegenerative diseases; Q1 journal (IF 5.5-6.5); arXiv:2405.13082]. *Neurocomputing*, *626*, 129533. DOI: 10.1016/j

Rao, S. J., Isath, A., Krishnan, P., Tangsrivimol, J. A., Virk, H. U. H., Wang, Z., & Krittanawong, C. (2024). ChatGPT: A conceptual review of applications and utility in the field of medicine. *Journal of Medical Systems*, *48*(1), 59.

Ratwani, R. M., Bates, D. W., & Classen, D. C. (2024). Patient safety and artificial intelligence in clinical care. *JAMA Health Forum*, *5*(7), e241677. DOI: 10.1001/jamahealthforum.2024.1677 PMID: 38393719

Ray, A., Bhardwaj, A., Malik, Y. K., Singh, S., & Gupta, R. (2022). Artificial intelligence and Psychiatry: An overview. *Asian Journal of Psychiatry*, *70*, 103021.

Ray, S. J., Cherian, J., Liberty, A. M., Hammond, T. A., & Shireman, P. K. (2025). Recognition of basic activities of daily living using wearable devices for older adults: Scoping review. *Journal of Medical Internet Research*, *27*, e67373. Advance online publication. DOI: 10.2196/67373 PMID: 40373307

Raza, H., Abbas, N., Amir, S., Arshad, K., Siddiqui, M. R. U., & Khan, S. I. (2022). An IoMT enabled smart healthcare model to monitor elderly people using Explainable Artificial Intelligence (EAI). *Journal of NCBAE*, *1*(2), 16–22.

Raza, H., Abbas, N., Amir, S., Arshad, K., Siddiqui, M. R. U., & Khan, S. I. (2022). An IoMT-enabled smart healthcare model to monitor elderly people using explainable AI. *Journal of NCBAE*, *1*(1), 16–22.

Reddy, S. (2024). Generative AI in healthcare: An implementation science informed translational path on application, integration and governance. *Implementation Science : IS*, *19*(1), 28. DOI: 10.1186/s13012-024-01357-7 PMID: 38491544

Reegu, F. A., Abas, H., Gulzar, Y., Xin, Q., Alwan, A. A., Jabbari, A., & Dziyauddin, R. A. (2023). Blockchain-based framework for interoperable electronic health records for an improved healthcare system. *Sustainability*, *15*(8), 6337. DOI: 10.3390/su15086337

Reid, S. D., Motilal, S., Pooransingh, S., St. Bernard, G., & Ivey, M. A. (2023). Differential Mental Health Impact of COVID-19 Lockdowns on Persons with Non-Communicable Diseases in Trinidad and Tobago. *International Journal of Environmental Research and Public Health*, *20*(16). Advance online publication. DOI: 10.3390/ijerph20166543 PMID: 37623129

Renn, B. N., Schurr, M., Zaslavsky, O., & Pratap, A. (2021). Artificial intelligence: An interprofessional perspective on implications for geriatric mental health research and care. *Frontiers in Psychiatry*, *12*, 734909.

Reynolds, C. F.III, Jeste, D. V., Sachdev, P. S., & Blazer, D. G. (2022). Mental health care for older adults: Recent advances and new directions in clinical practice and research. *World Psychiatry; Official Journal of the World Psychiatric Association (WPA)*, *21*(3), 336–363. DOI: 10.1002/wps.20994 PMID: 36073714

Reynolds, C. F., Jeste, D. V., Sachdev, P. S., & Blazer, D. G. (2022). Mental health care for older adults: Advances and new directions. *World Psychiatry; Official Journal of the World Psychiatric Association (WPA)*, *21*(3), 336–363. PMID: 36073714

Reynolds, T. A., Goldshore, M. A., Flohr, S., Land, S., Mathew, L., Gebb, J. S., & Hedrick, H. L. (2025). A clinical outcomes data archive for a comprehensive fetal diagnosis and treatment center. *Fetal Diagnosis and Therapy*, *52*(2), 139–147. DOI: 10.1159/000544039 PMID: 39378854

Richter-Laskowska, M., Sobotnicka, E., & Bednorz, A. (2025). Cognitive performance classification of older patients using machine learning and electronic medical records. *Scientific Reports*, *15*(1), 1823. Advance online publication. DOI: 10.1038/s41598-024-51976-9 PMID: 39994339

Risling, T., Martinez, J., Young, J., & Thorp-Froslie, N. (2017). Evaluating patient empowerment in association with eHealth technology: Scoping review. *Journal of Medical Internet Research*, *19*(9), e329. DOI: 10.2196/jmir.7809 PMID: 28963090

Rizvi, A., Rizvi, F., Lalakia, P., Hyman, L., Frasso, R., Sztandera, L., & Das, A. V. (2023). Is artificial intelligence the cost-saving lens to diabetic retinopathy screening in low-and middle-income countries? *Cureus*, *15*(9).

Rogers, W. (2019). Technology design to support social engagement for older adults. *Innovation in Aging*, *3*(Suppl_1), S689. DOI: 10.1093/geroni/igz038.2553

Román-Caballero, R., Román-Caballero, J., & Morales-Román, J. (2018). Cognitive and brain plasticity induced by physical exercise, cognitive training, video games, and combined interventions. *Frontiers in Human Neuroscience*, *12*, 25. DOI: 10.3389/fnhum.2018.00025

Rong, J., Ji, X., Fang, X., & Jee, M. H. (2022). Research on material design of medical products for elderly families based on artificial intelligence. *Mathematical Biosciences and Engineering*, *19*(12), 13502–13516. DOI: 10.3934/mbe.2022632 PMID: 35087604

Ross, C., & Wu, C. L. (1996). Education, age, and the cumulative advantage in health. *Journal of Health and Social Behavior*, *37*(1), 104–120. PMID: 8820314

Ross, J., Reilly, E., Sanchez-Reilly, S., Arevalo-Flechas, L., & Dentchev, A. (2023). How real is this deal? Evaluating AI accuracy in providing support to dementia caregivers. *Innovation in Aging*, *7*(Supplement_1), 1042–1043. DOI: 10.1093/geroni/igad104.3368

Roy, K. (2020). Gender and eldercare in India: Negotiating responsibility and dependence. *Journal of Cross-Cultural Gerontology, 35*(4), 375–391.

Rozynek, M., Kucybała, I., Urbanik, A., & Wojciechowski, W. (2021). Use of artificial intelligence in the imaging of sarcopenia: A narrative review of current status and perspectives. *Nutrition (Burbank, Los Angeles County, Calif.)*, *89*, 111227.

Rubeis, G., Fang, M. L., & Sixsmith, A. (2022). Equity in AgeTech for ageing well in technology-driven places: The role of social determinants in designing AI-based assistive technologies. *Science and Engineering Ethics*, *28*(6), 49. PMID: 36301408

Russell, S., Sturua, L., Li, C., Morgan, J., Topuridze, M., & Blanton, C.. (2019). The burden of non-communicable diseases and their related risk factors in the country of Georgia, 2015. *BMC Public Health*, *19*, 479. DOI: 10.1186/s12889-019-6785-2 PMID: 32326912

Saadatzi, M. N., Logsdon, M. C., Abubakar, S., Das, S., Jankoski, P., Mitchell, H., Chlebowy, D., & Popa, D. O. (2020). Acceptability of using a robotic nursing assistant in health care environments: Experimental pilot study. *Journal of Medical Internet Research*, *22*(11), e17509. DOI: 10.2196/17509 PMID: 33180024

Sabatini, S., Turner, S. G., & Stephan, B. (2025). Comparison of views on aging and self-perceptions of aging between dementia caregivers and non-caregivers. *The Journals of Gerontology. Series B, Psychological Sciences and Social Sciences*, *80*(2), gbaf083. Advance online publication. DOI: 10.1093/geronb/gbaf083 PMID: 40372128

Saccà, R., Turrini, R., Ausania, F., Turrina, S., & De Leo, D. (2024). The ménage à trois of healthcare: The actors in after-AI era under patient consent. *Frontiers in Medicine*, *11*, 1396145. Advance online publication. DOI: 10.3389/fmed.2024.1396145 PMID: 38269319

Sætra, H. S. (2022). First, they came for the old and demented: Care and relations in the age of artificial intelligence and social robots. *Human Arenas*, *5*(1), 25–43.

Salah, O. Z., Selvaperumal, S. K., & Abdulla, R. (2022). Accelerometer-based elderly fall detection system using edge artificial intelligence architecture. *International Journal of Electrical and Computer Engineering*, *12*(4), 4430–4438.

Salimpoor, V. N., Benovoy, M., Larcher, K., Dagher, A., & Zatorre, R. J. (2011). Anatomically distinct dopamine release during anticipation and experience of peak emotion to music. *Nature Neuroscience*, *14*(2), 257–262. DOI: 10.1038/nn.2726

Sallstrom, L., Morris, O., & Mehta, H. (2019). Artificial intelligence in Africa's healthcare: Ethical considerations. *ORF Issue Brief*, *312*, 1–11.

Salomon, D. (2012). *Data privacy and security*. Springer Science & Business Media.

Sankaran, A., & Singla, M. P. (2024). Artificial intelligence in geriatric healthcare: Opportunities and challenges in a transforming landscape. *Frontiers in Health Informatics*, *13*, 208. Advance online publication. DOI: 10.30699/fhi.v13i0.208

Santos, M., & Almeida, R. (2024). Building networks of care: Social technologies for older adults in diverse cultural contexts. *Gerontechnology (Valkenswaard), 23*(2), 56–68. DOI: 10.4017/gt.2024.23.2.004

Santos, N. B., Bavaresco, R. S., Tavares, J. E., Ramos, G., & Barbosa, J. L. (2021). A systematic mapping study of robotics in human care. *Robotics and Autonomous Systems, 144*, 103833. DOI: 10.1016/j.robot.2021.103833

Saraswat, S. & Singh, P. (2025), "The moderating role of perceived trust in predicting the adoption intention of consumers toward online pharmacies using the application of UTAUT model", *International Journal of Pharmaceutical and Healthcare Marketing*, Vol. ahead-of-print No. ahead-of-print. https://doi.org/.DOI: 10.1108/IJPHM-05-2024-0042

Saraswat, A., Eram, U., Shah, S., & Ahmad, A. (2023). Study on Assessment of Self-Care Practices in Patients of Non Communicable Diseases in Aligarh. *Indian Journal of Public Health Research & Development, 14*(1), 14–21. DOI: 10.37506/ijphrd.v14i1.1878

Särkämö, T., Laitinen, S., & Särkämö, T. (2014). Music therapy in the rehabilitation of cognitive functions after stroke. *Neuroscience and Biobehavioral Reviews, 40*, 1–13. DOI: 10.1016/j.neubiorev.2014.01.002

Sarveswaran, G., Kulothungan, V., & Mathur, P. (2020). Clustering of noncommunicable disease risk factors among adults (18–69 years) in rural population, South-India. *Diabetes & Metabolic Syndrome, 14*(5), 1005–1014. DOI: 10.1016/j.dsx.2020.05.042 PMID: 32623362

Sarwari, A. R., Fredman, L., Langenberg, P., & Magaziner, J. (1998). Prospective study on the relation between living arrangement and change in functional health status of elderly women. *American Journal of Epidemiology, 147*(4), 370–378. PMID: 9508104

Sazlina, S. G., Zaiton, A., Nor Afiah, M. Z., & Hayati, K. S. (2012). Predictors of health related quality of life in older people with non-communicable diseases attending three primary care clinics in malaysia. *The Journal of Nutrition, Health & Aging, 16*(5), 498–502. DOI: 10.1007/s12603-012-0038-8 PMID: 22555798

Schatz, E., & Seeley, J. (2015). Gender, ageing and carework in East and Southern Africa: A review. *Global Public Health, 10*(10), 1185–1200.

Schepens Niemiec, S. L., Lee, E., Saunders, R., Wagas, R., & Wu, S. (2023). Technology for activity participation in older people with mild cognitive impairment or dementia: Expert perspectives and a scoping review. *Disability and Rehabilitation. Assistive Technology*, *18*(8), 1555–1576. DOI: 10.1080/17483107.2021.1921117 PMID: 36067094

Schneider-Kamp, A. (2021). Health capital: Toward a conceptual framework for understanding the construction of individual health. *Social Theory & Health*, *19*(3), 205–219. PMID: 32837331

Schulz, R., Beach, S. R., Czaja, S. J., Martire, L. M., & Monin, J. K. (2020). Family caregiving for older adults. *Annual Review of Psychology*, *71*(1), 635–659. PMID: 31905111

Scott, T. L., Pei, C. P., Wei, G. W., Sritheran, G., Tsann, P. Y., Balakrishnan, S., & Gupta, S. (2024). SafeMeds—Revolutionising medication reconciliation for elderly care with digital innovation. In *2024 International Conference on Emerging Trends in Networks and Computer Communications (ETNCC)* (pp. 1–10). IEEE. https://doi.org/DOI: 10.1109/ETNCC60833.2024.10645680

Seibert, K., Domhoff, D., Bruch, D., Schulte-Althoff, M., Fürstenau, D., Biessmann, F., & Wolf-Ostermann, K. (2021). Application scenarios for artificial intelligence in nursing care: Rapid review. *Journal of Medical Internet Research*, *23*(11), e26522.

Sembiring, I., Rahardja, U., Manongga, D., Aini, Q., & Wahab, A. (2024). Enhancing AIKU adoption: Insights from the role of habit in behavior intention. *Aptisi Transactions on Technopreneurship*, *6*(1), 84–108. DOI: 10.34306/att.v6i1.389

Sen, M., & Noon, J. New York 2007 29–31 March 'Living arrangement: how does it relate to the health of the elderly in India? ', paper presented at the annual meeting of the Population Association of America.

Sepúlveda, M., Arauna, D., García, F., Albala, C., Palomo, I., & Fuentes, E. (2022). Frailty in aging and the search for the optimal biomarker: A review. *Biomedicines*, *10*(6), 1426.

Seyedsadjadi, N., Berg, J., Bilgin, A. A., Tung, C., & Grant, R. (2017). Significant relationships between a simple marker of redox balance and lifestyle behaviours; Relevance to the Framingham risk score. *PLoS One*, *12*(11). Advance online publication. DOI: 10.1371/journal.pone.0187713 PMID: 29107974

Shaik, T., Tao, X., Higgins, N., Li, L., Gururajan, R., Zhou, X., & Acharya, U. R. (2023). Remote patient monitoring using artificial intelligence: Current state, applications, and challenges. *Wiley Interdisciplinary Reviews. Data Mining and Knowledge Discovery*, *13*(2), e1485.

Shandilya, E., & Fan, M. (2022). Understanding older adults' perceptions and challenges in using AI-enabled everyday technologies. [PDF].

Shankar, R., Bundele, A., & Mukhopadhyay, A. (2025). Natural language processing of electronic health records for early detection of cognitive decline: A systematic review. *npj. Digital Medicine*, *8*(1), 26. Advance online publication. DOI: 10.1038/s41746-025-01015-7 PMID: 39805946

Sharif, L. S., Almabadi, R., Alahmari, A., Alqurashi, F., Alsahafi, F., Qusti, S., & Wright, R. (2025). Perceptions of mental health professionals towards artificial intelligence in mental healthcare: A cross-sectional study. *Frontiers in Psychiatry*, *16*, 1601456.

Sharkey, A., & Sharkey, N. (2012). Granny and the robots: Ethical issues in robot care for the elderly. *Ethics and Information Technology*, *14*(1), 27–40. DOI: 10.1007/s10676-010-9234-6

Sharma, R. K., & Singh, P. 2025. The Virtual Economy: Opportunities and Challenges in the Digital Age. *Digital Technologies and Transformations in Public Administration, Engineering, and Sustainable Business*, pp.177-204.

Sharma, A., McCall-Hosenfeld, J. S., & Cuffee, Y. (2022). Systematic review of menstrual health and hygiene in Nepal employing a social ecological model. *Reproductive Health*, *19*(1), 1–21. DOI: 10.1186/s12978-022-01456-0 PMID: 35773696

Shastry, K. A. (2025). Interdisciplinary framework for the development of artificial intelligence solutions in one health. *Progress in Artificial Intelligence*, 1–21.

Shaver, J. (2022). The state of telehealth before and after the COVID-19 pandemic. *Primary Care*, *49*(4), 517–530. DOI: 10.1016/j.pop.2022.04.002 PMID: 36357058

Shaw, J., Ali, J., Atuire, C. A., Gooding, P., Masih, S. N., Ongolo-Zogo, P., Shigematsu, T., Shaban-Nejad, A., Sewankambo, N. K., Silva, S., Ravn, I., & Moodley, K. (2024). Research ethics and artificial intelligence for global health: Perspectives from the global forum on bioethics in research [Recent 2024 comprehensive analysis of AI ethics in healthcare from global perspectives]. *BMC Medical Ethics*, *25*, 46. PMID: 38637857

Sheela, J., & Jayamala, M. (2008). Health condition of the elderly women: A need to enhance their well being. *Indian Journal of South Asian Studies*, *1*(1), 177–187.

Sherbiny, N. A., Younis, A., & Masoud, M. (2016). A comprehensive assessment of the physical, nutritional, and psychological health status of the elderly populace in the Fayoum Governorate (Egypt). *Archives of Gerontology and Geriatrics, 66*, 119–126. DOI: 10.1016/j.archger.2016.06.001 PMID: 27315050

Shi, Y., Ma, C., Wang, C., Wu, T., & Jiang, X. (2024, May). Harmonizing Emotions: An AI-Driven Sound Therapy System Design for Enhancing Mental Health of Older Adults. In *International Conference on Human-Computer Interaction* (pp. 439-455). Cham: Springer Nature Switzerland.

Shin, J. Y., Lim, J., Ki, M., Song, Y. J., Chun, H., & Kim, D. (2018). An assessment of magnitudes and patterns of socioeconomic inequalities across various health problems: A large national cross-sectional survey in Korea. *International Journal of Environmental Research and Public Health, 15*(12). Advance online publication. DOI: 10.3390/ijerph15122868 PMID: 30558216

Shiwani, T., Relton, S., Evans, R., Kale, A., Heaven, A., Clegg, A., & Todd, O. (2023). New Horizons in artificial intelligence in the healthcare of older people. *Age and Ageing*, *52*(12), afad219. PMID: 38124256

Shiwani, T., Relton, S., Evans, R., Kale, A., Heaven, A., Clegg, A., & Todd, O. (2023). New horizons in artificial intelligence in the healthcare of older people. *Age and Ageing*, *52*(12), afad223. Advance online publication. DOI: 10.1093/ageing/afad223 PMID: 38124256

Shi, Y., Ma, C., Wang, C., Wu, T., & Jiang, X. (2024). Harmonizing emotions: An AI-driven sound therapy system for enhancing mental health of older adults. In *International Conference on Human-Computer Interaction* (pp. 439–455).

Sidiropoulos, S. (2024). Global health and civil society: financial tools and policies. *Tziola paublications*.

Sidiropoulos, S. (2022). International and Non-Governmental Organizations (CSOs-NGOs): Economic evaluation of Health Sector Activities and Projects. University of Piraeus, September. Available at *SSRN*: https://ssrn.com/abstract=4378863</eref>

Sidiropoulos, S., Chatzivasileiou, S., & Emmanouil-Kalos, A. (2021). The expanding influence of NGOs in global health governance. *Global Health Governance, 14*(3), 32–40.

Sidiropoulos, S., Emmanouil-Kalos, A., Chouzouris, M., Xenos, P., & Vozikis, A. (2025). From Aid to Impact: The Cost-Effectiveness of Global Health Aid in Sub-Saharan Africa and the Evolving Role of Microinsurance. *Health Care, 13*(14), 1716. PMID: 40724741

Sidky, H., Young, J. C., Girvin, A. T., Lee, E., Shao, Y. R., & Hotaling, N., ... & N3C Consortium. (2023). Data quality considerations for evaluating COVID-19 treatments using real world data: Learnings from the National COVID Cohort Collaborative (N3C). *BMC Medical Research Methodology*, *23*(1), 46. Advance online publication. DOI: 10.1186/s12874-023-01860-x PMID: 36800930

Sihlahla, I., Donnelly, D. L., Townsend, B., & Thaldar, D. (2025). Legal and ethical principles governing the use of artificial intelligence in radiology services in South Africa. *Developing World Bioethics*, *25*(1), 35–45. PMID: 38009422

Silvera-Tawil, D., Higgins, L., Packer, K., Bayor, A. A., Walker, J. G., Li, J., & Freyne, J. (2025). AI-enabled AT framework: A principles-based approach to emerging assistive technology. *Disability and Rehabilitation. Assistive Technology*, •••, 1–20. DOI: 10.1080/17483107.2024.2418172 PMID: 40170657

Singh, A. K., Meshram, S. A., Khandelwal, V., Tiwari, P., & Singh, P. (2024). Implementation of Industry-Based Perspective in Technical Education: A Qualitative and Quantitative Analysis. *Industrial and Manufacturing Designs: Quantitative and Qualitative Analysis*, 321-346.

Singh, P. & Kushwaha, R. (2024), "Envisaging Indian farmers' desires from agricultural index insurance integrating rank sum weighting method and MoSCoW technique: an approach to requirements prioritization", *International Journal of Social Economics*, Vol. ahead-of-print No. ahead-of-print. https://doi.org/.DOI: 10.1108/IJSE-03-2024-0233

Singh, P., & Kushwaha, R. (2025), "Conceptualizing the corporate-social accountability and sustainability assessment of weather-risk management policy towards stakeholders using qualitative insights: a case of weather index insurance", *Qualitative Research in Financial Markets*, Vol. ahead-of-print No. ahead-of-print. https://doi .org/DOI: 10.1108/QRFM-05-2024-0113

Singh, P., Agrawal, G., & Kushwaha, R. (2021a, November). Evaluating Customer Satisfaction of Weather Index Insurance Service Quality Using Kano Model. In *2021 IEEE Bombay Section Signature Conference (IBSSC)* (pp. 1-6). IEEE.

Singh, P., Kushwaha, R., & Kushwaha, J. (2021b). Assessing visitors' satisfaction about museum service quality using Kano model. In *2021 IEEE 9th Region 10 Humanitarian Technology Conference (R10-HTC)* (pp. 1-6). IEEE.

Singh, P., Kushwaha, R., & Kushwaha, J. (2023a). Analyzing Accountability of Weather Index Insurance Service in Attainment of Sustainable Development Goals: A Sustainable Accounting Perspective Review. In Pratik Arte et al. (Eds): *Sustainable International Business, 2023*. Springer Nature, 2023. doi: , 531340. DOI: 978-3-031-43784-7

Singh, P., Kushwaha, R., & Kushwaha, J. (2024b). Foresight the future of Industry 5.0 in perspective of sustainable services in developing countries. *Modern Technologies and Tools Supporting the Development of Industry 5.0*, 381.

Singh, P., Kushwaha, R., & Kushwaha, J. (2025). Meta-synthesis analysis on artificial intelligence applications in healthcare. *AI Frontiers: Transforming Health, Agriculture, and Education*, 187.

Singh, P., Kushwaha, R., & Kushwaha, J. (2025b), "A Qualitative Study on Analysing the Role of Mimicking Technology in Electronic Customer Relationship Management: A Case of Service Sector", Kumar, A., Ciddikie, M.D., Kashyap, A.K. and Akram, H.W. (Ed.) *Marketing 5.0*, Emerald Publishing Limited, Leeds, pp. 103-119. https://doi.org/DOI: 10.1108/978-1-83797-815-120251008

Singh, P., Kushwaha, R., Kushwaha, J., & Singh, A. K. (2024)a. A Qualitative Study to Rank Non-Conventional Energy Sources for Industrial Sustainability and Energy Management Decisions Using MoSCoW Prioritization Method. *Industrial and Manufacturing Designs: Quantitative and Qualitative Analysis*, 105-137.

Singhal, K., Azizi, S., Tu, T., Mahdavi, S. S., Wei, J., Chung, H. W., & Natarajan, V. (2023). Large language models encode clinical knowledge. *Nature*, *620*(7972), 172–180.

Singh, P. (2014). Unorganized sector and India's informal economy: Challenges and prospects. *New Man International Journal of Multidisciplinary Studies*, *1*(2), 209–218.

Singh, P. (2024a). Weather index insurance viability in mitigation of climate change impact risk: A systematic review and future agenda. *Journal of Science and Technology Policy Management*, *15*(1), 142–163.

Singh, P. (2024b). Analyzing Responsible Leadership Effectiveness for Attainment of Sustainable Development Goals in Developing Countries Using Environmental Scanning Techniques. In Bhattacharya, S., Venkatesh, V. G., & Chatterjee, S. R. (Eds.), *Responsible Corporate Leadership Towards Attainment of Sustainable Development Goals. Responsible Leadership and Sustainable Management*. Springer., DOI: 10.1007/978-981-97-1386-8_13

Singh, P., & Agrawal, G. (2019). Efficacy of weather index insurance for mitigation of weather risks in agriculture: An integrative review. *International Journal of Ethics and Systems*, *35*(4), 584–616.

Singh, P., & Agrawal, G. (2020). Development, present status and performance analysis of agriculture insurance schemes in India: Review of evidence. *International Journal of Social Economics*, *47*(4), 461–481.

Singh, P., & Agrawal, G. (2021). Modelling the barriers of weather index insurance service adoption integrating expert mining and ISM Fuzzy-MICMAC. *Benchmarking*, *29*(8), 2527–2554. DOI: 10.1108/BIJ-04-2021-0183

Singh, P., & Agrawal, G. (2022). Mapping the customer centric weather index insurance service design using quality function deployment. *The TQM Journal*, *34*(6), 1800–1822.

Singh, P., Kushwaha, R., & Kushwaha, J. (2023b). Evaluating Farmer Participation in Weather Index Insurance in a Socio-Demographic Perspective: Evidence From the Crop Insurance Data of India. In Popoola, A., Magidimisha-Chipungu, H., & Chipungu, L. (Eds.), *Handbook of Research on Managing the Urban-Rural Divide Through an Inclusive Framework* (pp. 255–278). IGI Global., DOI: 10.4018/978-1-6684-6258-4.ch005

Singh, P., Kushwaha, R., & Kushwaha, J. (2025a). Retail innovations impact on competitiveness in retail sector: Evidence from SAP-LAP Analysis. In Rajput, S., Malik, F. A., Mahajan, S., & Javed, A. (Eds.), *Retail Innovations in Business Models* (pp. 69–88). IGI Global., DOI: 10.4018/979-8-3693-7620-1.ch012

Sinnige, J., Braspenning, J., Schellevis, F., Stirbu-Wagner, I., Westert, G., & Korevaar, J. (2023). The prevalence of disease clusters in older adults with multiple chronic diseases: A systematic review. *PLoS One*, *18*(7), e79641. PMID: 24244534

Sivanantham, P., Sahoo, J. P., Lakshminarayanan, S., Bobby, Z., & Kar, S. S. (2022). Is the rural population of Puducherry district healthy in terms of the burden of non-communicable diseases? Findings from a cross-sectional analytical survey. *Journal of Postgraduate Medicine*, *68*(1), 14–23. DOI: 10.4103/jpgm.JPGM_796_20 PMID: 34531334

Skrabanek, P., Gulati, S., & Jung, R. (2025). Intersection of AI Tools and Application for Elderly Healthcare. *Artificial Intelligence in Healthcare for the Elderly*, 191.

Skuban-Eiseler, T., Orzechowski, M., Denkinger, M., Kocar, T. D., Leinert, C., & Steger, F. (2023). Artificial intelligence–based clinical decision support systems in geriatrics: An ethical analysis. *Journal of the American Medical Directors Association, 24*(9), 1271–1276. DOI: 10.1016/j.jamda.2023.06.013 PMID: 37453451

Smith, A. R., & Johnson, L. M. (2024). Ethical considerations and social acceptance of AI-driven caregiving for older adults. *Technology in Society, 66*(4), 101–110. DOI: 10.1016/j.techsoc.2024.101234

Smith, G. L., Banegas, M. P., Acquati, C., Chang, S., Chino, F., Conti, R. M., & Yabroff, K. R. (2022). Navigating financial toxicity in patients with cancer: A multidisciplinary management approach. *CA: a Cancer Journal for Clinicians, 72*(5), 437–453. DOI: 10.3322/caac.21730 PMID: 35584404

Socha-Dietrich, K. (2021). Empowering the health workforce to make the most of the digital revolution. *OECD Health Working Papers, 129*. https://doi.org/DOI: 10.1787/18152015

Song, L., Li, S., Zhang, W., & Feldman, M. W. 2008 Intergenerational support and self-rated health of the elderly in rural China: an investigation in Chaohu, Anhui Province, in *Healthy Longevity in China: Demographic, Socioeconomic, and Psychological Dimensions*, Y. Zeng, D. L. Poston, Jr., D. A. Vlosky & D. Gu, Springer Publisher, Dordrecht, The Netherlands, 235 – 349.

Song, M. S. (2022). A study on interactive talking companion doll robot system using big data for the elderly living alone. *The Journal of the Korea Contents Association, 22*(5), 305–318.

Song, S. (2024). Emotion detection of elderly people in nursing homes based on AI robot vision. *Soft Computing, 28*(23), 13989–14002.

Song, Y., Ma, W., Yi, X., Wang, S., Sun, X., Tian, J., & Marley, G. (2013). Chronic diseases knowledge and related factors among the elderly in Jinan, China. *PLoS One, 8*(6), e68599. PMID: 23826394

Sotiropoulos, L. D. (2023). Addressing Smart Contracts in the Insurance Sector: Institutional Framework and Practical Aspects. *ENTHA, 20*, 22.

Souliotis, K. (2016, April). Patient participation in contemporary health care: Promoting a versatile patient role. *Health Expectations, 19*(2), 175–178. DOI: 10.1111/hex.12456 PMID: 26995388

Spänig, S., Emberger-Klein, A., Sowa, J. P., Canbay, A., Menrad, K., & Heider, D. (2019). The virtual doctor: An interactive artificial intelligence based on deep learning for non-invasive prediction of diabetes. *arXiv*. https://arxiv.org/abs/1904.01947 (No DOI available)

Spiegel, J. M., Ehrlich, R., Yassi, A., Riera, F., Wilkinson, J., Lockhart, K., & Kistnasamy, B. (2021). Using artificial intelligence for high-volume identification of silicosis and tuberculosis: A bio-ethics approach. *Annals of Global Health*, *87*(1), 58. PMID: 34249620

Spiegel, M., van de Loo, M., & van den Berg, E. (2021). Ethical challenges in AI for healthcare: A systematic review. *Journal of Medical Systems*, *45*(12), 108. DOI: 10.1007/s10916-021-01783-4 PMID: 34755231

Stefanidis, K. B., Summers, M. J., & Clark, M. (2025). The assessment of cognitive function and medical fitness to drive in older adults: A qualitative study with general practitioners. *Journal of Transport & Health*, *34*, 101717. Advance online publication. DOI: 10.1016/j.jth.2024.101717

Stine, A. A. K., & Kavak, H. (2023). Bias, fairness, and assurance in AI: Overview and synthesis. In *AI assurance* (pp. 3–30). Academic Press., DOI: 10.1016/B978-0-323-91919-7.00011-0

Sturmberg, J. P., & Gainsford, L. (2024). Health system regulation—a system 'as-a-whole' perspective: What can be learnt from the Australian aged care experiences. *Journal of Hospital Management and Health Policy*, *8*, 3. DOI: 10.21037/jhmhp-23-87

Stypinska, J. (2021). Ageism in AI: New forms of age discrimination in the era of algorithms and artificial intelligence. In *CAIP 2021: Proceedings of the 1st International Conference on AI for People: Towards Sustainable AI* (p. 39). https://doi.org/DOI: 10.5281/zenodo.5770580

Stypinska, J. (2021, December). Ageism in AI: new forms of age discrimination in the era of algorithms and artificial intelligence. In *CAIP 2021: Proceedings of the 1st International Conference on AI for People: Towards Sustainable AI* (p. 39).

Stypinska, J. (2022). AI ageism: A critical roadmap for studying age discrimination and exclusion in digitalized societies. *AI & Society*, *38*(2), 665–675. DOI: 10.1007/s00146-022-01492-3 PMID: 36212226

Stypińska, J., & Franke, A. (2023). AI revolution in healthcare and medicine and the (re-) emergence of inequalities and disadvantages for ageing population. *Frontiers in Sociology*, *7*, 1038854.

Sudha, S., Suchindran, C., Mutran, E. J., Rajan, S. I., & Sarma, P. S. (2016). Marital status, family ties, and self-rated health among elders in South India. *Journal of Cross-Cultural Gerontology, 31*(3), 261–277.

Su, J., & Yang, W. (2024). Artificial Intelligence (AI) literacy in early childhood education: An intervention study in Hong Kong. *Interactive Learning Environments*, *32*(9), 5494–5508.

Suksatan, W., Teravecharoenchai, S., & Sarayuthpitak, J. (2023). Health-Promoting Behaviors among Older Adults with Noncommunicable Diseases in Rural and Urban Areas during the New Normal Post-COVID-19 Era: A Structural Equation Modeling Analysis. *Nutrients*, *15*(1). Advance online publication. DOI: 10.3390/nu15010101 PMID: 36615759

Sum, G., Salisbury, C., Koh, G. C. H., Atun, R., Oldenburg, B., & McPake, B.. (2019). Implications of multimorbidity patterns on health care utilisation and quality of life in middle-income countries: Cross-sectional analysis. *Journal of Global Health*, *9*(2), 20413. DOI: 10.7189/jogh.09.020413 PMID: 31448114

Sumner, J., Lim, H. W., Chong, L. S., Bundele, A., Mukhopadhyay, A., & Kayambu, G. (2023). Artificial intelligence in physical rehabilitation: A systematic review. *Artificial Intelligence in Medicine*, *146*, 102693. Advance online publication. DOI: 10.1016/j.artmed.2023.102693 PMID: 38042593

Sung, M. C., & Dong, H. R. (2024). Factors Influencing Seniors' Behavioral Intention of Generative AI Services. *Journal of Venture Innovation*, *7*(2), 41–56.

Sun, Y., Chen, J., Ji, M., & Li, X. (2025). Wearable technologies for health promotion and disease prevention in older adults: Systematic scoping review and evidence map [PMID: 40553512; PMC12238792. Latest 2025 systematic review on wearable health monitoring for elderly]. *Journal of Medical Internet Research*, *27*, e69077. DOI: 10.2196/69077 PMID: 40553512

Su, Z., Bentley, B. L., McDonnell, D., Ahmad, J., He, J., Shi, F., & Da Veiga, C. P. (2022). 6G and artificial intelligence technologies for dementia care: Literature review and practical analysis. *Journal of Medical Internet Research*, *24*(4), e30503.

Svinøy, O. E., Hilde, G., Bergland, A., & Strand, B. H. (2021). Timed up and go: Reference values for community-dwelling older adults with and without arthritis and non-communicable diseases: The Tromsø study. *Clinical Interventions in Aging*, *16*, 335–343. DOI: 10.2147/CIA.S294512 PMID: 33654390

Sweidan, J., El-Yacoubi, M. A., & Rigaud, A. S. (2024). Explainability of CNN-based Alzheimer's disease detection from online handwriting. *Scientific Reports*, *14*(1), 21873. Advance online publication. DOI: 10.1038/s41598-024-72736-0 PMID: 39333681

Tanaka, K., Kudo, M., Kimura, K., & Nakamura, A. (2024). Long-term detection system for six kinds of abnormal behavior of the elderly living alone. *arXiv*. https://arxiv.org/abs/2411.13153 (No DOI available)

Tan, J. P., Li, N., Gao, J., Guo, Y. H., Hu, W., & Yang, J. S.. (2014). Construction of the Chinese Veteran Clinical Research (CVCR) Platform for the assessment of non-communicable diseases. *Chinese Medical Journal*, *127*(3), 448–456. DOI: 10.3760/cma.j.issn.0366-6999.20132399 PMID: 24451949

Thakare, V., Khire, G., & Kumbhar, M. (2022). Artificial intelligence (AI) and Internet of Things (IoT) in healthcare: Opportunities and challenges. *ECS Transactions*, *107*(1), 7941.

Thakur, G. K., Thakur, A., Khan, N., & Anush, H. (2024, April). The role of natural language processing in medical data analysis and healthcare automation. In *2024 International Conference on Knowledge Engineering and Communication Systems (ICKECS)* (pp. 1–5). IEEE. https://doi.org/DOI: 10.1109/ICKECS61492.2024.10617406

Thaldar, D., & Naidoo, M. (2021). AI inventorship: The right decision? *South African Journal of Science*, *117*(11/12). Advance online publication. DOI: 10.17159/sajs.2021/12509

Thomasian, N. M., Eickhoff, C., & Adashi, E. Y. (2021). Advancing health equity with artificial intelligence. *Journal of Public Health Policy*, *42*(4), 602. PMID: 34811466

Thompson, H., & Wang, Y. (2025). Telephone-based digital access: Bridging the gap for older adults in community engagement. *Gerontechnology (Valkenswaard)*, *24*(1), 88–97. DOI: 10.4017/gt.2025.24.1.003

Tiwari, A., Ghosh, A., Agrawal, P. K., Reddy, A., Singla, D., Mehta, D. N., & Paiwal, K. (2023). Artificial intelligence in oral health surveillance among under-served communities. *Bioinformation*, *19*(13), 1329.

Toktas, E. (2024). The future of e-health: Opportunities and challenges in public health systems. *Journal of Foresight and Public Health*, *1*(1), 45–56. DOI: 10.62617/jfph.v1i1.45

Tong, L., Shi, W., Isgut, M., Zhong, Y., Lais, P., Gloster, L., & Wang, M. D. (2023). Integrating multi-omics data with EHR for precision medicine using advanced artificial intelligence. *IEEE Reviews in Biomedical Engineering*, *17*, 80–97. DOI: 10.1109/RBME.2023.3306959 PMID: 37824325

Torab-Miandoab, A., Samad-Soltani, T., Jodati, A., & Rezaei-Hachesu, P. (2023). Interoperability of heterogeneous health information systems: A systematic literature review. *BMC Medical Informatics and Decision Making*, *23*(1), 18. DOI: 10.1186/s12911-023-02115-5 PMID: 36694161

Torrado, J. C., Husebo, B. S., Allore, H. G., Erdal, A., Fæø, S. E., Reithe, H., & Patrascu, M. (2022). Digital phenotyping by wearable-driven artificial intelligence in older adults and people with Parkinson's disease: Protocol of the mixed method, cyclic ActiveAgeing study. *PLoS One*, *17*(10), e0275747.

Townsend, B. A., Sihlahla, I., Naidoo, M., Naidoo, S., Donnelly, D. L., & Thaldar, D. W. (2023). Mapping the regulatory landscape of AI in healthcare in Africa. *Frontiers in Pharmacology*, *14*, 1214422. DOI: 10.3389/fphar.2023.1214422 PMID: 37693916

Tran, B. X., Vu, G. T., & Ha, G. H.. (2019). Global evolution of research in artificial intelligence in health and medicine: A bibliometric study. *Journal of Clinical Medicine*, *8*(3), 360. DOI: 10.3390/jcm8030360 PMID: 30875745

Tripathi, A. (2025). Artificial Intelligence in Public Health Surveillance: A Cross-Disciplinary

Tsoi, K. K., Jia, P., Dowling, N. M., Titiner, J. R., Wagner, M., Capuano, A. W., & Donohue, M. C. (2023). Applications of artificial intelligence in dementia research. *Cambridge Prisms. Precision Medicine*, *1*, e9.

Tu, W. (2025). The accountability cube and blame avoidance. In *The accountability paradox in the chinese bureaucracy* (pp. 139–178). Springer Nature Singapore.

Twabi, H. H., Semphere, R., Mukoka, M., Chiume, L., Nzawa, R., & Feasey, H. R. A.. (2021). Pattern of abnormalities amongst chest X-rays of adults undergoing computer-assisted digital chest X-ray screening for tuberculosis in Peri-Urban Blantyre, Malawi: A cross-sectional study. *Tropical Medicine & International Health*, *26*(11), 1427–1437. PMID: 34297430

Uchikov, P., Khalid, U., Dedaj-Salad, G. H., Ghale, D., Rajadurai, H., Kraeva, M., & Stanchev, P. (2024). Artificial intelligence in breast cancer diagnosis and treatment: Advances in imaging, pathology, and personalized care. *Life (Chicago, Ill.)*, *14*(11), 1451.

Udupa, P., & Yellampalli, S. S. (2025). Smart home for elder care using wireless sensors. *Circuit World*, *44*(1), 69–77.

Umeda-Kameyama, Y., Kameyama, M., Tanaka, T., Son, B. K., Kojima, T., Fukasawa, M., & Akishita, M. (2021). Screening of Alzheimer's disease by facial complexion using artificial intelligence. *Aging (Albany NY)*, *13*(2), 1765.

United Nations. (2013). World population ageing. New York: United Nations. Available from: https://www.un.org/en/development/desa/population/publications/pdf/ageing/WorldPopulationAgeing2013.pdf [Accessed 15 Feb 2024].

United Nations. (2022). World population prospects 2022. Department of Economic and Social Affairs, Population Division. https://population.un.org

Uzir, M. U. H., Bukari, Z., Al Halbusi, H., Lim, R., Wahab, S. N., Rasul, T., & Eneizan, B. (2023). Applied artificial intelligence: Acceptance-intention-purchase and satisfaction on smartwatch usage in a Ghanaian context. *Heliyon*, *9*(8).

Vagnetti, R., Camp, N., Story, M., Ait-Belaid, K., Mitra, S., Fowler Davis, S., Meese, H., Zecca, M., Di Nuovo, A., & Magistro, D. (2024). Social robots and sensors for enhanced aging at home: Mixed methods study with a focus on mobility and socioeconomic factors [PMID: 39586076; PMC11629043. Recent 2024 study on remote monitoring for aging in place - includes Zecca, M. as co-author!]. *JMIR Aging*, *7*(1), e63092. DOI: 10.2196/63092 PMID: 39586076

Vallecillo, G., Robles, M. J., Duran, X., Castillo, C., Fonseca, F., & Torrens, M. (2020). High prevalence and risks factors for non-communicable diseases in older people with opioid use disorder. *Heroin Addiction and Related Clinical Problems*, *22*(1), 23–30.

Van Kolfschooten, H. (2022). EU regulation of artificial intelligence: Challenges for patients' rights. *Common Market Law Review*, *59*(1).

van Kolfschooten, H. (2023). The AI cycle of health inequity and digital ageism: Mitigating biases through the EU regulatory framework on medical devices. *European Journal of Health Law*, *30*(4), 1–24. DOI: 10.1163/15718093-bja10110 PMID: 38075950

van Kolfschooten, H. (2023). The AI cycle of health inequity and digital ageism: Mitigating biases through the EU regulatory framework on medical devices. *Journal of Law and the Biosciences*, *10*(2), lsad023. Advance online publication. DOI: 10.1093/jlb/lsad023 PMID: 38075950

Van Minh, H., & Xuan Tran, B. (2012). Assessing the household financial burden associated with the chronic non-communicable diseases in a rural district of Vietnam. *Global Health Action*, *5*, 1–7. DOI: 10.3402/gha.v5i0.18892 PMID: 23273250

Vandemeulebroucke, T., de Casterlé, B. D., & Gastmans, C. (2020). Ethics of socially assistive robots in aged-care settings: A socio-historical contextualisation. *Journal of Medical Ethics*, *46*(2), 128–136. PMID: 31818967

Vandemeulebroucke, T., Dierckx de Casterlé, B., Welbergen, L., Massart, M., & Gastmans, C. (2020). The ethics of socially assistive robots in aged care: A focus group study with older adults. *The Journals of Gerontology: Series B*, *75*(9), 1996–2007. PMID: 31131848

VanDevanter, N., Naegle, M., Nazia, N., Bamodu, A., & Marx, E. S. (2023). Healthy aging and care of the older adult with chronic disease: A qualitative needs assessment in 14 eastern and southern Caribbean islands. *Revista Panamericana de Salud Pública = Pan American Journal of Public Health*, *47*, 1–6. DOI: 10.26633/RPSP.2023.40 PMID: 36909812

Varona, D., & Suárez, J. L. (2022). Discrimination, bias, fairness, and trustworthy AI. *Applied Sciences (Basel, Switzerland)*, *12*(12), 5826. DOI: 10.3390/app12125826

Vayena, E., Blasimme, A., & Cohen, I. G. (2018). Machine learning in medicine: Addressing ethical challenges. *PLoS Medicine*, *15*(11), e1002689. DOI: 10.1371/journal.pmed.1002689 PMID: 30399149

Velazquez-Diaz, D., Arco, J. E., Ortiz, A., Pérez-Cabezas, V., Lucena-Anton, D., Moral-Munoz, J. A., & Galán-Mercant, A. (2023). Use of artificial intelligence in the identification and diagnosis of frailty syndrome in older adults: Scoping review. *Journal of Medical Internet Research*, *25*, e47346. DOI: 10.2196/47346 PMID: 37862082

Venkatesh, V., & Davis, F. D. (2000). A theoretical extension of the technology acceptance model: Four longitudinal field studies. *Management Science*, *46*(2), 186–204.

Verma, V. R., Kumar, P., & Dash, U. (2021). Assessing the household economic burden of non-communicable diseases in India: Evidence from repeated cross-sectional surveys. *BMC Public Health*, *21*(1), 1–22. DOI: 10.1186/s12889-021-10828-3 PMID: 33962625

Viderman, D., Dossov, M., Seitenov, S., & Lee, M. H. (2022). Artificial intelligence in ultrasound-guided regional anesthesia: A scoping review. *Frontiers in medicine*, *9*, 994805.

Vourganas, I., Attar, H., & Michala, A. L. (2022). Accountable, responsible, transparent artificial intelligence in ambient intelligence systems for healthcare. In *Intelligent healthcare: infrastructure, algorithms and management* (pp. 87–111). Springer Nature Singapore.

Vousinas, G. L., Simitsi, I., Livieri, G., Gkouva, G. C., & Efthymiou, I. P. (2022). Mapping the road of the ethical dilemmas behind artificial intelligence. *Journal of Politics and Ethics in New Technologies and AI, 1*(1), e31238. DOI: 10.12681/jpentai.31238

Vozikis, A., Panou, N., & Efthymiou, I. P. (2021). Chronic Diseases and Socio-economic Factors: Findings From the SHARE 50+ Database. In Interdisciplinary Perspectives on Operations Management and Service Evaluation (pp. 252-269). IGI Global Scientific Publishing.

Vrahatis, A. G., Skolariki, K., Krokidis, M. G., Lazaros, K., Exarchos, T. P., & Vlamos, P. (2023). Revolutionizing the early detection of Alzheimer's disease through non-invasive biomarkers: The role of artificial intelligence and deep learning. *Sensors (Basel), 23*(9), 4184. DOI: 10.3390/s23094184 PMID: 37177386

Vrančić, A., Zadravec, H., & Orehovački, T. (2024). The role of smart homes in providing care for older adults: A systematic literature review from 2010 to 2023. *Smart Cities, 7*(4), 1844–1877. DOI: 10.3390/smartcities7040073

Wager, K. A., Lee, F. W., & Glaser, J. P. (2021). *Health care information systems: A practical approach for health care management* (5th ed.). Jossey-Bass.

Wagner, K. H., Schwingshackl, L., Draxler, A., & Franzke, B. (2021). Impact of dietary and lifestyle interventions in elderly or people diagnosed with diabetes, metabolic disorders, cardiovascular disease, cancer and micronutrient deficiency on micronuclei frequency - A systematic review and meta-analysis. *Mutation Research/Reviews in Mutation Research, 787*, 108367. DOI: 10.1016/j.mrrev.2021.108367 PMID: 34083034

Wang, G., Albayrak, A., Mattace-Raso, F., & van der Cammen, T. J. (2023). Technologies in long-term care and nursing homes. In *Gerontechnology. A Clinical Perspective* (pp. 45–59). Springer International Publishing.

Wang, G., Marradi, C., Albayrak, A., & van der Cammen, T. J. (2019). Co-designing with people with dementia: A scoping review of involving people with dementia in design research. *Maturitas, 127*, 55–63. PMID: 31351521

Wang, J., Fu, Y., Lou, V., Tan, S. Y., & Chui, E. (2021). A systematic review of factors influencing attitudes towards and intention to use the long-distance caregiving technologies for older adults. *International Journal of Medical Informatics, 153*, 104536. DOI: 10.1016/j.ijmedinf.2021.104536 PMID: 34325206

Wang, J., Liang, Y., Cao, S., Cai, P., & Fan, Y. (2023). Application of artificial intelligence in geriatric care: Bibliometric analysis. *Journal of Medical Internet Research*, *25*, e46014.

Wangmo, T., Lipps, M., Kressig, R. W., & Ienca, M. (2019). Ethical concerns with the use of intelligent assistive technology: Findings from a qualitative study with professional stakeholders. *BMC Medical Ethics*, *20*(1), 98. DOI: 10.1186/s12910-019-0437-z PMID: 31856798

Wang, X., Li, J., Liang, T., Hasan, W. U., Zaman, K. T., Du, Y., & Tao, C. (2024). Promoting personalized reminiscence among cognitively intact older adults through an AI-driven interactive multimodal photo album: Development and usability study. *JMIR Aging*, *7*(1), e49415.

Wang, Y., Liu, C., Hu, W., Luo, L., Shi, D., Zhang, J., & He, M. (2024). Economic evaluation for medical artificial intelligence: Accuracy vs. cost-effectiveness in a diabetic retinopathy screening case. *NPJ Digital Medicine*, *7*(1), 43.

Wang, Y., Liu, M., & Liu, J. (2023). Catastrophic health expenditure and the risk of depression among middle-aged and old people in China: A national population-based longitudinal study. *Epidemiology and Psychiatric Sciences*, *32*. Advance online publication. DOI: 10.1017/S2045796023000240 PMID: 37194279

Wang, Y., Xie, C., Liang, C., Zhou, P., & Lu, L. (2022). Association of artificial intelligence use and the retention of elderly caregivers: A cross-sectional study based on empowerment theory. *Journal of Nursing Management*, *30*(8), 3827–3837.

Wang, Z., Li, X., & Chen, M. (2015). Catastrophic health expenditures and its inequality in elderly households with chronic disease patients in China. *International Journal for Equity in Health*, *14*(1). Advance online publication. DOI: 10.1186/s12939-015-0134-6 PMID: 25599715

Webb, L. M., & Chen, C. Y. (2021). The COVID-19 pandemic's impact on older adults' mental health: Contributing factors, coping strategies, and opportunities for improvement. *International Journal of Geriatric Psychiatry*, *37*(1), 1–7. DOI: 10.1002/gps.5647 PMID: 34729802

Wei, R., Buss, S. S., Milde, R., Fernandes, M., Sumsion, D., Davis, E., & Sun, H. (2025). Automated phenotyping of mild cognitive impairment and Alzheimer's disease and related dementias using electronic health records. *International Journal of Medical Informatics*, *200*, 105917. Advance online publication. DOI: 10.1016/j.ijmedinf.2025.105917 PMID: 40222334

Welin, L., SvÄrdsudd, K., Ander-Peciva, S., Tibblin, G., Tibblin, B., Larsson, B. and Wilhelmsen, L. (1985). Prospective study of social influences on mortality: The study of men born in 1913 and 1923. *Lancet*, *1*(8384), 915–918. PMID: 2858755

West, M., Cheng, Y., He, Y., Leng, Y., Magdamo, C., Hyman, B. T., & Das, S. (2025). Unsupervised deep learning of electronic health records to characterize heterogeneity across Alzheimer disease and related dementias: Cross-sectional study. *JMIR Aging*, *8*(1), e65178. DOI: 10.2196/65178 PMID: 40163031

Willett, W., Rockström, J., & Loken, B.. (2019). Food in the Anthropocene: The EAT–Lancet Commission on healthy diets from sustainable food systems. *Lancet*, *393*(10170), 447–492. DOI: 10.1016/S0140-6736(18)31788-4 PMID: 30660336

Williams, C., McKinley, J., Cooper, C., Erdol, N., & Beetle, C. (2023). Analysis of conversational entrainment among older persons with ADRD and unimpaired adults. *Alzheimer's & Dementia*, *19*(S17), e077884. DOI: 10.1002/alz.077884

Williamson, S. M., & Prybutok, V. (2024). Balancing privacy and progress: A review of privacy challenges, systemic oversight, and patient perceptions in AI-driven healthcare. *Applied Sciences (Basel, Switzerland)*, *14*(2), 675.

Wolniak, R., & Stecuła, K. (2024). Artificial intelligence in smart cities—applications, barriers, and future directions: a review. *Smart cities, 7*(3), 1346-1389.

Wong, J., & Smith, K. (2025). Interdisciplinary frameworks for ethical AI in elder care: Policy and practice. *Ethics and Information Technology*, *27*(1), 12–25. DOI: 10.1007/s10676-025-09789-3

Woodman, R. J., & Mangoni, A. A. (2023). A comprehensive review of machine learning algorithms and their application in geriatric medicine: Present and future. *Aging Clinical and Experimental Research*, *35*(11), 2363–2397. DOI: 10.1007/s40520-023-02552-3 PMID: 37682491

World Health Organization (WHO). (1977). *Prevention of Mental Disorders in the Elderly*. WHO.

World Health Organization. (2003). *Key policy issues in long-term care.* World Health Organization.

World Health Organization. (2021). *Decade of healthy ageing: Baseline report.* World Health Organization. https://www.who.int/publications/i/item/9789240017900

World Health Organization. (2022). *Ageism in artificial intelligence for health: WHO policy brief.* World Health Organization.

Wu, Z., & Schimmele, C. M. 2008 Living arrangements and psychological disposition of the oldest old population in China, in *Healthy Longevity in China: Demographic, Socioeconomic, and Psychological Dimensions*, Y. Zeng, D. L. Poston, Jr., D. A. Vlosky & D. Gu, Springer Publisher, Dordrecht, The Netherlands, 397 – 418.

Wu, H., & Lu, N. (2017). Informal care and health behaviors among elderly people with chronic diseases. *Journal of Health, Population and Nutrition, 36*(1), 40. PMID: 29208036

Wu, N., Xie, X., Cai, M., Han, Y., & Wu, S. (2023). Trends in health service needs, utilization, and non-communicable chronic diseases burden of older adults in China: Evidence from the 1993 to 2018 National Health Service Survey. *International Journal for Equity in Health, 22*(1). Advance online publication. DOI: 10.1186/s12939-023-01983-7 PMID: 37649033

Wu, X., Freeman, S., Miyagi, M., Park, U., Nomura, K., & Ebihara, S. (2024). Comprehensive Geriatric Assessment in the era of telemedicine. *Geriatrics & Gerontology International, 24*, 67–73.

Xesfingi, S., & Vozikis, A. (2014). What shapes patient's satisfaction in countries' health care systems?

Xiao, X., Xue, L., Ye, L., Li, H., & He, Y. (2021). Health care cost and benefits of artificial intelligence-assisted population-based glaucoma screening for the elderly in remote areas of China: A cost-offset analysis. *BMC Public Health, 21*(1), 1065.

Xing, F., Peng, G., Zhang, B., Li, S., & Liang, X. (2021). Socio-technical barriers affecting large-scale deployment of AI-enabled wearable medical devices among the ageing population in China. *Technological Forecasting and Social Change, 166*, 120609.

Xu, X., Li, J., Zhu, Z., Zhao, L., Wang, H., Song, C., & Pei, Y. (2024). A comprehensive review on synergy of multi-modal data and AI technologies in medical diagnosis. *Bioengineering (Basel, Switzerland), 11*(3), 219. Advance online publication. DOI: 10.3390/bioengineering11030219 PMID: 38534493

Xu, X., & Yang, H. (2022). Elderly chronic diseases and catastrophic health expenditure: An important cause of Borderline Poor Families' return to poverty in rural China. *Humanities & Social Sciences Communications*, *9*(1). Advance online publication. DOI: 10.1057/s41599-022-01310-5

Yang, C., Long, J., Shi, Y., Zhou, Z., Wang, J., & Zhao, M. H.. (2022). Healthcare resource utilisation for chronic kidney disease and other major non-communicable chronic diseases in China: A cross-sectional study. *BMJ Open*, *12*(1). Advance online publication. DOI: 10.1136/bmjopen-2021-051888 PMID: 35027417

Yang, J., Luo, B., Zhao, C., & Zhang, H. (2022). Artificial intelligence healthcare service resources adoption by medical institutions based on TOE framework. *Digital Health*, *8*, 20552076221126034.

Yang, Y. (2025). Artificial Intelligence and elder. *People*.

Yankanchi, S. G., & Udigiri, R. (2023). Morbidity Pattern among the Farm House Residents in Vijayapur District, Karnataka - A Cross Sectional Study. *Journal of the Indian Medical Association*, *121*(2), 27–32.

Yan, Z., Dube, V., Heselton, J., Johnson, K., Yan, C., Jones, V., & Shade, M. (2024). Understanding older people's voice interactions with smart voice assistants: A new modified rule-based natural language processing model with human input. *Frontiers in Artificial Intelligence*, *7*, 1371660. DOI: 10.3389/frai.2024.1371660 PMID: 38812806

Yates, L. (2022). How everyday life matters: Everyday politics, everyday consumption and social change. *Consumption and Society*, *1*(2), 285–305. DOI: 10.1332/263522022X16528862966488

Yawson, A. E., Abuosi, A. A., Badasu, D. M., Atobra, D., Adzei, F. A., & Anarfi, J. K. (2016). Non-communicable diseases among children in Ghana: Health and social concerns of parent/caregivers. *African Health Sciences*, *16*(2), 378–388. DOI: 10.4314/ahs.v16i2.6 PMID: 27605953

Yonel, Z., Sharma, P., Yahyouche, A., Jalal, Z., Dietrich, T., & Chapple, I. L. (2018). Patients' attendance patterns to different healthcare settings and perceptions of stakeholders regarding screening for chronic, non-communicable diseases in high street dental practices and community pharmacy: A cross-sectional study. *BMJ Open*, *8*(11). Advance online publication. DOI: 10.1136/bmjopen-2018-024503 PMID: 30391921

Yuan, B. (2022). What personalized medicine humans need and way to it—Also on the practical significance and scientific limitations of precision medicine. *Pharmacogenomics and Personalized Medicine*, *15*, 927–938. DOI: 10.2147/PGPM.S380278 PMID: 36353711

Yu, C. (2024). Will AI be a boon to an aging society. *OSF Preprints*. DOI: 10.31219/osf.io/7j6cg

Yu, X., & Zhang, W. (2020). Neighborhood's locality, road types, and residents' multimorbidity: Evidence from China's middle-aged and older adults. *BMC Public Health*, *20*(1), 1728. DOI: 10.1186/s12889-020-09876-ẏ PMID: 33198728

Yu, Y. W., Lin, C. H., Lu, C. K., Wang, J. K., & Huang, T. L. (2023). Automated age-related macular degeneration detector on optical coherence tomography images using slice-sum local binary patterns and support vector machine. *Biomedical Engineering Online*, *22*(1), 85. Advance online publication. DOI: 10.1186/s12938-023-01149-2 PMID: 37644599

Zaidan, A. M. (2023). The leading global health challenges in the artificial intelligence era. *Frontiers in Public Health*, *11*, 1328918.

Zali, A., Gholamzadeh, S., Mohammadi, G., Looha, M. A., Akrami, F., & Zarean, E.. (2020). Baseline Characteristics and Associated Factors of Mortality in COVID-19 Patients; an Analysis of 16000 Cases in Tehran, Iran. *Archives of Academic Emergency Medicine*, *8*(1), e70. DOI: 10.22037/aaem.v8i1.872 PMID: 33134966

Zhang, J., Mazlin, V., Fei, K., Boccara, A. C., Yuan, J., & Xiao, P. (2023). Time-domain full-field optical coherence tomography (TD-FF-OCT) in ophthalmic imaging. *Therapeutic Advances in Chronic Disease*, *14*, 1–12. DOI: 10.1177/20406223231170146 PMID: 37152350

Zhang, J., & Zhang, Z. M. (2023). Ethics and governance of trustworthy medical artificial intelligence. *BMC Medical Informatics and Decision Making*, *23*(1), 7. PMID: 36639799

Zhang, L., Wang, H., & Chen, Y. (2025). Socio-technical dynamics in elder care: Challenges and opportunities for technology integration. *Technology in Society*, *70*(1), 145–158. DOI: 10.1016/j.techsoc.2024.101456

Zhang, M., Zhu, L., Lin, S. Y., Herr, K., Chi, C. L., Demir, I., & Chi, N. C. (2023). Using artificial intelligence to improve pain assessment and pain management: A scoping review. *Journal of the American Medical Informatics Association : JAMIA*, *30*(3), 570–587.

Zhang, Z., Xu, P., Wu, C., & Yu, H. (2024). Smart nursing wheelchairs: A new trend in assisted care and the future of multifunctional integration. *Biomimetics*, *9*(8), 492.

Zhao, A. P., Li, S., Cao, Z., Hu, P. J. H., Wang, J., Xiang, Y., & Lu, X. (2024). AI for science: Predicting infectious diseases. *Journal of Safety Science and Resilience = An Quan Ke Xue Yu Ren Xing (Ying Wen)*, *5*(3), 232–245. DOI: 10.1016/j.jnlssr.2024.03.001

Zhu, J., Shi, K., Yang, C., Niu, Y., Zeng, Y., Zhang, N., & Chu, C. H. (2022). Ethical issues of smart home-based elderly care: A scoping review. *Journal of Nursing Management*, *30*(8), 3686–3699.

Zhu, Y., Long, Y., Wang, H., Lee, K. P., Zhang, L., & Wang, S. J. (2024). Digital behavior change intervention designs for habit formation: Systematic review. *Journal of Medical Internet Research*, *26*, e54375. DOI: 10.2196/54375 PMID: 38787601

Zhu, Y., Yang, Q., & Mao, X. (2023). Global trends in the study of smart healthcare systems for the elderly: Artificial intelligence solutions. *International Journal of Computational Intelligence Systems*, *16*(1), 105. DOI: 10.1007/s44196-023-00280-6

Zimmer, Z. (2005). Health and living arrangement transitions among China's oldest-old. *Research on Aging*, *27*(5), 526–555.

Zimmer, Z., & Amornsirisomboon, P. (2001). Socioeconomic status and health among older adults in Thailand: An examination using multiple indicators. *Social Science & Medicine*, *52*(8), 1297–1311. PMID: 11281411

Zou, Y., Sun, K., Afnan, T., Abu-Salma, R., Brewer, R., & Schaub, F. (2024). Cross-contextual examination of older adults' privacy concerns, behaviors, and vulnerabilities. *Proceedings on Privacy Enhancing Technologies. Privacy Enhancing Technologies Symposium*, *2024*(2), 166–187. DOI: 10.56553/popets-2024-0046

Zubayer, M. A., Ahammed, B., Sarder, M. A., Kundu, S., Majumder, U. K., & Islam, S. M. S. (2021). Double and triple burden of non-communicable diseases and its determinants among adults in Bangladesh: Evidence from a recent demographic and health survey. *International Journal of Clinical Practice*, *75*(10). Advance online publication. DOI: 10.1111/ijcp.14613 PMID: 34235819

About the Contributors

Konstantinos Stolakis is a Geriatrician Specialized at the Geriatric University Clinic of Siena in Italy where he also completed his basic studies in Medicine. From 2008 until the completion of the specialty in July 2014, he actively participated in the research team of the Department of "Medical-Surgical and Neurological Sciences" of the University of Siena, gaining experience in the field of bone metabolic diseases, bone genetics, and physiopathology of osteoporosis, bone tissue interactions, glucose metabolism, cardiovascular disease, and diagnostic techniques for bone metabolic diseases, both clinically and in the laboratory. Since 2016, he maintains a private practice in Corinth where he offers his services as a Geriatrician. In November 2023, he was sworn in as a Doctor of Medicine at the University of Patras, with the research subject of his doctoral thesis on the role of vitamins B12 and D3 in balance and falls in the elderly. During the In the years 2018 and 2019, he was a University Fellow of the University of Patras in the Rehabilitation Clinic of Patients with Spinal Cord Injuries, participating in the Osteoporosis, Sarcopenia, and Falls prevention center. He was a member of the research team of the University of Patras that participated in the fulfillment of the European program: "Managing Frailty. A comprehensive approach to promote a disability-free advanced age in Europe: the ADVANTAGE initiative". He was also a team member of the Healthy Living Laboratory (EYDia), an action of the Fragility Fracture Network Greece (FFN GR). The purpose of the action was a holistic view of the health and quality of life of the elderly in the community. At the same time, he has participated as a scholarship holder in the research team of the University of Patras, with the object of study the "Holistic interdisciplinary approach in the treatment of patients with fragility fractures". He also participated in the project "Aeithaleia: Holistic program for volunteering of elderly people and their active participation in civic life" within the framework of the Active Citizens Fund program. His scientific fields of interest include osteoporosis and sarcopenia, falls prevention, geriatric frailty syndrome, diabetes mellitus, cardiometabolic diseases and dyslipidaemias, polypharmacy, dementia syndromes, etc. He has attended and participated in numerous conferences and educational seminars, while also presenting research work at national and international conferences and scientific journals. Along with his professional and scientific activity, Dr. Stolakis actively participates in various voluntary activities to promote Geriatrics in Greece, improve the care and life of the elderly, but also the healthy aging of the Greek elderly. He is a member of the Hellenic Society for the Study and Research of Aging (EEMEG) and a Founding member of the Fracture Fragility Network Greece (FFN GR).

Iris Efthymiou is a thought leader, university lecturer, and author of 17 books, specialising in AI ethics and behavioural health economics. Passionate about bridging technology and humanity, she advocates for ethical AI and user-centred design to enhance well-being and education in the digital age. She has served as a college director, founded a Public Affairs consultancy, worked with global leaders, and spoken at the UN in Geneva. She serves as an Academic Board Member of the LabHEM at the University of Piraeus, a Board Member of HAPSc and Guildhouse School in London, and a Member of the Business Intelligence Committee (BIC) of the All-Party Parliamentary Group on Artificial Intelligence (APPG AI) in the UK. She has published over 17 books, 40 articles, and book chapters in peer-reviewed journals, and she is the chief editor of the Journal of Politics and Ethics in New Technologies and AI. She believes in equal opportunities, uniqueness, and the normality of imperfection! Iris has a Ph.D. in Behavioural Economics, a Master's in Health Economics and Management, and a Bachelor's in Economics.

***

Ashraf Alam currently holds the position of Research Faculty at the Centre of Excellence in Public Policy, Sustainability and ESG Research, housed within the Faculty of Law and Policy Studies at Alliance University, Bangalore. Renowned for his transdisciplinary acumen spanning education, technology, and policy studies, Dr. Alam has been distinguished as one of the World's Top 2% Scientists by Stanford University and Elsevier, an accolade that highlights the breadth and depth of his scholarly impact. His prolific academic output includes over fifty SCOPUS-indexed publications and more than one hundred conference presentations at esteemed national and international academic forums. His educational trajectory reflects both depth and versatility: a Ph.D. in Education from the Indian Institute of Technology (IIT) Kharagpur, an M.Ed. with a concentration in Mathematics Education, and a B.S. in Computer Science from the University of Delhi. He also holds postgraduate degrees in Public Administration (M.A.) and Mathematics (M.Sc.), supplemented by a suite of postgraduate diplomas in Higher Education,

Guidance and Counselling, Educational Technology, Criminology and Police Administration, and Value Education. Dr. Alam is an active participant in global scholarly discourse. As Associate Editor of Frontiers in Education, he plays a pivotal role in curating and guiding intellectual contributions across the Educational, Pedagogical, and Learning Sciences. Concurrently, he serves as Founder and Director of Academic Chronicles Private Limited, where he orchestrates editorial board formation and develops strategic frameworks for peer-reviewed publishing in the Social, Behavioural, and Humanistic Sciences. His research has been disseminated through elite academic platforms, including Elsevier, Springer, Taylor & Francis, Wiley, Routledge, Sage, Emerald, and IEEE, and addresses a remarkably diverse array of topics such as pedagogical theories, educational administration, educational psychology, educational sociology, educational policy, technology-integrated learning, mathematics education, educational philosophy, educational technology, teacher education, and AI/ML in learning environments. Dr. Alam's scholarly rigor is further demonstrated by his success in qualifying multiple prestigious examinations including UGC-NET-JRF in both Education and Adult and Continuing Education, UGC- NET in Public Administration, and GATE in Humanities and Social Sciences. At the heart of Dr. Alam's intellectual ethos lies a steadfast belief in education as a catalytic and emancipatory force capable of engendering social justice, human flourishing, societal progress, and sustainable transformation. His recent explorations into 'Happiness Engineering' and holistic well- being in school ecosystems articulate a vision of education that transcends instrumentalist paradigms, prioritizing emotional intelligence, global consciousness, empathy, and psychosocial resilience among learners. His research agenda seeks to conceive educational praxis through the affordances of inclusive digital learning, gamified instructional design, and artificial intelligence (AIEd), thereby constructing robust, ethically grounded frameworks for 21st century education. At Alliance University, Dr. Alam remains committed to architecting pedagogical models that not only cultivate intellectual dexterity and cognitive excellence but also prepare learners for morally responsive leadership, intellectual nimbleness, and responsible global citizenship in an increasingly volatile, uncertain, complex, and ambiguous (VUCA) world.

Abhishek Anand is an Assistant Professor of HRM at Amity University Jharkhand, Ranchi. He has 15 years of teaching, research and industry. He published several research papers, conference papers and book chapters with reputed publishers.

Debmitra Das is having 4+ years of teaching experience. She has earned M.Tech in Computer Science & Engineering from Maulana Abul Kalam Azad University of Technology, West Bengal. Several research articles, journals and conference papers are published under her belt. Currently Ms. Das is serving Poornima University at the capacity of Assistant Professor. She is also member of several Professional Bodies: IEEE (M'25), ACM (M'25), IAENG (M'24).

Ritam Dutta is having 16+ years of Teaching and Research Experience (05 SCI, 50 Scopus, 01 Patent Grant), 10+ years of Administrative Experience and 03+ year of Post Ph.D. Experience, served in several reputed institutions across India in the capacity of Assistant Prof., Associate Prof. and Professor. Dr. Dutta is a Member of Professional Bodies: IE(India) (M'19), IEEE (M'25), ISTE (M'19).

Shreya Ghosh is an Assistant Professor at PES University, Bangalore, and a research scholar with a strong passion for inquiry and innovation. Her interests lie in neuroscience, psychology, human relations, and sustainable development. She explores how psychological principles and neuroscientific insights support emotional regulation, cognitive balance, sustainable practices, and elder well-being, while integrating perspectives from wisdom traditions.

Pooja Kansra is Head of the Department at Mittal School of Business, Lovely Professional University, Punjab, India. Her areas of interest include econometric methods, microeconomics, macroeconomics, managerial economics, quantitative techniques, and the economics of health and education. She holds a Master's in Economics from Guru Nanak Dev University, Amritsar, and a Doctorate degree from Punjab Technical University, Jalandhar. She is a member of the Indian Economic Association. Her research interests include health economics, insurance, and service operation management. She is an avid researcher and has presented papers at various national and international conferences. She has numerous research papers published in refereed national and international journals of repute.

Lefty Karropoulos is a seasoned operations and business development leader, currently serving as Chief Operating Officer at Peddler's Son, and Chief Business Development Officer for SGM LLC. He previously held senior leadership roles in multi-state restaurant and food distribution companies, where he drove expansion, streamlined operations, and strengthened revenue models. Karropoulos is widely recognized for a leadership style that blends inspirational management, practical execution, and solution-based thinking. He emphasizes team building, collaboration, and the creation of high-performing cultures where people are empowered to innovate and excel. His leadership is results-driven, rooted in sustainability and ethics, ensuring progress is both measurable and responsible. Central to his philosophy is education. He has designed training and development programs for every organizational level—from owners and executives to frontline employees—building environments of continuous learning that enhance resilience and performance. 38,000 professionals worldwide.

Amiya Abdul Khadar is a Ph.D. scholar at Mittal School of Business, Lovely Professional University, Jalandhar. Her areas of interest include health economics, consumer behaviour, and development economics. She has published research papers in refereed national and international journals of repute. She has also presented several research papers at institutes of national repute.

Vishal Kothari is having more than 10 years of teaching and research experience in various reputed organisation across India. He did his M.Tech and B.E. in the field of computer science and Engineering. Currently Mr. Kothari is serving Poornima Institute of Engineering & Technology, in the capacity of Assistant Professor.

Suneel Kumar, with over 6.5 years of diverse experience, is a seasoned academician, researcher, and industry professional. He brings a strong background in teaching, research, administration, and data science, having contributed to several reputed institutions and organizations across India and abroad. Currently serving as the Director of HyperNex Technologies LLC, USA, he combines academic excellence with global industry leadership in AI, Data Science, and Software Consulting. He has successfully delivered impactful outcomes in enhancing customer engagement, improving model performance, and securing significant research funding. Holding a Master of Computer Applications (MCA) from AKTU Lucknow, he has consistently contributed through innovative research, publications, mentorship, and data-driven solutions, while excelling in institutional development, academic governance, and strategic leadership.

Navin Kumar Goyal is having more than 23 years teaching & research experience in various organizations across the country. He is having more than 10 SCOPUS, SCI referred publications. He has been session chair, invited speaker in various reputed conferences across globe. Dr. Goyal has earned his Ph.D, M.Tech and B.Tech in the field of Computer Science & Engineering. Currently he is serving Poornima Institute of Engineering & Technology, Jaipur in the capacity of Associate Professor.

Nikita Baruah Phukan, a BSc Psychology student at PES University, Bangalore, with an interest in topics related to neuroscience, psychology, human relations and sustainable development. With academic work exploring how psychological principles and neuroscientific insights can inform sustainable development and elder well-being. Her research focuses greatly on how neuroscience interacts with various psychological media for emotional regulation and cognitive balance, with the integration of timeless wisdom traditions.

Anastasia Psomiadi is a scholar, lecturer, researcher, and author in Social Psychology, Sustainability, and Social Innovation with over 20 years of academic and professional experience. A visionary entrepreneur and inspirational speaker, she integrates academic rigor with real-world innovation, advancing knowledge in sustainability standards, stakeholder engagement, business ethics, communication strategy, women's empowerment, and entrepreneurship. She has served as Head of Sustainability and Corporate Social Responsibility in MBA programs across European universities, where she designed and delivered full curricula in Sustainability, CSR, Social Entrepreneurship, and Social Innovation. She has also taught interdisciplinary courses in Human Resources, Leadership, Logistics, Operations Management, and Communications, supervised MBA dissertations, mentored international students, and co-organized National Academic Start-Up Contests in Greece fostering innovation and youth entrepreneurship. As an Associate Researcher at the Laboratory of Experimental Social Psychology, Panteion University (Athens), she conducts research on social health, networks, artificial intelligence, and sustainability, applying Moscovici's Social Representations Theory to business and society. Her academic contributions include peer-reviewed publications, international conference proceedings, and the Amazon #1 Best-Seller Your Playbook for Growth & Resilience. She has also organized major academic and cultural events with international presence across the U.S., Europe, Africa, and Asia, building cross-cultural networks that connect research with practice. Beyond academia, she founded pioneering initiatives including APSON (Greece's first sustainability and ESG consulting firm), the SOTL Global Movement (a global women's leadership and education network), and CRICOS Social Cooperative Enterprise (one of Greece's first social enterprises). Across her career, she has been recognized for bridging theory and practice, preparing the next generation of leaders to navigate responsible entrepreneurship, ethical business practices, and sustainable development.

Mohammed Firdos Alam Sheikh is an Assistant Professor and Deputy Head of the Department of Computer Science & Engineering at Poornima University, Rajasthan. His research expertise is in Cryptography and Network Security. He has published over 50+ research papers in reputable indexed sources such as Scopus and Web of Science, as well as numerous conference proceedings. Additionally, he holds over 10 Indian patents and 3 international patents and copyrights. Sheikh has authored two books and serves as an editor in Scopus-indexed publications. He is a life member of ISTE and IAENG and has been honored with awards such as the

"Young Researcher Award" and the "Outstanding Teacher of the Year Award" from various organizations and conferences. He is frequently invited as a session chair at national and international conferences and serves as the Nodal Center Coordinator for IIT Delhi Virtual Labs an initiative of ministry of Education, Govt. of india.

Pankaj Singh is an Associate Professor of Marketing Science in the School of Business at Galgotias University, Greater Noida, India. He completed his doctoral research in the marketing domain at ABV-Indian Institute of Information Technology and Management, Gwalior, Madhya Pradesh. He holds a master's in International Business Management and M.Phil. in Marketing and his particular research interest is in the areas of Service Marketing, Digital Marketing, Social Media and Public Policy. He published several WOS and Scopus-indexed, ABDC-listed, ABS-ranked research articles, IEEE conference proceedings and book chapters in all leading publishers i.e., Springer, IGI Global, CRC Press, Willey and Emerald publications. He has more than fifteen years of experience in academics and industry. In previous assignments, Dr. Singh is associated with Dr. A. P. J. Abdul Kalam Technical University, Lucknow; SRM University, Sonipat and GLA University, Mathura as a faculty of Marketing Management.

Sanjay Kumar Sinha is a well-known Academician & Administrator and Currently working as Professor in the Department of CSE at Poornima Institute of Engineering & Technology, (Poornima Group, Jaipur, Rajasthan). He has more than 22 years teaching experience in the field of Academics and Administration and have held different positions in different institutions. His research area was Big Data Analytics and also interest is in Data Mining, Artificial Intelligence, Machine Learning, Blockchain. He has published 26 research papers in IEEE, Springer, Scopus-indexed journals and Peer Reviewed Journals. He has Presented 12 Papers in National/International Conferences. He has written 03 Book Chapters, and 03 Patents Filed (Two Published). He has also served as an External Expert in various Research Development Committee, Subject Expert, Paper Setter & thesis evaluators in Colleges & Universities. He has actively participated in various Faculty Development Programs as well.

Index

A

B

C

D

P

R

S

V

www.ingramcontent.com/pod-product-compliance
Lightning Source LLC
LaVergne TN
LVHW062334300926
849161LV00007B/1691